Applied Knowledge in Paediatrics

MRCPCH Mastercourse

Martin Hewitt
BSc BM MD MRCP FRCPCH

Consultant Paediatric Oncology & Paediatric Medicine
Nottingham Children's Hospital
Nottingham University Hospital NHS Trust
Nottingham UK
Senior Theory Examiner (AKP)
RCPCH
London UK

Roshan Adappa
MB BS MD FRCPCH

Senior Attending Physician Neonatology
Sidra Medicine
Doha Qatar
Honorary Senior Lecturer Cardiff University
Cardiff UK

ELSEVIER

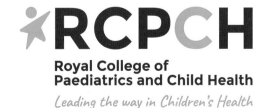

**Royal College of
Paediatrics and Child Health**

Leading the way in Children's Health

First edition 2022

Notices

Practitioners and researchers must always rely on their own experience and knowledge in evaluating and using any information, methods, compounds or experiments described herein. Because of rapid advances in the medical sciences, in particular, independent verification of diagnoses and drug dosages should be made. To the fullest extent of the law, no responsibility is assumed by Elsevier, authors, editors or contributors for any injury and/or damage to persons or property as a matter of products liability, negligence or otherwise, or from any use or operation of any methods, products, instructions, or ideas contained in the material herein.

ISBN: 978-0-7020-8037-1

Content Strategist: Alexandra Mortimer
Content Project Manager: Shivani Pal

Printed in China

Last digit is the print number: 9 8 7 6 5 4 3 2 1

Working together
to grow libraries in
developing countries

www.elsevier.com • www.bookaid.org

Contributors

Ibtihal Abdelgadir, MB BS MD MSc FRCPCH
Attending Physician Paediatric
Emergency Medicine
Sidra Medicine
Assistant Professor
Weill Cornell Medicine
Doha Qatar

Roshan Adappa, MB BS MD FRCPCH
Senior Attending Physician Neonatology
Sidra Medicine
Doha Qatar
Honorary Senior Lecturer Cardiff
University
Cardiff UK

Sudhakar Adusumilli, MB BS DCH, MRCP FRCPCH
Senior Attending Physician Paediatric
Emergency Medicine
Sidra Medicine
Doha Qatar

Shakti Agrawal, MB BS MRCP MRCPCH
Consultant Paediatric Neurology
Birmingham Children's Hospital
Birmingham UK

Juliana Chizo Agwu, MB BS MSc MRCP FRCPCH PCME
Consultant Paediatric Medicine &
Diabetes
Sandwell and West Birmingham NHS
Trust
West Bromwich UK

Rulla Al-Araji, MB ChB MRCPCH
Consultant Paediatric Gastroenterology
Great Ormond Street Hospital for
Children
London UK

Usama Al-Kanani, MB ChB FRCEM PEM Dip
Attending Physician Paediatric
Emergency Medicine
Sidra Medicine
Doha Qatar

Louise Allen, MB BS MD FRCOphth
Consultant Paediatric Ophthamology
Cambridge University NHS Trust
Associate Lecurer
University of Cambridge
Cambridge UK

Roona Aniapravan, MB BS FRCPCH
Attending Physician Paediatric
Emergency Medicine
Sidra Medicine
Assistant Professor Weill Cornell Medical
College
Doha Qatar

Karen Aucott, MB ChB MRCPCH
Consultant Paediatric Medicine
Nottingham Children's Hospital
Nottingham University Hospital NHS
Trust
Nottingham UK

Ramnath Balasubramanian, MB BS DNB MRCPCH
Consultant Paediatric Nephrology
Birmingham Children's Hospital
Birmingham UK

Srini Bandi, MB BS MD MSc FRCPCH
Consultant Paediatric Medicine
Leicester Royal Infirmary
Leicester UK

Sybil Barr, MB BCh MSc FRCPCH
Senior Attending Physician Neonatology
Sidra Medicine
Doha Qatar

Barbara Blackie, MD MEd FRCPC
Senior Attending Physician Paediatric
Emergency Medicine
Sidra Medicine
Assistant Professor
Weill Cornell Medicine
Doha Qatar

Gillian Body, BSc MB BS MMedSci FRCPCH
Consultant Paediatric Medicine
Noah's Ark Children's Hospital for Wales
Cardiff UK

Subarna Chakravorty, MB BS PhD MRCPCH FRCPath
Consultant Paediatric Haematology
King's College Hospital
London UK

Vince Choudhery, MB ChB FRCS MRCPCH
Consultant Paediatric Emergency
Medicine
Royal Hospital for Children
Glasgow UK

Angus Clarke, BM BCh DM MA FRCP FRCPCH
Professor Medical Genetics
University of Cardiff
Cardiff UK

Lucy Cliffe, MB ChB FRCPCH
Consultant Paediatric Immunology &
Infectious Diseases
Nottingham Children's Hospital
Nottingham University Hospital NHS
Trust
Nottingham UK

Madhumita Dandapani, MB BS
PhD MRCPCH
Clinical Associate Professor
University of Nottingham
Honorary Consultant Paediatric Oncology
Nottingham Children's Hospital
Nottingham University Hospital NHS Trust
Nottingham UK

Corinne de Sousa, BSc MB BS
MRCPsych
Consultant Child Psychiatry
Hopewood CAMHS
Nottinghamshire Healthcare NHS Trust
Nottingham UK

David Devadason, MB BS FRCPCH
Consultant Paediatric Gastroenterology
Nottingham Children's Hospital
Nottingham University Hospital NHS Trust
Nottingham UK

Yazeed Eldos, MD
Senior Attending Physician Paediatric
Emergency Medicine
Sidra Medicine
Doha Qatar

Elhindi Elfaki, MB BS, FRCPCH
Senior Attending Physician Neonatology
Sidra Medicine
Doha Qatar

Lucy Foard, BSc MBPsS
Psychometric Analyst
RCPCH
London UK

Sohail Ghani, MB BS FCPS FRCPCH
FRCPE
Attending Physician Paediatric
Emergency Medicine
Sidra Medicine
Doha Qatar

Graeme Hadley, MB ChB DCH
FRCPCH
Consultant Paediatric Medicine and
Emergency Mediine
Rondebosch Medical Centre
Cape Town South Africa

Richard Hain, MB BS MSc MD
FRCPCH FRCPE DipPalMed PGCert FHEA
Consultant Paediatric Palliative Care
Children's Hospital for Wales
Cardiff UK
Honorary Professor Clinical Ethics
Swansea University
Swansea UK

Martin Hewitt, BSc BM MD MRCP
FRCPCH
Consultant Paediatric Oncology &
Paediatric Medicine
Nottingham Children's Hospital
Nottingham University Hospital NHS Trust
Nottingham UK
Senior Theory Examiner (AKP)
RCPCH
London UK

Syed Haris Huda, MB BS IMRCS
FRCEM ACEP
Attending Physician Paediatric
Emergency Medicine
Sidra Medicine
Doha Qatar

Matthew Hurley, BSc MB BCh PhD
MRCPCH
Consultant Paediatric Respiratory
Medicine
Nottingham Children's Hospital
Nottingham University Hospital NHS Trust
Nottingham UK

Amna Hussain, BSc MB BS MRCPCH
Attending Physician Paediatric
Emergency Medicine
Sidra Medicine
Doha Qatar

Muhammad Islam, MB BS MRCEM
Attending Physician Paediatric
Emergency Medicine
Sidra Medicine
Doha Qatar

Nadya James, BSc MB BS MRCPCH
Consultant Community Paediatrics
Nottingham Children's Hospital
Nottingham University Hospital NHS Trust
Nottingham UK

Elisabeth Jameson, BSc MB BCh
MSc MRCPCH
Consultant Paediatric Metabolic Disease
Willink Biochemical Genetics Unit
St Mary's Hospital
Manchester UK

Sundaram Janakiraman, MB BS
FRCPCH
Consultant Neonatology
James Cook University Hospitals
Middlesbrough
Associate Lecturer
Newcastle University UK

Agnieszka Jarowska-Ganly, BSc
MSc
Pychometric Analyst
RCPCH
London UK

Nicola Jay, MB BS BSc MSc MRCPCH
PGDip Ethics
Consultant Paediatric Allergy
Sheffield Children's Hospital
Sheffield UK

Tawakir Kamani, MD MSc DOHNS
FRCS
Consultant Surgeon Ear Nose Throat
Nottingham University Hospital NHS Trust
Nottingham UK

Rohit Kumar, MB BS MRCPCH
Consultant Neonatology
James Cook University Hospital
South Tees Hospitals NHS Trust
Middlesbrough UK

Mithilesh Lal, MD MRCP FRCPCH
Consultant Neonatology
James Cook University Hospital
South Tees Hospitals NHS Trust
Middlesborough UK
Senior Theory Examiner
RCPCH
London UK

Prakash Loganathan, MB BS MD
Consultant Neonatology
James Cook University Hospital
South Tees Hospitals NHS Trust
Middlesbrough UK

Kah Yin Loke, MB BS MMed(Paed) MD MRCP FRCPCH
Associate Professor Paediatric
Endocrinology
National University of Singapore
Singapore

Andrew Lunn, BM MRCPCH
Consultant Paediatric Nephrology
Nottingham Children's Hospital
Nottingham University Hospital NHS Trust
Nottingham UK

Prashant Mallya, MB BS MD
MRCPCH
Consultant Neonatology
James Cook University Hospital
South Tees Hospitals NHS Trust
Middlesborough UK

Stephen Marks, MB ChB MD MSc
MRCP DCH FRCPCH
Reader Paediatric Nephrology
University College London
Consultant Paediatric Nephrology
Great Ormond Street Hospital for
Children
London UK

Eleanor Marshall, BSc MB BCh PhD
MRCPCH
Consultant Paediatric Allergy
Sheffield Children's Hospital
Sheffield UK

Katherine Martin, BSc MB ChB
MRCPCH
Consultant Paediatric Neurodisability
Nottingham Children's Hospital
Nottingham University Hospital NHS Trust
Nottingham UK

Flora McErlane, MB BCh MSc
MRCPCH
Consultant Paediatric Rheumatology
Great North Children's Hospital
Newcastle upon Tyne UK

Nazakat Merchant, MBBS MD DCH
FRCPCH
Consultant Neonatology
West Hertfordshire NHS Trust
Hon Senior Clinical Lecturer
King's College London
London UK

Moriam Mustapha, BSc RD
Neonatal Dietitian
Sidra Medicine
Doha Qatar

Vrinda Nair, MB BS MD FRCPCH
Consultant Neonatology
James Cook University Hospital
South Tees Hospitals NHS Trust
Middlesborough UK

Khuen Foong Ng, MB BS MRCPCH
Registrar Paediatric Infectious Diseases &
Immunology
Bristol Royal Hospital for Children
University Hospitals Bristol NHS
Foundation Trust
Bristol UK

Amitav Parida, BSc MB BS MRCPCH
Consultant Paediatric Neurology
Birmingham Children's Hospital
Birmingham UK

Sathya Parthasarathy, MB BS
MRCOG
Consultant Obstetrician (Fetal Medicine)
James Cook University Hospital
South Tees Hospitals NHS Trust
Middlesbrough UK

Colin Powell, MB ChB MD DCH
FRACP MRCP FRCPCH
Senior Attending Physician Paediatric
Emergency Medicine
Sidra Medicine
Doha Qatar
Honorary Professor of Child Health
Cardiff University
Cardiff UK

Andrew Prayle, BMedSci BM BS
PhD MRCPCH DipStat
Clinical Associate Professor
Paediatric Respiratory Medicine
University of Nottingham
Nottingham UK

Ruth Radcliffe, BMedSci BM BS
MRCPCH
Consultant Paediatric Medicine
University Hospitals of Leicester NHS
Trust
Leicester UK

Jane Ravescroft, MB ChB MRCGP
MRCP
Consultant Paediatric Dermatology
Nottingham Children's Hospital
Nottingham University Hospital NHS Trust
Nottingham UK

Muthukumar Sakthivel, MB BS
MD FRCPCH
Attending Physician Paediatric
Emergency Medicine
Sidra Medicine
Assistant Professor
Weill Cornell Medicine
Doha Qatar

Nafsika Sismanoglou, Ptychio
Iatrikes, (MD) MSc MRCPCH
Registrar Paediatric Immunology &
Allergy
Northern General Hospital
Sheffield, UK

Elisa Smit, MD FRCPCH
Consultant Neonatology
Cardiff and Vale University Health Board
Clinical Senior Lecturer Cardiff University
Cardiff UK

Alan Smyth, MA MB BS MD MRCP
FRCPCH
Professor of Child Health
University of Nottingham
Honorary Consultant Paediatric
Respiratory Medicine
Nottingham University Hospitals NHS
Trust
Nottingham UK

Sibel Sonmez-Ajtai, MD MSc
MRCPCH Dip Clin Ed
Consultant Paediatric Allergy
Sheffield Children's Hospital
Sheffield UK

Jothsana Srinivasan, MB BS DCH
MRCPCH
Consultant Paediatric Medicine &
Paediatric Dermatology
Nottingham Children's Hospital
Nottingham University Hospital NHS Trust
Nottingham UK

Richard Stewart, MB BCh BAO MD
FRCS FRCS(Paed)
Consultant Paediatric Surgery
Nottingham Children's Hospital
Nottingham University Hospital NHS Trust
Nottingham UK

Amy Taylor, BMedSci MB ChB
MRCPCH
Consultant Paediatric Neurodisibility
Nottingham Children's Hospital
Nottingham University Hospital NHS Trust
Nottingham UK

Robert Tulloh, BA BM BCh DM
FRCPCH FESC
Professor Congenital Cardiology
University of Bristol
Consultant Congenital Cardiology
University Hospitals Bristol and Weston
NHS Trust
Bristol UK

Sunitha Vimalesvaran, MB BS
MSc MRCPCH
GRID Registrar Paediatric Hepatology
King's Colle Hospital
London UK

Joanna Walker, MBE BA FRCP
FRCPCH
Consultant Paediatric Endocrinology
Portsmouth Hospitals University NHS
Trust
Portsmouth UK
Senior Theory Examiner (AKP)
RCPCH
London UK

Timothy Warlow, MB ChB, BMedSc,
FRCPCH DipPallMed
Consultant Paediatric Palliative Medicine
University Hospitals
Southampton UK

Lisa Whyte, MB ChB MSc MRCPCH
Consultant Paediatric Gastroenterology
Birmingham Children's Hospital
Birmingham UK

Kate Adel Wilson, MNutrDiet BSc
Dietitian
Sidra Medicine
Doha Qatar

Damian Wood, MB ChB DCH FRCPCH
Consultant Paediatric Medicine
Nottingham Children's Hospital
Nottingham University Hospital NHS Trust
Nottingham UK

Acknowledgements

The editors would like to thank the following individuals for their helpful comments on the text or their contribution of images and clinical scenarios.

Dr Gillian Body
Dr Will Carroll
Dr Mark Fenner
Dr Amy Kinder
Sheran Mahal (Question Bank and Quality Assurance Manager RCPCH)
Dr Eloise Shaw
Professor Harish Vyas
Dr Joanna Walker
Dr David White
Dr Nigel Broderick provided many of the radiological images and appropriate explanations of the appearances.

We are also grateful to Sue Hampshire (Director of Clinical and Service Development Resuscitation Council UK) for her support and the permission to use the management flow-charts produced by the Resuscitation Council UK.

Some of the images used in this book are taken from MRCPCH Mastercourse (volumes 1 and 2), edited by Professor Malcolm Levene published by Churchill Livingstone/Elsevier in 2007. We are grateful to the many paediatricians who sourced the images in that publication and trust that the images continue to contribute to their educational aims.

Martin Hewitt
Roshan Adappa

Foreword

This book forms part of the Mastercourse in Paediatrics series produced by the Royal College of Paediatrics and Child Health with each book aimed at covering the topics outlined in the relevant RCPCH examination syllabus. It has been written by experienced specialist authors and outlines core information of presentation, assessment and management of conditions affecting all systems plus information on ethics, UK law, clinical governance and evidence-based paediatrics. Although written for candidates preparing for the Applied Knowledge in Paediatrics examination, the book will also provide useful information and knowledge for the practicing paediatrician.

Supporting children and young people and helping them achieve their full potential requires many skills. These include the ability to engage with the patient and their carers, the need to assess the extent and type of problems presented and the knowledge to provide current and effective treatments.

The training of a paediatrician must, therefore, aim to develop these skills and ensure a sound knowledge of clinical conditions and their management. The practicalities of such management also require the recognition of the urgency and priority of any proposed investigation and treatment. This book covers many of these important topics.

The authors have provided a presentation of many of the common conditions seen in clinical practice at an appropriate level for the paediatric trainee. It is well recognised, however, that such basic knowledge requires continued revision. Consequently, every encounter with a child or young person must be seen as an opportunity for the paediatrician to learn and improve their understanding of the patient and their family, the problem presented and the appropriate management for that problem.

This book, therefore, contributes to that growth of clinical skills and professional development of the paediatric trainee and will help them as they prepare for the AKP exam.

Dr Camilla Kingdon
President of the Royal College of Paediatrics and Child Health

Preface

This book, *Applied Knowledge of Paediatrics: MRCPCH Mastercourse*, has been written specifically for trainees in paediatrics who have around 18–24 months of clinical experience and who may be preparing for the Applied Knowledge in Practice (AKP) examination. It forms part of the Mastercourse in Paediatrics series that was established by the RCPCH and joins the *Science of Paediatrics* book edited by Lissauer and Carroll. Both books are written with the prime aim of helping trainees prepare for specific RCPCH theory examinations but they will also be of value to paediatric trainees as part of their everyday practice.

Membership of the Royal College of Paediatrics and Child Health (MRCPCH) is a postgraduate qualification in Paediatric Medicine that is recognised in the UK and internationally. The award of the qualification indicates that a trainee has achieved a high standard of practice and is able to start Higher Specialist Training.

The AKP examination assesses the candidate's knowledge of the presentation, investigation and management of a wide range of conditions affecting children and young people. This level of understanding comes from clinical exposure to patients, reading about the details of the clinical conditions presented and taking the opportunity to discuss issues with experienced colleagues.

The chapters in *Applied Knowledge of Paediatrics* cover all the systems and each starts with the points listed in the RCPCH **AKP syllabus**. The subsequent chapter was then written by the specialist authors to ensure these topics were addressed.

Within each chapter there are **Practice Points** that capture important issues relevant to clinical practice or that may include explanations using examples.

Clinical Scenarios are also presented and are based on known, but modified, clinical stories to outline some of the issues that may present themselves to the clinician. Some of the issues presented are not resolved and so reflect the reality of current practice.

At the end of each chapter there are **Important Clinical Points** that provide a list of some of the significant points raised in the chapter.

Images are used throughout the chapters. These will demonstrate many important features that may appear in the examination but they should also act as a prompt to the reader to seek out further examples of the appearances shown. The adage 'One swallow doesn't make a summer' could be adapted to make the point that 'One image doesn't capture all the relevant features'.

Each chapter finishes with a short list for **Further Reading** to allow the reader to explore reviews and topics in more detail. Many chapters have drawn information from current guidelines published by the National Institute for Health and Care Excellence (NICE). Clearly these guidelines may change over time and it is the responsibility of every clinician to ensure that the most up-to-date version is consulted.

The first chapter provides some advice on preparing for the AKP examination including some insight into the process of producing the actual exam papers, assessing the questions and the post-examination review. The aim is that by understanding how the papers are constructed from items in the RCPCH Question Bank and how the results are reviewed after the exam, the candidate will gain some understanding of the structure of the examination.

The final chapter provides 50 AKP exam-style questions presented in random order along with itemised answers that aim to provide clarification on how answers can be assessed and the correct ones chosen. The reader may wish to use this as a practice examination but must remember that questions in the real examination have different weightings allocated depending on various factors such as length, complexity and format.

We would like to thank all the authors of each of the chapters for sharing their knowledge and expertise, and for their understanding as we made changes and requested further reviews of their text.

Our thanks also to Alexandra Mortimer, Shivani Pal and the larger team at Elsevier for their support and guidance during the production of this book.

Finally, our thanks must go to our families for their patience and tolerance as we committed time to working on this project.

We hope the book proves valuable to all trainees and contributes to the improvement in the care and treatment of the many children who will come under their care.

Martin Hewitt
Roshan Adappa

Contents

Chapter | 1 |

Preparing for the AKP exam

Martin Hewitt

After reading this chapter you should understand:
- the structure and format of the AKP examination
- the range of topics covered by the syllabus
- the style of questions presented in the examination
- how each question is produced and reviewed
- advice on some aspects of examination preparation

The Applied Knowledge in Practice (AKP) examination is one of the three theory exams that must be passed before a candidate is allowed to present themselves for the clinical examination—Foundation of Practice (FoP) and Theory and Science (TaS) being the other two. Passing all four examinations leads to the award of Membership of the Royal College of Paediatrics and Child Health.

This chapter will describe the exam format and so allow the candidate to prepare in an appropriate manner. Some details of the exam may change over time and it is therefore imperative that the candidate consults the RCPCH exam website at an early stage to identify possible updates and new advice.

This book is not a comprehensive paediatric textbook. It does, however, aim to cover practically all of the topics outlined in the RCPCH Examination Syllabus and therefore forms the basis of questions in the examination. Although the syllabus and examination aim to cover the main topics of clinical paediatric practice that a Specialist Trainee with 18 months of experience might encounter, it should also be expected that some less-common conditions will appear. A paediatrician should be able to identify uncommon conditions within common presentations, which is a point illustrated by the phrase "all that wheezes isn't asthma."

Preparation

Candidates can sit the RCPCH theory examinations in any order although most progress from FoP though TaS to the AKP exam. After six attempts, further attempts are only permitted if evidence of further study is provided. The AKP exam is usually first attempted by trainees who have accrued at least 12 months of paediatric training. However, for those in UK training schemes, there is a pressure to complete the theory exams during 3 years of full-time training as failure to do so will usually require an extension of training time. The AKP exam assesses clinical knowledge and decision-making skills, and an exposure to a broad range of general and specialty clinical paediatrics is therefore needed.

This is a UK examination and assesses understanding of UK laws, expectations and clinical practice. Question writers aim to produce questions that can be supported by published evidence, national guidelines of accepted practice and information in established and respected textbooks and journals.

It is important to remember that much of the AKP exam is aimed at assessing clinical understanding of paediatric medical practice encountered by candidates during their normal daily duties. Questions will ask about the presentation of clinical problems, possible differential diagnoses, appropriate common investigations and the interpretation of results. Answers to other questions will require a knowledge of management and long-term consequences of a broad range of conditions. The examination will also test the ability of candidates to establish clinical priorities and ensure that time-critical decisions are recognised and acted upon. All paediatricians will recognise that care occurs within the context of the family, and therefore an understanding of professional and legal obligations is necessary and assessed in the examination.

Candidates will obviously need to build their knowledge base by further background reading.

Examination structure

The examination is a curriculum-driven, computer-based assessment that takes place three times each year. There are two separate papers sat on the same day with each paper lasting 2.5 hours. In total there are 120 questions across the two papers. The exam does not use negative marking—a wrong answer scores zero. The allocation of topics across the various syllabus headings is set by the "Theory Examination Blueprint" that allows specific mapping of questions to the syllabus and aims to provide a balanced selection of questions across the entire syllabus in each exam.

Question journey

The development of questions used and the building of each exam involves many separate steps to ensure that the questions are **relevant** and **current** and that the exam is well balanced. Before appearing in an exam, each and every question will have been individually scrutinised by at least nine separate, experienced paediatricians and will be reviewed again by a panel of another six to eight paediatricians after the exam has taken place.

The questions are generated at Question Setting Group meetings that occur throughout the year at various locations in the UK and abroad. The meetings are organised by RCPCH staff and are open to all paediatricians who already hold the MRCPCH diploma. Senior exam facilitators are part of the meeting and guide small groups to create the questions. Each question is then assessed by the Senior Theory Examiner for AKP and is reviewed again by two senior clinicians at RCPCH Examination Board. Following this review, the approved question is placed in the question bank for future use.

Following every exam, and before the results are finalised, a panel of paediatricians meet with the RCPCH psychometrician at the "post examination Angoff meeting" and review the performance of every question. This meeting scores the level of difficulty for each question and reviews any possible discrepancies or problem questions identified in the exam. If,

for example, most candidates choose an answer different from the allocated correct answer, this suggests that the phrasing of the question is ambiguous and points to more than one acceptable valid answer. The panel would review that question in detail and, if it is agreed that phrasing of any part of the question is ambiguous and therefore unfair, then the question is removed from that examination. The question is sent for review rather than returned to the question bank.

Question types

There are different question types used in the examination. Examples of these can be seen on the RCPCH website and in Chapter 35 of this book. Some information on each question type is offered here.

Single best answer (SBA)

Most of the questions in the exam follow this format. The stem may include a clinical history, examination, results and images and the question is posed. There are then five answers offered with only one being correct. The most important point for a candidate to understand is that all answers shown will be plausible but only one is the most appropriate for the question asked. If the candidate reads a question and concludes that all answers are correct then the question is a good example of the single best answer format. In this situation, the candidate is advised to re-read the question and clarify the exact phrase of the question posed. Examples of the different types of phrasing are:
..the **next** most appropriate step in management
..the **most appropriate** initial management
..the treatment to be given **immediately**
..the test which will **provide a diagnosis**
..the **most likely** diagnosis

For example, a question may describe a child presenting in extremis to the emergency department and, in real life, multiple interventions will be undertaken. Each of these interventions will be appropriate and necessary and therefore will be listed in the answer list. The question may then ask which one intervention from this list must be undertaken as a priority.

Multiple best answer (MBA)

Some questions will ask for more than one answer such as needing two investigations to support a diagnosis. The questions do not ask for more than three answers and the list of options provided will be up to a maximum of 10 answers available.

Multipart question (MPQ)

This question structure follows the format of the single best answer but there are usually two questions joined to the initial scenario and each question is independent of the other. The answer to part one does not give a clue to the answer of part two.

Extended matching questions (EMQ)

This format provides an introductory statement that explains the general topic for the question. Examples would include cardiac diagnoses, drugs for epilepsy or investigations for hypernatraemia.

The question then presents the first statement or clinical scenarios followed by a list of 10 potential answers. The second scenario is then presented followed by the same list of 10 answers and finally the third question with the same 10. It is possible that one of the answers may be chosen for more than one of the questions—each question is independent of the other two.

Detailed advice

Some questions may seem to have one or two obvious answers and the candidate needs to look for further clues in the question stem to support one or the other. For questions where there is no obvious answer, one approach would be to ask the 'reverse question' and identify those answers which clearly do not fit the clinical scenario in the question stem. Having removed these answers, the candidate can then work on those remaining to identify the appropriate and correct answer.

All questions in the examination that include results of laboratory investigations will also show the normal ranges for each of the listed test. These ranges may be slightly different from those used at the candidate's institution but these are the ones agreed for examination. In practice, this is not a problem as the provided results, where appropriate, are obviously abnormal or obviously normal.

The candidate should read the stem very carefully as it often contains specific details to guide the candidate towards particular conditions that may occur more commonly in certain ethnic groups or in certain geographical locations.

An awareness of the indications, contraindications and long-term consequences of some of the drugs administered to children is important. Candidates are advised to use the BNFc during their normal working day as part of their revision and to look at contraindications and common side effects.

Many questions will contain images such as clinical photos, radiographs and ECGs.

Clinical photographs will cover a range of features including specific syndromes and disease-related abnormalities. The ability to identify a series of clinical features in a child and recognise the underlying syndrome is a skill that many geneticists and paediatricians take many years to develop. However, recognising the features of a small group of syndromes is required for the AKP exam and these are presented in this book. Trainees are advised to review as many images as possible of these syndromes to ensure they can identify the major features. Similarly, wherever a condition which has recognised clinical features is described in the text, the candidate should seek out example images or descriptions.

There are questions that require the ability to interpret radiographs although it is accepted practice that it is the radiologist who will provide the definitive opinion and final report. Trainees, however, do need to identify common radiological abnormalities that require an immediate response and management such as the presence of a pneumothorax, a pneumonia, or necrotising enterocolitis. MRI and CT scans must be reported by radiology staff but an AKP candidate must have an understanding of the common abnormalities to allow explanation of the findings to patients, carers and colleagues usually following a discussion with the radiologist. Trainees should attend as many radiology meetings as possible and be prepared to ask radiologists to explain important features.

Evidence-based paediatrics

The AKP examination will contain two questions about evidence-based practice in each paper. The questions usually present information from a published paper but with the methodology and results summarised. The data can be complex and each answer should be compared in turn with the given results to determine whether the answer statement can be supported.

IMPORTANT CLINICAL POINTS

Marking

- marks awarded for each question are different and weighted for complexity
- a wrong answer scores zero

Single best answer

- understand the exact phrase of the question being asked

Multi-part question

- answer to each question is independent of any other part

Extended matching question

- the same answer may apply to more than one of the three questions

Results

- normal ranges are shown for each test

Images

- review as many images as possible of syndromes
- review as many images as possible of clinical signs and described lesions

Radiographs

- attend as many radiology meetings as possible

Further reading

RCPCH Theory Examinations. https://www.rcpch.ac.uk/resources/theory-examinations-structure-syllabus.

Chapter | 2 |

Neonatology

Authors: *Mithilesh Lal, Elisa Smit, Nazakat Merchant*

Contributions from: *Sunitha Vimalesvaran, Vrinda Nair, Prakash Loganathan, Prashant Mallya, Rohit Kumar, Janakiraman Sundaram, Sathya Parthasarathy*

After reading this chapter you should be able to diagnose and manage:
- birth injury
- short and long-term consequence of preterm birth
- common medical conditions
- common surgical conditions
- congenital anomaly
- common postnatal problems

and
- know the effect of prenatal and perinatal events on neonates

Antenatal assessment of fetal growth

Antenatal assessment of the mother and fetus requires a comprehensive history and examination, investigations for potential congenital infections and chromosomal anomalies and ultrasound monitoring. Ultrasonography will assess the breathing pattern, muscle tone, body movement and amniotic fluid volume. The main aim is to identify early intrauterine growth restriction—IUGR—(also referred to as fetal growth restriction [FGR]).

IUGR is defined as the failure of the fetus to achieve its full growth potential and could be due to maternal, fetal or neonatal causes. It is the biggest risk factor for stillbirth, perinatal and neonatal morbidity and mortality.

Definition and classification

The most common obstetric definition of IUGR is an estimated weight below the 9th centile for gestational age in the second half of pregnancy. This definition does not distinguish the normal, constitutionally small fetus (small for gestational age [SGA]) from the small fetus whose growth potential is restricted. The latter fetus is at increased risk of perinatal morbidity and mortality whereas the former is not.

IUGR may be:

Symmetrical IUGR (20%–30% of small fetuses) that refers to a growth pattern in which all fetal organs are decreased proportionally and is thought to result from a pathological process **manifesting early in gestation.**

Asymmetrical IUGR (70%–80 % of small fetuses) where there is a relatively greater decrease in abdominal size (liver volume and subcutaneous fat tissue) than in head circumference and is thought to occur late in gestation.

Screening for intrauterine growth restriction

Fundal height (FH) measurement

Measurement of the distance between the upper edge of the pubic symphysis and the top of the uterine fundus is performed during antenatal care to detect IUGR.

Selective ultrasonography

Indications for a growth scan are:
- first FH measurement below 9th centile at between 26–28 weeks
- no increase in sequential measurements

5

Table 2.1 Indications for serial growth measurements during pregnancy.

Current pregnancy	Past medical history	Past obstetric history
maternal age over 40 years	chronic hypertension	previous birth weight <9th centile
maternal smoking	diabetes	previous stillbirth
drug misuse	renal impairment	
maternal BMI > 35		
multiple pregnancy		
hypertension or preeclampsia		
unexplained APH		
concerns related to growth measurements		

- sequential measurements do not follow the expected growth
- sequential measurements cross centiles in an upward direction

All women should be assessed at booking for risk factors to identify those who need increased surveillance. Some will be at increased risk of developing fetal growth restriction because of factors in the current pregnancy, in the past medical history or the past obstetric history. Those women with such risk factors will need serial scans at least every 3 weeks from 26–28 weeks until delivery (Table 2.1).

Growth indices

Estimated fetal weight is the most common method of identifying the growth-restricted fetus as it combines multiple biometric measurements including abdominal circumference, biparietal diameter, head circumference and femur length.

Customised growth charts are used to plot both fundal height measurements obtained during clinical examination and estimated fetal weight following an ultrasound examination. They are customised to each individual taking into account the height, weight, ethnicity, and parity of the mother.

Amniotic fluid volume assessment can identify pregnancies with the most severe oligohydramnios as these have high rates of perinatal mortality, congenital anomalies and IUGR.

Doppler velocimetry looks for abnormal doppler wave forms in maternal uterine arteries and fetal vessels (umbilical arteries, middle cerebral arteries, ductus venosus) that will indicate poorer neonatal outcomes.

Abdominal circumference is the most sensitive single biometric indicator of IUGR and is usually performed at approximately 34 weeks of gestation.

Perinatal events and birth injury

Hypoxic-ischaemic encephalopathy

Hypoxic-ischaemic encephalopathy (HIE) is the result of a significant lack of oxygen and reduced blood flow to the fetal brain and other organs during labour and delivery.

Causes include:
- underlying conditions producing circulatory compromise in the mother
- utero-placental problems—umbilical cord prolapse, placental abruption
- fetal conditions—cardiac failure, feto-maternal haemorrhage

Sometimes the insult is more prolonged and chronic in nature, but both acute and chronic asphyxia can lead to HIE.

Infants with HIE are often in poor condition at birth and invariably require resuscitation, and the condition is described as mild, moderate or severe encephalopathy (see Sarnat stages in Table 2.1).

Relevant information contributing to the diagnosis of HIE includes:
- evidence of fetal distress
- sentinel events—cord prolapse, antepartum haemorrhage, shoulder dystocia
- low Apgar scores
- placental report indicating dysfunction
- Kleihauer-Betke test—if feto-maternal haemorrhage is suspected

Investigations

- blood gas—identify degree of acidosis
- electrolytes, glucose, calcium if seizures
- amplitude integrated electroencephalography (aEEG)
- infection screen
- cranial ultrasound (oedema or areas of parenchymal or basal ganglia/thalamic damage)
- doppler studies of cerebral flow velocity

Table 2.2 **Stages of hypoxic-ischaemic encephalopathy (Sarnat)**		
mild – stage 1	**moderate – stage 2**	**severe – stage 3**
hyperalert	lethargic	coma
eyes wide open	reduced tone	weak or absent respiratory drive
does not sleep	diminished brainstem reflexes (pupil/gag/suck)	no response to stimuli
irritable	clinical seizures	floppy
seizures absent		diminished brainstem reflexes (pupil/gag/suck)
usually lasts <24 hours		diminished tendon reflexes
		EEG severely abnormal

Treatment and managment

Supportive treatment is required for those babies with multisystem involvement including ventilation in view of poor respiratory effort. Periods of hypo- and hyperoxia as well as hypo- and hypercapnia may develop and indicate a worse neurological outcome.

Therapeutic hypothermia is the only neuroprotective treatment effective in term infants with moderate or severe HIE. This involves a reduction of core body temperature to 33.5°C for 72 hours followed by a slow rewarming phase (0.5°C/hour increase) over 6 hours. The treatment must be initiated within 6 hours after birth for it to be beneficial.

Infants with HIE may develop overt seizures, whilst others will have seizures on aEEG without a clinical component—'electrical seizure activity'. There is no clear consensus on management, but many would treat seizures with a duration of over 3 min or greater than 3 seizures in 1 hour.

Cardiac dysfunction may require inotropic support and the issue may become evident during cooling when many infants show a hypothermia-induced bradycardia of around 70–90 bpm.

Transient renal impairment is common and careful fluid management is required. Potential hypoglycaemia should be avoided by an adequate glucose infusion rate. Liver dysfunction can cause coagulopathy and severe bleeding, which may require treatment with blood and clotting products. Hepatic and renal drug clearance is often impaired and doses may need adjustment and monitoring.

Important sequelae

Moderate and severe HIE have a high mortality and morbidity rate and many who do survive have significant intellectual disability and poor motor function. Despite therapeutic cooling, the combined outcome of death or disability at 18–24 months is around 50% with 25% mortality and 25% disability.

Several features can help to define the prognosis and those with poor feeding and decreased tone at 2 weeks will have a poor neurodevelopmental outlook. MRI of the brain between day 5–14 can identify abnormal signals in the posterior limb of the internal capsule, which again is indicative of a poor outcome. Epilepsy, vision or hearing difficulties, as well as behaviour and learning difficulties are all recognised consequences of hypoxic ischaemic encephalopathy.

Brachial plexus injury

Brachial plexus palsy is flaccid paralysis of the upper limb seen at birth, due to stretching, rupture or avulsion of some, or all, of the cervical and first thoracic nerve roots (Table 2.3).

Risk factors:
- shoulder dystocia
- birth weight over 4 kg
- maternal diabetes—associated with macrosomia
- breech delivery—difficulty in extracting the trailing arm
- instrumental delivery

Other findings which may be seen are:
- fracture of humerus or clavicle with crepitus or swelling
- Horner's syndrome—sympathetic nerve damage
- respiratory distress—phrenic nerve injury resulting in diaphragmatic paralysis
- encephalopathy—associated hypoxic ischaemic event

Investigations

Usually limited to chest x-ray to identify a clavicle or humeral fracture or diaphragmatic palsy. Nerve conduction studies or MRI may be required if surgical intervention is indicated.

Table 2.3 Types of brachial palsy and diagnostic features

	Erb's palsy	Klumpke's palsy	total palsy
nerve roots	C5, 6 and sometimes T1	C8, T1	C5-T1
clinical presentation	weakness of arm decreased arm movements arm is adducted and internally rotated with elbow extended, forearm is in pronation and wrist is flexed ('waiter's tip') (Figure 2.1).	weakness of intrinsic muscles of hand leading to 'claw hand'	weakness of entire arm
Moro reflex	absent	present	absent
biceps reflex	absent	present	absent
radial reflex	absent	present	absent
grasp reflex	present	absent	absent

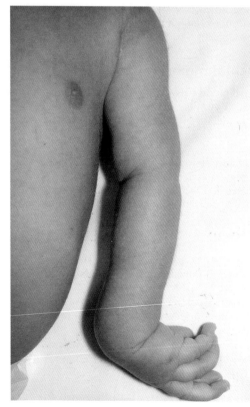

Fig. 2.1 Brachial plexus injury (Erb's palsy) following shoulder dystocia. Image shows internal rotation at shoulder and flexion of digits

Treatment and management

Parents are advised of the need for careful handling of infants in the first 1–2 weeks till the inflammation subsides but after this time, a formal exercise programme will be initiated by the physiotherapy team. About 70% to 80% of infants make a full recovery without intervention in 6 weeks to 3 months. The child should be referred to colleagues with expertise in nerve injuries if there is no improvement by 6 weeks.

Antenatal management of preterm labour

Accurate identification of women in true preterm labour allows appropriate application of interventions that can improve neonatal outcome such as the administration of antenatal corticosteroid therapy, prophylaxis against group B streptococcal infection or necessary transfer to a facility with an appropriate level of newborn care.

Risk factors for preterm labour include:
* previous preterm delivery
* multiple pregnancy
* advanced maternal age
* teenage mother
* smoking or drug abuse
* deprivation

Interventions aimed at reducing the risk of preterm birth include:
* education and health promotion programmes including smoking cessation, treatment of drug misuse,

maintenance of a normal body mass index and longer intervals between pregnancies
- low-dose aspirin may reduce the risk of spontaneous preterm birth
- cervical cerclage placement may prolong gestation for women with a history of preterm birth

Management of preterm labour

The diagnosis of preterm labour is based on clinical criteria of regular painful uterine contractions accompanied by cervical dilation or effacement. Tocolytics can be used to try and delay preterm labour so that antenatal steroids and magnesium sulphate can be given.

Management of the high-risk pregnancy

Preterm birth can result in significant health consequences in both the short and long term. Pregnancies that are likely to produce infants at high risk of problems include those with:
- intrauterine growth restriction—from maternal, placental or fetal causes
- prolonged preterm rupture of membranes, presenting as infection or risk of infection or related poor lung growth
- congenital malformations from syndromic association
- chronic maternal illness—maternal diabetes and other medical conditions
- acute fetal compromise—placental abruption, cord prolapse
- twin or higher order pregnancy
  Initial assessment and intervention in the delivery room:
- pregnancies at risk of difficulties should occur in a hospital with a level 3 NICU. Antenatal steroid administration for lung maturation and magnesium sulphate for neuroprotection should also be administered to the expectant mother.
- delivery room temperature needs to be kept above 25°C and the use of a plastic covering for the preterm infant will help maintain better thermal control. Each degree below 36.5°C is associated with increased mortality in preterm babies of about 28%.

Following birth

Most preterm or term infants will not need any intervention. The management outlined in the Resuscitation Council UK algorithm should be followed if intervention is required (Figure 2.2).

Specific aspects of the assessment of the newborn require consideration.

Clamping of the cord can be delayed for up to 3 minutes in the preterm infant, although there is good evidence that clamping the cord after a good respiratory effort is established is more effective than time based delayed cord clamping. Positive End Expiratory Pressure (PEEP) support has been shown to be beneficial by establishing a functional residual capacity in the lungs. Routine airway suction with or without meconium has no benefit and is therefore not recommended.

Medical conditions in the preterm neonate

Respiratory distress syndrome

Respiratory distress syndrome (RDS) is primarily seen in premature babies and is the result of surfactant deficiency and immature lung development and therefore the incidence decreases with increasing gestational age. Risk factors for RDS include prematurity, maternal diabetes, absence of labour and lack of antenatal steroids. Antenatal steroids, surfactant therapy and noninvasive respiratory support have resulted in reduced mortality from RDS.

The preterm infant with RDS will have tachypnoea, grunting, chest wall retractions, nasal flaring and 'head bobbing'. As the condition becomes more severe the baby becomes cyanotic and pale and may have apnoeic episodes.

Differential diagnosis
- transient tachypnoea of newborn (TTN)
- aspiration
- pneumonia or sepsis
- cyanotic congenital heart disease

Investigations

The chest x-ray will show the recognised changes of RDS with the reticulogranular pattern (ground glass) in the lung fields, an air bronchogram and low lung volumes (Figure 2.3).

Treatment and management

Antenatal steroids reduce the incidence and severity of RDS and the consequent need for mechanical ventilation. Current recommendation is for them to be offered to all women between 24+0 and 33+6 weeks of pregnancy who are at risk of preterm delivery within 7 days. The ideal therapeutic window for administration is when delivery is expected 1 to 7 days after a complete course of treatment.

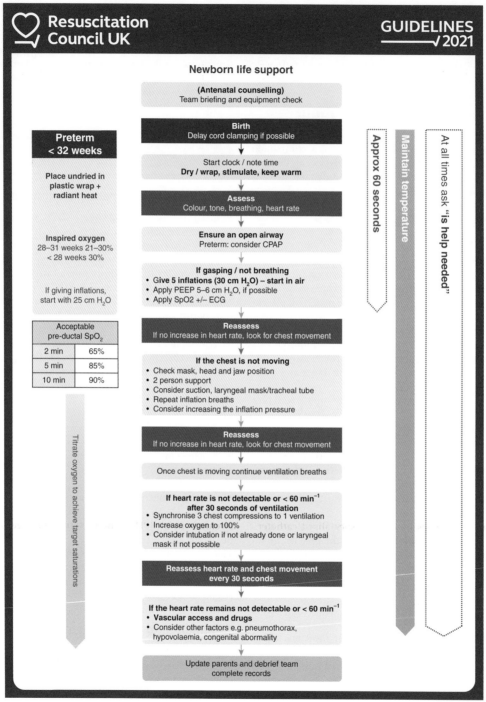

Fig. 2.2 Newborn Life Support algorithm (Reproduced with permission from the Resuscitation Council UK 2021)

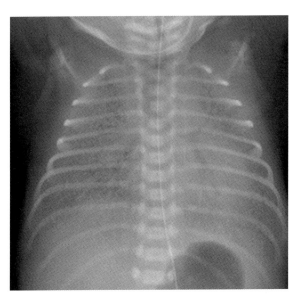

Fig. 2.3 Chest x-ray of 28-week gestation neonate with clinical signs suggestive of respiratory distress syndrome (Copyright – Dr Mithilesh Lal - used with permission)

Surfactant can be given prophylactically to those infants who are at risk of RDS, even before signs of RDS develops, and is usually given within 10–30 mins of delivery. Rescue surfactant treatment is usually given within 12 hours when specific criteria for RDS severity are met (e.g., receiving noninvasive support and FiO_2 over 30%–40%). Both animal-derived and synthetic surfactants are available, although the former is usually used. New techniques for surfactant administration are minimally invasive surfactant therapy (MIST) and less invasive surfactant administration (LISA). These techniques administer surfactant in spontaneously breathing, nonintubated neonates by using a specialised catheter. These methods are associated with reduced incidence of BPD, duration of invasive ventilation and incidence of pneumothorax.

Mechanical respiratory support

Continuous positive airway pressure (CPAP) is a form of noninvasive respiratory support which delivers constant positive pressure and is delivered through fitted nasal devices. CPAP can be used from birth in a preterm baby to aid respiratory effort or after extubation following a period of ventilation.

Noninvasive positive pressure ventilation (NIPPV) provides support using a face mask or prongs and provides a positive pressure at preset intervals. It is thought to be superior to CPAP in small neonates.

High flow nasal cannulae (HFNC) have a similar efficacy as other forms of noninvasive respiratory support.

Indication for use of invasive mechanical ventilation include deteriorating respiratory function, recurrent apnoea, increasing oxygen requirement and worsening of hemodynamic status. Volume-targeted ventilation results in reduction of broncho-pulmonary dysplasia (BPD), pneumothorax and days of ventilation when compared to pressure limited modes. Early extubation to noninvasive respiratory support should be planned if a ventilated neonate has a good response to surfactant, but if conventional support fails then high frequency ventilation is used as rescue mode.

Ventilatory support aims to maintain oxygen saturations between 91% to 95%, but the high oxygen flows required leads to an increase in the incidence of retinopathy of prematurity and BPD. The use of caffeine citrate in preterm infants under 31 weeks reduces ventilation days, the incidence of BPD and cerebral palsy.

Bronchopulmonary dysplasia

Bronchopulmonary dysplasia (BPD) is defined as the need for respiratory support and supplemental oxygen at 36 weeks postmenstrual age, and its development is inversely proportional to gestational age and birth weight.

The most important risk factors for BPD are prematurity and low birth weight although some antenatal risk factors include maternal smoking and maternal hypertension. Neonates with persistent ductus arteriosus or who need mechanical ventilation with high pressures and volumes are also at risk of developing the condition.

Treatment and management

Antenatal interventions including the administration of antenatal steroids will make a significant impact of the development of BPD. If the preterm baby needs ventilatory support then noninvasive techniques should be considered, whilst surfactant, caffeine and steroids will all have a protective effect although the potential side effects of each needs to be considered.

The long-term management of BPD will vary depending upon the extent of residual lung dysplasia. Those babies with mild BPD may only require supplemental oxygen for a short period of time and may be discharged with a home oxygen supply. Those with more severe disease may require continued oxygen and home ventilation supported by a dedicated community respiratory team. Further information is presented in Chapter 17, Respiratory.

The aim of any such treatment will be to ensure maximal growth and development with the intention that developing lung tissue will be sufficient to allow the child to dispense with ventilator support.

Patent ductus arteriosus

The ductus arteriosus in term babies usually closes within 1–3 days after birth but in the preterm neonate about 40% fail to close spontaneously and usually leads to clinical problems. Neonates at risk of developing a clinically significant patent ductus arteriosus (PDA) include those who are small for gestational age, those with late onset sepsis and those who are given excessive fluids during the first days after birth.

A **persistent** ductus arteriosus is defined as one that is still present one month after the baby should have been born and therefore excludes preterm babies who are still within their due dates. This persistence is associated with BPD, NEC and intraventricular haemorrhage.

Echocardiography is required to assess the presence and impact of a PDA.

The symptomatology of PDA is dependent on ductal size, shunt volume, and the extent of a 'circulatory steal' effect. Clinical features of a hemodynamically significant PDA include:

- pan-systolic, pan-diastolic murmur (continuous, machinery murmur)
- active precordium with a wide pulse pressure
- features of cardiac failure
- pulmonary oedema
- high oxygen requirement

Treatment and management

There is limited consensus regarding the treatment of a PDA. Conservative management includes fluid restriction, diuretics and the application of positive end-expiratory ventilatory pressure.

Prophylactic treatment refers to treating all babies within 24 hours, without any screening and prior to any symptoms or signs. Treatment is usually started after 6 hours but before 24 hours of birth with medications such as indomethacin, ibuprofen or paracetamol. However, there is no difference in mortality or composite outcome of death or neuro-disability at 18–36 months with this approach. It is estimated that up to 60% of these infants would close their duct spontaneously.

Though there are advantages of prophylactic treatment in avoiding unnecessary drug exposure, the concern is that the damage could have already been done by the time the PDA becomes symptomatic. Both indomethacin and ibuprofen have been reported to have similar effectiveness for ductal closure (60%–80%), and ibuprofen has been reported to have a better side effect profile. Paracetamol can be used for ductal closure if there is contraindication (NEC, IVH) to use indomethacin or ibuprofen.

Surgical ligation of the PDA is performed in infants with hemodynamically significant PDA where medical treatment has failed or is contraindicated, particularly if the baby remains ventilated and weaning is difficult.

Necrotising enterocolitis (NEC)

Necrotising enterocolitis describes an inflammatory process in the small and large bowel that can affect preterm and, occasionally, term babies. The pathogenesis remains unclear but is multifactorial although there are recognised risk factors that include IUGR, prolonged resuscitation with low APGAR scores and neonatal sepsis. Some factors have been identified that reduce the risk of developing NEC and these include antenatal steroids, breast milk feeding and probiotics.

In preterm neonates, NEC presents around 2–3 weeks of age with features suggestive of sepsis and gastrointestinal obstruction. Abdominal distension, bilious aspirates and blood with mucus in the stool are all characteristic findings. Disease progression leads to peritonitis, hypotension, DIC and shock.

A differential diagnosis would include spontaneous isolated intestinal perforation, congenital bowel anomalies and a food-protein induced enterocolitis.

Investigations

An abdominal x-ray will identify bowel wall oedema and thickening along with intramural and portal venous gas (Figure 2.4). Pneumatosis intestinalis is a pathognomonic finding and indicates that the mucosal surface is damaged

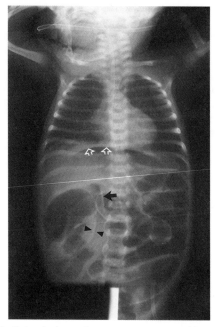

Fig. 2.4 Abdominal x-ray in a preterm neonate with necrotising enterocolitis. Air is visible below the diaphragm (open arrows), on either side of the bowel wall (black triangles) and outlining the falciform ligament (black arrow)

and bowel gases have tracked along the tissue planes. Sentinel bowel loops (fixed loops) may indicate bowel necrosis without pneumatosis.

Treatment and management

Conservative management includes pain relief and sedation, cessation of all oral intake and use of parenteral nutrition to allow resting of the bowel. Broad spectrum antibiotics with anaerobic cover for 10–14 days should be given along with circulatory and ventilatory support if needed. Bowel perforation is the only absolute indication for surgery in the acute phase. Failure of conservative management also warrants surgery and is considered with extensive NEC prior to impending bowel perforation. Surgery usually involves laparotomy with resection of necrotic bowel, with or without stoma formation.

Germinal matrix and intraventricular haemorrhage (GM-IVH)

Intracranial haemorrhage occurs mainly in the germinal matrix or extends into ventricular system and is an important cause for neurological morbidity in the preterm neonate. The haemorrhages tend to develop within the first 6 hours after birth and almost 90% have appeared by day 4. Consequently, perinatal and delivery room interventions and early neonatal care are likely to have impact on incidence of IVH.

Risk factors for intraventricular haemorrhage include hypoxia, severe RDS and hypotension. Practice aimed at preventing intraventricular haemorrhage include antenatal steroids, maintaining normal oxygenation, volume ventilation to avoid hypocapnia, in-utero transfer to tertiary centre and indomethacin prophylaxis.

The neonate with a GM-IVH may be asymptomatic and the bleed is then detected incidentally on cranial ultrasound examination (Figure 2.6a and 2.6b). Most, however, will be recognised by the onset of apnoeic episodes, seizures, or cardiovascular collapse with significant acidosis due to the acute blood loss.

Treatment and management

Once identified, the initial management is mainly supportive. The appearance of posthaemorrhagic hydrocephalus may require surgical intervention in the form of insertion of a ventricular reservoir or ventriculo-peritoneal shunt.

Neurodevelopmental outcome

Infants with severe GM-IVH had increased risk of cerebral palsy, cognitive delay and moderate to severe neurodevelopmental impairment. Preterm babies born before 32 weeks' gestation are at particular risk of developing long term neuro-developmental problems.

Most neonatal units will follow preterm babies under 32 weeks' gestation until 24 months corrected age to monitor neurodevelopmental progress. These babies will often require the ongoing support of all members of the community neurodevelopmental team.

Periventricular leukomalacia

Periventricular leukomalacia (PVL), or white matter injury (WMI), represents one of the most common forms of brain injury in the preterm infants resulting from focal necrosis and gliosis of white matter around lateral ventricles. Risk factors include NEC, significant hypotension, neonatal sepsis, severe hypoxia, hypocapnia and chorioamnionitis.

Three common forms of PVL are described:
- cystic PVL—most severe type due to focal cystic necrosis
- microcystic PVL—cystic lesions are only detected on high resolution MRI
- diffuse WMI—the most frequent type of injury

Table 2.4 Grading systems for germinal matrix and intraventricular haemorrhage	
Severity	
grade 1	germinal matrix haemorrhage with or without IVH (less than 10% of ventricle filled with blood) (Figure 2.5).
grade 2	IVH (10%–50% of ventricle filled with blood), typically without ventricular dilation.
grade 3	IVH (greater than 50% of ventricle filled with blood) typically with ventricular dilation (Figure 2.6a and 2.6b).
grade 4	periventricular haemorrhagic infarction.

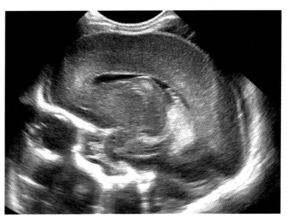

Fig. 2.5 Para-sagittal view of a small GMH-IVH (grade 1 IVH) (Copyright – Dr Mithilesh Lal - used with permission)

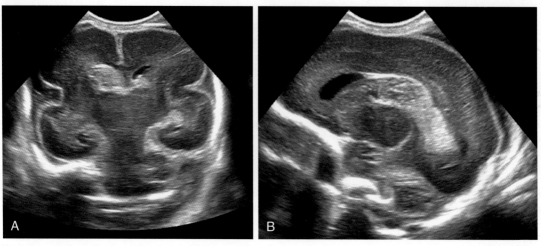

Fig 2.6a and Fig. 2.6b. Coronal and parasagittal view of grade 3 IVH (Copyright – Dr Mithilesh Lal - used with permission)

The condition is initially asymptomatic and only identified on routine cranial USS but can later lead to abnormalities of tone, poor feeding and seizures.

Treatment and management

Strategies to prevent PVL include antenatal steroids and antenatal magnesium sulphate given to the mother when preterm delivery is imminent. Once born, management will include delayed clamping of cord, optimum resuscitation and stabilisation and gentle ventilation to avoid extremes in CO_2 and O_2 levels. Adequate management to maintain normal levels of blood pressure, temperature and blood glucose are important steps in early management that help prevent neurological damage.

Neurodevelopmental outcome

Cystic PVL often leads to spastic diplegia. It is easier to predict neuromotor outcomes than other domains of neurodevelopmental problems, including cognitive and behavioural issues relating to more common and widespread diffuse WMI.

Retinopathy of prematurity (ROP)

Retinopathy of prematurity is a disease of immature and developing retinal vasculature and was associated with increasing use of supplemental oxygen and improved survival in the preterm infant. Restrictive use of supplemental oxygen led to reduction in ROP but an increase in deaths and disability due to cerebral palsy. Up to 60% to 70% of VLBW babies can develop ROP, 5% require treatment for severe ROP, and 1% will develop blindness. Classification of ROP is based on anterior-posterior location (zone), severity (stage), extent (number of clock hours of ROP along the circumference of retina), dilation and tortuosity of posterior pole vessels.

Signs indicative of ROP activity including increased venous dilation and arteriolar tortuosity of the posterior retinal vessels. These features may later increase in severity to include iris vascular engorgement, poor pupillary dilation (rigid pupil) and vitreous haze.

Screening criteria in UK advise that all babies less than 32 weeks gestational age (up to 31 weeks and 6 days) or less than 1501 g birth weight should be screened for ROP.

Treatment and management

Laser ablation is the current treatment of choice as this prevents progression of the lesions to retinal detachment and blindness. Intraocular injections of anti-VEGF agents such as bevacizumab are considered as first-line treatment for localised central ROP as laser ablation is ineffective in the prevention of retinal detachment.

Medical conditions in the term neonate

Meconium aspiration syndrome

This condition is a relatively common cause of respiratory distress in term or near-term infants born through

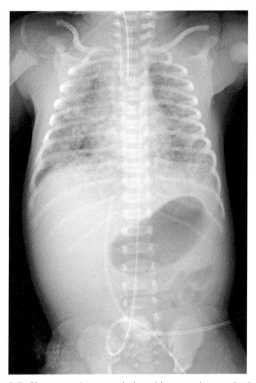

Fig. 2.7 Chest x-ray in a term baby with meconium aspiration.

meconium-stained amniotic fluid. The newborn will have features of respiratory distress with low oxygen saturations that respond poorly to supplemental oxygen and mechanical ventilation. Chest x-ray will show heterogenous lung fields with a combination of atelectasis, coarse patchy lung infiltrates, air trapping and pneumothorax (Figure 2.7).

Treatment and managment

Routine tracheal suctioning and intubation is not recommended in vigorous infants or for infants with poor respiratory effort and low tone. Intubation should only be considered if bag mask ventilation is not effective or there is concern about airway obstruction.

Following transfer to the NICU, the goal is to provide optimum oxygenation and ventilation. Surfactant should be considered for ventilated infants with a high supplemental oxygen requirement along with any required circulatory support. Pulmonary vasodilators such as inhaled nitric oxide can be considered once the diagnosis of pulmonary hypertension is confirmed on

echocardiography. In babies with severe hypoxaemic respiratory failure and a high oxygenation index, extra corporeal membrane oxygenation (ECMO) should be considered.

Transient tachypnoea of the newborn (TTN)

Transient tachypnoea occurs in term babies and develops immediately after birth but has resolved by 48 to 72 hours. It is commonly seen in babies born to mothers with diabetes and to those delivered by a planned elective caesarean. The baby develops tachypnoea, nasal flaring, chest wall recession and grunting.

Treatment and management

Supportive care is provided with only a small number requiring supplemental oxygen and ventilatory support usually with CPAP. Antibiotics may be given if there is any doubt about early sepsis.

Persistent pulmonary hypertension of the newborn (PPHN)

Persistent pulmonary hypertension of the newborn causes severe and refractory hypoxaemic respiratory failure in the term infant. Primary PPHN is mainly due to pulmonary vascular changes but secondary PPHN may develop due to:
- meconium aspiration syndrome
- severe sepsis
- congenital pneumonia
- respiratory distress syndrome
- congenital diaphragmatic hernia

The newborn will present within a few hours of birth with cyanosis and respiratory failure.

Investigations
- chest x-ray—in primary PPHN the lung fields appear dark due to reduced pulmonary blood flow
- arterial blood gas analysis—differential saturations in the upper and lower extremities is suggestive of PPHN due to right to left shunt across the PDA
- echocardiogram—to confirm structurally normal heart and identify elevated right-sided pressures

Clinical severity of PPHN is evaluated using oxygenation index (OI). An OI value below 15 is classed as mild hypoxaemic respiratory failure, whereas a value OI over 40 indicates severe hypoxic respiratory failure with a predictive mortality of up to 50%.

Treatment and management

Mechanical ventilation is needed if severe hypoxia and respiratory failure are identified and high-frequency oscillatory ventilation is invariably required. Pulmonary vasodilators such as inhaled nitric oxide have improved outcomes in PPHN and are usually started at 20 parts per million and then weaned as tolerated. Other pulmonary vasodilators include sildenafil and milrinone. ECMO would be indicated if the OI remains over 30 for more than 4 hours, particularly if there is no response to optimised ventilation, ionotropic support and inhaled nitric oxide.

Neonatal hypoglycaemia

Hypoglycaemia is a common finding in the newborn and can cause long-term neurodevelopmental impairment.
Common associations include:
- infants of diabetic mothers
- IUGR
- moderate to late preterm infants

Clinical presentation

- apnoea
- altered level of consciousness
- seizures
- abnormal feeding behaviour
- jitteriness—although common, is not always due to low blood sugars

Investigations

More detailed investigations in a neonate should be undertaken if the hypoglycaemia is persistent, profound (<1.0 mmol/l at any time) or the infant develops signs of acute neurological dysfunction. Investigations should be completed during the period of hypoglycaemia and include:
- blood glucose, insulin, cortisol, growth hormone, fatty acids, ketone bodies, carnitine, acylcarnitine profile, amino acids, ammonia, lactate.
- urine ketones and organic acids

Treatment and management

Preventative measures include maintaining normothermia, early feeding and encouraging establishment of breast feeding. Further management depends on gestation and degree of hypoglycaemia. In the term infant:
- if blood sugars are over 1.0 mmol/l and the baby is asymptomatic then help to establish feeding should be provided along with buccal dextrose gel for those with a blood glucose between 1.0—1.9 mmol/l
- if blood sugars fall below 1.0 mmol/l, or clinical signs become evident, then the baby requires an IV bolus of 10% dextrose
- IV dextrose and breast or bottle feeds should be continued unless the baby is too ill to feed
- if glucose infusion rates remain high, the investigations for hyperinsulinemia should be undertaken

Hyperbilirubinemia

Clinically identifiable hyperbilirubinemia in first 24 hours of life is pathological and serum bilirubin level should be measured within 2 hours.

Unconjugated hyperbilirubinaemia

A prolonged unconjugated hyperbilirubinemia may be physiological and is usually related to breastfeeding. Unconjugated jaundice can also be secondary to some pathological conditions:
- haemolytic diseases—isoimmune haemolysis, blood group incompatibility, red cell membrane defects, G6PD deficiency
- congenital hypothyroidism
- urinary tract infection
- inherited syndromes including Crigler-Najjar or Gilbert syndromes

Crigler-Najjar syndromes (two variants) are autosomal recessive disorders of bilirubin conjugation leading to a very high unconjugated hyperbilirubinemia. There is a high risk of kernicterus.

Gilbert syndrome is an inherited condition of reduced ability to conjugate bilirubin and is usually an incidental finding on bloods taken for other reasons or from the diagnosis being made in other family members. It does not lead to chronic liver disease and no treatment is required.

Treatment and management

Further monitoring is required and should be continued until safe levels of bilirubin are reached and maintained.

Phototherapy is started if standard treatment thresholds by gestation and age are exceeded or if serum bilirubin levels are rising rapidly. Usually, serum bilirubin measurement is repeated 12–18 hours after stopping phototherapy to identify a marked rebound.

Double volume exchange transfusion is indicated for bilirubin levels above the exchange treatment line, for rapidly rising levels or if signs of acute bilirubin encephalopathy develop.

Complications

Acute bilirubin encephalopathy can present with seizures and variations in tone. Some infants will go on to develop a kernicterus-spectrum disorder with an athetoid cerebral palsy, sensorineural hearing loss and cognitive delay.

Conjugated hyperbilirubinemia

This is usually identified in those neonates who remain jaundiced at 2 weeks of age and have a conjugated bilirubin over 25 micromol/litre. The cause is always pathological and requires further investigations. A differential diagnosis would include:
- bacterial sepsis
- biliary obstruction
- hypothyroidism and hypopituitarism
- metabolic disease—galactosaemia and tyrosinaemia

The infant with jaundice and pale stools is likely to have a biliary obstruction whilst those with jaundice without obviously pale stools are likely to have elevated liver enzymes and have a neonatal hepatitis syndrome. Important extrahepatic signs that will aid a diagnosis include dysmorphic features, cardiac murmurs (babies with Alagille syndrome have a peripheral pulmonary artery stenosis) and hypoplastic male genitalia which are seen with panhypopituitarism. An ill infant with liver failure will develop a coagulopathy unresponsive to intravenous vitamin K.

Investigations

Clarification of the underlying aetiology for the conjugated hyperbilirubinaemia requires a broad range of investigations including:
- FBC and clotting profile
- liver function tests
- metabolic screen—amino acids, organic acids, gal1-put, alpha-1-antitrypsin
- congenital infection screen
- thyroid function and cortisol
- US scan liver and biliary system

Treatment and management

Most disorders affecting the major bile ducts require surgical correction and, in particular, surgery for biliary atresia must occur before 6 weeks of age to minimise the chance of liver cirrhosis. Liver dysfunction is managed medically by preventing bleeding disorders and hypoglycaemia.

Neonatal sepsis

Neonates with evolving sepsis usually present with non-specific signs although certain features in the history should raise the suspicion of an infective cause for the clinical signs. These include:
- parenteral antibiotic treatment to the mother during labour or postpartum period
- invasive group B streptococcal infection in a previous baby
- maternal group B streptococcal in current pregnancy
- premature rupture of membranes more than 18 hours in preterm and 24 hours in term baby
- preterm birth
- intrapartum fever higher than 38°C
- chorioamnionitis

Clinical indicators of possible early-onset neonatal infection are respiratory distress starting within 4 hours after birth, seizures or signs of shock, whilst more subtle indicators of sepsis would include temperature instability, glycaemic instability, episodic cyanosis, apnoea, early jaundice, early signs of encephalopathy, abnormal coagulation and metabolic acidosis.

Investigations

A full infection screen including blood culture, CRP and lumbar puncture is required.

Treatment and management

The administration of antibiotics will follow local protocols. Intravenous benzylpenicillin with gentamicin is the first-choice antibiotic regimen for empirical treatment of suspected infection. If there is microbiological evidence of gram-negative bacterial sepsis, cefotaxime should replace benzylpenicillin. If meningitis is suspected and the causative pathogen is unknown, then intravenous penicillin and cefotaxime is advised.

Late-onset sepsis occurs at 4–90 days of life and may be caused by coagulase-negative staphylococci, group B streptococci or gram-negative organisms.

Neonatal seizures

Seizures are seen with relative frequency in neonatal practice and may be the result of a wide range of conditions. Prompt assessment and treatment is important as continued seizure activity may lead to further neurological insult.

Causes of seizures include:

- HIE—most common cause in term infants
- intracranial haemorrhage—most common cause in pre-term infants
- infection
- metabolic disturbances
- maternal drug withdrawal
- epilepsy syndromes

Clinical presentation

Subtle seizure activity presents with transient bradycardias, oxygen desaturations or apnoeas. More overt signs include repetitive oral and tongue movements, jerking or cycling leg movements or peddling arm movements, eye deviation, staring or blinking. Benign sleep myoclonus can be confused with seizure activity and is a term describing jerking movements that are seen in clusters during active sleep. They can be suppressed by gentle restraint and the EEG is normal. It is a diagnosis of exclusion.

Investigations

- electrolyte and metabolic screen including lactate, ammonia and blood glucose
- infection screen
- cranial ultrasound—to identify IVH
- amplitude-integrated EEG (aEEG)—simplified EEG but may miss focal seizure activity. A conventional EEG would still be needed.
- urine toxicology—if neonatal abstinence syndrome suspected

Treatment and management

Phenobarbital is the preferred first-line treatment for acute seizures and may be repeated if limited response to a first dose. Phenytoin is usually used as a second-line treatment whilst benzodiazepines, lidocaine and off-label drugs such as levetiracetam and topiramate are also being used.

Neonatal abstinence syndrome

Neonatal abstinence syndrome (NAS) describes a drug withdrawal syndrome seen in neonates who are exposed to opioids in utero although some other drugs may produce similar neuro-behavioural dysregulation.

Onset of symptoms depends on the length of drug exposure, the half-life of drug in question and last maternal dose prior to delivery. NAS presents with:

- hyperirritability, anxiety and sleep deprivation
- yawning and sneezing
- tremors
- tachycardia

Common drugs causing NAS include opioids (including methadone), benzodiazepines, barbiturates, amphetamines and alcohol.

Investigations

NAS is a clinical diagnosis although toxicological confirmation is necessary to identify the substance taken. Urine for toxicology should be collected as soon as possible after birth, as many drugs are rapidly metabolised.

Treatment and management

When substance misuse is identified in a mother then an MDT meeting should be organised as early as possible in the pregnancy. Alternative medications can then be considered and offered to the mother along with a plan for postnatal management agreed between the team members and the mother. Naloxone should be avoided following the birth as it may induce respiratory depression, acute withdrawal and seizures. Babies should only be separated from their mothers if there are social, legal or medical reasons identified antenatally.

Infants at risk of NAS should be observed closely and assessments undertaken at frequent intervals using standardised scoring charts. If the withdrawal scores are low, then soothing techniques can be used. Pharmacotherapy is initiated if supportive therapy fails to control clinical manifestations and includes oral morphine, phenobarbitone, clonidine, buprenorphine and methadone.

Neonatal thrombocytopenia

Neonatal thrombocytopaenia with a platelet count of less than 150×10^9/l mainly occurs in preterm, IUGR or sick neonates. In most situations, it is mild and does not warrant intervention.

Causes include:

- asphyxia
- alloimmune thrombocytopenia
- autoimmune conditions
- viral infections (HSV, cytomegalovirus)
- thrombotic events—renal, catheter related
- sepsis and DIC
- Kasabach-Merritt syndrome

Treatment and management

Levels above 25×10^9/l are considered safe in asymptomatic well babies, but platelet transfusions can be given to treat or prevent bleeding although they may be ineffective in conditions causing platelet consumption.

Common surgical conditions affecting the term neonate

Thoracic and abdominal abnormalities requiring surgical assessment and intervention may be identified on antenatal scans. Respiratory compromise, abdominal distension and bilious vomiting are common presenting features after birth.

Practice Point – common causes of bilious vomiting in neonates

- malrotation with or without midgut volvulus
- meconium ileus
- duodenal atresia and duodenal web
- jejunal or ileal atresia
- Hirschsprung disease
- necrotising enterocolitis
- incarcerated inguinal hernia
- sepsis

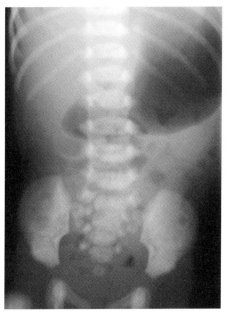

Fig. 2.8 Abdominal x-ray in term baby with malrotation showing air in the stomach and duodenum but asymmetric gas pattern elsewhere.

Malrotation with or without midgut volvulus

Bilious vomiting in the term neonate is a surgical emergency as malrotation with midgut volvulus can obstruct the superior mesenteric vessels and lead to bowel necrosis and the consequent short gut. In an infant with bilious vomiting a plain abdominal x-ray will show gastric distension and paucity of distal bowel gas (Figure 2.8). The most informative investigation for malrotation is an upper gastrointestinal contrast study. Blood gas analysis may show a metabolic acidosis and a raised lactate.

Treatment and management

All enteral feeds should be stopped and a free draining, large-bore nasogastric tube inserted. Intravenous fluids should be commenced and any losses from the gastric tube replaced with a potassium-containing fluid. Monitoring of hydration status, urine output, renal function and electrolytes should be undertaken. Sepsis and necrotising enterocolitis are important differential diagnoses and antibiotics should be administered after blood cultures have been taken.

Meconium ileus

Meconium ileus is characterised by thick plugs of meconium and mucous blocking the bowel and leading to obstruction. The most likely cause is cystic fibrosis and this is the underlying aetiology in over 90% of infants with meconium ileus. Hypothyroidism can also lead to slow gut motility and plugs. Meconium ileus can be suspected on antenatal scans when dilated bowel loops are identified or, if antenatal perforation has occurred, intraabdominal calcification. The newborn will present on day one with bilious vomiting and abdominal distension.

An abdominal x-ray will show distended bowel loops whilst lower gastrointestinal contrast study will show distended loops proximal to the plug. An atretic colon may be seen due to nonuse in utero.

A bowel washout will help to clear the obstructing plugs when the condition is uncomplicated but urgent surgical intervention is required for those with signs of bowel perforation or atresia.

Duodenal atresia and duodenal web

Duodenal atresia is a congenital obstruction of the second part of the duodenum. The condition can be isolated or associated with other congenital anomalies such as Down syndrome, cardiac disease, malrotation or imperforate anus. A duodenal web leads to a partial obstruction at the level of the duodenum and symptoms may be less obvious or occur later.

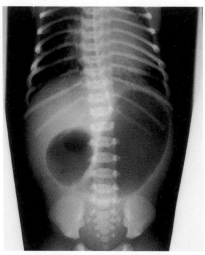

Fig. 2.9 Abdominal x-ray in term baby with duodenal atresia showing 'double bubble' appearance. No gas patterns in remaining bowel.

The diagnosis may be suspected antenatally if poly-hydramnios was present, although the usual presentation is with vomiting, which may be bilious. An abdominal x-ray will show the typical 'double bubble' appearance of the stomach and dilated proximal duodenum (Figure 2.9). Surgical resection of the atretic section or web with re-anastomosis of the duodenum is required.

Tracheo-oesophageal fistula and oesophageal atresia

Oesophageal atresia is associated with a tracheo-oesophageal fistula in 90% of affected newborns and most fistulae connect the distal part of the oesophagus to the trachea. Tracheo-oesophageal fistula commonly forms part of the VACTERL or VATER condition.

Infants born to mothers with polyhydramnios should have a nasogastric tube passed following birth that will coil back into the pharynx if an oesophageal atresia is present. Typically, the baby will present on day one with choking, coughing and cyanosis during feeding whilst copious oral secretions may be evident.

Investigations

Chest and abdominal x-rays show a proximal oesophageal pouch with the coiled nasogastric tube in the upper half

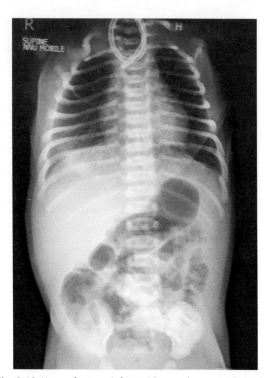

Fig. 2.10 X-ray of a term infant with a tracheo-oesophageal fistula. Note nasogastric tube coiled in pharynx and presence of air in stomach indicating fistula connection.

of the chest. Air will be visible in the stomach if there is a connecting fistula from the trachea to the distal oesophageal pouch. The abdomen will remain gasless is a distal fistula is absent (Figure 2.10).

Treatment and managment

A wide-bore, double-lumen suction catheter (Replogle tube) is placed in the blind-ending oesophageal pouch to allow the continuous suction of secretions and regular flushing. Prompt surgical referral is required and early intervention will take place to ligate the fistula and anastomose the oesophagus. When it is not possible to bring the two ends of the oesophagus together due to the long atretic section, the repair is delayed to allow a period of growth or to facilitate a 'gastric pull-up' if the gap remains too long. The level of the oesophageal anastomosis can form strictures or narrowing which require repeated dilatations. Gastro-oesophageal reflux symptoms are very common and problematic along with difficulty in eating 'lumpy' food and choking.

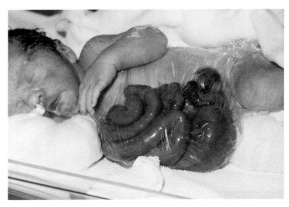

Fig. 2.12 Term infant with gastroschisis showing intestines without covering sac, plastic film wrap and towelling to support intestines.

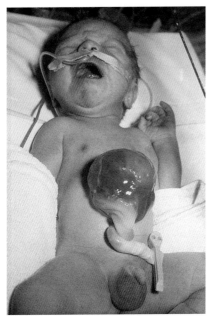

Fig. 2.11 Term infant with exomphalos showing midline position and peritoneal sac covering of intestines.

Anorectal malformations

An imperforate anus is usually identified during the newborn physical examination and can be isolated or part of the VACTERL association. The passage of meconium does not exclude an anorectal malformation as fistulas can occur between the bowel and vagina or urethra. Surgical repair is required and may be staged with an early colostomy and a later reconstruction.

Vacterl association

The acronym describes a recognised cluster of congenital anomalies that may be found together in a newborn. It is usual to identify at least three of the characteristic features before the term is used.

- vertebral anomalies—hemi- or fused vertebrae, rib anomalies, sacral agenesis
- anal atresia
- cardiac defects—VSD, Tetralogy of Fallot
- tracheo-oesophageal fistula
- renal anomalies—absent, dysplastic ectopic or horseshoe kidney
- limb abnormalities—radial hypoplasia or agenesis, poly- or syndactyly

Exomphalos

An exomphalos is protrusion of the abdominal content through the umbilical ring and are therefore midline abnormalities. They are usually covered by peritoneum although this may tear during delivery (Figure 2.11). It is usually diagnosed during the 20-week anomaly scan. Other congenital abnormalities are common. Surgical repair is required and may take place over multiple stages.

Gastroschisis

The abdominal wall defect in gastroschisis is para-umbilical and the exposed abdominal contents lack a peritoneal covering (Figure 2.12). The bowel wall is thickened, often scarred and covered with a thick fibrous peel containing multiple adhesions.

Treatment and management

At birth the defect should be covered immediately to prevent fluid and heat loss and the eviscerated organs supported to avoid twisting. Plastic film wrap is commonly used to achieve this.

The abdominal wall opening is usually relatively small compared to the protruding intestine and there is a risk of compromised blood flow to the bowel. Urgent surgical correction is therefore performed to protect the exposed intestine and reduce fluid losses. Many infants show delayed gut motility and take many weeks to establish full enteral feeds.

Congenital diaphragmatic hernia

Congenital diaphragmatic hernia (CDH) is a defect usually in the left diaphragm allowing the abdominal organs to enter the chest cavity. Pulmonary hypoplasia develops due to compression within the chest cavity (Figure 2.13). The diagnosis is often made antenatally during the 20-week anomaly scan. Right-sided hernias are usually significant before being detected as the smaller defects are occluded by the liver.

Those affected infants who are not identified on the antenatal scan will usually present with significant respiratory distress at birth and examination will reveal cardiac displacement and a scaphoid abdomen.

Treatment and managment

Immediate insertion of a nasogastric tube allows decompression of the stomach and bowel, which will be part located within the chest cavity. Bag and mask ventilation should be avoided at birth and intubation is undertaken if respiratory distress is present. Most infants will require invasive ventilatory support with conventional ventilation or high frequency oscillation due to the pulmonary hypoplasia and consequent persistent pulmonary hypertension. Definitive surgery to close the diaphragmatic defect is required.

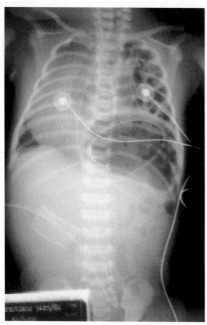

Fig. 2.13 Chest x-ray of a term infant with left-sided diaphragmatic hernia. Note stomach with nasogastric tube in chest, absence of gas in the abdomen and mediastinal shift to the right.

IMPORTANT CLINICAL POINTS

Hypoxic-ischaemic encephalopathy
- therapeutic hypothermia to be initiated within the first 6 hours
- death or disability following cooling treatment is seen in 50% of infants bronchopulmonary dysplasia

Bronchopulmonary dysplasia
- antenatal and postnatal factors contribute to neurodevelopment
- respiratory symptoms and signs can persist into adulthood jaundice

Jaundice
- jaundice within the first 24 hours of life should be considered pathological
- conjugated hyperbilirubinaemia is pathological
- suspected biliary atresia requires immediate assessment and referral surgical presentation

Surgical presentation
- bilious vomiting is a surgical emergency
- malrotation with midgut volvulus can rapidly lead to bowel necrosis
- upper gastrointestinal contrast study is required to diagnose malrotation

Further reading

Therapeutic hypothermia for neonatal encephalopathy BAPM Framework for Practice. Published December 2020. https://www.bapm.org/resources/237-therapeutic-hypothermia-for-neonatal-encephalopathy

Identification and Management of Neonatal Hypoglycaemia in the Full-Term Infant BAPM Framework for Practice. Published December 2020. https://www.bapm.org/resources/40-identification-and-management-of-neonatal-hypoglycaemia-in-the-full-term-infant-2017

Neonatal infection: antibiotics for prevention and treatment. NICE guideline [NG195] Published 20 April 2021.

Chapter | 3 |

Adolescent medicine

Damian Wood, Karen Aucott

After reading this chapter you should be able to:
- manage transition of adolescents with chronic health needs to adult services
- assess and diagnose risk-taking behaviours including non-adherence, self-harm, alcohol and substance misuse and make appropriate referral to specialist services
- to assess, diagnose and manage eating disorders and know the risks and complications of treatment
- to assess, diagnose and manage problems relating to sexual health including contraception, sexually transmitted disease and teenage pregnancy

Adolescent health needs

Adolescence is defined as the transition from childhood to adulthood and is characterised by typical physical, psychological and social changes that do not occur at any other time during a person's life. The onset of adolescence is heralded by the physical changes of puberty, whereas in later adolescence key psychosocial transitions signal the emergence into adulthood. The key events of adolescence are:
- completion of growth and sexual development
- development of a personal identity which is distinct from that of their carers
- formation of intimate relationships with members of their peer group
- development of autonomy and independence

The WHO defines adolescence as 10–19 years and youth defined as up to 25 years. However, it is increasingly argued that there are biological, psychological and social reasons to extend the definition of adolescence beyond 19 years of age and even up to 25 years as the neurobiological changes of adolescence continue into the third decade of life.

Adolescence is a time of great opportunity where the individual develops interests, friendships, lifestyles and belief systems that form a basis for their adult lives. It is also a time of great health vulnerability with an increased risk of death and morbidity from injury, an increased susceptibility to mental illness and poorer outcomes from any pregnancy.

Control of long-term conditions such as asthma, epilepsy, arthritis and diabetes often deteriorates during adolescence, and risks from acute infections (such as meningococcal disease), allergic disease (fatal anaphylaxis) and cancer are also increased compared to school-age children. Young people with neurodevelopmental disorders are at increased risk of health-related problems as they navigate the psychological and social transitions to adulthood. When considering young people aged 10–19 years, it is important to recognise that the patterns of mortality, morbidity and presentation of illness are very similar to those of young adults and therefore the needs of young people in relation to healthcare providers are similar to those of young adults. Increasingly, the two age groups are considered together as adolescents and young adults (AYA) in a healthcare context.

Risk-taking behaviours during adolescence contribute to mortality and morbidity during this key developmental stage. It is now understood, however, that the risk-taking behaviours which create health vulnerabilities are a key and necessary aspect of development which facilitate the transition to adulthood.

The challenge for paediatricians is to:
- understand the unique patterns of illness and injury during adolescence and their social determinants
- provide developmentally appropriate healthcare services for young people and support their transition to adulthood with an improvement rather than a deterioration in their health
- work with young people, families, other health providers and governments to ensure services and policies are

in place which promote the health needs of adolescents and young adults

- research and innovate to enhance the health of young people and improve access to developmentally appropriate healthcare through meaningful and ethical participation
- promote the health and safety of young people, respect their individual rights, reduce health inequalities and tackle the social determinants of health as this is likely to have important health and economic consequences into the future.

The use of formal interview tools can help discussions with adolescents and ensure that important areas that may impact on health are addressed. One such tool is the structured HEEADSSS method of interview developed by Drs Goldenring and Rosen that provides introductory phrases for each of the listed topics.

PRACTICE POINT – the HEEADSSS structured interview

- H - Home environment
- E - Education and Employment
- E - Eating
- A - Activities (peer related)
- D – Drugs
- S – Sexuality
- S - Suicide/depression
- S - Safety

Legal framework

As young people acquire independence during the transition to adulthood, they are permitted greater rights as citizens and this includes the right to vote, the right to work and the right to make decisions for themselves free from parental involvement. They are also granted the right to participate in a range of activities that are prohibited for children such as consensual sexual intercourse, getting married, driving motor vehicles, buying alcohol and tobacco, gambling and obtaining financial credit.

In England and Wales, the Children Act 1989 applies to all children and young people up to their 18th birthday and outlines the responsibility of the state and parents in this regard. There is, however, other UK legislation that permits young people to receive adult responsibilities at ages younger than 18yrs. For example, young people can apply for a provisional driving licence at 17yrs of age, can legally have consensual sex from 16yrs of age and are assumed to have mental capacity to make some decisions from age 16ys or earlier.

The key to understanding the legal framework is the issue of context. There is no single piece of UK legislation that defines adulthood, rather a series of different pieces of legislation that define when a young person can acquire the right to adult responsibilities. From a healthcare perspective, it is crucial that paediatricians have expertise in the legal framework of consent and confidentiality in relation to children and young people. This topic is presented in more detail in Chapter 32 on Ethics and Law.

Risk-taking behaviour

Substance abuse

Substance misuse by adolescents and young adults is a major public health concern as it contributes to morbidity and mortality in adolescence. Over the lifetime of an individual, much of the morbidity and mortality attributed to alcohol, tobacco and other drugs can be traced to behaviours that begin during adolescence. Substance use is also associated with risks of abuse, poor educational and employment outcomes, criminality, disrupted peer and family relationships as well as a range of mental and physical health disorders.

Alcohol, tobacco and cannabis are the substances most often used by adolescents although trends in drug use do vary over time. There have been recent reductions in prevalence of adolescent alcohol use and smoking in the UK but with increases in the use of cannabis, novel psychoactive substances and vaping. Shifting trends in drug use are predictable and cyclical, although they are influenced by population level factors such as legislation, taxation and law enforcement activity.

The period of adolescence includes the ongoing state of brain development and is a time of risk-taking and sensation-seeking behaviours. Such behaviour would include substance use that may lead to permanent changes. The CRAFFT screen is a brief screening tool that has been validated in the adolescent primary care setting to identify problematic substance use and uses a series of six questions to explore the topic and help identify those young people who may need support.

Alcohol

Alcohol is the drug most commonly used by adolescents and is a CNS depressant that stimulates the endorphin and dopaminergic reward systems. It is rapidly absorbed and has physical, mood and cognitive effects.

Recent UK data show that although rates of alcohol use continue to rise with increasing age, the number of young people who drink and the amount that they drink appears to be decreasing gradually over time. Similarly rates of hospitalisation of young people for alcohol-related conditions are falling.

Alcohol use increases with age and, among 15 year olds in England, 18% report drinking in the previous week. Alcohol use in young people remains a serious public health concern as alcohol contributes to preventable deaths and injury and alcohol use established in adolescence tracks into adulthood.

Alcohol use in young people has been associated with the following:
- injury—motor vehicle accidents, falls, interpersonal violence
- victim of physical/sexual assault
- sexual risk behaviours
- criminality
- self-harm and suicidality

Alcohol is neurotoxic and whilst the extent of the effects on the developing adolescent brain have not been fully elucidated, it is known that binge drinking and heavy alcohol use in adolescence has effects on brain structure and function including impaired learning, impaired memory and disruption of the sleep-wake cycle. Young people do appear to be more tolerant of the acute intoxicating effects of alcohol and show fewer acute withdrawal effects than adults.

Children of parents with an alcohol use disorder are four to ten times more likely to develop the same problem. The perceptions of parental approval of alcohol use and the parents' use of alcohol have been identified as risk factors for adolescent initiation of drinking behaviours. Early initiation of alcohol before 14 years of age is associated with an increased risk of alcohol use disorder.

Marketing and media influences have a substantial effect on alcohol use by young people. This includes alcohol industry–sponsored advertising but also the depiction of alcohol use in media and exposure to alcohol use by peers and older adults through the internet and social media.

Alcohol use disorders

The diagnostic criteria for alcohol use disorders describe a maladaptive pattern of substance use leading to clinically significant impairment or distress, as manifested by two or more of the following, occurring at any time in the same 12-month period:
- alcohol often taken in larger amounts or over a longer period than was intended
- persistent desire or unsuccessful efforts to cut down or control alcohol use
- excess time is spent in obtaining alcohol, using alcohol or recovering from its effects
- craving for, or a strong desire to use alcohol

- recurrent alcohol use resulting in a failure to fulfil major role obligations
- continued alcohol use despite having social or interpersonal problems caused by alcohol
- important social, occupational or recreational activities are given up because of alcohol use
- recurrent alcohol use in situations in which it is physically hazardous

If alcohol misuse is identified as a potential problem, then a brief assessment of the duration and severity of the alcohol misuse is required. Young people under 16 years of age with alcohol use disorder should be referred to a specialist child and adolescent mental health service (CAMHS).

Tobacco and vaping

Smoking is the primary cause of preventable morbidity and mortality in the UK, accounting for one in six of all deaths. One in five young people try smoking at some point; however, regular smoking is less common and there has been recent and significant downward trend in smoking by young people.

Risk factors for smoking in adolescence include
- low socioeconomic status
- low educational attainment
- parental, sibling or peer smoking
- those with low self-esteem or depression
- lesbian, gay and bisexual young people

Nicotine is a highly addictive substance and abstinence leads to withdrawal symptoms:
- cravings
- increased appetite
- depression
- poor concentration
- irritability/aggression
- sleep disruption

All young people who smoke should be advised to stop and should be offered referral to a local smoking cessation service or given information on how to access such services. Interventions can increase the chances of smoking cessation and generally fall into two categories: medication and psychological support. The evidence suggests that smokers are four times more likely to quit successfully by using a combination of pharmacological and psychological intervention.

Nicotine replacement therapy

Nicotine replacement therapy (NRT) works by substituting the nicotine provided in cigarettes, alleviating nicotine withdrawal symptoms and allowing users to gradually reduce their dependence on nicotine. NRT includes nicotine-containing chewing gum, transdermal patches, lozenges, mouth spray, inhalator and nasal spray and is usually taken for 8 to 12 weeks.

E-cigarettes and vaping

Electronic cigarette use (also known as vaping) is increasing amongst adolescents and young adults and there is emerging evidence that they may be effective in helping adult smokers to quit. NICE advises that young people wishing to stop smoking should be advised that whilst the safety and quality cannot be assured, e-cigarettes are likely to be less harmful than cigarettes. Recent reports of vaping-associated lung injury have added to concerns regarding their safety.

Illicit drugs

Cannabis

Marijuana is derived from the dried seeds, stems, leaves and flowering tops of the plant *Cannabis sativa* and is the most commonly used illegal substance in the UK. It may be smoked, vaped or ingested with smoking being the most common route (table 3.1).

Table 3.1 Cannabis names and methods of intake		
Methods	**Names**	
smoked:	weed	hash or hashish
spliff or joint – rolled in a	pot	ganja
cigarette paper	dope	bud
blunt – a hollowed out cigar	grass	pollen
bowl – a pipe	skunk	bhang
bong – a water pipe	resin	sensi
ingested: (brownies/cakes)	puff	sensimiella

Onset of use typically occurs in adolescence although the peak prevalence of use is among young adults. Adolescents and young adults are more susceptible than adults to the adverse effects of marijuana use and more likely to develop cannabis use disorders.

The effects of inhalation are usually apparent within 30 minutes and typically lasts 2–3 hours, but with ingestion the effect-onset is delayed and lasts longer. The recognised effects of acute intoxication from cannabis are:

- euphoria
- distorted perception
- reduced inhibition
- anxiety
- psychotic symptoms
- cognitive impairment
- processing difficulties
- sedation
- increased appetite
- tachycardia
- orthostatic hypotension
- supine hypertension
- conjunctival injection

Short-term effects may include impairments of
- short-term memory which will affect learning and retention of information
- motor coordination—increasing the risk of injury through accidents
- judgment and risk perception—increasing the risk of injury, assault and potentially harmful or risky sexual behaviours

Repeated use of cannabis leads to tolerance, and a cannabis withdrawal syndrome has been described with symptoms of withdrawal being similar to those of nicotine withdrawal. They typically appear within one day of cessation, peak after one week, and may last up to two weeks. Withdrawal symptoms include irritability, depression, anxiety, restlessness, reduced appetite, sleep problems and weight loss.

Repeated exposure to cannabis in adolescence leads to neurotoxic effects in brain structure and function which persist into adulthood and may not be entirely reversible. This includes an association between frequent use of cannabis and a significant decline in IQ whilst heavy cannabis use has also been associated with poor educational and social outcomes. Given the importance of educational attainment to adolescent development and outcomes, the cognitive effects of cannabis are of particular concern.

Adolescent-onset cannabis use is associated with mental disorders including a risk of developing a psychotic disorder (including schizophrenia) which is increased in those with a family history. Regular use in adolescence is also associated with anxiety, depression, suicidality and deterioration in symptoms in those who already have depression, bipolar disorder or schizophrenia.

Assessment should include enquiring about cannabis use in the past year and this may be incorporated into adolescent psychosocial screening tool such as HEEADSSS. If the young person endorses use in the last year, then the CRAFFT questions can help to elicit problematic substance misuse. Cannabis use is detectable on urine toxicology testing although this is not true for synthetic cannabinoids. Emergency presentations related to cannabis are rare. For those with acute marijuana intoxication, supportive care is all that is required.

There are no specific pharmacotherapies available to treat cannabis use disorder and intervention is based on motivational enhancement and cognitive behavioural therapies, which may be delivered in individual or group settings.

Other drugs of abuse

Use of other drugs of abuse such as opioids, MDMA (ecstasy), benzodiazepines, amphetamines, LSD, ketamine and novel psychoactive substances is much less common in adolescence, but they are all associated with significant potential harms.

Novel psychoactive substances are synthetic drugs that are designed to mimic the effects of other psychoactive substances. They can be grouped into four main categories—stimulants, cannabinoids, hallucinogens and depressants—and all can be taken in a number of ways. Toxicity is a significant concern for novel psychoactive substances and they are not "safe" alternatives.

Inhalants

Inhalants are most frequently used by younger adolescents (10–12yrs) and use decreases with age. The four groups of inhalants are volatile solvents, aerosols, nitrites and medical gases. They have a rapid onset of action, low cost and are often readily available in legal products such as spray paint, glues, cleaning fluid, permanent markers and deodorants. They are typically inhaled from a plastic bag ("bagging") or saturated cloth ("huffing").

Indicators of inhalant abuse may be subtle and it may only be suspected when potential inhalants are discovered by parents/carers. Abusers may have chemical odours on the breath or clothes, show a change in behaviour or develop a marked decrease in appetite. Young people may exhibit confusion, poor concentration, depression, irritability, hostility and paranoia and inhalation of solvents may lead to peri-nasal and peri-oral rashes and epistaxis. Social and educational decline and neglect of personal care are commonly seen. Initially they cause stimulation progressing to depression and their use often escalates as the 'high' is short lived. Inhalant abuse can lead to sudden death and for chronic users may lead to irreversible neurological, renal, cardiac or hepatic injury.

Nitrites including amyl, butyl and isobutyl nitrites are known as 'poppers'. They lead to vasodilatation, increased sexual pleasure and a mild high or 'rush'.

In recent years, abuse of 'laughing gas'—nitrous oxide—has increased as the drug is sold in balloons or canisters and is inhaled for a rapid onset. Inhalants are not detected by routine urine drug screenings.

Self-harm

Self-harm is defined as self-poisoning or self-injury irrespective of the apparent purpose of the act and includes any form of behaviour that leads to self-injury. National guidance avoids the use of the term 'deliberate' and other descriptions that imply the presence or absence of suicidal intent such as 'attempted suicide', 'parasuicide', 'non-suicidal self-injury'.

Community-based studies estimate around 10% of young people reported self-harm whilst other UK and European studies have suggested rates between 15% to 22%. Young females report two to four times higher rates of self-harm than young males and there has been a trend of increasing hospitalisations in young people for self-harm (Figure 3.1). Most young people who do self-harm do not attend hospital and many do not seek or access medical or psychological treatment. Suicide is a leading cause of death in young people and the risk is greater for boys than girls.

Young people may not be able to explain why they self-harm and this is not surprising when self-harm itself is a way of communicating, coping or adapting to intense emotional or psychological distress. The act of self-harm may serve a number of purposes in relation to the intense distress including distracting, self-punishing, communicating, controlling and distracting.

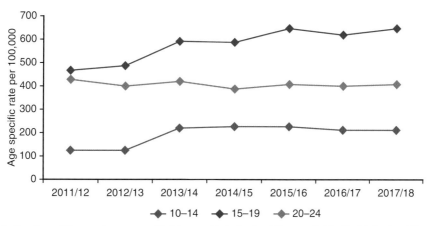

Fig. 3.1 Hospitalisation for self-harm rates among 10–24 year olds in England (Source: Public Health England Hospital Episode Statistics 2017/18. Permission to use via Open Government Licence.)

Risk factors for self-harm
- female gender
- affective or depressive symptoms
- onset of sexual activity
- sexual and gender identity
- adverse childhood experiences such as abuse, bullying, parental separation or death
- mental health disorders
- drug and alcohol use

The focus of paediatric management is:
- emergency assessment of the method, extent, timing and context of the self-harm
- emergency management of the injury or poisoning
- initial assessment of psychosocial risks and resilience and risk of abuse or neglect
- establishing whether the young person is fit for a comprehensive psychosocial assessment and any issues relating to legal framework such as consent and confidentiality
- ensuring a comprehensive psychosocial assessment of risk and need is undertaken and the results shared appropriately between professionals, young person and parents/carers
- a care plan is established with the young person to promote their safety and well-being and reduced the risk of death or serious harm

Working with young people who self-harm can induce a range of negative emotions (including anger, frustration and sadness), and paediatricians and other health professionals need to be aware of the potential for this and to understand how it may influence a professional response.

Assessment of risk

Certain aspects of the history may indicate an increased risk of later completed suicide or repetition of the attempt. These include:
- specific plan for suicide or suicidal intent
- final acts—writing a note
- no regret or a regret that attempt has failed
- potentially fatal method of self-harm
- known mental illness—depression
- repeated attempts with escalation of frequency or risk
- lack of engagement with professional response
- suicide attempts in a first-degree relative or completed suicide in any relative
- friend who has died by suicide
- making a suicide pact with another

The young person should be referred to a specialist child and adolescent mental health service that can offer an urgent comprehensive psychosocial assessment of both risk and need. If there are safeguarding concerns, a referral should be made to child protection services. The assessment of risk should include the risk of a future completed suicide and the risk of repetition as well as to document any other risks to the young person.

In addition to identifying the current resources, coping abilities and protective factors of the young person and family the assessment should also consider the needs of the young person and family in relation to safeguarding risks, mental health issues, drug or alcohol use and financial needs. It is important that paediatric and CAMHS services collaborate closely with colleagues in social care and health professionals with safeguarding expertise.

Safety planning

Parents and carers should be advised regarding safe storage of medicines and removal of sharps and provided with contacts for local and national crisis support services.

Outcomes

Suicide is uncommon before 15 years of age but increases in prevalence with age, and it is clear that rates of death from suicide are increasing in young people. The strongest predictors of suicide in young people are self-harm, cannabis and other drug use, exposure to self-harm in others and personality type. Specific groups who are at increased risk are:
- children looked after
- bereaved young people (especially those bereaved by suicide)
- LGBT+ young people
- university and college students

Eating disorders

Eating disorders are psychological disorders characterised by a preoccupation with weight and shape leading to unhealthy eating behaviours. They are relatively common and cause significant physical and psychosocial morbidity. The causes of eating disorders are complex and are likely to be multifactorial but include:
- biological—possibly genetic
- psychological—low self-esteem
- cultural—peer pressure to be a particular weight or shape
They can be categorised as:
- restrictive eating disorders—anorexia nervosa
- binge-purge type eating behaviours—bulimia nervosa

Anorexia nervosa

Diagnosed in a patient by identifying:
- restriction of energy intake
- fear of gaining weight
- disturbance of body image

All three features must be present to make the diagnosis, but the presence of two would lead to a diagnosis of atypical anorexia nervosa.

The young person with anorexia nervosa will restrict their energy intake relative to requirements which leads to a significantly low body weight in the context of age, sex, development and physical health.

They demonstrate a fear of gaining weight or becoming fat or display persistent behaviour that interferes with weight gain, even though they are underweight. They are often worried that if they eat normally they will become fat, so they often start altering their diet by avoiding fatty foods and carbohydrates with the aim of losing weight. They may also change behaviours to achieve weight loss such as excessive exercise, self-induced vomiting and laxative abuse.

They also display a disturbance of body image, with undue influence of body weight or shape on self-evaluation or denial of the seriousness of the current low body weight. Young people with anorexia nervosa will often see themselves as being overweight despite being a healthy weight or underweight. They see themselves as being good or bad depending on how much they have eaten and how much they weigh and may also feel that others are judging them in the same way.

Bulimia nervosa

People with bulimia nervosa can appear perfectly healthy. Usually, they maintain a normal body weight but are very worried about what people think of them and are preoccupied with dieting and losing weight.

Bulimia can be a way of dealing with difficult feelings. When a person with bulimia feels sad, angry, unloved or depressed, they may binge on large quantities of food. They often feel ashamed after a binge and try to counteract it by making themselves sick, taking large amounts of laxatives or starving for a few days.

Clinical presentation

Young people with an eating disorder may present in a variety of ways. Their difficulties often come to light after family or friends raise concerns or they present with physical manifestations of the eating disorder (table 3.2). The physical manifestations of anorexia nervosa result from weight loss and malnutrition. With starvation, there is:
- loss of tissue mass from internal organs (brain, heart)
- metabolic rate slows down
- hormonal systems are suppressed

Whilst people with bulimia are often not underweight, physical manifestations are related to the mode and degree of purging.

The initial assessment includes:
- assessment of the degree of malnutrition—height, weight, BMI centile, rate of weight loss
- identification of abnormal cognitions around food and weight
- evaluation of the potential medical complications
- psychosocial assessment (HEEADSSS)
- identification of associated conditions such as depression or obsessive-compulsive disorders
- assessment for other medical conditions which may account for the weight loss

Investigations

When a young person presents with a suspected eating disorder, initial investigations should be focused on:
- excluding other causes for weight loss
- seeking evidence of malnutrition
- seeking acute medical complications—bone marrow suppression, renal and liver impairment, electrolyte abnormalities.

Initial investigations should include a full blood count, inflammatory markers, thyroid function, coeliac serology, renal function, liver function, bone profile and magnesium.

Treatment and management

Treatment of eating disorders is best managed in the community by a multidisciplinary team including psychiatrists, psychologists, dieticians, and medical and nursing staff, and the initial treatment will be aimed at weight restoration and nutritional stabilisation. Psychological therapies include:
- family therapy (preferred treatment anorexia nervosa)
- cognitive behavioural therapy (preferred for bulimia nervosa)

Paediatricians also have a role for those young people who are medically unstable and for assessment and management of complications of chronic illness such as growth, pubertal development and bone health.

Acute admissions should be reserved for those who are severely malnourished, medically unstable, have acute complications from being underweight or have acute food refusal. The aim of an acute admission is to achieve medical stabilisation and begin weight restoration and the Junior MARSIPAN Tool (Royal College of Psychiatrists) can be used to assess the level of risk for a young person with an eating disorder. Weight restoration should be achieved by the oral route where possible but if nasogastric feeding is needed then consideration needs to be given as to whether the young person has the capacity to consent to such an intervention. Nasogastric feeding can be implemented for those who do not consent, depending on their age, under

Table 3.2 Physical manifestations of eating disorders

	Anorexia nervosa	Bulimia nervosa
metabolic	fatigue bradycardia, hypothermia, poor peripheral perfusion	fatigue
cardiovascular	postural changes in heart rate and blood pressure leading to dizziness and syncope reduced myocardial contractility, arrythmias, heart failure and prolonged QTc	postural changes in heart rate and blood pressure leading to dizziness and syncope arrythmias and cardiomyopathy
respiratory		aspiration pneumonia
gastrointestinal	delayed gastric emptying leading to early satiety, pain and bloating constipation raised liver transaminases	tooth decay parotid swelling, oesophagitis, Mallory-Weiss tears, oesophageal rupture acute pancreatitis ileus secondary to laxative use
renal	dehydration elevated creatinine	dehydration elevated creatinine
neurological	poor concentration and recall	seizures
endocrine	sick euthyroid syndrome suppression of the hypothalamic-gonadal axis leading to delayed or arrested puberty primary or secondary amenorrhoea faltering growth	oligomenorrhoea
musculoskeletal	weakness muscle wasting low bone mineral density and increased fracture risk	muscle weakness and cramps
haematological	anaemia, leucopenia, neutropenia, thrombocytopenia	
dermatological	lanugo hair, dry skin, hair loss	calluses on the dorsum of the hand (secondary to induced vomiting)

the Children Act 1989 with parental consent (best interests) or by use of the Mental Health Act.

Food and nutrition are the treatments for all of the manifestations associated with being underweight and medications are not used routinely to treat eating disorders. Occasionally anxiolytics will be prescribed for a young person with an eating disorder with the aim of decreasing the eating disorder cognitions, and the prescribing is usually led by CAMHS.

Potential complications

Young people who have been starved and had restricted intake for a period of time are at risk of refeeding syndrome which is a serious and potentially fatal complication. During starvation, the body is energy depleted and once glycogen stores have been consumed, the body starts to break down fats, protein and muscle as an alternative energy source. With refeeding, the body changes from a catabolic to an anabolic state and carbohydrates become the primary energy source again. The subsequent insulin secretion leads to a rapid shift of electrolytes from extracellular to intracellular compartments. Phosphate is needed for glucose metabolism, and the increased use of phosphate combined with total body depletion leads to extracellular hypophosphataemia (the hallmark of biochemical refeeding syndrome). Low phosphate levels impact on metabolic processes and can affect all systems, leading to clinical refeeding syndrome. Potassium moves into cells to give hypokalaemia. Clinical features of the syndrome include:

- delirium with visual and auditory hallucinations
- dyspnoea
- paraesthesia
- generalized weakness and fatigue
- peripheral oedema
- seizures
- coma

Clinical refeeding syndrome can be prevented by:
- correction of hypophosphataemia
- gradual introduction of nutrition
- monitoring of electrolytes—phosphate, sodium, potassium, magnesium and calcium
- monitoring of ECG (evidence of prolonged QTc)

Important sequelae

Being chronically underweight can lead to suppression of the hypothalamic-gonadal axis, and the reduction in gonadal hormones leads to delayed or arrested puberty. Low oestrogen levels, along with other hormones, leads to decreased bone mineral deposition and increased resorption; this can affect both linear growth of the bones (implications for height) and final bone density (leading to brittle bones and increased fracture risk). Restoring a healthy weight is the primary treatment for both of these sequelae.

Sexual health

For a young person to enjoy good sexual health, they need to avoid unplanned pregnancy and sexually transmitted infections (STIs). A positive approach to relationships and sex requires self-esteem, an understanding of themselves and the ability to make informed choices. To make informed choices, they need to:
- understand the risks associated with different sexual practices
- have the communication skills to be able to negotiate and engage in safer sex (such as the ability to say no to sex without condoms)
- have access to contraceptive advice and the skills needed to be able to use this effectively (knowing how to use a condom)

It is important to utilise opportunities when young people present to health care settings to assess risk-taking behaviours in sexual health and give advice and health promotion on safe sexual practices. Discussions should focus around behaviour change and provision of information about local services.

In order to be effective, sexual health services need to be accessible, convenient and confidential. They should provide:
- testing for STI and pregnancy
- contraceptive advice and provision
- contact tracing and partner notification
- vaccinations

It is important that services are able to offer confidentiality and to consider the possibility of child sexual abuse or exploitation.

PRACTICE POINT - teenagers and sex: some facts

- the average age of first sex in the UK is 16 years for both males and females
- 31% of boys and 29% of girls have sex before they are 16 years old
- 6.9% of young people aged between 16–24 report being pressured into sex
- average age when child sexual abuse (CSE) is first identified is suggested to be 12–15 years
- the rates of teenage pregnancy are falling in the UK
- the proportion of conceptions in young people under 18 years that result in termination is just over 50%
- in England, sexually transmitted infections are highest in 15–24 year olds for both sexes

Teenage pregnancy

Risk factors

Rates of teenage pregnancy are higher in certain vulnerable groups:
- young people in care
- those living in a deprived neighbourhood
- those who have poor school attendance and poor educational attainment
- those with learning difficulties
- those with poor mental health
- those involved in crime
- those with history of sexual abuse

There is an association between alcohol consumption and the likelihood of high-risk sexual behaviours such as unprotected sex. In addition, adolescents are at a higher risk of becoming young parents if their fathers were from the lowest two socioeconomic groups or their mother was pregnant at a teenager.

Consequences of teenage parenthood

Teenage parents are at a higher risk of obstetric complications and maternal mortality. They are more likely to have insufficient social support, experience relationship breakdown, live with relative poverty and face the stigma associated with being a teenage parent. There is a higher risk of postnatal depression and poor mental health and many end up being 'not in education, employment or training (NEET)'.

Health outcomes of child born to young parents

Infants born to teenage parents have a 40% risk of higher mortality and a higher risk of being born prematurely or small for gestational age. They are less likely to be breast fed and are at an increased risk of poor nutrition. They are twice as likely to be hospitalised due to accidental injuries up to the age of 5 years and are in the highest risk group for behavioural problems.

Reducing teenage pregnancy

It is important that young people receive high quality education about sex and relationships in primary and secondary school and out of school settings. This should focus on providing knowledge and skills such as delaying age of first sex, the risks of unprotected sex and effective contraception and condom use. Parents also need to be provided with information and skills to be able to talk to their children about sex and relationships. Health practitioners working with young people require training on sexual health and relationships.

Paediatricians should be able to provide information to young people on their contraceptive choices and to consider their specific contraceptive and sexual health needs. In particular, paediatricians should know how to facilitate access to contraceptive and sexual health services including timely access to emergency contraception and management of unplanned pregnancy.

Young people need easy access to confidential, youth-friendly, sexual health services. NICE guidance recommends targeted prevention for more vulnerable groups as well as coordinated support for young parents, including contraceptive advice.

Sexually transmitted infection

- helping all young people to protect themselves is a major public health issue
- in England, sexually transmitted infections in heterosexuals are highest in 15–24 year olds (Figure 3.2)
- those under 25 years accounted for 63% of all new chlamydia cases in 2016
- chlamydia is the most frequent STI diagnosis, followed by genital warts and gonorrhoea
- the introduction of the HPV vaccinations in adolescent girls may potentially have had an impact on recent trends in new diagnoses of genital warts. This is now being offered to adolescent boys as well
- in 2017, there was a reduction of 40% of new HIV diagnoses among those aged 15–24 years

Reinfection with acute STIs is a particular problem with young people, but the risk decreases with increasing age.

Chlamydia causes an infection that is often symptomless but may be associated with vaginal bleeding, discharge, abdominal pain, fever and inflammation of the cervix in women and watery discharge from the penis in men. Long-term complications may be severe, particularly

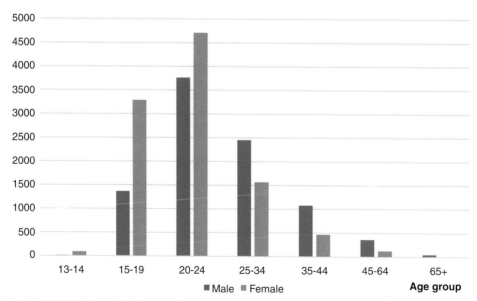

Fig. 3.2 Rates (per 100,000) of new STI diagnoses by age group and gender in England 2019 (Source: Public Health England annual report. Permission to use via Open Government Licence.)

in women, as it can lead to pelvic inflammatory diseases, ectopic pregnancy and infertility.

Gonorrhoea has an incubation period of only a few days, and males and females may experience a urethral discharge. Women are at risk of long-term serious complications such as infertility and ectopic pregnancy and it is possible to have long-term infection without obvious symptoms.

Syphilis has an incubation period ranging from a few days to 3 months. Symptoms are nonspecific, though illness usually begins with painless, highly infectious sores anywhere around the body but usually at the site of infection.

Genital warts are caused by the human papillomavirus (HPV) and are found around the penis, anus and vagina. Certain types of HPV are associated with cervical cancer and head and neck cancers. Warts often disappear without treatment but can also be removed by freezing, burning and laser treatment.

Genital herpes is a common infection caused by *Herpes simplex virus type 2 or 1*. Symptoms include small blisters in the genital area, which break down to give painful ulcers. Herpes may cause pain on urination.

Acne

Acne vulgaris is a common problem in adolescence and is a multifactorial inflammatory disease affecting the pilosebaceous follicles of the skin.

Increasing androgen production associated with puberty stimulates sebum production, and this can block the pores and result in inflammation of the surrounding skin. The spots are caused by *Propionibacterium acnes*, a common bacterium on the skin that colonises sebaceous areas. This bacteria feeds on sebum and produces waste products and fatty acids that irritate the sebaceous glands and make them inflamed.

The clinical features include
- seborrhoea—increased grease production
- noninflammatory comedomes—open (blackheads) and closed (whiteheads)
- inflammatory lesions (papules, pustules and cysts)

Acne can be painful, itchy and sore and can lead to irreversible scarring if not treated appropriately. In addition to the physical morbidity, it can also have a significant impact on the psychological well-being of a young person, leading to poor self-esteem, depression and anxiety. It can lead to young people avoiding meeting up with friends and leave them relatively isolated.

Factors which can exacerbate acne include:
- stress or emotional tension
- picking at spots

- hormones—exogenous: progesterone-only pill; endogenous: polycystic ovarian syndrome
- menstruation
- drugs—steroids, anticonvulsants, ciclosporin
- greasy emollients

Clinical assessment should address the distribution of acne, type and severity of lesions and the impact on well-being and quality of life. Young people will often underestimate the impact that the condition has and may not volunteer this information. It is good practice to use the HEEADSSS assessment to open up conversations on this issue.

Management

There is no proven evidence to suggest that hygiene, diet or sweating cause acne.
- lifestyle advice:
  - wash face twice daily with a mild cleanser
  - avoid squeezing or picking at spots as this may cause scarring
  - oil-free moisturisers are advised
- medications

Treatment of acne varies depending on the severity and the lesion type.

Those with mild acne are treated with topical treatments such as benzoyl peroxide, topical retinoids and topical antibiotic.

The management of moderate acne requires the addition of oral tetracycline or a macrolide. For young females the combined oral contraceptive pill is another alternative if there are no contraindications.

Topical treatment needs to be applied to the acne-prone areas and not just individual spots and should be continued for at least 6 weeks to see benefit. If a response is seen, the treatment should be continued for at least 6 months.

For those with severe, scarring or resistant acne, treatment with oral isotretinoin is usual. In the UK this treatment should only be delivered by a specialist dermatology service with expertise in monitoring therapy with oral retinoids. Young people usually receive treatment for around 6–8 months, and the treatment requires monitoring of mood, blood count, liver function and serum lipids. The major safety concerns are the potential effect on mood and teratogenicity. Young people with the potential for pregnancy need careful discussion regarding the need for effective contraception. A referral to a dermatology service should be undertaken if the acne is extensive, nodulocystic, scarring or shows no improvement to the initial treatment

CLINICAL SCENARIO

A 15-year-old female who was known to have epilepsy and dyslexia presents to clinic for a routine review. She reports that her seizures have been well controlled but she is feeling fed up and tearful. Her acne is becoming worse and she is embarrassed to go out with her friends. Her mother is concerned about her daughter's appetite and feels that she may have lost weight. The family are also concerned about a change in her mood and increased anxiety about school. Her periods started when she was 12 years of age and she had established a regular pattern but has now not had a period for 2 months.

On examination, she looked thin and had lost 2 kgs since her appointment 3 months previously. She was dressed in a baggy long-sleeved hoody despite it being a warm day. Her blood pressure was 94/55 and her heart rate was 46 bpm. She had cold hands with a capillary refill of 3 seconds peripherally, a low volume pulse and a scaphoid abdomen. She made little eye contact throughout the consultation and had a flat affect. Her BMI was 14.6 which was below the 0.4 centile for her age.

A differential would include an eating disorder, depression, potential side effects of medication and possible underlying medical illnesses such as inflammatory bowel disease, coeliac disease or thyroid abnormalities.

The issues that need consideration are multiple and interrelated. Initially it is important to establish a healthcare appropriate for her maturity and development including the need for an independent consultation and reassurance about confidentiality. A formal HEEADSSS assessment would be important along with obtaining details about her mental health, nutritional intake and attitudes to food which would all allow a comprehensive approach to be developed. Active treatment of her acne would also all help her to regain her self-confidence.

Early investigations were undertaken and excluded some of the listed medical conditions. It became clear that she had developed thoughts and behaviours typical of anorexia nervosa and was significantly restricting her calorie intake.

She was admitted for acute management of her condition by the multidisciplinary team and a comprehensive care plan was developed in collaboration with the patient and her parents. This included ensuring that all the issues identified were addressed.

It was recognised that her problems were likely to require longer term support and therefore planning for transition to adult services would need to be considered.

IMPORTANT CLINICAL POINTS

Illicit drugs

- use of illicit drugs should be considered in young people presenting with abnormal or erratic behaviour
- novel psychoactive substance use may be undetectable on routine urinary drug screening

Anorexia nervosa

- restriction of energy intake, fear of gaining weight and disturbance of body image are cardinal features of anorexia nervosa

- refeeding syndrome is a serious and potentially fatal complication
- hypophosphataemia is the hallmark of biochemical refeeding syndrome and monitoring and correction is vital
- consent for treatment can use the Children Act 1989 (best interests) or the Mental Health Act

Further reading

Eating disorders: recognition and treatment NICE guideline [NG69]. Published: May 2017. Updated: December 2020. https://www.nice.org.uk/guidance/ng69/chapter/Recommendations

Junior MARSIPAN: Management of Really Sick Patients under 18 with Anorexia Nervosa Royal College of Psychiatrists. London. https://www.rcpsych.ac.uk/docs/default-source/improving-care/better-mh-policy/college-reports/college-report-cr168.pdf

Contemporary Pediatrics. Published January 2014.

HEEADSSS 3.0: The psychosocial interview for adolescents updated for a new century fuelled by media https://www.contemporarypediatrics.com/view/heeadsss-30-psychosocial-interview-adolescents-updated-new-century-fueled-media

Suicide and suicide attempts in adolescents. Benjamin Shain and Committee on adolescence Pediatrics. 2016; 138(1) https://pediatrics.aappublications.org/content/138/1/e20161420

Chapter 4

Growth and puberty

Joanna Walker

After reading this chapter you should:
- know the causes of problems relating to growth and puberty
- be able to assess, diagnose and manage problems relating to growth and puberty

Disorders of growth

Growth is an excellent clinical tool to help distinguish between health and disease in any child in any setting and can be affected by genetics, nutrition and pathology in any system. It is a dynamic process so the position of a child on a growth chart matters less than how they arrived there, and sourcing and plotting previous growth data is invaluable.

Children who are short for expected family height and relatively overweight are likely to have an endocrine or syndromic cause for their short stature, especially if there is evidence of slow growth. Constitutional early puberty is the commonest cause of unusually tall stature in children and is often related to overnutrition. Such children enter puberty relatively early and therefore reach their expected height early compared with their healthy weight peers. Pathological causes of tall stature are rare and are often syndromic.

Short stature

In the UK, it is possible to obtain previous growth measurements from the Personal Child Health Record and the National Childhood Measurement Programme which measures height and weight of all children entering a reception class (aged 4–5 years) and all leaving primary school (Year 6—aged 10–11 years). These measurements can be used to establish the pattern of growth.

Clinical presentation

The key point when assessing any child with concerns about short stature is to seek any of the 'red flags' that help distinguish the minority with an identifiable or treatable cause from the majority with familial short stature. To do so necessitates a broad and detailed history and examination since growth can be affected by pathology in any system.

Important features in the history include:
- general health—whether the child is otherwise healthy and active
- whether the child has always been small or growth is a new concern
- whether siblings are overtaking them in height
- past medical history including pregnancy, birthweight, early feeding and growth in infancy. Some syndromic causes are linked to feeding difficulties in infancy, e.g., Turner, William, Noonan, 22q.11 deletion, Silver Russell and Prader-Willi
- history of prolonged conjugated neonatal jaundice or neonatal hypoglycaemia that may point to hypothalamo-pituitary problems
- history of any chronic illness such as asthma or inflammatory bowel disease that can slow growth
- family history including the health and heights of parents, grandparents and wider family along with a family history suggestive of constitutional growth delay with later than average puberty
- full systems review—particularly any history suggestive of malabsorption or gut inflammation, headaches or visual problems that might suggest a pituitary tumour and any symptoms of hypothyroidism such a cold intolerance or constipation

35

- any symptoms suggestive of an undiagnosed chronic illness such as coeliac disease
- history of developmental, education or behaviour problems
- current and previous drug history especially of steroid use to include dose, mode of delivery and adherence to treatment
- psychosocial history as short stature may be the result of emotional abuse
- Important features in the examination include:
- height, weight and, if indicated, BMI plotted on an age and sex appropriate chart. Previous data will help to establish the growth pattern
- height centiles of both parents and target centile range should be calculated. The target range is the mid-parental centile (the midpoint between the parents' centiles) ± 8.5cm and further assessment is required if the child falls outside this range
- sitting height or crown rump length is compared with leg length. Disproportionate short stature suggests a skeletal dysplasia, possibly inherited from a parent especially if they too are exceptionally small
- head circumference is measured and plotted as patients with some skeletal dysplasias have relatively large heads
- BMI is calculated and plotted on a UK Standard chart
- full examination to include general health and appearance as disease of any system can present with poor growth

---

PRACTICE POINT – short stature: 'red flags' suggesting pathological cause

- extreme short stature—the further below the 0.4th centile the greater the chance of identifiable pathology
- short and greater than one major centile below target range for normal parents although many will be constitutional
- dysmorphic features
- skeletal disproportion
- evidence of slow growth with downwards crossing of the centiles
- short and overweight—suggests an endocrine cause
- evidence of chronic illness

Investigations

These will be dictated by the differential diagnosis that emerges after the history and examination. If a child is healthy, falls within an acceptable range for their parents and there is no evidence of growth slowing, further tests may not be necessary. A system-related condition such as inflammatory bowel disease should be investigated if there is clear evidence found in the history.

The following tests should be requested when there are concerns about the growth pattern with no obvious cause:

- full blood count, indices and film—to exclude anaemia
- CRP—to exclude undiagnosed inflammation
- urea, electrolytes and creatinine—assessing renal function
- liver function tests—low albumin can be seen in many chronic conditions
- bone profile—calcium, phosphate and ALP
- IgA and anti-TTG antibodies—screening tests for coeliac disease
- thyroid function tests—FT4 and TSH—TSH without the FT4 may miss secondary hypothyroidism
- IgF-1 and IgF-BP3—limited value in screening for growth hormone deficiency but reassuring if normal. Varies with age, so age-related values should be used
- karyotype in girls—to exclude Turner Syndrome and possibly DNA for SHOX (Short stature Homeobox-containing gene) mutations in both sexes
- bone age estimation for skeletal maturity

Further investigations will depend on the results and the clinical scenario but could include:

- skeletal survey (modified)—to exclude a skeletal dysplasia
- formal pituitary functions tests—to assess growth hormone production

Important sequelae

There are many publications supporting the view that short stature is a source of psychological and behaviour problems in affected children but many of these studies risk bias as they only include patients seen in a growth service. Population studies show very little impact on adult functioning and this may be important when counselling families.

Specific conditions
Familial short stature

Familial short stature is the most common diagnosis in children referred to a growth clinic. A healthy child whose height is within expectation for parents, who are themselves of normal height, and without evidence of slow growth should be discharged after explanations and reassurance.

Small for gestational age (SGA)

Definitions of SGA vary but the UK cut-off is a birthweight below minus 2.0 SDS on the centile charts. Length is not routinely measured at birth. About 80% of babies who are born SGA show catch-up growth and in those who remain small, other pathology might be identified such as:

- Silver Russell syndrome
- Turner syndrome
- Prader-Willi syndrome
- Fetal alcohol spectrum disorder

Growth hormone is licensed in the UK for those who have not shown catch up and remain short for expected family size by the age of 4 years. Early studies show a modest increase in final height.

Chronic conditions

Any disorder associated with poor health—physical or emotional—can impair growth, and management should be directed at correcting the underlying pathology. Examples include:

- coeliac disease—introducing a gluten-free diet
- juvenile idiopathic arthritis—using disease-modifying agents
- asthma control—addressing inadequate treatment or reducing doses of inhaled steroids
- psychosocial short stature—by a successful change of environment

Chronic renal impairment is the only such condition where growth hormone is part of the management although higher than replacement doses are needed due to growth hormone resistance.

Endocrine causes

The impact on growth is presented here, but further details of these conditions can be found in Chapter 25 Endocrinology.

Growth hormone deficiency

Clinical presentation

The age at which growth hormone deficiency (GHD) presents depends on the extent of the deficiency. Unless there are obvious midline anomalies, undescended testes or micropenis, GHD in neonates is usually identified during investigations for hypoglycaemia and GH should be part of a 'hypoglycaemia screen' at any age.

Growth during the first 2 years is predominantly nutritionally driven, so in older children GHD tends to manifest with slowing of growth with increased body fat—the child who is overnourished yet short. There might also be symptoms or signs of skeletal immaturity, e.g., slow tooth eruption or delayed puberty. This might be isolated GHD, part of evolving hypopituitarism or as the result of a midline brain tumour such as a craniopharyngioma or optic nerve glioma. GHD is also one of the consequences of high-dose cranial irradiation needed for some brain tumours.

Investigations

Children with possible GHD should undergo standard formal pituitary function 'stress' tests (Table 4.1) ensuring that thyroid function is normal in advance to avoid a false-positive diagnosis (the GH response can be blunted if metabolism is slow due to hypothyroidism). A TRH test is rarely indicated because thyroid involvement can usually be detected from standard tests of Free T4 and TSH. Similarly, an LHRH test as puberty is best assessed clinically.

All neonates and children diagnosed with clinical and biochemical evidence of GHD should undergo an MRI scan and most will have an abnormality of varying severity. They should also be screened and then monitored for the development of other pituitary hormone deficiencies.

Treatment and management

Treatment is with daily injections of recombinant GH until final height is achieved when all patients should be retested. In adults, lower doses are needed to maintain normal body composition, bone health and to avoid cardiovascular risk factors.

Pharmacological agents used

Growth hormone is manufactured using recombinant technology and is administered by daily subcutaneous injection using a choice of device although adherence to

TABLE 4.1 Results of pituitary function stress testing with glucagon in a 6 year old with slow growth. The 'stress' response is as a result of an initial increase in blood glucose that stimulates insulin release and thus a rapid drop in glucose. These results show severe GHD but no evidence of cortisol deficiency.

Time (minutes)	Glucose mmol/l (3.5–6.5 mmol/l)	Growth Hormone (>8.3 ng/dl)	Cortisol (>550 nmol/l)
0	4.5	2.8	450
30	6.4	3.4	320
60	2.9	2.1	685
90	3.7	3.7	420
120	4.9	3.3	330
150	4.7	3.2	295

treatment can be a problem. Headache is the commonest side effect but rarely severe enough to stop treatment, and idiopathic intracranial hypertension has been reported. Starting GH can also unmask latent deficiencies of ACTH and thyroid hormone.

Hypothyroidism

Untreated hypothyroidism whatever the cause will slow growth, and a history that the child's peer group or sibs are overtaking is probably the commonest presentation as this is noticed more than the other insidious classic features. Treatment is with thyroxine replacement in a dose that increases with body size.

Cushing syndrome or disease

Excess steroids can impair growth and lead to excess weight gain, and children usually have very few of the other characteristic signs. The commonest cause is iatrogenic and, as an example, the guidelines in the UK are that all children on regular inhaled steroids should have their height and weight measured and plotted every 6 months.

Syndromic causes

The impact on growth is presented here but further details on each of these syndromes can be found in Chapter 5 Genetics.

Turner syndrome

Endocrine features invariably include short stature and almost invariably primary ovarian failure. GH use is licensed, but the recommended dose is about twice the standard replacement dose to help overcome the growth hormone resistance linked to the bone dysplasia. The features of TS are variable, partly dependent on karyotype, and may be very mild so chromosome analysis should be requested on all girls with significant short stature irrespective of parental heights. Primary ovarian failure is managed with induction of puberty at an appropriate age and monitoring through adulthood. Further details are provided below in the section on primary gonadal failure.

SHOX mutations

The short stature homeobox-containing gene (SHOX) has an important role in long bone growth. The frequency of SHOX-deficient short stature is thought to be relatively common (estimated at 6%–22%), and analysis of the gene should be considered in all children with significant short stature. Growth hormone is licensed in the UK for children with SHOX mutations.

Noonan syndrome

Noonan syndrome is inherited in an autosomal dominant fashion, and the phenotypic features can be mild and include short stature plus other features. The use of GH to improve final height in Noonan syndrome is controversial and it is not currently licensed in the UK.

Silver Russell syndrome (SRS)

This rare imprinting disorder is characterised by severe pre- and postnatal growth restriction, no catch up and typical dysmorphic features (see Chapter 5 Genetics). These children have marked feeding difficulties, low muscle mass, excessive sweating and are at risk of hypoglycaemia well beyond the neonatal period. Older children with SRS are at risk of exaggerated adrenarche and subsequently other complications of insulin resistance. It is primarily a clinical diagnosis but an underlying molecular cause can currently be identified in around 60% of patients. Again, the use of GH is controversial but it may help prevent hypoglycaemia, improve appetite and motor development.

Fetal alcohol spectrum disorder

There is a wide spectrum of teratogenic effects of alcohol on an unborn baby, but one cardinal feature in severe toxicity is impaired childhood growth.

Skeletal dysplasias

There are numerous skeletal dysplasias described that are associated with short stature and slow growth. Many children or affected adults will show disproportionate limb or spinal growth that might not be obvious on clinical examination. There is therefore a need to measure sitting height or crown rump length, calculate leg length and then plot both on the relevant chart in all significantly short children. The more obvious skeletal dysplasias include achondroplasia and hypochondroplasia. Growth hormone has been trialled but is ineffective.

Tall stature

Referrals of children with unusually tall stature are much less common than short stature and most do not have a pathological cause. The commonest causes are overnutrition or normal, but early, puberty in a child with tall parents. These children will complete their growth phase and reach their predicted height earlier than their peers and within expectations for their parents.

All children and young people with unusually tall stature should be weighed, measured and plotted on the appropriate growth chart along with sitting height and calculated leg length. This will help identify the rare child with disproportionate, long-limbed tall stature. The presence of other dysmorphic features may help identify any recognised syndromes.

Investigations are rarely indicated although an estimation of bone age can be reassuring for final height if it confirms advanced skeletal maturity. In a rapidly growing child, any signs of abnormally early puberty, growth hormone excess or symptoms and signs of thyrotoxicosis should be investigated.

Syndromic causes with disproportionate long-limbed tall stature

Marfan syndrome

The clinical diagnosis of this autosomal dominant connective tissue disorder condition relies on a set of defined criteria but ectopia lentis or a significant aortic root abnormality are cardinal. Skeletal disproportion, including arachnodactyly (Figure 4.1), contributes to the 'systemic score' of other typical features used when one of the above signs is absent and there is no positive family history. The diagnosis and decision to analyse the FBN1 gene should almost always be made by a clinical geneticist as a diagnosis of Marfan syndrome has

potentially serious repercussions for future health of the patient and their family.

Klinefelter syndrome

Presented below in section on Puberty.

Syndromic causes without disproportionate long-limbed tall stature

The overgrowth conditions or cerebral gigantism (as opposed to pituitary gigantism due to GH excess) include:

Beckwith–Wiedermann syndrome

The classical features include macrosomia at birth, macroglossia and hemi-hypertrophy plus others which are outlined in Chapter 5 Genetics.

Neonates are at risk of hypoglycaemia due to hyperinsulinism caused by pancreatic hyperplasia. Children also have a predisposition to childhood tumours, particularly nephroblastoma, and need regular renal ultrasound screening until the age of about 6 years.

Sotos syndrome

Characterised by tall stature and accelerated growth through childhood with an advanced bone age so final height is within the normal range. Classical features include large head with a prominent forehead and sparse frontal hair, down-slanting palpebral fissures,

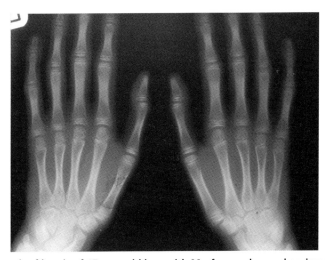

Fig. 4.1 **Radiograph of hands of 17-year-old boy with Marfan syndrome showing arachnodactyly.**

pointed chin and facial flushing and variable degrees of behaviour and learning difficulties—often in speech and language.

Disorders of puberty

Clinical assessment of **timing** and **sequence** are the mainstays when seeing a child with concerns about puberty. The two commonest referrals to clinic are early puberty in girls and late puberty in boys and both tend to run in families. In children with sexual precocity, it is important to consider what hormone or hormones are responsible for the clinical changes as this will help distinguish between gonadotrophin-dependent and gonadotrophin-independent development and direct any investigations and management.

Children may have normal timing but an abnormal sequence of puberty due to the development of endocrine pathology such as autoimmune hypothyroidism. Even when there is no pathological cause for early or late puberty in either sex, treatment may be appropriate due to the psychological and social impact of the changes on the child or young person.

Normal puberty is defined in girls as having the onset between the ages of 8–13 years and in boys between 9–14 years, and the average duration of puberty in both sexes is about 3 years. It is a gradual process that follows a sequence of development shown Tanner staging charts (Figure 4.2).

In girls, the first signs of puberty are nipple enlargement, 'breast buds', sometimes with a palpable small disc or plate of tissue beneath the nipple. This is followed by progressive breast development with the onset of pubic hair usually a few months later. Oestrogen is an excellent growth promoter

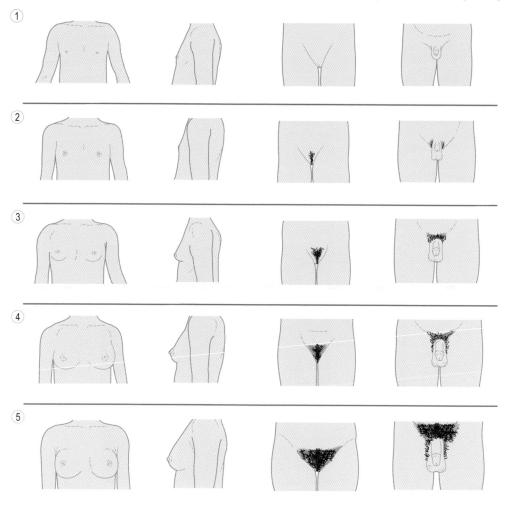

Fig. 4.2 Tanner stages of puberty.

in low concentrations so the growth spurt of puberty comes relatively early with peak height velocity reached at about Stage 3 breast development. Menarche occurs as the growth rate is declining and is a good marker that puberty and the growth phase is nearing completion. This explanation that menarche comes later on in puberty is often important reassurance for families of girls with sexual precocity.

In boys, the earliest sign of puberty is testicular enlargement to 4 mls with progressive further enlargement to the 15–25 mls of the adult male. The majority of testicular volume is a marker of sperm production and therefore abnormally small testes in an otherwise normally functioning adult man may be a marker of infertility or subfertility. Testicular volume is generally less helpful in pubertal assessment than the assay of their testosterone production, i.e., staging of genital and pubic hair development plus evidence of secondary sexual characteristics. Testosterone is not a significant growth promoter until present in high concentrations, hence the growth spurt in boys comes later with peak height velocity reached at around Stage 4 for genital development, some 2–3 years after the onset of puberty. This is important when seeing boys with constitutional delay of growth and puberty (CDGP). Voice breaking and shaving come towards the completion of puberty.

Sexual precocity

Sexual precocity is best divided into:
- normal sequence, gonadotrophin dependent (or central),
- abnormal sequence, gonadotrophin independent

Clinical presentation

Important features in the history and examination include:
History
- physical symptoms of hormone production—pubic hair or breast
- age of onset and whether they are progressing
- any history of a growth spurt—a rapid increase in shoe size
- family history—age mother start her periods
- history of any underlying brain disorder or injury
- past medical history including birth history and weight
- how problem affects the child and family—any hormone-driven behaviour problems
Examination
- height, weight and, if indicated, BMI plotted on an age- and sex-appropriate chart. Search for and plot previous data to help establish growth pattern
- height centiles of both parents, target centile range calculated and identification whether the child falls outside this range
- general examination—including skin for café-au-lait pigmentation suggestive of NF1 or McCune-Albright syndrome
- pubertal staging according to Tanner standards
- testicular volume in boys using a Prader orchidometer (Figure 4.3)

CLINICAL SCENARIO

A 5-year-old boy presents with concerns about rapid growth. Plotting his growth data his height has moved from 50th to 90th centiles over the 12 months since he started school and he is tall for his parents. The mid-parental centile is 9th–25th. He is otherwise well. Examination shows Tanner Stage 3 genital development but prepubertal testes (≤3mls).

This assessment acts as a 'clinical bioassay' and identifies what development is present and what hormone or hormones must be responsible. Both the **timing** of pubertal development (premature) and the **sequence** of events is abnormal. This is most likely to be gonadotrophin-independent sexual precocity and the hormone responsible is most likely to be testosterone being produced from somewhere other than the testes.

The likeliest source is the adrenal glands with the most likely diagnosis being a form of congenital adrenal hyperplasia, probably 21-hydroxylase deficiency (95% of CAH). These clinical findings then drive the investigations and subsequent management.

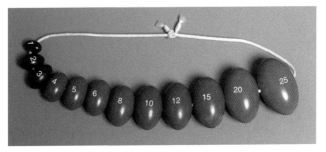

Fig. 4.3 The Prader Orchidometer.

Gonadotropin-dependent sexual precocity

This is common and rarely pathological in
- girls
- certain racial groups—Afro-Caribbean
- children with a positive family history
- children who are overweight or obese

Some girls struggle socially with their early development and therefore merit treatment. A pathological cause should be suspected in **all** boys and in girls who are very young (under 7 years) or who do not fit any of the groups listed above. Pathological gonadotrophin-dependent precocity is often rapidly progressive and risk factors include any underlying current (hypothalamo-pituitary axis tumours) or previous (periventricular hypoxia in the neonatal period) brain disorder and not just those involving the hypothalamo-pituitary axis. Even a minor head injury can precipitate abnormally early puberty, especially in girls. Children with neurofibromatosis type 1 are known to progress through puberty earlier than unaffected children and are at high risk of sexual precocity if found to have an optic nerve glioma on their routine MRI scans.

Breast development in overweight girls is sometimes difficult to distinguish from simple adiposity. Consequently, evidence of other signs of oestrogen effect such as changes to the external genitalia should be sought.

Investigations

The choice of investigations should be driven by the history and examination and the following should be considered:
- pelvic USS to assess ovarian volume and the development of follicles plus the size and shape of the uterus and the presence of endometrial lining. It can confirm whether puberty is underway in overweight girls where breast development is difficult to judge and also give some idea if menarche is imminent
- left wrist and hand radiograph for skeletal maturity 'bone age' assessment
- baseline LH and FSH—LH must be measurable to make a biochemical diagnosis of puberty but a low level does not exclude it as secretion is nocturnal until mid-puberty. A GnRH test might be needed where there is doubt about the clinical diagnosis or where sex hormones are high but baseline LH levels are low, suggesting a diagnosis of gonadotrophin-independent precocity
- androgens if there is clinical evidence of early virilisation in boys or girls
- oestrogen should be interpreted with caution due to reliability of assay at low levels

- urine steroid profile will confirm excess androgens and identify any block in the androgen pathway in CAH or the likelihood of an androgen-secreting tumour
- cranial MRI scan is mandatory in boys with any evidence of gonadotrophin-dependent sexual precocity. In girls an MRI should be considered if the child has a lean build, is young (under 7 years), has rapidly progressing features and no relevant family or racial history. In both sexes, an MRI should be undertaken if there is any evidence of current or previous intracranial pathology
- abdominal USS to help rule out an adrenal tumour although MRI may be needed
- tumour markers

Treatment and management

Most causes of gonadotrophin-independent sexual precocity need no treatment or follow-up. Children with CAH are managed with oral steroid replacement and careful follow-up. Their final height prognosis might be impaired if the diagnosis is delayed or if normal puberty is precipitated. The latter might need treatment.

Children with gonadotrophin-dependent sexual precocity needing treatment receive a gonadotrophin-releasing hormone analogue that abolishes the pulsatile pattern of secretion essential for most peptide hormone function. This is given by a slow-release injection every few weeks and aims to halt pubertal progress. Puberty cannot be halted indefinitely because of the detrimental effects on bone mineralisation.

Potential complications

Early puberty can cause significant psychosocial and behaviour problems for affected children

Important sequelae

Untreated pathological sexual precocity can impair final height due to shortening of the projected growth phase. Early recognition and appropriate treatment should minimise this.

Gonadotrophin-independent sexual precocity

Premature thelarche

This describes isolated breast development and is usually seen in toddlers. There is fluctuating or even cyclical unilateral or bilateral breast enlargement in an otherwise healthy girl starting soon after birth with no other symptoms or signs of puberty including growth acceleration.

The aetiology is still not clear but may be linked to tissue sensitivity to oestrogens or functioning ovarian cysts. Tests are rarely needed and the parents can be reassured that the development is benign and will eventually resolve, usually by the age of 2–3 years. Any additional signs of puberty require further investigation.

Exaggerated adrenarche

Adrenarche is a normal event in all children between the ages of about 5–8 years when the adrenal gland starts to produce androgens. In most children this goes unnoticed, but in some there is adult sweat odour, acne, axillary hair and/or sparse, long, pubic hair confined to the vulva in girls and the base of the penis in boys. This relatively common disorder is termed 'Exaggerated Adrenarche'. It is a diagnosis of exclusion from significant testosterone production, assessed clinically by the absence of virilisation or growth acceleration plus normal biochemistry and no significantly advanced bone maturity. It is seen much more often in girls. It was considered a benign condition but is now known to be a marker of insulin resistance, so children, especially those who are overweight or obese, in whom it is more common, are at risk of metabolic syndrome as adults. There is often a family history of this condition including polycystic ovarian syndrome in women. Families should be warned about this risk and advised to keep their children as slim and fit as possible.

McCune–Albright syndrome

This is characterised by the triad of irregular-outline, café-au-lait pigmentation, polyostotic fibrous dysplasia and risk of endocrine hyperfunction such as early puberty, Cushing syndrome or thyrotoxicosis.

Delayed puberty

Delayed puberty is best divided into causes mediated by disorders of:
* hypothalamo-pituitary function ('central')
* gonadal failure

Clinical presentation

Important features in the history and examination include:

History

* general health—whether the young person is otherwise healthy and active

* whether short stature is present or any history of growth cessation
* family history of delayed puberty, e.g., age mother started periods or father's voice broke
* symptoms suggestive of an undiagnosed chronic illness such as coeliac disease
* history of education or behaviour problems
* any gonadal surgery or irradiation
* current and previous drug history especially of steroid use
* normal sense of smell—absence suggests Kallmann syndrome
* how this issue is affecting the young person

Examination

* height, weight and, if indicated BMI, plotted on an age- and sex-appropriate chart. Previous data will to help establish growth pattern
* height centiles of both parents and target centile range calculated and plotted on chart
* evidence of skeletal disproportion
* dysmorphic features suggestive of Turner or Klinefelter syndrome
* pubertal staging according to Tanner standards
* presence of gynaecomastia in boys
* testicular volume in boys using a Prader orchidometer
* fundoscopy and visual fields if intracranial pathology suspected

Central delayed puberty

A common referral to an endocrine clinic is a young male aged 14–16 years with relative short stature and delayed puberty who comes from a short family where one or both parents have a similar history. Typically, they are of slim build but otherwise healthy and they are often acutely aware of standing out amongst their peer group. The history and examination are normal apart from the delayed development. Apart from a bone age estimation, investigations are unlikely to be necessary and the diagnosis is that of constitutional delay of growth and puberty (CDGP).

Any chronic illness can delay the onset of puberty, particularly those associated with chronic inflammation such as inflammatory bowel disease or impaired food intake or absorption as found in anorexia nervosa or coeliac disease. This is probably due to downregulation of growth by the hypothalamus until overall health improves. It is important to control the underlying condition and correct any nutritional deficiency before considering hormone treatment. In the amenorrhoea of chronic anorexia nervosa, supplementary hormones have no beneficial effect on bone mineral density.

Permanent hypogonadotrophic hypogonadism may be one component of multiple pituitary hormone deficiency.

Primary gonadal failure
Primary ovarian failure

- genetic—e.g., Turner syndrome
- acquired—autoimmune or following radiotherapy

Testicular failure

- genetic—e.g., Klinefelter syndrome
- acquired—radiotherapy or surgery for maldescent of the testes

Both Turner and Klinefelter may present for the first time during adolescence as features may be subtle and are easily missed. Boys with Klinefelter may present with gynaecomastia (although most boys with gynaecomastia do not have Klinefelter) that can be a significant source of distress. Some have behaviour and/or education difficulties.

Investigations

The choice of investigations should be driven by the history and examination. The following list is similar to that in sexual precocity but for different reasons:
- pelvic USS to assess any ovarian and uterine maturation
- left wrist and hand radiograph for bone age in CDGP
- baseline LH and FSH should be interpreted with caution. If grossly elevated, they are diagnostic of primary gonadal failure but low levels do not diagnose hypogonadotrophic hypogonadism because secretion is nocturnal until mid-puberty. A GnRH test might be needed where there is doubt.

- karyotype if LH and FSH high suggesting primary gonadal failure
- baseline testosterone in boys and oestrogen in girls
- cranial MRI scan if evidence of hypogonadotrophic hypogonadism or intracranial pathology

Treatment and management

Reassurance of their normality for boys with CDGP may be adequate. If they are willing to attend a clinic to discuss such a personal issue, then they are likely to be seeking treatment and will benefit psychosocially from a short course of supplementary testosterone. This will boost their growth and development whilst their own system matures. The dose and the length of the course depends on their stage of puberty at outset and their age and is usually given as an injection of slow-release testosterone esters (Sustanon) every 4 weeks for 3–12 months from the age of 14 years onwards. The treatment is safe and has no adverse effect on final height. This diagnosis is much less common in girls but they may also benefit from very low dose oestrogen treatment for up to 12 months although it is less effective.

In both hypogonadotrophic hypogonadism and primary gonadal failure, puberty is induced with gradually increasing doses of either oestrogen or testosterone over about 3 years to mimic normal puberty and hormone replacement treatment will be lifelong. For these young people, the discovery during adolescence of a diagnosis that can impact on puberty and fertility can be devastating and they are likely to need significant psychosocial support.

IMPORTANT CLINICAL POINTS

Short stature
- previous growth measurements can be obtained from Child Health Records
- familial short stature is the most common diagnosis in children referred to a growth clinic
- population studies show very little impact of short stature on adult functioning
- GHD in neonates is usually picked up during investigations for hypoglycaemia
- GHD in over 2 years presents with slowing of growth with increased body fat

Tall stature
- commonest causes are overnutrition or normal, but early, puberty in a child with tall parents
- assessment of limb length will identify those with disproportionate tall stature

Sexual precocity
- defined in girls as any signs under 8 years—common and unlikely to be pathological
- defined in boys as any signs under 9 years—rare and pathology should be excluded
- sexual precocity can be gonadotrophin dependent or gonadotrophin independent

Delayed puberty
- defined in girls as no signs over 13 years—rare and may merit investigation
- defined in boys as no signs over 14 years—common and unlikely to be pathological
- primary gonadal failure can be genetic or acquired

Further Reading

Faltering growth: recognition and management of faltering growth in children NICE guideline [NG75]. Published: 27 September 2017 https://www.nice.org.uk/guidance/ng75.

Human growth hormone (somatropin) for the treatment of growth failure in children Technology appraisal guidance [TA188]. Published: 26 May 2010 https://www.nice.org.uk/guidance/ta188.

Practical Endocrinology and Diabetes in Children. Donaldson M C; Gregory JW; Van-Vliet G; Wolfsdorf JI . Wiley. 4th Edition April 2019

Chapter | 5 |

Genetics and dysmorphology

Angus Clarke, Martin Hewitt

After reading this chapter you should:
- be able to explain and provide advice regarding patterns of inheritance
- be able to diagnose and manage common genetic and dysmorphological conditions
- be able to discuss the role of pre- and postnatal genetic investigations
- understand the effects of environmental factors affecting the fetus

Patterns of inheritance

Chromosomal abnormality and mutations

There are many conditions seen in paediatric practice that are the result of a genetic mutation, and these range from structural chromosome changes to single nucleotide alterations. These mutations may result in disease and are referred to as pathogenic mutations whilst others, non-pathogenic mutations, are not implicated in disease causation.

Chromosomal abnormalities can be classified as either numerical or structural.

Numerical abnormalities:

- polyploid—additional sets of 23 chromosomes as in triploidy
- aneuploidy—presence or absence of one or more chromosome
- trisomy—presence of three copies of a chromosome
- monosomy—presence of only one member of the chromosome pair

Structural abnormalities

Translocations, most inversions and large (microscopic) deletions, duplications or insertions will be visible on karyotype. Chromosome microarray analysis will detect even small changes in copy number (sub-microscopic deletions and duplications) but will fail to detect other rearrangements, such as translocations and inversions, unless there are associated alterations in copy number of nearby sequences. The recognised types of structural abnormalities (Figure 5.1) include:

- translocation—transfer of material from one chromosome to another
- balanced translocation—transfer of material between chromosomes but no loss of genetic material
- reciprocal translocation—chromosome breaks and exchange of material between chromosomes
- Robertsonian translocation—breaks close to the centromere of acrocentric chromosomes and subsequent fusion with another acrocentric chromosome. This leads to the loss of both short arms of the chromosomes involved but without adverse consequences as the missing regions contain no protein-coding genes
- insertion—insertion of segment into another position in a chromosome
- deletion—loss of part of chromosome
- duplication—duplication of part of a chromosome
- inversion—section of a chromosome rotated by 180° and reinserted
- ring chromosome—chromosome break, with the two ends joining together to form a ring. There is loss of chromosomal material.

Sex chromosome abnormalities

- loss of part or all of one of the sex chromosomes as in Turners syndrome (45X0)

46

a) Reciprocal chromosomal translocation

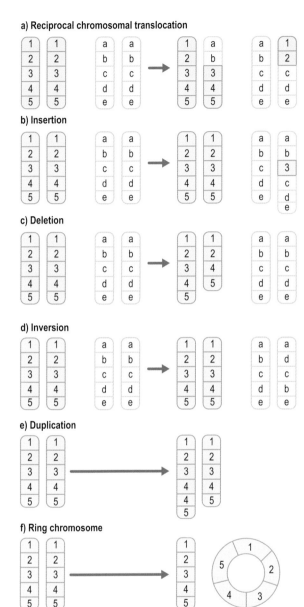

b) Insertion

c) Deletion

d) Inversion

e) Duplication

f) Ring chromosome

Fig. 5.1 Diagrammatic representation of chromosomal rearrangements

- duplication of one the sex chromosomes as in Klinefelter syndrome (47 XXY)

Genetic sequence variants (point mutations)

- alterations of one or several contiguous nucleotides, usually within a gene and often within the coding sequence or nearby, so that RNA splicing is affected.

These alterations can be complex. The simplest categories are:

- substitutions—replacement of one nucleotide by another
- insertions—addition of one or more nucleotide
- deletions—loss of one or more nucleotide

The brief description of the nucleotide alteration within the coding sequence of a gene is preceded by 'c.' (for coding) and then followed by the associated change in the amino acid sequence of the relevant protein product, itself preceded by 'p.' (for protein). Thus, the commonest pathogenic variant in the CFTR gene, causing cystic fibrosis in homozygotes and formerly known as ΔF508, is now presented as: c.1521_1523delCTT; p.Phe508Del.

Such alterations in DNA sequence are now classified by their pathogenicity as definitely benign (class 1), probably benign (class 2), of uncertain significance (class 3), probably pathogenic (class 4) or definitely pathogenic (class 5). There are multiple factors to be taken into account in deciding whether or not a variant is pathogenic. This is complex and involves bioinformatic analysis according to national and international standards and comparisons with international reference databases. It may also require a comparison with test results on parents, siblings and other members of the family.

Autosomal dominant conditions

The disorder is expressed completely in the heterozygote individual, and all offspring of an affected person will have a 50% chance of inheriting the mutation, giving rise to vertical transmission in the pedigree. Variable expression and incomplete or age-dependent penetrance can complicate recognition of autosomal dominant inheritance.

Autosomal recessive conditions

The disorder is expressed in the affected homozygote individuals and may arise de novo or be recognised if

---

Conditions with autosomal dominant inheritance

- achondroplasia
- hereditary elliptocytosis
- hereditary spherocytosis
- Huntington's disease
- Marfan syndrome
- myotonic dystrophy
- neurofibromatosis NF1 and NF2
- Noonan syndrome
- tuberous sclerosis complex
- von Willebrand disease

there are affected siblings. When both parents are carriers, each of their offspring has a 25% risk of being homozygous affected and a 50% risk of being a heterozygous carrier.

> **PRACTICE POINT – conditions with autosomal recessive inheritance**
>
> - alpha-1 antitrypsin deficiency
> - ataxia telangiectasia
> - beta thalassaemia
> - cystic fibrosis
> - Fanconi anaemia
> - galactosaemia
> - glycogen storage disorders
> - homocystinuria

X chromosome linked conditions

These conditions result from mutations in a gene carried on the X chromosome and therefore males are usually affected as they only have one copy of the gene. Female carriers of X-linked conditions are often unaffected but may show some features of the disease, although usually less severely than an affected male.

Features of this X-linked form of inheritance are:
- no male-to-male transmission
- all daughters of an affected male will be carriers
- half of all daughters of a carrier female will be carriers

X chromosome gene disorders are occasionally separated into X-linked recessive, which tend not to manifest significantly in females, and X-linked dominant in which females are commonly affected. In some of these conditions, males may be so severely affected as to die in utero or in early infancy. The distinction between X-linked recessive and X-linked dominant can help in assessing patterns of inheritance in a family, although the random and variable nature of X chromosome inactivation will often blur the distinction.

> **PRACTICE POINT – conditions with X-linked inheritance**
>
> - Becker muscular dystrophy
> - Duchenne muscular dystrophy
> - Glucose-6-phosphate dehydrogenase deficiency
> - haemophilia A and B
> - hypohidrotic ectodermal dysplasia
> - incontinentia pigmenti
> - Rett syndrome
> - Wiskott-Aldrich syndrome

Mitochondrial mutations

Mitochondrial DNA mutations are transmitted by maternal inheritance and are passed down from mother to child but not from father to child. In most people, all mitochondria contain identical copies of the mitochondrial genome (homoplasmy), but in those with mitochondrial disorders there may be a mix of mitochondria with normal and mutated DNA within each cell (heteroplasmy), especially if the mutation would be lethal if it were present in all copies of the genome (that is, if there were homoplasmy for the mutation).

Imprinting conditions

For most autosomal genes, both alleles are expressed in a cell but, for some, only one allele is expressed and the other is switched off. Whether an allele is expressed or repressed is determined by the sex of the parent contributing that gene and the phenomenon is termed imprinting (see Figure 5.2). The terms used are:
- maternally imprinted gene—the maternally derived allele is inactivated
- paternally imprinted gene—the paternally derived allele is inactivated

> **PRACTICE POINT – conditions due to genetic imprinting abnormalities**
>
> - Prader-Willi syndrome (PWS)—maternally imprinted factors; syndrome arises when the paternal copy is absent (by deletion or maternal disomy) or defective
> - Angelman syndrome—UBE3A gene, paternally imprinted gene; syndrome arises when the maternal allele is absent or defective
> - Beckwith-Wiedemann syndrome—there is cluster of growth-regulating genes at distal 11p15 that are subject to a complex pattern of imprinting; the condition can arise when the balance of gene activity is disturbed through a variety of mechanisms, including paternal 11p15 duplication, paternal uniparental disomy, or point mutation in one of the imprinting control regions or in a specific gene
> - Silver Russell syndrome—has a number of causes including maternal uniparental disomy for chromosome 7 or for 11p15 (the converse of Beckwith-Wiedemann syndrome, above)
> - pseudohypoparathyroidism type 1a—GNAS1 gene, paternal allele suppressed
> - pseudopseudohypoparathyroidism—GNAS1 gene, maternal allele suppressed

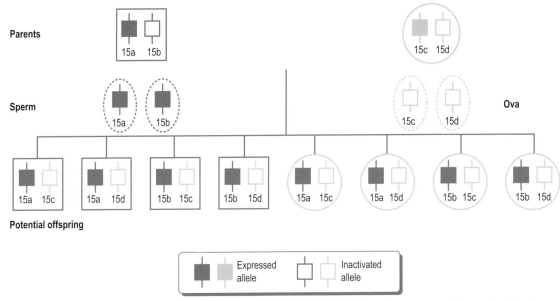

Fig. 5.2 The inheritance of a maternally imprinted gene. Father represented in blue. Mother represented in purple. Only the paternally derived copies are expressed. In the ova, imprinting inactivates all maternally derived copies of the allele.

Common genetic and dysmorphological conditions

The number of conditions which have a clear genetic basis is extensive and ever expanding, and a detailed knowledge of the vast majority is beyond the scope of the AKP exam. Clinical features that may suggest an underlying genetic disorder include:

- multiple individuals of the same family being affected by the same problem
- multiple problems in the same individual including congenital abnormalities, growth problems, neuro-developmental problems and unusual tumours

Certain features on their own may raise suspicion of a genetic condition and examples of such features are:

- eyes—unusual shape, different coloured irises
- hair—brittle, sparse, white patches
- tongue—large or small tongue
- teeth—misshapen, extra, primary oligodontia
- extremes of stature
- digits—webbed
- birthmarks that are unusual

There are, however, a core of conditions which may be seen by the paediatric team due to specific abnormalities such as neurodisability, congenital cardiac abnormalities or specific facial or somatic features. Some of these conditions are presented here to illustrate recognised inheritance patterns and some identifiable clinical features and it would be important for candidates to review as many images as possible for each of these recognised diagnoses. This section will show the diagnosis and the associated phenotypic features, but further details about associated clinical problems and their management will be presented in the chapters indicated.

Confirmation of the clinical suspicion through more detailed investigations should be undertaken by clinical genetics teams who will have access to the most appropriate investigations, the required understanding to interpret the results and the appropriate team members to explain the findings and implications to the patient and their family members.

Down syndrome

Trisomy 21—most arise through nondisjunction
Common phenotypic features

- eyes—up-slanting, epicanthic folds, Brushfield spots, cataracts
- midface hypoplasia, small mouth and jaw
- brachycephaly
- hand abnormalities—single palmar crease, (short broad) hands, clinodactyly
- hypotonia and hypermobility
- intellectual disability common (usually mild-moderate)
- cardiac abnormalities—AVSD most common then VSD then ASD

Antenatal screening is offered to all pregnant women and is outlined in further detail below. Details of management are to be found in Chapter 27 Neurodevelopmental Medicine

Patau syndrome

Trisomy 13
    Common phenotypic features include
- cleft lip and palate
- polydactyly
- eye abnormalities—microphthalmia, anophthalmia, coloboma
- cardiac anomalies—VSD, ASD
- CNS defects, including holoprosencephaly and meningomyelocoele
- death usually within the first 12 months

Edward syndrome

Trisomy 18
    Common phenotypic features include
- significant defects in brain development
- eye abnormalities—microphthalmia, anophthalmia, coloboma
- cardiac anomalies—VSD, ASD
- characteristic hand position at birth (see Figure 5.3)
- death usually within the first 12 months, but survival has improved over the past few decades

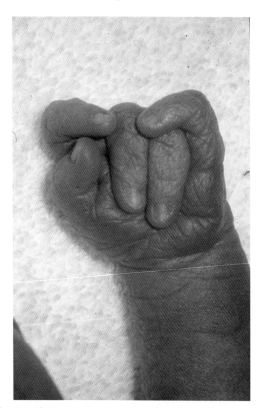

Fig. 5.3 Characteristic appearance of the hand in Edward syndrome

Turner syndrome

45,X (also 45,X0) or 45,X with mosaicism
    Common phenotypic features
- short stature
- lymphoedema in the neonate
- low hair line
- webbing of neck (Figure 5.4)
- wide-spaced nipples
- shield-shaped chest
- cubitus valgus
- cardiac defects—bicuspid aortic valve, coarctation
- usually intellectually normal
    Details of management are to be found in Chapter 4 Growth and Puberty.

Klinefelter syndrome

47 XXY
    Common phenotypic features in babies and young children
- hypospadias
- micropenis
- cryptorchidism
- mild-moderate neurodevelopmental problems (not in all)
- incomplete pubertal development
- gynaecomastia
- small testes
    Details of management are to be found in Chapter 4 Growth and Puberty.

Wiskott-Aldrich syndrome

X-linked recessive
    Common phenotypic features
- thrombocytopenia
- eczema
- combined immunodeficiency
    Details of management are to be found in Chapter 15 Immunology.

Chromosome 22q11.2 deletion (Di George syndrome, Velo-cardio-facial syndrome)

Common phenotypic features
- cyanotic and acyanotic cardiac anomalies:
    ○ truncus arteriosus, tetralogy of Fallot, ASD and VSD, vascular rings
- hypoplastic thymus—giving leucopenia and recurrent infections
- parathyroid hypoplasia—leading to hypocalcaemia—may present with seizures
- developmental delay
- cleft lip and palate
- distinctive facial dysmorphism

Aspects of management are to be found in Chapter 25 Endocrinology and Chapter 27 Neurodevelopmental Medicine

Williams syndrome

Autosomal dominant
  Common phenotypic features (see Figure 5.5)
- short stature
- facial dysmorphism (broad forehead, short nose, long philtrum),
- large mouth, widely spaced teeth, full lips
- cardiac—supravalvular aortic or pulmonary stenosis
- renal artery stenosis
- high calcium levels
- hypothyroidism
- sociable and language skills comparatively good ('Cocktail Party Chatter')
  Details of management are to be found in Chapter 27 Neurodevelopmental Medicine.

Prader-Willi syndrome

Absence of a functioning paternal copy of 15q11; usually either by deletion of this region of the paternal chromosome 15 or by maternal uniparental disomy
  Common phenotypic features
- reduced fetal movements, small for dates, polyhydramnios
- severe neonatal hypotonia with poor feeding with a weak cry
- thin upper lip, downturned mouth; almond-shaped eyes and hypotelorism
- boys often have cryptorchidism with maldescended testes
- short stature often linked to abnormalities in growth hormone production
- uncontrolled appetite with rapid development of obesity from 2 years of age
- learning impairment common
  Details of management are to be found in Chapter 27 Neurodevelopmental Medicine.

Angelman syndrome

Absence of a functioning (maternal) copy of the *UBE3A* gene on 15q. This is usually caused by deletion of the maternal chromosome 15q11-13 or by paternal disomy for chromosome 15, or by point mutation in *UBE3A*.
  Common phenotypic features (see Figure 5.6).
- manifests between 6 and 12 months of age
- physical features include wide mouth, wide-spaced teeth
- significant developmental delay and later microcephaly
- smiling, laughter and hand clapping
- motor features include ataxia, fine tremors, stiff-legged, wide-based gait

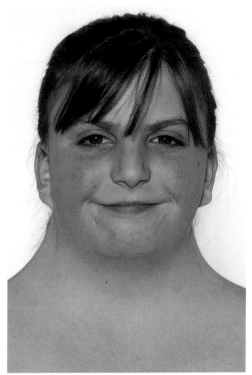
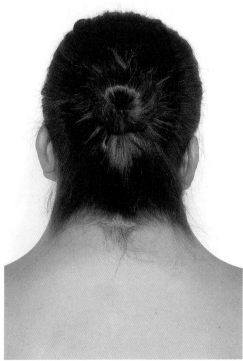

Fig. 5.4 Turner syndrome. Note webbing of the neck, low set ears and low posterior hair line

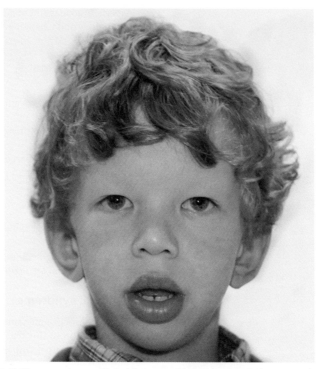

Fig. 5.5 A 6-year-old boy with Williams syndrome. Clinical features of broad forehead, short nose, long philtrum, large mouth, widely spaced teeth, full lips (Reprinted with permission from Collins, T. [2013]. Cardiovascular Disease in Williams Syndrome. Circulation, 127:21, 2125-2134.)

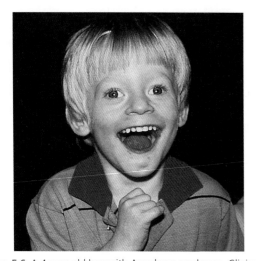

Fig. 5.6 A 4-year-old boy with Angelman syndrome. Clinical features of smiling child with stiff-legged, wide-based gait (Image use with permission from Rapid Review Pathology: First South Asia Edition. Ed. Goljan, EF. Chapter 6. Elsevier Inc.)

Details of management are to be found in Chapter 27 Neurodevelopmental Medicine.

Peutz-Jeghers syndrome

Autosomal dominant with mutation in *STK11* on Chromosome 19p

Common phenotypic features (see Figure 5.7)
- multiple polyps in gastrointestinal tract
- polyps are premalignant and can undergo malignant change
- mucocutaneous pigmentation of lips

Beckwith–Wiedemann syndrome

Imprinted gene abnormality 11p15

Common phenotypic features
- hemi-hypertrophy
- macrosomia
- macroglossia
- omphalocoele
- crease on pinna of ear (see Figure 5.8)

Details of management are to be found in Chapter 4 Growth and Puberty.

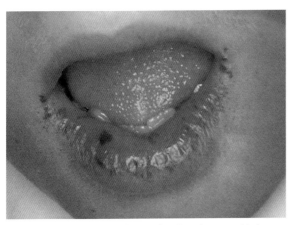

Fig. 5.7 Peutz-Jeghers syndrome showing pigmented lesions on lips (Image use with permission from Zitelli and Davis' Atlas of Pediatric Physical Diagnosis, Zitelli BJ et al. 7th. Edition. Chapter 18. Authors Katz A, Richardson W. Elsevier Inc.)

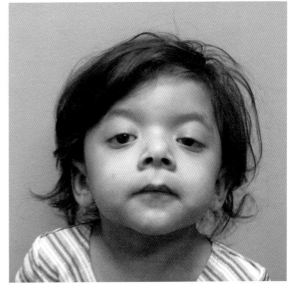

Fig. 5.9 A 3-year-old girl with Noonan syndrome. Clinical features of broad forehead, hypertelorism, downward slanting eyes, epicanthic folds, low set ears (Image use with permission from Zitelli and Davis' Atlas of Pediatric Physical Diagnosis, Zitelli BJ et al. 7th. Edition. Chapter 1. Authors Madan-Khetarpal, Arnold G. Elsevier Inc.)

Noonan syndrome

autosomal dominant—50% new mutations
Common phenotypic features (see Figure 5.9)
- short stature and dysmorphic features (broad forehead, hypertelorism, downward slanting eyes, epicanthic folds, low-set ears)
- congenital cardiac defects and risk of cardiomyopathy
- lymphoedema
- variable coagulopathy and bruising
Details of management are to be found in Chapter 4 Growth and Puberty.

Fragile X syndrome

Mutation of FMR1 gene on X chromosome
Common phenotypic features
- long narrow face with prognathism and prominent forehead
- large ears
- testicular enlargement (post-puberty)
- intellectual disability
- motor delay
- behavioural issues—hyperactive, social anxiety, inattention, stereotypic movements
- phenotype associated with pre-mutation in *FMR1* is late onset and distinct from the fragile X syndrome phenotype

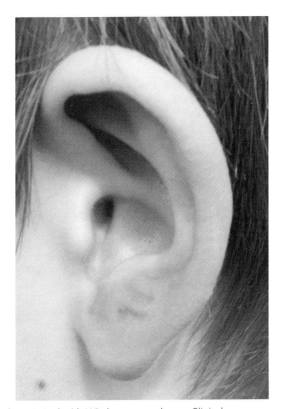

Fig. 5.8 Beckwith-Wiedemann syndrome. Clinical appearance of characteristic creases on the ear lobes

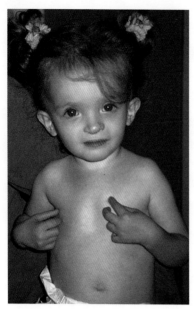

Fig. 5.10 A 2-year-old girl with Silver Russell syndrome. Clinical features of bossed forehead and triangular face (Image use with permission from Emery's Elements of Medical Genetics. 7thEdition. Editors Turnpenny PD, Ellard S. Chapter 6. Elsevier Ltd)

Marfan syndrome

Autosomal dominant. De novo in 25% to 30%
   Common phenotypic features
- tall stature
- skeletal abnormalities—arachnodactyly, long limbs, pectus deformity, scoliosis
- malar hypoplasia
- aortic abnormalities—valve regurgitation, dissection, dilatation
- ocular abnormalities—upward dislocation of lens
   Details of management are to be found in Chapter 4 Growth and Puberty.

Silver Russell syndrome

Various causes including loss of imprinting at 11p15 that controls IGF2 (60% of patients) and
maternal uniparental disomy for Chromosome 7 (10% of patients).
   Common phenotypic features (see Figure 5.10)
- severe pre- and postnatal growth restriction, sometimes with asymmetry
- feeding difficulties, swallowing problems
- developmental delay
- dysmorphic features include relative macrocephaly broad forehead triangular face micrognathia
   Details of management are to be found in Chapter 4 Growth and Puberty.

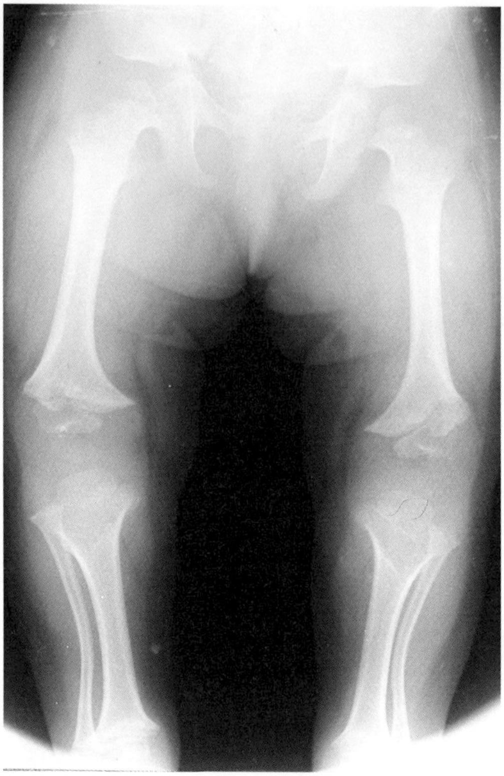

Fig. 5.11 Radiological appearances of lower limbs in achondroplasia

Rett syndrome

Mutation of *MECP2* gene on Xq28. Usually sporadic.
   Common phenotypic features
- predominantly in females
- growth failure, progressive microcephaly
- initial normal development but then regression typically at 12–18 months of age; later social reemergence but severe problems of communication and cognition
- low tone, motor delay, feeding problems, speech delay, disturbance of motor function, often with spasticity from late childhood
- stereotypical midline 'hand-wringing' movements and unprovoked screaming episodes
- seizures
- bruxism (teeth grinding)
   Details of management are to be found in Chapter 27 Neurodevelopmental Medicine.

Achondroplasia

Autosomal dominant
   Common phenotypic features
- short stature
- proximal long bone shortening (see Figure 5.11)

- shortened digits
- macrocephaly
- facial features—frontal bossing, flattened nose
- risk of cervical spine compression

Albright's Hereditary Osteodystrophy (also known as pseudohypoparathyroidism type 1a)

Most likely autosomal dominant with genetic imprinting affecting some of the endocrine features but not the dysmorphism or disturbance of growth

Common phenotypic features
- short stature
- shortened fourth and fifth metacarpals
- rounded facies
- mild mental retardation
- hypocalcaemia, hypophosphataemia and raised PTH and additional endocrine features in some patients

Details of management are to be found in Chapter 4 Growth and Puberty.

Genetic testing

There are many ways in which genetic diseases can be investigated once the suspicion of such a diagnosis is raised. Direct analysis of genetic material takes two main forms:
- assessing the copy number of sections of chromosome in a microarray analysis
- determining DNA sequence information

Microarray analysis is used to detect chromosomal deletions and duplications. (The karyotype now has fewer indications, such as when a complex structural rearrangement is suspected.) Sequence variants may be sought in a single gene, in a panel of several or many genes, in the exome or in the whole genome.

Screening of individuals

Genetic testing is used in order to confirm an ever-increasing range of diagnoses by identifying the underlying cause, and it can also be used to look for possible causes of other, undiagnosed conditions. Other investigations, such as measurement of biochemical constituents known to be associated with particular gene defects or the identification of structural defects by imaging, can all support the diagnosis. Whatever the method of confirming a genetic diagnosis, it is important to understand the consequences for the individual and their family. These consequences can be deep and personal and lead to enduring sadness and distress.

PRACTICE POINT – types of genetic testing

- **diagnostic genetic test**—the individual has features of a genetic disease and is tested to confirm or exclude the diagnosis
- **predictive genetic test**—an otherwise healthy person is tested to see if they carry a genetic alteration that may lead to a particular genetic disease in the future
- **genetic carrier test**—identifies unaffected carriers of an autosomal recessive disorder or of a sex-linked disorder or a balanced chromosomal rearrangement

The nature of genetic disorders, along with the incomplete understanding of their complexities in our current state of knowledge and the limitations of the techniques used to carry out genetic testing, mean that caution must be applied when interpreting test results and explaining the implications to children and their families.

PRACTICE POINT – genetic test results

Six types of result may be returned from a diagnostic genetic investigation. The clinician should be aware of these possibilities, which may all need to be discussed with the patient or parents in advance of testing:
- **positive result**: a clear and definite explanation for the child's disease or condition
- **negative (completely normal) result:** no explanation found for the child's illness. This does not prove that the underlying genetic cause is not genetic, just that the cause has not been recognised
- **variant of uncertain significance:** such as an alteration in a gene in which other variants have been associated with the condition in the child. The uncertainty concerns whether **this** genetic variant in **that** specific gene would be able to cause the particular phenotype in the child
- **incidental finding:** a finding that is not relevant to the reason for the investigation but would count as an unanticipated finding that relates to a completely different disease but one which may be relevant to the child's future health or reproduction, or to the health of other members of the family
- **additional sought finding:** a finding that is relevant to the child's future health or reproduction but not to the principal reason for testing. This is especially relevant in the context of exome or genome sequencing
- **additional or altered result may arise in the future** after reanalysis or after reinterpretation of the initial findings, leading to the need to recontact the patient's family and their health professionals, perhaps after an interval of some years. Variants interpreted initially as being definitely pathogenic or definitely benign may be subject to re-interpretation over time

For many types of genetic analysis, a negative test result must be interpreted with care in case it is a false negative and the genetic abnormality is actually present but has not been detected by the test.

When performing any testing it is important to be aware that the diagnosis of a genetic disease will not only have implications for the affected individual but may have ramifications for other family members, who may be at risk of being affected or being carriers for the condition.

Diagnostic genetic testing

Genetic testing will help if there are issues around growth and development of a child, and a greater understanding of a clinical condition would allow improved management or surveillance for possible complications of a condition. For a child or young person who is acutely unwell, the detailed understanding provided by genetic studies could also provide important information that may direct treatment options.

Predictive genetic testing

The decision to undertake genetic testing in an otherwise healthy person is particularly important in paediatric practice and requires careful consideration. Such testing may be warranted in those at increased risk of developing a genetic condition that would impact on the health and well-being of the child. If a condition can be prevented or ameliorated by an intervention at an earlier stage, then genetic testing will be considered worthwhile.

Predictive genetic testing will usually be considered in an individual already known to be at risk for a specific condition due to their family history and the test will usually be considered in the context of genetic counselling. It is not always beneficial to carry out pre-symptomatic testing in children, particularly for those conditions that become evident in adult life and for which little or no treatment is available. Children tested for Huntington disease, for example, lose the opportunity to decide for themselves whether to be tested as adults (only 15% to 20% of adults at risk of Huntington disease decide to be tested). Adults retain control of the confidentiality over a test result and how this information is used, whilst a child who is tested will lose that control. Knowledge of the test result could lead to emotional and social problems in the child, altering both relationships within the family and expectations for the future in a variety of areas such as education, employment, life and health insurance, long-term relationships and reproduction.

Genetic carrier testing

It is not usually necessary to identify unaffected carriers of genetic disorders as the implications are largely for their reproductive decisions in the future. However, it may be appropriate in particular circumstances.

There are two broad categories of genetic carrier. With autosomal recessive disorders, the chance that a carrier will have an affected child depends on whether their partner is also a carrier. For the other types of conditions—sex-linked disorders and balanced chromosomal rearrangements, such as translocations—the risk to a child arises purely from the carrier parent; the genetic constitution of the other parent usually plays little part. This second category of 'carrier' may also be significant for the child as there may be disease-related phenotypes.

Population screening

Genetic population screening involves testing apparently unaffected individuals in order to detect unrecognised genetic disease, its precursors or carrier status, when there are no particular reasons to suspect that the individual is at increased risk. Screening programmes may include the whole population or a large subgroup, such as the screening of all pregnant women or newborn babies for a range of conditions.

There are four major categories of a population genetic screening programme
- carrier screening
- prenatal screening
- newborn screening
- disease susceptibility screening

Population carrier screening

This responds to the wishes of some individuals and couples to understand the potential risks in a future pregnancy when one or both of them may be carriers of a known genetic disease. Carrier screening is made available in many populations to identify carriers of the haemoglobinopathies, especially beta-thalassaemia and sickle cell disease. Such screening programmes are sometimes established in countries where it is difficult or impossible to meet the costs of care for affected individuals. In such situations, carrier screening leads to the termination of affected pregnancies and so makes it possible to provide care for those patients who are born with the condition. Carrier screening has been extended in some countries to include a range of other autosomal recessive disorders and sometimes also certain sex-linked disorders. It is ideally made available before a pregnancy but it may be offered in the antenatal period.

A very different situation arises when one or both members of a couple are at higher than population risk because of a family history of a genetic disorder. If the variant that causes disease in the family is known, then testing the individual with the positive family history can then give very accurate information. If the variant is not known, then it can be helpful to arrange testing for the affected family member, if they are available and agree to be tested. This is a form of family cascade testing, and the probability calculations (of whether an individual or a pregnancy—a future child—is at risk) need to be assessed for each specific family context.

The details of a genetic variant may have already been made available as follow-up of the family of the affected proband, when the extended family may be offered testing to track the genetic variants and see who else may be carriers. A couple may seek more information, and perhaps testing, if they are both healthy and each had a sibling with, for example, cystic fibrosis, or if one individual has an affected sibling and the other comes from a population with a known frequency for being a carrier.

Similarly, those with family members affected by haemoglobinopathies or other specific conditions may wish some guidance on future risks to their children when planning a family. The chances that a couple will have an affected child are increased if they are related to each other, especially if they are also both related to an individual affected by an autosomal recessive disorder.

Prenatal screening

The current UK antenatal screening programme includes the screening of a range of conditions, both genetic and nongenetic. Enquiry is made concerning family history of disease and the consumption of alcohol, cigarettes and recreational drugs. Blood tests are performed for congenital infection, blood group and red cell allo-antibodies and the three autosomal trisomies compatible with survival beyond the perinatal period. Fetal ultrasound scans are used to assess fetal and placental position, to monitor fetal growth and development and to identify anatomical defects in the fetus.

Screening for Down syndrome, Edward syndrome and Patau syndrome is offered at the end of the first trimester to all mothers or couples but is different from the other screening tests in that it should very much be offered on the basis of a considered parental choice rather than as a routine procedure, as not all will wish to partake for a variety of reasons. Assessment of nuchal translucency via ultrasound, beta-HCG and the Pregnancy Associated Plasma Protein A are collated to provide information about the chance that the fetus has one of these autosomal trisomies. In those pregnancies found on this initial screen to have an above average chance of an affected fetus, the pregnant woman will usually be offered noninvasive prenatal testing, on the basis of DNA sequences present in maternal blood. The crucial measures of the performance of this test are the sensitivity and the positive predictive value (PPV) of the initial screening test. If noninvasive prenatal testing is performed as

a stand-alone test, the PPV is about 80%; if performed as a second-tier test, after an increased chance found on preliminary screening, it has a PPV of about 90%. A confirmatory (diagnostic) test is still required after a positive NIPT screening test result, whether first tier or second tier.

Newborn screening

Every newborn baby in the UK is included in the standard screening programme. This includes:

- medical examination—to identify structural anomalies and address parental concerns
- hearing assessment—usually undertaken before discharge from hospital or within 4–5 weeks. The initial test, known as the automated otoacoustic emission (aOAE) test, plays a click and looks for a response in the baby, and those who fail to respond are referred for a further assessment with the automated auditory brainstem response (AABR) test.
- blood test—a heel prick blood spot sample is taken on day 5 and analysed for nine conditions, most of which are of genetic origin. Molecular genetic testing is performed on small numbers of samples as a second-tier investigation, when indicated, such as tests for common mutations in the CFTR gene when the IRT (trypsin) level is high. Note that the commonest condition detected on the blood spot, congenital hypothyroidism, is not primarily of genetic origin

It is important to remember that children born in other countries and who then move to the UK may not have been part of a national screening programme and could therefore present with some of the conditions usually identified here.

PRACTICE POINT – UK Newborn Screening Programme

- sickle cell disease
- cystic fibrosis
- hypothyroidism
- phenylketonuria
- medium-chain acyl CoA dehydrogenase deficiency (MCADD)
- maple syrup urine disease
- isovaleric acidaemia
- glutaric aciduria type 1
- homocystinuria

Developments in newborn screening are likely over the next few years, including extended metabolic screening and perhaps, more controversially, sequencing of parts or the whole of the genome.

Disease susceptibility screening

There is a very definite role for disease susceptibility screening in two contexts:

(i) population screening of adults for hypertension, hypercholesterolaemia, glaucoma and cancers of the breast, cervix and bowel

(ii) targeted surveillance for the development of complications in those with conditions that put them at particular risk, as with numerous rare inherited disorders (e.g., neurofibromatosis type 1, Marfan syndrome and many familial cancer syndromes)

However, there is no evidence of clinical utility for genome-based screening for susceptibility to the common, complex diseases. A role for polygenic risk scores for these disorders may, in the future, in at least some specific contexts, be identified in adults, but there are grounds for concern that should lead to a substantial degree of caution about such screening in children.

Effects of environmental factors affecting the foetus

The normal development of the foetus *in utero* is a complex process but one which can be adversely affected by influences of the maternal lifestyle and environment. An understanding of these factors will allow the clinician to advise and support a mother who may wish to eliminate or reduce such effects.

Smoking

Tobacco products in their various forms have a significant and adverse effect on foetal development and neonatal health. Cigarettes are the most common modality of nicotine absorption and therefore the most studied, but electronic cigarettes have become more popular over recent years and their impact is yet to be fully understood. Current advice would be to discourage the use of all forms of nicotine during pregnancy. Maternal smoking is known to increase the risks of:

- preterm delivery (increased risk x2)
- low birthweight babies (increased risk x3)
- stillbirth (increased risk by 50%)
- neonatal death (increased by 20%)

Education of both the mother and her partner about the effects of active and passive smoking must be included in antenatal sessions and active support offered for those who are determined to curtail their smoking habit.

Drugs

Drugs taken during pregnancy may be legitimately prescribed for medical conditions of the mother or may be consumed by her for recreation. Many prescribed medications are known to have potential teratogenic effects on the developing foetus, and their use during pregnancy needs careful consideration and planning where possible.

The current advice for women who are already receiving medication that is known to have a potential for teratogenicity is that they either change away from that medication when they move into the childbearing age or ensure that they know of the risks and have access to appropriate contraception. Sodium valproate is associated with significant risk of birth defects and developmental disorders and the medication should not be prescribed for any young woman who is fertile without a discussion of risks and the need for contraception. Similarly, sodium valproate should not be prescribed to girls who are likely to remain on the medication as they move into puberty. The prescription of some antidepressants will also need review if pregnancy is a possibility.

Substance misuse during pregnancy will also have a significant effect on the health of the mother and thereby the health of the baby, both *in utero* and following delivery. Some aspects will have lifelong implications for the child. Screening for substance abuse is part of the antenatal assessment in the UK and involves history taking rather than biochemical investigations. A supportive and understanding approach should be adopted.

The most commonly encountered substances used for recreation by mothers during pregnancy include opioids (morphine, methadone), MDMA, amphetamines and cannabis. All may lead to a neonatal withdrawal syndrome seen after delivery although for others the direct effects are uncertain.

Alcohol

There is a wide spectrum of teratogenic effects of alcohol on an unborn baby and they are described as being part of the Foetal Alcohol Spectrum Disorder. The amount and timing of alcohol consumed by the mother will affect the baby in different ways, but for those who are most severely affected these effects include:

- impaired childhood growth
- microcephaly
- characteristic facies—small palpebral fissures, flattened philtrum and thin upper lip (see Figure 5.12)
- neurocognitive problems—poor concentration, behaviour and learning difficulties

Details of management are to be found in Chapter 27 Neurodevelopmental Medicine.

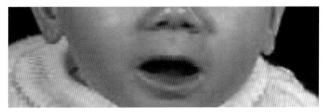

Fig. 5.12 Eight-month-old child with foetal alcohol syndrome. Image shows flattened philtrum and thin upper lip

---

Important Clinical Points

X-Linked inheritance shows
- no male-to-male transmission
- all daughters of an affected male will be carriers
- half of all daughters of a carrier female will be carriers

Imprinting conditions
- maternally imprinted gene—the maternally derived allele is inactivated
- paternally imprinted gene—the paternally derived allele is inactivated

Common genetic and dysmorphological conditions
- important to recognise common syndromes

Newborn screening
- every newborn baby in the UK is included in the standard screening programme
- examination, hearing bloods for nine conditions

Further reading

Firth HV, Hurst JA. Oxford desk reference–Clinical genetics. 2nd edition. Oxford: Oxford University Press; 2017.

Read A, Donnai D. New clinical genetics: a guide to genomic medicine (4th edition). Scion Press. Unique (rare chromosome disorders charity) http://www.rarechromo.org.
Has much useful information for parents and clinicians, including printable disorder guides.

Chapter | 6 |

Nutrition

Moriam Mustapha, Kate Wilson, Sybil Barr

After reading this chapter you should be able to assess, diagnose and manage:
- problems arising during the establishment of infant feeding regimes
- malnutrition, obesity and their complications
- specific vitamin, mineral and micronutrient deficiencies

The assessment of nutrition in paediatric practice requires an understanding of the requirements through the periods of growth and development along with an appreciation of the actual intake and content of fluids and foods. There is a need to recognise that energy, fat, protein, carbohydrate, vitamins and minerals must be sufficient to meet the changing needs of the growing child. Growth in the first year of life is rapid, particularly of the brain, and a normal infant requires around three times more energy per kilogram than an adult reflecting the added energy requirements needed for growth.

Infant feeding

Breast feeding

Breast milk is the most appropriate food for newborn infants and every mother should be encouraged and supported to establish this method of infant nutrition. No breast milk substitute can completely replicate the physiological role of breast milk as a source of nutrition and immunoprotection, and the inappropriate use of breast milk substitutes remains one of the most important worldwide causes of preventable mortality in infancy.

The UK has one of the lowest rates of breastfeeding in Europe although the trend is towards an improvement in uptake, and the most recent UK figures for 2019/2020 report that 48% of mothers are breastfeeding at 6–8 weeks. These rates, however, fall over the following weeks and months such that only about 30% of infants are receiving breast milk at 6 months. The prevalence of breastfeeding is particularly low among very young mothers and disadvantaged socioeconomic groups.

Women most commonly give up breastfeeding early due to perceptions that they are failing to provide adequate nutrition for their child. Confidence in breastfeeding is severely undermined when supplementary formula milk feeds are recommended by health care staff and supplementation is strongly associated with secondary lactation failure and premature cessation of breastfeeding in mothers. Many maternity units operate a nonformula supplementation policy (a fundamental component of the UNICEF Baby Friendly Initiative) and medical staff should actively support this approach.

PRACTICE POINT – breast milk content

- approximate content per 100 ml; carbohydrate 7g; fat 4g; protein 1.3g
- protein—70% whey, 30% casein (whey is easier to digest; cow's milk is 80% casein)
- protein—lactoferrin, lysozyme, secretory IgA—role in host defence
- carbohydrate—lactose and oligosaccharides
- fat—triglycerides, essential fatty acids, sterols and phospholipids
- enzymes that aid digestion (e.g., lipase) and may also be bactericidal (e.g., lysozyme)
- vitamins and minerals
- growth factors—insulin-like factors; epidermal growth factors
- immunological factors; leukocytes; macrophages; stem cells; IgA; lactoferrin
- Prebiotics including human milk oligosaccharides

Formula feeding

For some mothers, breastfeeding may be contraindicated, and some may elect to use formula feeds. These milks must meet the current UK laws pertaining to formula and follow-on milks that define their composition and marketing. These laws clarify that the essential composition of these formula milks 'must satisfy the nutritional requirements of infants in good health, as established by generally accepted scientific data and that the labelling allows the proper use of such products and promotes and protects breastfeeding'.

All formula milks recommended for general use are made from modified cow's milk. Whey-based infant formulae ('first milks') are all that is required for the first year of life. Manufacturers are keen to promote casein-dominant formulas ('second milks') which are nearer to cow's milk as this requires less modification, but they are less physiologically similar to breast milk. Mothers should be advised to continue whey-based formulae until the child switches to full-fat whole cow's milk after the age of one.

Alternative milks and their clinical indications

The range of alternative milks is extensive and are proposed for a range of differing indications. Those available include:
- extensive hydrolysed formula—first-line treatment in both IgE and non-IgE cow's milk protein allergy
- amino acid formula—second-line treatment in both IgE and non-IgE cow's milk protein allergy under guidance from paediatric and dietetic colleagues
- soya-based formula - not recommended for infants under 6 months of age due to phytoestrogen levels. Can be used in older infants with cow's milk protein allergy when other formulas are rejected for palatability and may be chosen by families practicing veganism
- lactose-free formula—for secondary lactose intolerance (true lactose intolerance is very rare in babies)
- anti-reflux formula—thickened formula for regurgitation. Other causes for regurgitation should be ruled out and it may be contraindicated with certain anti-reflux medication which also thicken feeds
- low birthweight formula—for preterm infants typically born less than 35 weeks gestation
- high energy formula—for infants with increased energy requirements or fluid restrictions such as those with cardiac or pulmonary abnormalities

Goats' milk formula is compliant with current UK regulations but is no less likely to cause allergies than cows' milk formula due to a high level of cross-reactivity. Other milks available include 'hungry baby formula', comfort formula and follow-on formula but formal assessment does not reveal any significant benefits in using these milks for the problems described.

Complimentary feeding

This is also known as weaning and refers to the process by which solid foods are gradually introduced to the diet. The current UK advice to parents is that this should start around 6 months and not before 4 months corrected gestational age. It is recommended that all food groups be introduce to infants even if there is a history of atopy or a high risk of food allergy. Salt and sugar should not be added to solid food for infants.

Assessment of nutritional status

Accurate growth monitoring is a fundamental component for assessing the health, development and nutritional status of infants and children as disturbances in health and nutrition, regardless of their aetiology, almost always affect growth. Dietary assessment cannot be safely used to diagnose poor nutrition although food diaries can provide help and information about the range and type of food eaten and they act as a guide to dietary advice once the problem has been identified. The more comprehensive assessment of nutritional status requires information from the history and examination along with the plotting of growth parameters on population-based charts appropriate for patient characteristics.

Weight, height (or length) and body mass index (BMI) provide a measure of nutritional status. These features should be accurately measured and plotted over time as it is important to incorporate more than one measurement for a complete assessment. BMI must be interpreted in the light of body habitus as an athletic teenager may have a high BMI value due to increased muscle bulk. Head circumference is measured in infants and toddlers up until the age of 2 years. Recumbent length is measured in infants and toddlers under the age of 2 years and beyond this age their height is measured. Mid-upper arm circumference measurements are also used to assess nutritional status particularly in more rural settings where anthropometric equipment is not available or in medical conditions where weight and height measurements are inaccurate such as those with renal disease, liver disease or cerebral palsy.

All anthropometric measurements should be plotted on the correct corresponding growth chart and documented in the clinical notes.

Growth charts

Growth is an important indicator of health for infants and children, and growth charts provide a way to objectively assess and monitor growth from birth to 18 years of age, depending on the growth chart used.

The WHO growth standards describe optimal growth for healthy, breastfed (i.e., exclusively breastfed from 0–6 months of age) children from 0 to 5 years of age. As breastfeeding is considered the gold standard form of nutrition for infants, these data are regarded as a standard, rather than a reference. The most common growth charts used in countries around the world rely on local and WHO data on growth. Condition-specific growth charts are available for individuals with Down syndrome, Turner syndrome, homozygous sickle cell disease and Williams syndrome.

The use of growth charts allows the identification of individuals whose measurements lie some distance from the population mean using centile lines or, in some situations, z-scores. The latter are statistical scores that relate directly to standard deviations from the mean of the growth parameter under review. Z scores are particularly useful when growth measurements are at either extreme of the centile chart.

Malnutrition (undernutrition)

Faltering growth (previously known as failure to thrive) refers to a slowing of weight gain in childhood that is less than expected for age and sex. It is not a diagnosis but describes a problem and denotes the need to investigate and determine the aetiology. Faltering growth can be acute (present for less than 3 months) or chronic (present for more than 3 months). Early detection and simple interventions to increase nutritional intake can help prevent acute faltering growth becoming a chronic condition.

Malnutrition (undernutrition) is defined as an imbalance between nutrient requirements and intake that results in cumulative deficits of energy, protein or micronutrients that may negatively affect growth, development and other relevant outcomes. The term therefore describes undernutrition (inadequate intake) and poor nutrition (inappropriate intake) of calories and required nutrients and the term malnutrition will be used here to include both concepts (Table 6.1).

Observations in the table refer to centile ranges. The impact of chronic malnutrition leads to stunting.

The paediatric population is at higher risk of malnutrition-related complications such as poor wound healing, higher risk of infection, delayed recovery, prolonged hospitalisation and developmental delay. This is due to infants and children having a lower energy reserve and the higher nutritional requirements needed for growth.

When a child is assessed for suspected faltering growth, a thorough clinical, developmental and social assessment should be conducted that includes anthropometry,

Table 6.1 WHO criteria for the classification of malnutrition

	Moderate		Severe	
	acute	chronic	Acute	chronic
BMI	0.4 – 9th		less than 0.4	
length or height		0.4 – 9th		less than 0.4

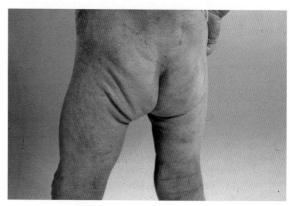

Fig. 6.1 Malnutrition (undernutrition) in a 3-year-old boy showing redundant skin folds.

nutritional intake and output and gastrointestinal symptoms. Initial assessment should look for evidence of dehydration or of an illness or disorder that might account for the weight loss. Other invasive investigations are only necessary if clinical symptoms or signs exist. Concern and further investigations are warranted if a newborn infant, younger than 2 weeks of age, loses more than 10% birthweight or does not regain birthweight within the first 7 to 14 days of life.

In infants and older children, faltering growth is usually defined as weight for age falling across two or more weight centiles. A BMI between 0.4 and the 9th centile is considered unusual and may reflect **moderate** malnutrition (undernutrition—Figure 6.1), but genetic factors such as a small build should be considered. A BMI less than 0.4th centile is considered outside the normal range and **severe** malnutrition can be diagnosed.

Feeding difficulties that cause growth to falter occur due to a range of factors and it may not be possible to identify a clear cause. Neurodevelopmental concerns and psychosocial factors, including postnatal depression or parental anxiety, can adversely affect growth. Referral to a trained professional who can observe feeding and

Table 6.2 Factors to consider when completing a nutritional assessment
Infants on milk feeds
ineffective sucking in breast feeding
ineffective bottle feeding
feeding routines being used
the feeding environment
parent and child interactions
parents' ability to recognise and respond to infants feeding cues
Older children
mealtime arrangements and practices
types of food offered
food aversion or avoidance
parent and child interactions
appetite
environmental factors (posture, seating)

complete a quantitative nutritional assessment might be needed (Table 6.2).

Assessment of gastrointestinal symptoms and signs is important in the investigation of faltering growth, and investigations will be needed in some children.

Investigation

- full blood count (anaemia, red cell indices)
- iron studies
- coeliac screen
- urine culture

Treatment and management

Treatment should focus on early detection and simple healthy eating and behavioural lifestyle changes. This would include eating together as a family, encouraging the child to self-feed, avoiding coercive feeding, establishing regular eating schedules, offering a wide range of foods from five food groups daily and rewarding the child with praise, attention and play rather than with food. Regular physical activity, at least 12 hours of sleep and limiting screen time should all be encouraged.

Oral nutritional supplementation should be considered for infants and children who are unable to obtain adequate nutrition through normal family meals. They are particularly useful for children with a chronic illness who have increased energy requirements or infants who are fluid restricted. Children prescribed oral nutrition support should be encouraged to drink these after normal meal times as they may suppress appetite.

Extra care should be taken when prescribing oral nutrition support for young children less than 5 years of age as consumption may displace healthy foods leading to:

- reduction in food intake (early satiety or preference for milk)
- constipation (drink less fluids as they are full)
- dental caries (bottle feeding beyond 12 months and high sugar formulas)
- delayed oral motor skills

If first two interventions have been unsuccessful and the child is unable to tolerate adequate oral nutrition, then parenteral nutrition should be considered.

CLINICAL SCENARIO

A 26-month-old boy was referred as his parents were concerned that he was pale and quiet. He did not like to eat with his family, preferring to drink fresh milk only from an infant bottle like his baby sister.

His height and weight followed the 50th centile until 6 months ago when his weight dropped to the 9th centile whilst his height remained on 50th centile. Assessment of growth at this review showed weight = 9th centile; height = 50th centile; BMI = 13.5 kg/m² (<2nd centile).

This showed faltering growth as his weight had fallen across two or more centiles and his BMI is less than 2nd centile, suggesting moderate malnutrition (undernutrition). A more thorough assessment was warranted.

Treatment was indicated as he was at risk of becoming clinically undernourished. His dietary preference for consumption of one food group—dairy product—placed him at risk of both macro- and micronutrient deficiency. Considering his pale completion and fatigue, iron studies were undertaken. His preference for drinking from an infant bottle also suggests that development of his oral motor skills was delayed which could affect his language skills. Referral to a multidisciplinary feeding therapies was recommended, including speech and language therapist and dietetics.

Advice was given to his parents to encourage him to sit at the table with his family for all meals and snacks and to teach him to drink from a cup. Parents were advised to provide soft textured, easy-to-eat meals to include foods from all of the five food groups on a daily basis, to enjoy mealtimes with their children and to focus on teaching eating skills (bite chew swallow) and how to drink from a cup.

Obesity

Obesity is the excessive accumulation of subcutaneous and visceral adipose tissue in the body and, according to the World Health Organisation (WHO), it is the fastest growing nutritional disorder in the world. Childhood obesity is defined as a BMI on or above the 98th centile for age, and the term 'overweight' is used for those with a BMI between the 91st and 98th centile. Whilst BMI is an easy and practical measure, it should be interpreted with caution, as it is not a direct measure of adiposity.

Obesity has a multifactorial aetiology with genetics making a contribution for some, but the most common causes are excessive energy intake and low physical activity levels. It is directly linked to serious comorbidities such as:

- type 2 diabetes
- hypertension
- fatty liver disease
- sleep apnoea
- cardiovascular disease

Obesity can be difficult to discuss with children and their families due to social perceptions surrounding the topic. Discussions about a "typical day" in the child's life to assess eating habits and patterns of activity, exploring family beliefs around weight gain, eating patterns and physical activity and recognising certain ethnic backgrounds can have different ideas of what constitutes a healthy weight. An understanding is required of previous attempts to make changes and identifying any various stressors such as poverty, learning difficulties or bullying which will impact on attempts at weight control.

Further investigations may be needed for children with a BMI in the obese category to rule out suspected comorbidities. A thorough family medical history can be helpful with determining which further investigations to conduct.

Treatment and management

Information should be provided to help the child and their family understand obesity and the associated health risks. Such information should be tailored to accommodate the age, ethnic background, cultural beliefs, socioeconomic circumstances and level of health literacy of the individual and their family.

Obesity management requires a variety of interventions, which rely upon a family-oriented holistic approach. Small and simple SMART (Specific, Measurable, Attainable, Relevant and Time-bound) goals could be developed and agreed with the family involving each of the following components:

- Behavioural strategies that encourage positive healthy changes for the whole family and for parents to act as role models for the desired behaviours. Emphasis should be placed on controlling and reducing stimuli that promote sedentary behaviour such as watching television or playing video games).
- Physical activity should be encouraged and all children need to aim for at least 60 minutes each day. The type of physical activity will vary depending on the age of the child and can focus on forms of exercise that the child and family enjoy.

- Dietary changes for the whole family should be discussed and the advantages of healthy eating promoted such as increasing the intake of fruits and vegetables and eating fewer takeaway foods. It is important to try and make changes for the whole family rather than just focusing on the child's diet.
- Referral to a paediatric weight management programme, where available, is recommended.

CLINICAL SCENARIO

A 12-year-old boy was referred after complaining of indigestion and heartburn. He had no other significant medical history. His mother had type 2 diabetes that was controlled with metformin. Assessment showed weight = 65 kg (98th–99.6th centile); height = 148 cm (50th centile); BMI = 29.7 kg/m² (>99.6th centile)—obese category.

A "typical school day" history was obtained which demonstrated that the child missed breakfast before he left for school, and at the mid-morning break, he had an energy drink and a chocolate bar. At lunch time he usually had pizza slices and drank water. On the way home from school, he would have a packet of crisps.

He would enjoy the home-cooked evening meal and would sometimes go for a second helping. Alternatively, the family would order a takeaway meal some 2–3 times a week. After dinner he would often have chocolate biscuits or crisps while playing video games. He had physical education at school twice a week, his least favourite class, and he was a keen video game player.

This diary helped recognise that his diet was not healthy and that he did not undertake sufficient physical activity. Investigations showed that his blood sugars and HbA1c were normal. Education about obesity and how healthy lifestyle changes would benefit the whole family was provided to the patient and his parents. This included advice on reducing the amount of time spent on video games, increasing physical activity, reduction in number of takeaway meals eaten each week and the encouragement of choosing healthy snacks. Healthy food choices at school were discussed along with the option of a packed lunch for several days.

Vitamin, mineral and micronutrient deficiencies

Micronutrients are substances required in trace amounts for optimal growth and development and they are an essential part of our diet, as they cannot be synthesised in vivo. They are typically divided into minerals and vitamins

Table 6.3 **Common vitamins seen in disease. (The mnemonic FAKED can help in recalling the fat-soluble vitamins)**

Fat-soluble vitamins	Water-soluble vitamins
vitamin A	thiamine (B1)
vitamin D (Ch 25)	riboflavin (B2)
vitamin E	niacin (B3)
vitamin K	pantothenic acid
	vitamin B6
	vitamin B12
	folate
	vitamin C

Vitamins

These are classified as fat soluble or water soluble and they have a major role in maintaining normal physiological functions. Patients with conditions that result in fat malabsorption are at significant risk of developing fat-soluble deficiencies. Once deficiencies are diagnosed, they will require correction by supplementation, and the dose and route of administration should be obtained from approved sources (Table 6.3).

Vitamin A

Vitamin A and its retinol equivalents are essential for cellular differentiation, integrity and photo-transduction in the eye. Common rich dietary sources include offal (liver, kidney), egg yolks, butter, fortified margarines, carrots and sweet potato.

Vitamin A deficiency is one of the most common micronutrient deficiencies globally, and up to 30% of children under the age of 5 years are estimated to be affected. Children with disorders of fat malabsorption are also at an increased risk. Clinical deficiency typically presents with night blindness, and in severe disease, complete blindness and xerophthalmia. Clinical findings can be supported by low serum retinol levels.

Thiamine (vitamin B₁)

Thiamine plays an important role in energy metabolism and acts as a coenzyme in the conversion of pyruvate to acetyl coenzyme A in the first step in the citric acid cycle. It is also involved in nerve impulse propagation. Thiamine is predominantly found in beans, lentils, wholegrain foods and pork.

Thiamine deficiency in those under 18 years is commonly seen in diets that are very high in refined grains or with protein-energy malnutrition, particularly those at risk of refeeding syndrome. Children with certain metabolic disorders such as maple syrup urine disease usually need routine supplementation to prevent deficiency.

Clinically, the deficiency can present as beriberi in children or as Wernicke-Korsakoff syndrome in teenagers and adults. Beriberi is often seen in infants of thiamine-deficient, breastfeeding mothers and presents with symptoms of cardiomegaly, tachycardia and oedema. Severely deficient mothers should avoid breastfeeding due to high levels of toxic methyl-glyoxal present in their breast milk.

Riboflavin (vitamin B₂)

Riboflavin is a water-soluble vitamin that plays an essential role in coenzymes involved in energy and drug metabolism, cellular growth and differentiation. It is also involved in the metabolism of other B vitamins including niacin and vitamin B₆. It is found in a wide variety of foods including milk, cheese, yogurt, eggs, meat, fish, green vegetables, almonds and yeast.

Riboflavin deficiency is referred to as ariboflavinosis and can present with a sore throat, angular stomatitis, glossitis and normocytic, normochromic anaemia.

Niacin (vitamin B₃)

Niacin plays an important role in energy metabolism and the maintenance of neurological functions and skin integrity. Good dietary sources include meat, fish, eggs, fortified wheat flour, cereals and seeds.

Niacin deficiency results in pellagra, characterised by dermatitis, glossitis, vaginitis, and oesophagitis, diarrhoea and dementia, and if left untreated can result in death. With routine fortification of flour, bread and breakfast cereals, the condition is incredibly rare in the UK. It can be seen in eating disorders such as anorexia nervosa and in alcohol abuse.

Pantothenic acid (vitamin B₅)

Pantothenic acid is necessary for the production of coenzyme A. It is found in a wide variety of foods including eggs, milk, meat, poultry, potatoes and whole grains. It is also produced by colonic bacteria.

Pantothenic acid deficiency is incredibly rare, particularly in isolation of other micronutrient deficiencies. When deficiency does occur, it produces a 'burning feet syndrome' characterised by paraesthesia and dysesthesia.

Pyridoxine (vitamin B₆)

Vitamin B₆ includes pyridoxine, pyridoxamine, pyridoxal and other derivatives which are all essential for gluconeogenesis, immune function and the synthesis of amino acids, haem and neurotransmitters. Rich sources of vitamin B_6 are meat, poultry, eggs, fish, nuts and seeds.

Deficiency is common in certain metabolic disorders such as homocystinuria and as a side effect with some medications including isoniazid and penicillamine. Symptoms include nonspecific stomatitis, glossitis, seborrheic dermatitis, microcytic anaemia and seizures.

Folate (vitamin B_9, folic acid)

Folate plays a crucial role in DNA and RNA synthesis as well as erythropoiesis. It is commonly found in dark leafy vegetables and meat products and is routinely fortified in breakfast cereals.

Patients with malabsorption disorders such as coeliac disease and other conditions including chronic haemolytic anaemias and renal failure are at increased risk of deficiency. Some medications are also known to increase risk of folate deficiency and include methotrexate, trimethoprim and sodium valproate. Deficiency will also result in megaloblastic anaemia whilst deficiency during pregnancy can also increase the risk of neural tube defects.

Vitamin B_{12}

Vitamin B_{12} is required for the formation of hematopoietic cells as well as maintaining cerebral and neurological functions. It is found in meat, fish, eggs, milk products and fortified cereals.

Vitamin B_{12} is not found in fruit and vegetables and consequently those following a vegan diet and patients with malabsorption are at increased risk of deficiency. Prolonged deficiency of vitamin B_{12} will result in a megaloblastic anaemia and obvious lethargy and pallor. Other symptoms will include stomatitis and glossitis. If left untreated it can result in neurological and psychological changes including depression, confusion, numbness and visual changes.

Ascorbic acid (vitamin C)

Vitamin C is essential for collagen production, iron absorption and functioning as an antioxidant. It is found in a wide variety of fruit and vegetables, particularly citrus fruits, tomatoes, broccoli and red peppers.

Chronic severe deficiency can result in scurvy with petechial and perifollicular haemorrhaging, impaired wound healing and abnormal bone and dentine formation.

Vitamin E

Vitamin E works predominantly as an antioxidant, protecting polyunsaturated fatty acids in cellular membranes from peroxidation and plays a role in inhibiting cell proliferation and platelet aggregation. Rich dietary sources include plant oils, nuts, seeds and whole wheat products.

As with all fat-soluble vitamins, patients with fat malabsorption are at increased risk of deficiency and presents with neuromuscular and haemolytic disorders.

Vitamin K

Vitamin K is an essential cofactor for the synthesis of clotting factors and also plays a role in bone metabolism by influencing osteoblast function. It is commonly found in olive oil, green leafy vegetables and whole grains but can also be synthesised by colonic bacteria.

Vitamin K deficiency presents as bruising or bleeding from any mucosal or subcutaneous site. Intramuscular injections of vitamin K1 are routinely given to all newborn infants shortly following delivery, in order to prevent neonatal vitamin K deficiency bleeding. As with other fat-soluble vitamins, patients with fat malabsorption are at increased risk of deficiency.

Micronutrients
Zinc

Zinc is a component of various enzymes and helps maintain structural integrity of protein molecules. It is widely distributed in many foods, with meat, fish and poultry being the main sources, but fortified breakfast cereals, nuts, whole grains and milk products are also a significant source.

Those at risk of zinc deficiency include children following a vegan diet and infants who are exclusively breast fed with delayed introduction of solid food. Acrodermatitis enteropathica (Figure 6.2) is a recessively inherited condition with defective intestinal zinc absorption.

Moderate and severe deficiency can result in significant weight loss, dermatitis, alopecia and diarrhoea. As serum

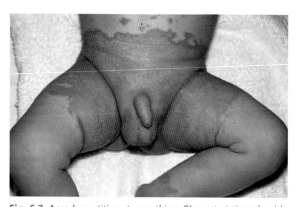

Fig. 6.2 Acrodermatitis enteropathica. Characteristic rash with well-demarcated borders. Alopecia usually present.

zinc levels are tightly regulated, mild deficiency cannot always be identified from plasma levels alone.

Iodine

This is an essential nutrient and is a major component of thyroxine and is found in seafoods and dairy products.

Individuals living in parts of the world with iodine poor soils may not have an adequate intake of iodine. Most resource-rich countries produce ionised table salt that provides supplemental iodine.

Deficiency will result in goitre which can be endemic in certain geographical areas.

IMPORTANT CLINICAL POINTS

Monitoring of growth

- measurement of growth is essential for health and developmental assessment
- use of correct chart for age and condition is essential
- interpreting measurements is vital for determining appropriate interventions

Faltering growth

- Focus should be on early detection and simple advice
- Referral on to specialist feeding services if problem persists or developmental feeding difficulties are identified
- Paediatric population is at higher risk of malnutrition and complications due to higher nutritional requirements of growth
- This is particularly important during infancy when growth and development are most rapid

Obesity

- common and preventable nutritional disorder linked with serious comorbidities

- BMI centile is measured for overweight and obesity
- BMI centile interpreted with caution as not a direct measure of adiposity
- multiple lifestyle strategies are needed to manage and treat childhood obesity

Micronutrients

- deficiency in those with feeding difficulties, metabolic and nutrition-related disorders
- deficiency in fat-soluble vitamins seen in those with conditions with fat malabsorption
- certain medications can also increase the risk of micronutrient deficiencies

Zinc deficiency

- acrodermatitis enteropathica presents in infants with chronic diarrhoea, dermatitis and alopecia

---

Further reading

Faltering growth: recognition and management of faltering growth in children NICE Clinical guideline [NG75]. Published September 2017. https://www.nice.org.uk/guidance/ng75

Obesity: identification, assessment and management NICE Clinical guideline [CG189]. Published September 2014. Accessed March 2021 https://www.nice.org.uk/guidance/cg189

Chapter 7

Behavioural medicine and mental health

Amy Taylor, Corinne de Sousa

After reading this chapter you should:
- be able to assess, diagnose and manage common emotional and behavioural problems
- know about the effects of physical diseases on behaviour and vice versa
- know and understand the presentation of conduct disorders and antisocial behaviour
- understand the role of Child and Adolescent Mental Health Services (CAMHS)
- be able to assess and diagnose important mental health problems
- be able to identify anxiety disorders, phobias, panic attacks, and obsessive-compulsive disorders

Behaviour is the way in which a person acts or conducts themselves, especially towards others. In general, we behave in certain ways for a reason, often to either gain an advantage or to guard against actions which may have an adverse effect. It is also important to consider any extrinsic factors that may affect an individual child and what the behaviour pattern might indicate about their lifestyle.

Common emotional and behavioural problems

Sleep Problems

It is well recognised that sleep is important in helping the overall quality of life and is thought to help lay down memories and filter what needs to be remembered. Lack of sleep affects concentration and attention and can therefore increase problems with behaviour.

Both settling to sleep and waking in the night are common problems seen throughout childhood. Parasomnias are behaviours that interrupt sleep and include nightmares and night terrors. These activities are most common in children under 5 and decrease in frequency over the following years. Children with neurodevelopmental problems and mental health difficulties are more likely to suffer sleeping difficulties.

The amount of sleep needed changes through childhood and adolescence. Babies will spend more of their time asleep than awake, usually waking for feeds but gradually increasing the periods of alertness between naps.

- 2-year-old will have nearly 12 hours sleep at night plus over an hour during the day
- 5-year-old needs 11 hours at night on average
- 9-year-old will have 10 hours
- 14-year-old will have 9 hours

It is normal for children to wake in the night for a few minutes, but those who experience difficulties with self-settling can find it difficult to go back to sleep when this occurs. The phases of sleep include periods of light, deep and REM sleep. Figure 7.1:

It is also important to consider the typical body clock for children and young people of different ages. Adolescents often do not feel tired until late in the evening and will choose to sleep into the later morning whilst some young children will wake early.

Some medical problems can present with sleeping difficulties.

Obstructive sleep apnoea and sleep disordered breathing will produce loud and excessive snoring in the child along with periods of apnoea. The snoring might wake the child or other family members and so draw the attention of the parents to the problem. A sleep study can help to determine oxygen saturations overnight and determine if the breathing appears disordered; in such situations, a referral to a respiratory physician or ENT surgeon can be helpful. Treatment will usually depend on the cause but can include treatment of comorbidities such as obesity, adenotonsillectomy and even noninvasive ventilation.

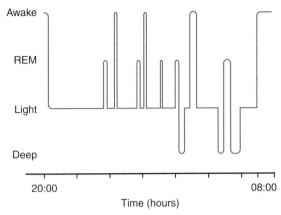

Fig. 7.1 Diagram of normal sleep architecture in an 8-year-old boy

Pain can be a recognised cause of interrupted sleep and underlying causes should be sought.

Restless leg syndrome is linked to iron deficiency.

Narcolepsy is a rare neurological condition characterised by excessive daytime somnolence and can be associated with cataplexy (drop attacks on laughing and suddenly fall to sleep). Diagnosis of narcolepsy is made with a multilatency sleep test and possibly a lumbar puncture to look at the level of orexin (a neuropeptide that regulates awakened state) in CSF.

Smith-Klein-Levin syndrome is a genetic neurological disorder and describes a child who falls asleep for prolonged periods. Like narcolepsy, the condition needs careful management by a specialist team.

Up to 30% of healthy children have problems with bedtime or nighttime waking at some point in their childhood and problems are usually related to:

- bedtime resistance or refusal
- delayed sleep onset
- prolonged night awakenings

Important factors in the child that may impact on patterns of sleep include neurodevelopmental disorders and anxiety. There are also environmental factors to consider such as a shared bedroom, parents working long hours, domestic violence or parental mental health problems.

Bedtime resistance or refusal

Children often refuse or resist going to bed and there can be many distractions in the family home which can contribute to this effect. Helping to minimise these and build a good bedtime routine are therefore helpful. A routine with three or four soothing activities is advised and should not involve screens, TV or electronic devices as these can inhibit melatonin production due to the emitted blue light.

Allowing a young child to cry themselves to sleep—controlled crying—can work for some whilst a gradual withdrawal from the room by the carer can help others. Gradual withdrawal is useful for those children who need the parent in the same room to fall to sleep. Older children who are anxious about falling to sleep may benefit from support to address the anxiety.

Delayed sleep onset

This is common in children with neurodevelopmental conditions such as autism spectrum disorder or ADHD. Some children do not feel tired until later in the night and implementing a planned 'bedtime fading' has been shown to be beneficial. This involves moving the bedtime to a time the child would naturally fall asleep and then bring it forwards by 15–20 minutes every few nights. For older children, the advice of using the bedroom as a place to sleep, rather than to relax, chat to friends and play games can also help.

Nightmares and night terrors

Nightmares and night terrors are common in children between the ages of 3 and 9 years. A nightmare is a vivid dream, and the child wakes and seeks reassurance from a caregiver. That is in contrast to a night terror, where the parent finds the child in a distressed, agitated state and yet may still appear to be asleep. Reassurance by the caregiver is usually the only course of action needed although anticipatory scheduled waking may help children with recurrent night terrors as they often occur at the same time each night.

Delayed sleep-wake cycle disorder

Adolescents and young adults can have a circadian rhythm that lasts more than 24 hours and so leads to a shift in their sleep-wake cycle and can impact on school attendance or other activities.

Relevant pharmacological agents used

Occasionally, when all sleep hygiene strategies have been tried, children with neurodevelopmental conditions or significant anxiety can be given a trial of melatonin. This has been found to be effective in helping reduce sleep latency (time taken to fall asleep) and can increase total duration of sleep by approximately 30 minutes. It should only be used in the short term, although those with neurodevelopmental conditions may need it for much longer. There are no long-term studies looking at its efficacy or safety.

Historically, children with neurodisability have also been prescribed chloral hydrate and sedating antihistamines such as promethazine. These are seen as less favourable options as they can cause adverse 'hangover' effects and so increase behavioural problems in the daytime.

Feeding difficulties

Food is an emotive subject and all parents are concerned when their child has difficulties with eating. There can be a number of different reasons for children presenting with feeding problems:

- pain or discomfort related to eating as with gastro-oesophageal reflux or respiratory conditions
- sensory processing difficulties result in certain tastes, textures and smells being overwhelming. This can often result in the child only eating a limited number of foods that they recognise and will accept
- negative feeding experiences (severe choking or reflux) that have led to anxiety about eating
- developmental stage—many toddlers go through a phase of fussy eating and this generally improves with time
- chronic medical conditions (malignancy, iron deficiency) may make eating unpleasant
  Management includes:
- ensuring that the child sits at a table to eat in an appropriate seat and is offered the same meal as the rest of the family
- ensuring that the child's growth follows the expected centile and referring to a dietician if needed
- ensuring that reflux medication is optimised
- encouraging the child to play with food
- offering the same food on many occasions
- referral to a speech and language therapist to help with oral desensitisation

Avoidant and Restrictive Feeding Intake Disorder (ARFID)

ARFID is a recognised feeding disorder and is diagnosed when there is an eating or feeding disturbance such as:

- lack of interest in eating or food
- avoidance of food due to the sensory characteristics of food
- concern about aversive consequences of eating

It can cause significant nutritional deficiency and weight loss such that some children require enteral feeding via an NG or PEG tube. The feeding disturbance is also not explained by a medical condition, lack of available food or concerns about body image.

People with an autism spectrum disorder, sensory processing difficulties and those who have suffered negative feeding experiences such as severe, painful gastro-oesophageal reflux, are all at risk of developing ARFID.

The condition is often linked to anxiety, indicating that such children are more at risk of other psychiatric disorders and they do not outgrow the typical 'picky' eating phase that occurs during early childhood.

ARFID is usually managed by a multidisciplinary team consisting of a combination of a paediatrician, speech and language therapist, occupational therapist, dietician and psychologist with advice given about trying to encourage feeding and improving a child's repertoire of foods.

Pica

The history of a child seeking out and eating soil, paint, soap or other items without any nutritional value will raise concerns in parents and carers and suggest a diagnosis of pica. Such activity can be seen in children with intellectual disability but can also be seen in elemental deficiency such as iron or zinc. Further assessment and possible investigations will usually be needed.

Behavioural manifestations in physical disease

Children show many behavioural manifestations of physical disease and they can often feel anxious when they are unwell. Anxiety can manifest as physical symptoms such as tachycardia, feeling faint, 'butterflies in the stomach', but it can also manifest as aggressive or violent behaviour.

It is also important to remember that diseases or treatment that affects the brain can cause problems with behaviour and examples include:

- children with brain tumours can present with personality changes and may appear as angry, aggressive or uncooperative.
- thyroid disorders can mimic psychiatric conditions; for example, those with hypothyroidism may present as depressed and lethargic whilst those with hyperthyroidism could be agitated and hyperactive.
- anti-epileptic drugs such as sodium valproate and levetiracetam can cause behavioural side effects.

Impact of chronic disease

There is a massive and complex interplay between physical and mental health and this is certainly the case when a child and family are facing the implications of living with a lifelong condition. Psychological support for children with any chronic illness is very important in helping to manage the situation and will improve their outcome.

CLINICAL SCENARIO

A 14-year-old girl was recently diagnosed with type 1 diabetes and was under the care of the Diabetic Team at the local hospital. She had been progressing well at school and was described as 'popular' with a close group of friends. Following the diagnosis, she became withdrawn and prone to outburst of temper.

A meeting with a team psychologist was able to identify the issues of concern to the girl and these included:

- initial response to diagnosis by child and family was one of upset and distress
- recognition and realisation that this was a disease that she would have for the rest of her life and this led to a grief reaction for the life she may not have
- the need for daily injections, treatment and pumps had a physical and psychological impact on her
- she described feelings of rebelliousness, unfairness, difference to peers and asking 'why me?', 'I didn't ask for this'.
- she expressed feelings of denial at becoming unwell suggesting 'it won't happen to me'
- the need to take responsibility for her condition rather than it resting with her parents led to family disputes
- the resentment that the illness occurred at the time she was developing her own independence

Once these issues were identified and discussed, it was possible to introduce measures which may help.

Somatic symptom disorders

Disorders where there are somatic symptoms include:

- somatic symptom disorder
- illness anxiety disorder
- conversion disorder (functional neurological symptom disorder)
- fabricated or induced illness by carers

In these conditions medical pathology is absent or, if present, the symptoms are unexplained or over-exaggerated and cause distress and impairment. These disorders are uncommon but they can cause significant demand on healthcare resources.

Somatic symptom disorder

Young people present with somatic symptoms that consistently disrupt daily life and spend a significant amount of time thinking about these symptoms or health concerns.

Illness anxiety disorder

The individual does not have somatic symptoms or, if present, are only mild in intensity, but the young person has a high level of anxiety about health and undertakes excessive health-related behaviours such as repeated body checks. They are preoccupied with the notion that they will develop a serious illness.

The main difference between a somatic symptom disorder and illness anxiety disorder is that the distress that occurs in an illness anxiety disorder is not from the physical symptoms but instead from the anxiety around illness itself.

Conversion disorder (functional neurological symptom disorder)

This describes presentations in children and young people where there are symptoms of altered voluntary motor or sensory function which are unexplained by recognised neurological or medical conditions. Physical examination and investigations are normal. The symptoms cause clinically significant distress or impairment in important areas of everyday life and comorbidities with anxiety and depression are common. Young people affected by this condition are often highly functioning individuals and the psychological trigger may be subconscious. Treatment is focussed on reassurance, support and explanation and it is important for the patient to understand that the symptoms they are experiencing are real.

Antisocial behaviour and conduct disorder

Aggressive and defiant behaviours are part of normal childhood and growing up and, in particular, teenagers are often defiant as they question boundaries set by their parents and find their own ideas developing.

Conduct disorders

These are characterised by:

- repetitive and persistent patterns of antisocial, aggressive or defiant behaviour
- behaviour that amounts to significant violations to everyday social expectations

Such conduct problems are relatively common and the number of children and young people demonstrating problems with antisocial behaviour increases into adolescence.

Conduct disorders are seen more commonly in those who are looked after, have been abused, are on a child protection plan or have ADHD.

Characteristic features of conduct disorders include:

- aggression to people and animals—lies, initiates fights, cruelty to others and to animals
- deliberate destruction of property—destroys the property of others, starts fires

- deceitfulness or theft—steals, burglary, shoplifting
- serious violations of the rules—truanting, runs away from home, bullies others

These behaviours are not simply 'one-offs' but must have been occurring consistently for at least 6 months.

Risk factors for developing a conduct disorder include:
- local community ('difficult' neighbourhoods)
- influence from friends
- physical abuse
- witness to domestic violence
- attachment difficulties
- intellectual disability and learning difficulties
- family disadvantage
- negative, harsh, inconsistent parenting style

Oppositional defiant disorder

This is a milder form of a conduct disorder and is usually seen in children younger than 11 years of age. It is characterised by:
- severe or frequent temper tantrums inappropriate for age
- doing things deliberately to annoy other people
- blaming others for own mistakes or misbehaviour
- being angry or resentful
- defiant and actively refuses to comply with the rules or adults' requests

Treatment and management

Parenting programmes and multisystemic therapy are the main forms of management and pharmacological treatments are not routinely used.

Challenging behaviour in children with intellectual disability

When considering a child with intellectual disability it is important to consider their developmental age rather than their chronological age when considering whether a particular behaviour may be 'normal'. Toddler-type tantrums may be expected and understandable in a child with severe autism who is 8 years of age but whose development is around age 2–3 years.

Some children with an intellectual disability may demonstrate significant challenging behaviour as a way of communicating their anxiety or distress. Some do not have verbal skills and are unable to use typical methods of communication. In these situations, it is very important to consider how a child communicates and what triggers unwanted behaviours. These behaviours can then be managed by avoiding triggers and using communication strategies that the child might be familiar with, such as images and symbols. When some children are feeling very distressed, they may communicate this by harming themselves or others people.

Many CAMHS services have a dedicated Intellectual Disability service whose members are able to offer specialist help and expertise in unpicking challenging behaviour with families and offering strategies to help.

It is uncommon to prescribe medication to help reduce challenging behaviour and this should only be done by specialists with expertise in intellectual disability and in conjunction with behavioural strategies.

Child and adolescent mental health services (CAMHS)

The structure and organisation of CAMH services varies widely across the UK and services are generally dependent upon the local commissioning arrangements in each area. This may generate issues if a young person should transfer from one area to another and they find that the way services are arranged is significantly different.

It is necessary, therefore, to be familiar with the local arrangements and in particular:
- service structures
- service organisation
- referral processes
- referral criteria
- interface between paediatric and mental health services

Assessment of mental health concerns recognises that changes in mood states or behaviours can affect everyone including young people although they may be more evident in this group as they pass through puberty and adolescence and mature. Any assessment should therefore consider whether these changes are:
- developmentally appropriate
- associated with impairment or distress
- adversely affecting daily functioning and activities

It is developmentally appropriate for a young person aged 15 years to become less communicative and want to spend time alone and away from family, even if their previous relationship with family was very close. This would not necessarily be indicative of a depressive disorder.

It is developmentally appropriate for toddlers to exhibit separation anxiety and for teenagers to encounter social anxiety and neither would be indicative of anxiety disorders unless they adversely impact on daily functioning.

Mental health conditions

Depressive disorder

The prevalence of depressive disorder increases from childhood to adolescence. It is equally common in girls and boys during childhood, but during adolescence the number of females affected is about twice the number of males. The aetiology of depressive disorder is multifactorial and potential risk factors are known as 'the 3 Ps':

- predisposing factors—genetic factors, early adversity
- precipitating factors—stressful life events
- perpetuating factors—continuing family dysfunction

Clinical presentation

- mood changes—low mood, irritability
- loss of enjoyment and interest in usual activities
- cognitive features—guilt, hopelessness, difficult concentrating, loss of confidence, suicidal thoughts
- biological features—changes in appetite, sleep disturbance, fatigue, loss of libido
- behavioural features—withdrawal, isolation, self-harm
- functional impairment—this may be seen at home, in school or with peers

Initial assessment will usually focus on mood changes but should also consider the features shown above and include current difficulties and any risk of self-harm.

Differential and comorbid diagnoses

Psychiatric comorbidity is common especially with anxiety disorders, conduct disorders and substance misuse whilst those with physical health disorders, particularly those that are long term or chronic (e.g., diabetes, epilepsy), may also develop clinical depression.

Treatment and management

Alongside treatment of a depressive episode, any comorbid psychiatric conditions may require specific interventions. A holistic approach to treatment will also aim to address problems in family relationships, school or with peers. The NICE guideline on depression in children and young people, recommends an initial 2-week period of 'watchful waiting' and, if symptoms fail to resolve or worsen, then referral to mental health services should be initiated.

Mild to moderate depression should initially be managed with psychological treatments. Cognitive behavioural therapy (CBT) is used to aid understanding of the issues, address behavioural issues and promote reassurance. Interpersonal psychotherapy is used to addresses problem relationship areas such as role conflicts, transitions or losses.

Relevant pharmacological agents used

Moderate to severe depression will most likely require treatment with antidepressant medication and input from specialist mental health services. Selective serotonin reuptake inhibitors (SSRIs), especially fluoxetine, are helpful for those in the adolescent age group. Close monitoring is necessary due to the slightly increased risk of suicidal events with SSRIs. Poor progress or a high risk of self-harm may signal the need for psychiatric admission.

Bipolar disorder

Bipolar disorder with an onset before the age of 18 years is a serious mood disorder and is regarded as an episodic illness with distinct periods (days to weeks) of mania or hypomania, depression and euthymia (normal mood state) (Figure 7.2). It can be a debilitating condition and is often associated with considerable functional impairment and suicidality.

Mania and hypomania are essentially defined by irritability or an abnormally elevated mood. The distinction between them is dependent on symptom severity and length of episode, with mania manifesting severe functional impairments or psychotic symptoms.

Peak onset for bipolar disorder is the 15- to 19-year-old age group, with males and females equally represented. The initial presentation is commonly depression with around 20% to 30% of depressed young people, particularly those with psychosis or a family history of bipolar disorder, eventually developing the condition.

Clinical presentation

- excitability, irritability or elevated mood
- inflated sense of self or grandiosity
- intensified speech—loud, rapid, difficult to interrupt, nonstop
- poor concentration, distractibility
- overfamiliarity, disinhibition or reckless behaviour
- overactivity, pacing, inability to sit still (psychomotor agitation)
- rapid jumping around of ideas, racing thoughts ('flight of ideas')
- excessive creativity

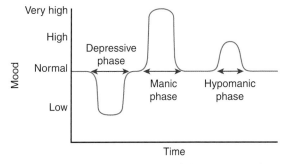

Fig. 7.2 Diagrammatic representation of changes in mood in bipolar disease

- unusual clothing choices (bright colours, inappropriate for season)
- psychotic symptoms

Differential and comorbid diagnoses

Bipolar disorder is particularly difficult to diagnose in children and young people because of the nature of its presentation and complex comorbidities including anxiety disorders, substance misuse, personality disorders and attention deficit hyperactivity disorder (ADHD).

Treatment and management

If bipolar disorder is suspected, referral to specialist mental health services would be indicated for treatment of the acute episode of mania or depression and then longer-term prophylaxis. Psychological treatments such as family psychoeducation are beneficial. However, pharmacotherapy is the main treatment for acute mania with aripiprazole recommended as a first line treatment. Second generation antipsychotics such as risperidone, quetiapine and olanzapine are increasingly used as mood stabilisers in the treatment of bipolar disorder. They may also be used along with lithium as longer term treatments.

Early onset psychosis and schizophrenia

Psychosis can essentially be defined as a loss of contact with reality and can be described by signs and symptoms that include:

- **Delusions**—falsely held beliefs, including paranoia and grandiosity
- **Hallucinations**—perceptions in the absence of a stimulus—including auditory and visual

  Simple auditory hallucinations are the most frequent symptom in young people whilst delusions, which occur less frequently, are usually thematically related to childhood experiences. A young person experiencing psychotic symptoms may go on to be subsequently diagnosed with schizophrenia.

Clinical presentation

The onset of schizophrenia in young people is usually insidious and, in hindsight, issues are evident in childhood. Typical features of schizophrenia include:

- disorganised thinking and speech with bizarre or unusual behaviour
- mood changes—sense of fear, making familiar places and people seem unfamiliar
- distortion of normal functioning—hallucinations, delusions, paranoia

- reduction of normal functioning—poverty of thought and speech, social withdrawal and self-neglect, emotional apathy

Treatment and management

A referral to a specialist mental health service should be made urgently when a young person experiences transient or attenuated psychotic symptoms or other experiences suggestive of possible psychosis. Treatment options for children and young people with first episode psychosis are oral antipsychotic medication in conjunction with psychological interventions (family intervention with individual CBT).

CLINICAL SCENARIO

A 16-year-old boy with quadriplegic cerebral palsy and intellectual disability was reviewed after his mental health deteriorated following neurosurgery to remove an intrathecal baclofen pump. He had had no previous psychiatric illnesses.

Following the surgery, his mother had noticed marked changes in his behaviour. He became suspicious and paranoid and was exhibiting bizarre speech. He appeared to be responding to unseen stimuli and experiencing auditory and visual hallucinations. This presentation was initially thought to be related to baclofen withdrawal but his symptoms continued after returning home. He displayed episodes of anxiety, agitation and aggression towards his mother. There were associated difficulties with sleep and mood.

It was felt that he was exhibiting signs and symptoms of psychosis and so antipsychotic treatment was started—a gradually increasing dose of aripiprazole along with a short course of diazepam to help with agitation. His symptoms slowly resolved and his behaviour became calmer, with no further episodes of bizarre speech. His sleep pattern and mood improved and he regained interest in his usual activities.

After remaining stable for one year, gradual withdrawal of aripiprazole was attempted. Unfortunately, his symptoms returned (suspicious and paranoid behaviours, alterations in sleep pattern and mood) and consequently his medication was reinstated. He remains well on low-dose aripiprazole.

Anxiety disorders

Anxiety is an unpleasant feeling of apprehension accompanied by physiological, cognitive and behavioural responses and is a normal human experience which aims to protect us from potential sources of danger. Anxiety disorders occur when this useful response becomes mal-adaptive and is triggered by a non-threatening stimulus (e.g., earthworms) or the response occurs in a manner that is disproportionate to the presenting threat (e.g., fear of flying).

Most anxiety disorders have a relatively early age of onset with symptoms that have often started in childhood or adolescence. Anxiety disorders in children and young people commonly run a chronic course and are associated with an increased risk of other serious mental health problems.

Clinical presentation

Physical symptoms include racing heart, tight chest, rapid breathing, nausea or vomiting, shaking, dry mouth, headaches, sweating, pins and needles and muscle pains. Psychological symptoms which are recognised are pacing, restlessness, constant worrying, irritability, difficulty concentrating, tiredness, sleep difficulties and low mood.

Anxiety disorders can be differentiated according to the feared situation or the pattern of anxiety seen.

Separation anxiety disorder

Excessive and developmentally inappropriate anxiety relating to separation from caregivers or worrying about the welfare of caregivers. This may result in school refusal.

Generalised anxiety disorder

Excessive worry about a number of different events, associated with heightened tension that tends to be generalised and persistent and not restricted to any particular situation. This 'free floating' anxiety is hard to control and usually accompanied by physical symptoms.

Social anxiety disorder

This is characterised by a marked and persistent fear of humiliation or embarrassment. This results in anxiety about social situations that involve interaction, observation and performance and may lead to avoidance behaviours resulting in social isolation.

Panic disorder

Recurrent and unexpected attacks of severe anxiety accompanied by physical symptoms that are unrelated to any particular situation are described as "panic attacks". During these discrete episodes, the young person may experience an intense fear of losing control or dying which leads them to avoid certain situations or places if they believe this would induce the panic attacks.

Specific or simple phobias

Excessive fears of discernible, circumscribed objects or situations that provoke an immediate anxiety response. These objects or situations are either avoided or tolerated with great discomfort. They can be grouped into animal, situational, nature or environment (e.g., water, heights).

Agoraphobia

These are an often overlapping cluster of phobias relating to crowds, public places, leaving home or travelling alone. Persistent avoidance behaviour may limit anxiety but result in isolation and impaired functioning.

Post-traumatic stress disorder

This can develop after experiencing a stressful event or situation of an exceptionally threatening or catastrophic nature that is likely to cause pervasive distress in almost anyone. In more recent times, such events have been most often experienced by young people who have come to the UK as refugees or asylum seekers.

Differential and comorbid diagnoses

Anxiety disorders are one of the most prevalent psychiatric conditions in young people so comorbidity with other psychiatric disorders is high. Making an early diagnosis is important as anxiety disorders can increase the risk of depression and substance misuse, but they often remain unrecognised and therefore untreated.

Assessment involves evaluating the aetiological factors and the resulting distress and impairment. Obtaining information from the young person, their family and their school can be helpful in ascertaining whether the anxiety displayed is developmentally appropriate.

Treatment and management

Initial treatment options are psychoeducation (to aid understanding and promote reassurance) and self-help strategies. These include information about relaxation techniques, breathing exercises and mindfulness but if this approach fails, then cognitive behavioural therapy or medication may be indicated.

Relevant pharmacological agents used

SSRIs can be effective and generally well-tolerated treatments for most of the anxiety disorders but may not always be indicated. Some clinical guidelines advise against offering pharmacological interventions and therefore advice from mental health services should be sought when considering such treatment for young people. Potential side effects of SSRIs include sedation, insomnia, agitation, abdominal discomfort and headaches whilst suicidal behaviour is an uncommon side-effect. Benzodiazepines are generally not recommended in young people as they have failed to demonstrate efficacy whilst behavioural disinhibition and dependency are risks. There is little paediatric data on beta blockers.

Obsessive compulsive disorders (OCD)

Many successful individuals have thoughts and behaviours that they manage effectively and which benefit, rather than hinder, their lives. This is sometimes considered 'perfectionism' and can be a valued attribute in many workplaces. If obsessions or rituals begin to adversely impact on the daily functioning of the individual, then it could be considered that they have an obsessive compulsive disorder.

Clinical presentation

OCD is characterised by the presence of obsessions or compulsions.
- obsessions—intrusive, repetitive and distressing thoughts, images, doubts or urges
  - contamination, symmetry, harm coming to others
- compulsions—repetitive, stereotyped and unnecessary behaviours or rituals
  - washing, cleaning, checking, repeating, ordering, reassurance-seeking

Young people with OCD usually have both obsessions and compulsions and sometimes there may be an obvious link between the two such as fears about germs and hand washing behaviour. In some instances, the young person may not be able to articulate the obsessions clearly but just 'feels bad' if they do not complete the rituals. Occasionally there are secondary consequences of compulsions, such as food avoidance (due to contamination fears) leading to restricted dietary intake, weight loss and nutritional concerns.

It should also be recognised that obsessions can be highly distressing and the young person may not recognise them as their own thoughts, describing them instead as 'voices'. These would then obviously need to be distinguished from psychotic phenomenon.

Treatment and management

Initial treatment options are psychoeducation and self-help strategies both for the young person and their family. Treatment must always involve family members in order to prevent 'accommodation', in which family members do not impede the ritualistic behaviour and may actually reinforce the behaviour. If symptoms remain after psychoeducation and self-help, then cognitive behavioural therapy incorporating exposure and response prevention could be offered. This involves facing up to the feared stimulus and resisting the urge to carry out a ritual in these circumstances.

Relevant pharmacological agents used

SSRIs have been shown to have a role in management and can be introduced if CBT proves to have had a limited effect. Full therapeutic effects may not be apparent for 8–12 weeks so waiting for a response is advised, as increasing the dose too quickly raises the risk of potential of side effects.

IMPORTANT CLINICAL POINTS

Sleep disorders
- obstructive sleep apnoea
  - produce excessive snoring and periods of apnoea
- narcolepsy
  - characterised by excessive daytime somnolence
  - associated with cataplexy
  - confirmed by a multilatency sleep test
- nightmare
  - vivid dream—child wakes and seeks reassurance
  - night terror—child distressed, agitated state and may appear to be asleep

Antisocial behaviour and conduct disorder
- somatic symptom disorder presents with symptoms that disrupt daily life
- illness anxiety disorder presents with minimal somatic symptoms but a high level of anxiety about health
- conduct disorders—aggressive actions towards people, animals and property
- oppositional defiant disorder—mild conduct disorder in children younger than 11 years of age

Mental health conditions
- mild to moderate depression should initially be managed with psychological treatments
- delusions are falsely held beliefs, including paranoia and grandiosity
- hallucinations are perceptions in the absence of a stimulus—including auditory and visual
- obsessions—intrusive, repetitive and distressing thoughts, images, doubts or urges
- compulsions—repetitive, stereotyped and unnecessary behaviours or rituals

Further reading

Depression in children and young people: identification and management NICE guideline [NG134]. Published 2019. Accessed 2021. https://www.nice.org.uk/guidance/ng134.

Bipolar Disorder: The Assessment and Management NICE Clinical Guideline [CG185]. Published 2014. Revised 2020. Accessed 2021. https://www.nice.org.uk/guidance/cg185.

Antisocial behaviour and conduct disorders: recognition and management NICE Clinical guideline [CG158]. Published 2013. Revised 2017. Accessed 2021. https://www.nice.org.uk/guidance/cg158.

Chapter | 8 |

Emergency medicine

Co-ordinators: *Colin Powell; Ibtihal Abdelgadir*

Authors: *Sohail Ghani, Sudhakar Adusumilli, Muthukumar Sakthivel, Roona Aniapravan*

After reading this chapter you should be able to assess diagnose and manage:
- cardiac arrest
- shock
- anaphylaxis and acute upper airways obstruction
- acute seizures
- acute neurological emergencies

Children and young people frequently present to emergency departments with overwhelming and life-threatening acute conditions. Prompt assessment and management is crucial and requires the coordinated effort of skilled paediatric practitioners.

Basic life support

When any vulnerable children (premature infants or children with life threatening chronic illness) are discharged home; the parents should be taught about basic life support (BLS) techniques. The majority of paediatric cardiac arrests out of hospital or even within the hospital are due to respiratory failure, and therefore, early recognition and management of the airway and breathing are extremely important. The provision of basic life support, even by a single rescuer, can support the vital respiratory and circulatory systems until definitive help and expertise arrive.

Initial assessment of a collapsed or unconscious child

The steps in BLS have been designed to help teach the parents and carers about the early recognition of an unresponsive child and describe the sequence as:

Safe environment—ensuring that it is safe to approach the child and that there is no risk to the rescuer is crucial in the first instance. The child should be moved to a nearest place of safety such as being removed from a bath or leaving a building where there is fire.

Stimulate—stimulating the child or infant and looking for a response and, if there is no response, help should be summoned. Stimulation can be by shouting or tapping the shoulders. Tapping the feet of infants is appropriate but shaking the baby must not be undertaken.

Check airway and breathing—ensuring that the airway is open and patent and whether there is any breathing effort over a period of 10 seconds should next be undertaken. The airway can be opened by gently tilting the head backwards and the chin lifted to check the mouth for any apparent obstruction. Any obvious foreign bodies should be removed but the fingers should not be pushed deep in the mouth.

Circulation—the initial response includes five rescue breaths followed by 30 chest compressions. After the first cycle, the airway should be rechecked and two more breaths given before continuing the 2:30 cycle, although if there are two rescuers, the cycle should be 2:15. This should be continued until help arrives or child shows signs of life ,and once the child is breathing, they can then be placed in the recovery position to facilitate any fluids or vomitus draining easily out of the mouth and airway. The recovery position should be maintained and the child should not be allowed to accidentally roll back to their back.

Choking child—supporting a choking child with simple techniques could save them from going into cardiorespiratory arrest, although the technique used depends on whether there is breathing effort or the child is unresponsive.

When a cough and breathing effort are present, the child should be supported and encouraged to cough up and bring out the foreign object blocking the airway. If the cough or the breathing effort is poor or absent, an urgent response is required to help push out or cough up the foreign object. Depending upon the age of the child, different techniques could be used.

In the child who is less than 1 year old, chest thrusts are advisable as abdominal thrusts can cause damage to abdominal organs. The infant is held on the knee with the head down and five back blows are given to the thoracic area. The child is then turned to face the rescuer and, still on the knee with head down, five thrusts are given to the sternum. The cycle of five blows and five thrusts is continued until the foreign object is dislodged, but if the child is not responding then CPR should be commenced.

In the child above 1 year, it is safe and more useful to apply abdominal thrusts. The child is held in standing position and five firm back blows to the middle of their back are given followed by five abdominal thrusts which are sharp and aimed upwards towards diaphragm. As long as the child is responsive, this cycle can be continued until the foreign object is expelled. If the child becomes unresponsive, then CPR should be started and help sought.

Paediatric cardiac arrest

Primary respiratory failure is the most common cause of cardiac arrest in the paediatric population, whereas in adults cardiac causes are more common. However, the terminal event seen in children is mainly due to arrhythmias including ventricular fibrillation or pulseless ventricular tachycardia. The cardiorespiratory arrest in children has poor prognosis

Table 8.1 Reversible causes of cardiac arrest

4 Hs	4 Ts
Hypoxia	Tension pneumothorax
Hypovolaemia	Tamponade (cardiac)
Hypothermia	Toxins
Hyperkalaemia	Thromboembolic phenomenon

Treatment and management

The APLS guidelines are taught to all trainees and can be summarised in the algorithm produced by the Resuscitation Council UK (Figure 8.1).

The key to management of cardiac arrest is its early recognition and call for help followed by systematic assessment (ABCDE). The immediate evaluation should be focused on identification and treatment of reversible causes along with assessment of cardiac rate and rhythm (Table 8.1).

The interventions are undertaken at every step of the ABCDE assessment, and each step of the management is not started until the preceding abnormality has been addressed, although there are some exceptions such as massive haemorrhage. In this situation, management of the circulatory problem is undertaken alongside assessment and management of airway and breathing.

Parental presence during cardiac resuscitation is known to be important and a dedicated member of the team should be allocated to support them and explain events taking place. The decision to stop resuscitation is made by the lead clinician when there is no spontaneous return of circulation after 30 minutes of effective resuscitation although children with primary hypothermia or those with poison ingestion may require longer periods of support.

Shock

Shock is an acute process in which the body is unable to deliver adequate oxygen to the vital organs and tissues to meet up their normal metabolic demands. As a result, the normal aerobic metabolism at cellular level is switched to anaerobic metabolism which is less effective. The poor tissue oxygenation will trigger multiple compensatory mechanisms in the body to preserve oxygenation to vital organs and this is manifested by poor capillary refill time seen especially in neonates and young children.

These compensatory mechanisms are initially very effective, hence the name *compensated shock*, during which time the blood pressure is maintained. The mortality rates in paediatric and neonatal shock, especially septic shock, are about 3% in healthy children and up to 9% in children with underlying chronic medical problems.

If the shock is not recognised and managed promptly, vital organs are further deprived of oxygen leading to metabolic and lactic acidosis. Early recognition and management of shock on presentation is vital to prevent the potentially rapid and irreversible or *uncompensated shock* that leads to multiorgan failure and death. Hypotension is a late sign of shock especially in the paediatric population.

Shock can be generally classified into five major types:
- **hypovolemic shock** is the most common type of shock seen in the paediatric population globally and is frequently caused by fluid losses through diarrhoea, vomiting or haemorrhage
- **cardiogenic shock** could be due to congenital or acquired heart diseases including myocarditis, cardiomyopathies and structural cardiac defects (pre- or postoperative)
- **distributive shock** occurs due to loss of vasomotor tone as seen in anaphylaxis, burns, acute spinal cord or brainstem injuries and ingestion of certain drugs

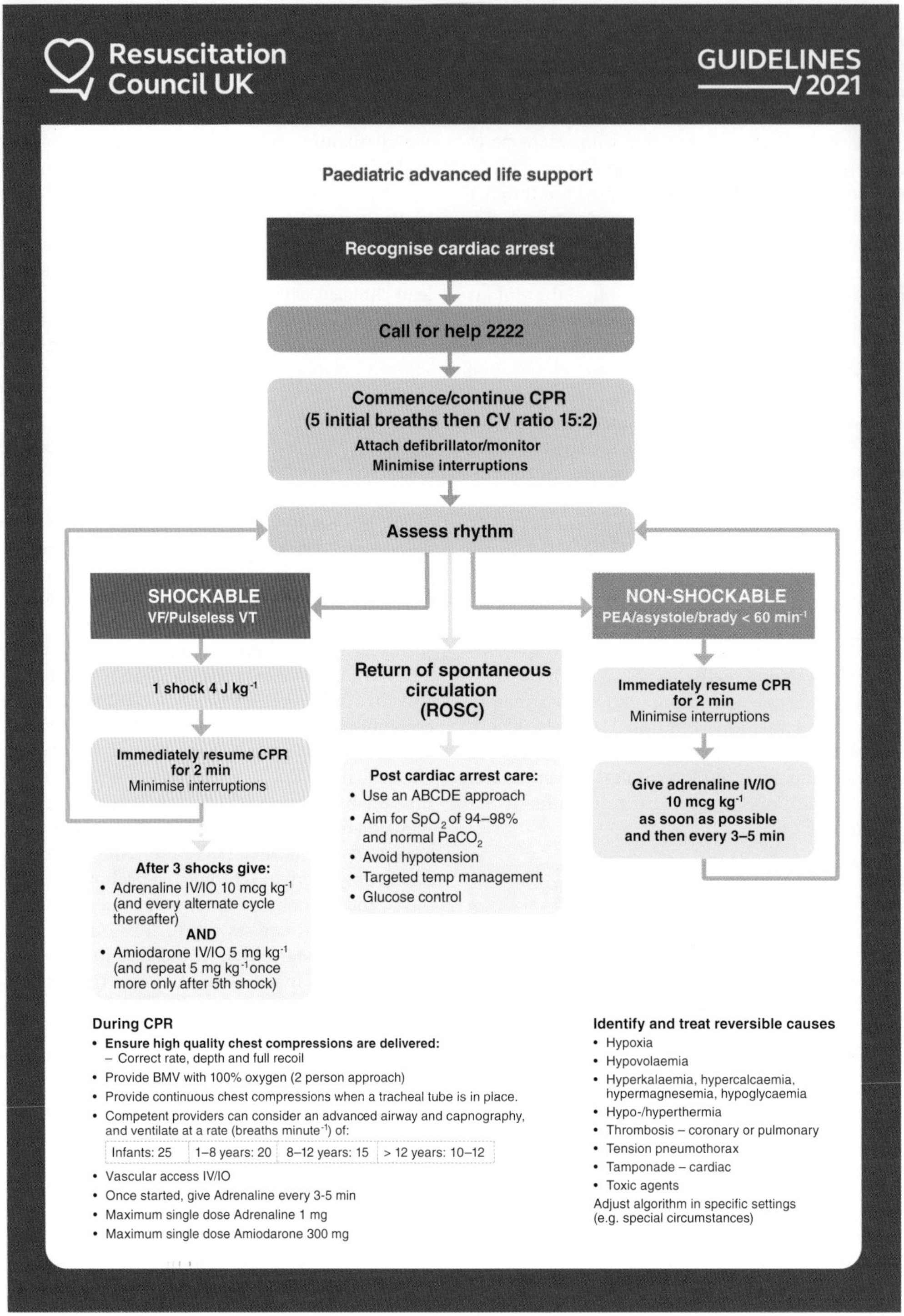

Fig. 8.1 Paediatric Advanced Life Support algorithm. (Reproduced with permission from the Resuscitation Council UK 2021)

- **obstructive shock** occurs due to obstruction to normal cardiac output as seen with tension pneumothorax, cardiac tamponade or pulmonary embolism
- **septic shock** is usually due to a combination of multiple types of shocks especially hypovolemic, distributive and cardiogenic. It could be caused by viral, bacterial or fungal infections and immunocompromised patients are at a particular risk of fulminant sepsis

Table 8.2 Important signs of different types of shock.	
type of shock	**Signs**
Hypovolaemic	dry mucous membranes, poor skin turgor, cool peripheries, delayed capillary refill time, poor volume pulses
Cardiogenic	tachypnoea, poor peripheral perfusion, gallop rhythm, hepatomegaly, reduced urine output, altering mental status
Distributive	increased cardiac output but ineffective due to vascular dilatation
Obstructive	poor peripheral pulses, low BP, tachypnoea, cool peripheries
Septic	tachypnoea, bradypnea, pyrexia, hypothermia, low BP, poor peripheral pulses

Clinical manifestations

The clinical manifestations of any type of shock depend partly on the underlying aetiology, but if not treated then all types of shock follow the common pathway of multiorgan failure and death. Tachycardia is usually the early sign of all types of shock, followed by tachypnoea. Hypovolemia is a late sign especially in paediatric population and usually manifests during the advanced phase of uncompensated sepsis (Table 8.2).

Investigations

The laboratory investigations, imaging and other studies depend on the suspected underlying cause and type of shock.

The common investigations to be considered in a child presenting with shock include:
- full blood count: may show leucocytosis or leucopenia, anaemia, thrombocytopenia
- serum electrolytes and renal function
- glucose
- blood gas including lactate level
- liver function tests and coagulation profile
- C-reactive protein
- blood and other tissue cultures
- chest x-ray
- ECG

Treatment and management

The key in management of any type of shock is its early recognition followed by stabilisation of airway, breathing and circulation and provision of specific therapy as indicated by the underlying aetiology. The guidelines and algorithms devised by the Advanced Paediatric and Neonatal Life Support groups should be followed.

Administration of IV sodium chloride 0.9% is usually required for volume expansion in the early phase of shock management, and a 20 ml/kg bolus is given and could be repeated up to 60–80 ml/kg. More cautious fluid resuscitation at 10 mls/kg per bolus may be more appropriate in some situations. Careful use in cardiogenic shock is required to avoid worsening of cardiac function. Refractory shock after 40–60 ml/kg fluid therapy will require the commencement of inotropes.

Relevant pharmacological agents used

Adrenaline increases cardiac contractility and heart rate although at high doses its vasoconstrictor effect may cause poor renal perfusion and arrhythmia.
Dopamine increases cardiac contractility and peripheral vasoconstriction may cause arrhythmias at higher doses.
Dobutamine is a cardio-selective inotrope that increases cardiac contractility and produces a peripheral vasodilator.
Antimicrobial therapy. Specific role in septic shock if the diagnosis of sepsis or septic shock is made then administration must occur within 1 hour of presentation.

Anaphylaxis

Anaphylaxis is a severe, life-threatening, generalised or systemic hypersensitivity. There is a range of symptoms and signs but anaphylaxis is likely when all of the following three criteria are met:
- sudden onset and rapid progression of symptoms
- life-threatening problems of the airway, breathing or circulation
- skin or mucosal changes including flushing, urticaria and angioedema

Exposure to a known allergen for the patient helps support the diagnosis but it is important to remember that

- skin or mucosal changes alone are not a sign of anaphylactic reaction
- skin and mucosal changes can be subtle or absent in up to 20% of reactions
- GI symptoms such as vomiting, abdominal pain and incontinence can also occur

Patients at risk of severe anaphylaxis include those with:

- food allergy
- history of asthma or current asthma exacerbation
- delayed administration of adrenaline
- previous biphasic or severe anaphylactic reactions

Biphasic anaphylaxis describes recurrence of symptoms that develop following the apparent resolution of the initial anaphylactic episode with no additional exposure to the trigger. They typically occur within 8 to 10 hours after resolution of the initial symptoms, although recurrences up to 72 hours later have been reported.

The child may feel and look unwell and occasionally describe a sense of 'impending doom'. Other symptoms and signs will include:

- airway swelling leading to difficulty in breathing and swallowing and a feeling that the throat is closing, hoarse voice, stridor
- breathing problems include increased respiratory rate, wheeze, hypoxia leading to confusion
- circulation compromise includes pale, clammy skin, tachycardia, low blood pressure leading to dizziness and collapse, decreased level of consciousness
- skin and mucosal signs are often the first feature and present in about 80% of children. Patchy or generalised erythema, urticarial rash—often itchy, angioedema of eyelids, lips, mouth and throat

Investigations

Anaphylaxis is essentially a clinical diagnosis and laboratory tests are not commonly required. Mast cell tryptase will help confirm a diagnosis of anaphylactic reaction but measurement should not delay initial treatment of anaphylaxis.

Management of acute episode

The ABCDE approach as described in the APLS guidelines (Figure 8.2) should be followed for all age groups

- early call for help
- follow Resus UK anaphylaxis algorithm
- IM adrenaline—if indicated, administered as soon as anaphylaxis identified
- investigation and follow up by an allergy specialist

Children younger than 16 years who have had emergency treatment for suspected anaphylaxis should be admitted to hospital under the care of a paediatric medical team and observed for 12 hrs after the episode. Longer periods of observations are recommended for those with risk factors or who have ingested an allergen. They should be reviewed by a senior clinician and a decision made about the need for further treatment or longer period of observation when:

- severe reactions with slow onset
- individual has severe asthma or with a severe asthmatic component
- possibility of continuing absorption of allergen
- previous history of biphasic reactions Figure 8.2

Management following acute episode

Adrenaline auto-injector are usually recommended to those at increased risk of idiopathic anaphylaxis or for anyone at continued high risk of reaction. Individuals provided with auto-injector on discharge from hospital must be given instructions and training and have appropriate follow up including contact with the patient's GP. All patients presenting with anaphylaxis should be referred to an allergy clinic to identify the cause and thereby reduce the risk of future reactions and prepare the patient to manage future episodes themselves.

Relevant pharmacological agents used

Adrenaline should be given early after the onset of the reaction and is best given via the IM route which is safer and is easy to learn how to administer
Antihistamines are given after initial resuscitation and may help counter histamine-mediated vasodilatation and bronchoconstriction. It can be given IV or IM
Steroids may help prevent or shorten protracted reactions

Acute airway obstruction

The upper airway extends from the nares and lips to the subglottis, and major causes of upper airway obstruction are infections (viral croup 80%, epiglottitis 5%) and foreign body aspiration.

Acute upper airway obstruction in paediatric patients is one of the most daunting emergency situations faced by clinicians and, unless promptly diagnosed and appropriately managed, it rapidly progresses to hypoxia and cardiac arrest. The acuteness of symptoms may not permit time for investigations and the diagnosis rests on clinical assessment. The potential for sudden occlusion of the airway is always present and all specialists involved in the care of the paediatric airway should be trained in emergency cricothyroidotomy.

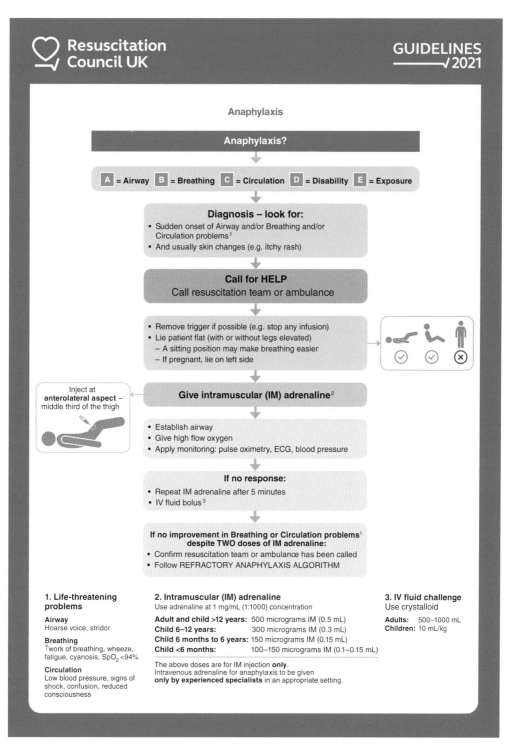

Fig. 8.2 Anaphylaxis Guideline 2021. (Reproduced with permission from the Resuscitation Council UK 2021)

Causes of airways obstruction include:

- infections—croup, epiglottitis, tonsillitis, abscess
- foreign body
- trauma
- anaphylactoid reactions
- neoplasia—lymphoma

Important details in the history include age, predisposing events, speed of progression of symptoms, associated symptoms such as fever and drooling, past medical history detailing neonatal history (birth trauma or prolonged and repeated intubations) and any history of previous neck or chest surgery.

Any examination should not disturb the child and ensure that they remain in a position of comfort—usually on the knee of the carer. Neck swelling with fever suggests peritonsillar or retropharyngeal abscess whilst stridor, particularly biphasic, is suggestive of an airway obstruction.

Investigations

A child with features suggestive of acute airways obstruction should simply be observed and no invasive investigations undertaken until the airway is assessed and secured. They should not attend the radiology department until the airway is safe due to risk of deterioration. A chest x-ray is useful in identifying any radio-opaque foreign bodies or suspected intrathoracic pathology.

Acquired acute upper airway obstruction

Acquired causes of upper airways obstruction are usually due to infections, foreign bodies and trauma.

Croup

Viral croup—acute laryngotracheobronchitis—is the most common cause of upper airway compromise in children and usually presents between the ages of 6 months and 3 years. Parainfluenza virus is the usual cause but other viruses such as influenza viruses, adenovirus and respiratory syncytial virus can be responsible.

Croup is usually diagnosed on clinical grounds with typical symptoms of 1–2 days of coryza, followed by barking cough, hoarse voice and stridor. Most children suffer mild, self-limiting illness and are successfully managed without any specific treatment.

Treatment and management

Mild croup can be managed at home with advice about fluid intake, antipyretics and safety net advice regarding when to seek help. Children with moderate to severe croup require hospital treatment and close observation.

Recommended treatments include oral dexamethasone or nebulised budesonide for those with mild disease along with antipyretics. Those children who are more severely affected may require nebulised adrenaline, inhaled oxygen and fluid management.

Patients should be observed for 3–4 hours after initial treatment and the majority can be safely discharged home. A small proportion of children with severe croup may need admission to intensive care units.

Peritonsillar abscess

It is the most common deep neck abscesses in children, usually in later childhood. The classical presentation is with a low-grade pyrexia, a severe sore throat, a muffled voice, drooling and trismus. Diagnosis can be made from history and inspection whilst a CT scan will provide further details once the airway is safe and secure. Appropriate antibiotic cover should be commenced promptly but surgical incision and drainage is usually needed.

Retropharyngeal abscess

The condition tends to occur in preschool age children and is due to the progression of bacterial pharyngitis or pharyngeal trauma. They present with pyrexia, drooling, asymmetrical neck swelling and extension of the neck. Appropriate antibiotic cover should be commenced promptly but surgical incision and drainage is usually needed.

Epiglottitis

Epiglottitis is a life-threatening, rapidly progressive condition characterised by local inflammation and oedema of the supraglottic area and epiglottis. While *Haemophilus influenzae* vaccination has practically eliminated other infections with this organism, 10% of children with epiglottitis still have *H. Influenzae* type b infection.

Clinical presentation

- high grade fever
- child appears toxic
- assume the 'tripod' position leaning forward with both hands on a surface
- breathing with open mouth with protrusion of tongue and extended neck
- anxious, with muffled voice and unable to cough

Treatment and management

Urgent intubation is required to protect the airway and this should be undertaken by the most experienced professional available. An ENT specialist should also be present in case of acute airways obstruction. Intravenous antibiotics are required.

Bacterial tracheitis

The most common organism causing bacterial tracheitis is *Staphylococcus aureus although Haemophilus influenzae* can also be identified. Children appear toxic and have a high-grade fever and can rapidly progress to upper airway obstruction. Management usually requires intubation and admission to intensive care unit and the direct laryngoscopy will reveal normal epiglottis but a trachea full of purulent debris. Appropriate antibiotic cover should be commenced promptly but dexamethasone and nebulised adrenaline are not effective (Table 8.3).

Airway foreign bodies

Inhaled foreign bodies can lodge at any level of upper airway from the supraglottic area to trachea and are a leading cause of accidental death in children under the age of 5 years. Common aspirated foreign bodies include nuts, seeds and popcorn in toddlers and clips, coins and pen caps in older children. Toy balloons, marbles and small balls can cause complete airway obstruction and be rapidly fatal.

The child will usually present with a sudden onset of respiratory symptoms having been previously well. Coughing and choking may be evident features of the history. Inspiratory and expiratory chest films should be obtained that may identify air-trapping due to a 'ball-valve' effect (Figure 8.3). The x-ray may also reveal radio-opaque items although normal studies do not exclude the presence of a foreign body

Treatment and management

Severe hypoxia suggests the need for immediate resuscitation and securing of the airway with rigid bronchoscopy then used to address suspected or conformed foreign body aspiration.

Table 8.3 Differences between croup, tracheitis and epiglottitis			
	croup	tracheitis	epiglottitis
Organism	viral	S. aureus streptococcus	haemophilus influenza b
age	6m–3yr	all ages	18m–6yr
temperature	low grade	over 38.5°C	over 38.5°C
cough	barking	barking	absent or muted
swallowing	normal	limited	drooling of saliva
position	lying down	sitting upright	tripod position, neck extended
appearance	settled	distressed	toxic

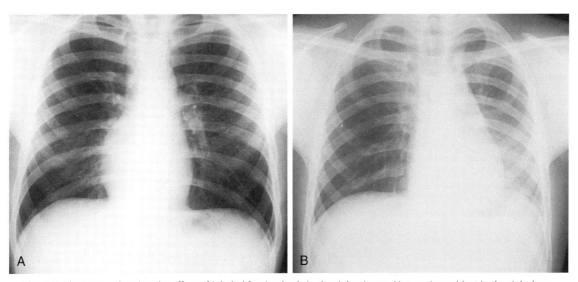

Fig. 8.3 Chest x-ray showing the effect of inhaled foreign body in the right airway. Air trapping evident in the right lung.

Acute seizures

Convulsive status epilepticus (CSE)

This is the most common paediatric neurological emergency and is defined as a tonic-clonic seizure lasting for 5 minutes or more or a series of separate seizures without the individual regaining consciousness between each episode. Febrile seizures are most commonly seen in children from 6 months to 6 years of age.

Investigations

Infants under 1 year of age have the highest incidence of acute symptomatic seizures and an underlying cause should be sought particularly for hypoglycaemia. Acute CNS infections and sepsis must be considered in children with a fever and seizures and blood cultures undertaken. Neuroimaging should be considered for the following clinical presentations:

- persistent altered mental status
- new onset focal neurological deficit
- suspected acute CNS infection
- suspected raised intracranial pressure
- history of head injury or coagulation abnormalities

Treatment and management

The priority in a child with active seizures is similar to all medical emergencies, with securing airway, supporting breathing and circulation. Convulsive seizures lasting 5 minutes or longer are unlikely to resolve spontaneously and therefore pharmacological treatment to stop seizure should be instituted at 5 minutes. Some children with epilepsy and recurrent convulsive status epilepticus may have their own individualised management plan.

Medication

The first line anticonvulsant for infants over 28 days of age and children with seizure lasting 5 minutes without any signs of abating is intravenous benzodiazepine. Buccal midazolam or rectal diazepam are the preferred benzodiazepines especially in prehospital setting or when an immediate intravenous or intraosseous access is unavailable. In children with vascular access, IV lorazepam is the preferred drug as it has a longer duration of action, is more effective and is less likely to cause respiratory depression.

If seizure activity is still present some 5 minutes after the first dose of benzodiazepine, then a second dose should be administered. It is preferable to administer the second dose as an intravenous preparation, but rectal diazepam or buccal midazolam can be given. No more than two doses of benzodiazepines (including prehospital treatment) should be administered to avoid the risk of respiratory depression.

The second-line anticonvulsant in children with ongoing seizures is intravenous phenytoin or levetiracetam. IV phenytoin administration may cause cardiac arrhythmias, hypotension and extravasation injury, and therefore ECG monitoring should be available.

If seizures continue after the second-line medication, then rapid sequence intubation with thiopental and admission to intensive care unit is required.

Acute neurological emergencies

A child being presented to the emergency department with reduced conscious level is a frequent occurrence and the underlying causes are extensive. These would include:

- seizures
- head injury causing intracranial bleed or swelling in the brain
- infection
- circulatory or respiratory failure leading to hypoxic ischemic brain injury
- intoxication from drugs or alcohol
- metabolic causes producing an encephalopathy
- brain tumours
- children with hydrocephalus and shunt malfunction

Infants can present with symptoms of vomiting, high-pitched cry, drowsiness or seizures. In older children symptoms include vomiting, headache, lethargy and seizures. Examination can reveal a reduced conscious level, fever, bulging fontanelle and hypertension.

Some findings will suggest an aetiology including fever in infections, pinpoint pupils with opiate poisoning, hypoglycaemia, hypertension or unexplained bruising caused by a nonaccidental injury.

Raised intracranial pressure may be identified if there is:

- bradycardia with hypertension
- unilateral or bilateral dilatation of pupils
- hyperventilation, Cheyne-Stokes breathing and apnoea
- papilloedema

Treatment and management

The obvious concern is that of reduced consciousness level and this indicates a need for management of airways and circulation in the first instance following APLS guidelines.

The Glasgow coma score (GCS) should be used to assess the conscious level of child and depth of coma and should be regularly undertaken to monitor the neurological status.

The child or young person who has a GCS of 8 or below needs immediate intubation to protect the airway and to avoid hypercapnia which can lead to significant increase in ICP. If signs of shock are present then a fluid bolus of 20 mls/kg of normal saline is required followed by prompt reassessment.

If a raised intracranial pressure is identified then:
• immediate intubation and ventilation are required
• patient should be nursed head up at 20 degrees to help cerebral venous drainage
• hypertonic saline 3% 3 mls/kg or mannitol 250 mg–500 mg/kg should be given
• dexamethasone, but only for oedema for surrounding space occupying lesion
Acute management of meningitis requires:
• IV ceftriaxone or cefotaxime
• IV acyclovir if herpes simplex suspected

• dexamethasone to start within 4 hours of antibiotics (except if less than 3 months)
If opiate poisoning is suspected then naloxone should be administered slowly.

Stroke

Though uncommon, stroke must be considered a neurological emergency and the most common risk factors are:
• congenital heart disease
• sickle cell disease
• meningitis
• trauma to head and neck
Children invariably present with headache, altered mental state and motor signs and the diagnosis is confirmed by MRI scan.

Treatment and management

Thrombolysis or antithrombotic therapy is required and haematological and neurological advice should be sought.

IMPORTANT CLINICAL POINTS

Cardiac arrest
• early recognition followed by systematic assessment (ABCDE)
• identify and treat reversible causes (4H and 4T)
• parental presence is an important aspect of management

Anaphylaxis
• identified by three criteria
    • sudden onset and rapid progression
    • life-threatening airway and circulation problems
    • skin or mucosal changes
• IM adrenaline administered as soon as anaphylaxis identified
• refer to specialist allergy clinic after recovery

Airway obstruction
• acute, severe or rapidly progressive airway obstruction needs urgent management
• defer examination and investigations until airway been assessed and secured
• maintain a position of comfort for optimal airway opening
• securing of airway should be done before significant hypoxia develops

Seizures
• status epilepticus—most common paediatric neurological emergency
• febrile seizures are common between 6 months to 6 years of age
• benzodiazepines are the first-line treatment for prolonged seizures

---

Further reading

The management of children and young people with an acute decrease in conscious level, RCPCH Guideline. Published: 2015. Revised: 2019. https://www.rcpch.ac.uk/sites/default/fil es/2019-04/decon_guideline_revised_2019_08.04.19.pdf
Head injury: assessment and early management. Clinical guideline [CG176]. Updated September 2019. https://www.nice.org.uk/ guidance/cg176

Sepsis: recognition, diagnosis and early management. NICE guideline [NG51]. Updated September 2017. https://www.nice.org.uk/ guidance/ng51?unlid=28010410720161191 7351

Chapter | 9 |

Unintentional injuries and poisoning

Co-ordinators: *Colin Powell; Ibtihal Abdelgadir*

Authors: *Muhammad Islam, Graeme Hadley, Amna Hussain, Barbara Blackie, Syed Haris Huda, Usama Al-Kanani, Vince Choudhery, Yazeed Eldos*

After reading this chapter you should be able to assess, diagnose and manage:
- unintentional injuries including trauma and drowning
- life-threatening haemorrhage
- head and spinal injuries
- burns and scalds
- life- or limb-threatening injuries
- injuries that can be managed less urgently and their x-ray appearances
- poisoning

PRACTICE POINT - Approach to assessment and management of individual with major injury

- Primary survey of patient and resuscitation
  - follow Airway, Breathing, Circulation, Disability, Environment steps
  - address bleeding, hypovolaemia, pain control
- Secondary survey of patient
  - detailed head-to-toe assessment to identify any other injuries or issues

Unintentional injuries

Children and young people can present to the emergency department with significant and life-threatening injuries. Their emergency care and management require prompt assessment and urgent action applying a structured approach by a well-rehearsed team of experienced clinicians.

The management of all those with significant injuries begins with a primary survey of the patient and their presenting problem with resuscitation using an ABCDE approach. Obvious life-threatening injuries will need immediate action whilst airway management and circulatory compromise may need special consideration in light of any injuries. Once stabilised, the injured children must then have a secondary survey to determine less urgent consequences of the insult.

Trauma

Trauma in the form of road traffic accidents, falls and non-accidental injury (NAI) remains the biggest cause of death in children worldwide.

Primary survey

Addressing an exsanguinating haemorrhage in a child must be the first priority in trauma and early use of pressure and tranexamic acid will improve outcomes. Endotracheal intubation is required if there are signs of airway compromise but a nasopharyngeal airway should be avoided if there is basal skull trauma or facial injuries. Any assessment must assume that there is a cervical spine injury and so immobilisation is crucial until the cervical spine is assessed and known to be without injury.

Those patients who present with rib fractures, especially flail chest, have been exposed to large forces and consequently serious internal damage is likely. Some chest injuries require immediate treatment including a tension pneumothorax (Figure 9.1), massive haemothorax, flail chest and cardiac tamponade.

Falling blood pressure in children indicates a decompensating shock and is a preterminal event. Consequently, obtaining venous access with high flow intravenous cannulae or intraosseous needles is a priority.

The initial assessment must consider the distress and pain evident in the patient and administer appropriate

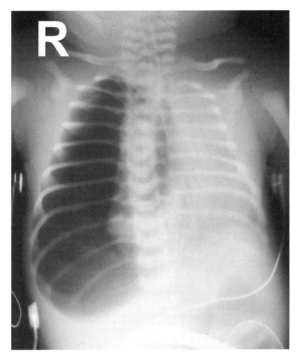

Fig. 9.1 Tension pneumothorax—chest x-ray of 6-week-old boy involved in a road traffic accident. Shows mediastinal displacement and lung fields without markings.

levels of analgesia. The type, dose and route of administration of any analgesia should be carefully monitored and titrated to the child's response particularly for those with a decreased level of consciousness. Intravenous morphine, intranasal diamorphine or intranasal fentanyl are the commonly used agents.

Drowning

Drowning is the commonest cause of traumatic death in children aged between 1–4 years and survival is dependent on immersion time, on-scene resuscitation and subsequent intensive care management. In those children who are competent swimmers, a medical cause such as seizures, arrhythmias, long QT syndrome and intoxication should be suspected as a cause for the drowning. In young children it is important to consider that the episode may be caused intentionally and that actions to safeguard the child may be necessary.

Treatment and management

Active management requires the maintenance of adequate oxygenation, prevention of aspiration and the stabilisation of body temperature. Hypothermia is common and wet clothes should be removed, the child dried and, if there is no cardiovascular instability, they should be rewarmed at a rate of at 0.5°C per hour to 34°C. The administration of warmed intravenous fluids will help in raising the core temperature particularly if it is less than 35°C. Active management should also aim to maintain cerebral perfusion and oxygenation with the administration of osmotic agents (hypertonic saline or mannitol) if there are signs of raised intracranial pressure.

Investigations

- electrolytes to aid fluid assessment and management
- ECG for prolonged QT syndrome
- consider drug and alcohol screen

CLINICAL SCENARIO

A two-year-old girl was unsupervised at a family party and was found floating face down in the outdoor swimming pool. The lifeguard pulled her out of the pool, called for help and started immediate basic life support. It was felt she had been missing for a maximum of three minutes. The emergency services team continued the cardiac massage, maintained adequate oxygenation and prevented aspiration. Her core temperature was 35.5°C but had she been hypothermic she needed rewarming at a rate of at 0.5°C per hour to 35°C. When she arrived at the emergency department, she was spontaneously breathing with high flow oxygen attached and her cardiovascular assessment was appropriate for her age. High flow oxygen was continued and she was given warmed intravenous fluids.

This child had a short immersion time, immediate resuscitation and basic life support and was then quickly taken to an emergency department. The most important indicator of a good outcome is the response to the initial resuscitation. Drowning can occur quickly even in a few inches of water and children should therefore always be supervised by a responsible adult.

Life-threatening haemorrhage

Severe hypovolemic shock is typically caused by the disruption of intrathoracic or intraabdominal organs or vessels although significant blood loss may result from long bone or pelvic fractures.

The clinical response to volume loss includes tachycardia, weak peripheral pulse, cool mottled peripheries and

Table 9.1 **Estimated circulating blood volumes by age**	
Infant	80 ml/kg
1–3 yrs of age	75 ml/kg
over 3 yrs	70 ml/kg

prolonged capillary refill time. A further clinical deterioration will lead to lethargy and poor urine output. A fall in systolic BP may not occur until there is a 30% decrease in circulating blood volume and consequently hypotension is a late sign of hypovolaemia.

Treatment and management

The initial control of haemorrhage is crucial and any obvious external sites of haemorrhage will require direct manual pressure to control the bleeding. If internal haemorrhage is suspected, tranexamic acid (antifibrinolytic) may be used to reduce the bleeding whilst urgent surgical assessment is obtained. Those with long bone fractures may require reduction and splinting to produce haemostasis whilst those with suspected pelvic fractures will benefit from a pelvic stabilisation device. Large scalp lacerations usually respond to surgical closure using sutures, surgical staples or scalp clips.

The need for fluid resuscitation will also be identified during the primary survey and the aim will be to rapidly replace the circulating volume to the level appropriate for the age of the patient. In an acute situation, calculations of the weight of the child can either come from the carers or from a length-based resuscitation tape available in all resuscitation rooms.

Blood products including packed red blood cells, fresh frozen plasma and platelets are preferred over crystalloids although an initial use 20 ml/kg of isotonic saline followed by 10–20 ml/kg of packed red cells, 10–20 ml/kg of fresh frozen plasma and platelets (Table 9.1).

Head and spinal injuries

Head injury

Trauma to the head is common in the paediatric population and although the majority are minor, about 5% have intracranial complications. The most common causes of severe head injury are road traffic collisions, falls from a height and, in the under 2-year age group, nonaccidental injury. Intracranial bleeds can occur at different anatomical sites leading to differences in management.

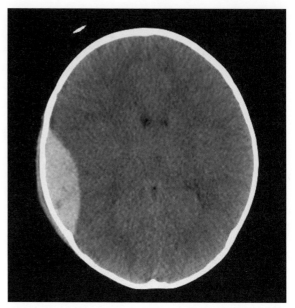

Fig. 9.2 CT scan of a 14-year-old-boy following head trauma showing the convex-shaped lesion in the extradural space (Image use with permission from Paediatric Surgery Ed. Coran AG. 7th edition. Chapter 24. Jea A, Luerssen TG. Elsevier Inc.)

Extradural

This is usually the result of a significant blow to the head with a loss of consciousness resulting in the laceration of the middle meningeal artery. The classical history sees the patient regaining consciousness (lucid period) before deteriorating over the next few hours as arterial blood accumulates under pressure in the extradural space (Figure 9.2). If left unchecked, there is coning and death, but if surgically decompressed in time, the prognosis is good.

Subdural haemorrhage

Shearing forces during trauma cause disruption of bridging veins over the sulci which then empty into the dural venous sinuses. In under 2-year-olds, the presence of subdural haemorrhage is highly suspicious of abusive head trauma.

Classification of head injury

The main measurements of severity used to classify head injury are the Glasgow Coma Score (GCS), duration of loss of consciousness (LOC) and posttraumatic amnesia (PTA) (Table 9.2).

Investigations

Skull x-rays are not useful in the investigation of acute trauma and they should not be requested. CT scanning is used for the assessment of the head injury, and the NICE guidelines indicate a need for such a scan within an hour of the injury in the following circumstances:

- suspicion of nonaccidental injury
- posttraumatic seizure but no history of epilepsy
- GCS less than 14
- suspected open or depressed skull fracture or tense fontanelle
- any sign of basal skull fracture
- focal neurological deficit
- laceration of more than 5 cm or bruising on the head of a child under 1 year
- further clinical deterioration

Treatment and management

A primary and secondary survey with an ABCDE approach is required although the special consideration for those with a head injury require a full assessment of the cervical spine in case of the need for intubation. Whilst such an assessment is being undertaken, the airway is maintained using a jaw thrust manoeuvre where the mandible is pushed anteriorly and the mouth opened manually. This draws the tongue forward and away from the pharynx. Nasopharyngeal airways or nasogastric tubes must be avoided if there are signs of a base of skull fracture.

The monitoring of the level of consciousness using the GCS scale and pupillary response will continue throughout the survey periods (Table 9.3).

There is a modified version of the GCS for nonverbal children, usually applied to those under 2 years old.

Seizures are a common feature in children with a significant head injury and they need aggressive management using standard protocols. It can, however, be difficult to detect seizure activity with a paralysed ventilated patient, so there should be a low threshold for introducing anticonvulsant treatment if there is tachycardia, hypertension and bilateral dilatation of the pupils.

Maintenance fluids in the form of isotonic saline will be required, but volumes should be restricted to 70% of normal maintenance as inappropriate ADH secretion can occur with severe head injury.

Uncal herniation may develop due to a critical rise in ICP that will lead to a sudden clinical deterioration with a unilateral pupillary dilation, hypertension and bradycardia and, if not treated urgently, will lead to death. This process can be reversed by hyperventilating the child, administering a bolus of mannitol or hypertonic saline and potential neurosurgical intervention.

Once stabilised, a focused neurological and physical examination is carried out during the secondary survey and includes:

- checking scalp for bruising, lacerations, swelling, and tenderness
- checking for bulging fontanelle (infants)
- signs of basal skull fracture:
- bruising around the eyes (panda eyes)
- bruising behind ear (Battle's sign)
- CSF leak from the nose or ears
- haemotympanum
- pupil size and reactivity to light
- tone, reflex and movement of all four limbs
- cranial nerve assessment where possible
- Glasgow Coma Scale score adapted to age

Table 9.2 **Levels of severity of head injury**			
	GCS	**LOC**	**PTA**
Mild	13–15	< 30 mins	< 1 hour
Moderate	9–12	30 mins–24 hrs	1–24 hrs
Severe	3–8	>24 hrs	>24 hrs

Table 9.3 **Standard Glasgow Coma Scale (GCS) for patients over 2 years old**					
Eye opening		**Best verbal response**		**Best motor response**	
spontaneous	4	Oriented	5	follows commands	6
to verbal stimuli	3	Confused	4	localized pain	5
to pain	2	inappropriate words	3	withdraws to pain	4
None	1	incomprehensible sounds	2	flexion to pain	3
		None	1	extension to pain	2
				none	1

Spinal injury

Paediatric spine injuries are rare and 60% to 80% involve the cervical spine. Road traffic accidents and incorrect positioning of seat belts and car seats are common reasons for these injuries in younger children whilst sporting injuries are a more common cause in older children and adolescents. Children with Down syndrome have atlanto-axial instability and, along with those with rheumatoid arthritis, are at risk of cervical spine injury. Clinical examination of the spine is best assessed by log rolling the patient and palpating the thoracic and lumbar spine for tenderness, swelling or step deformity over the length of the spine. A defined sensory level is a most important clinical sign and indicates the level of injury.

Treatment and management

Cervical spine injury must be assumed in all patients with head trauma or injury and the neck must be immobilised in the neutral position and movement minimised in the manner already described. Injuries to the cervical and high thoracic regions can lead to paralysis of the intercostal muscles and diaphragm and consequently ventilatory support may be required. The use of hard cervical collars, side blocks and overhead tape used to be standard practice for cervical spine immobilisation but these are now considered unsuitable in young children. Allowing the child to stay still in a position of comfort is recognised as the best option.

If stability of the cervical spine cannot be established clinically then imaging must be obtained using CT or, if there are neurological long tract signs, MR scanning.

Injuries of the thoracolumbar spine are exceptionally rare in children and compression fractures are the most common in the thoracic and lumbar areas. These often give rise to wedge appearance on lateral plain films and are usually stable.

Burns and scalds

Burns can be caused by heat, radiation, electricity, friction or contact with chemicals. Scalds are secondary to hot liquids and usually occur in the toddler age group within the home environment.

The clinical presentation of burns and the accompanying signs and symptoms vary depending on the causative agent, duration of contact and the sites involved. The severity of the burn is described by the depth and extent of the observed lesions (Figure 9.3).

The depth of a burn can be described as:
- **superficial or epidermal burns** that involve the epidermis alone. The skin appears red but is dry and intact with no blistering but is very painful.
- **partial thickness burns** involve the dermis and they can be:
  - superficial dermal burns–pale pink with blisters and usually a large amount of exudate. The burnt area blanches, has a brisk capillary refill and is very painful.
  - deep dermal burns—reddish with a mottled blotchy appearance and capillary refill is slow or absent. They are not painful and have limited sensation.
- **full thickness burns** involve tissues deep to the dermis. These burns are white, waxy or charred in appearance and there is no blistering and no capillary refill (Figure 9.4). Full thickness burns lack sensation due to the destruction of the dermal nerve endings.

The extent of the burn can be assessed by a variety of methods. One involves using the size of the patient's hand with fingers adducted and taking that as roughly 1% total body surface area. Alternatively, Lund-Browder Charts can be used (Figure 9.5). Only partial thickness (dermal) and full thickness burns are used in the calculation of total body surface area of a burn

Burns involving fire may result in inhalation injury producing stridor or a hoarse voice if the child is vocalising. Tachypnoea and hypoxia on presentation may be due to direct thermal injury to the lungs although associated injuries such as chest trauma need to be considered. Blast injuries and a fall from heights may result in blunt chest trauma with pneumothoraces or haemothoraces.

Burns over 10% partial thickness and significant full thickness burns result in increased fluids losses and those children with involved areas of more than 20% of the body surface area can develop significant hypovolemia. This usually appears a few hours after the injury but if the patient is hypotensive on initial presentation, an alternative cause such as an unrecognised tension pneumothorax or haemorrhage should be considered.

Carbon monoxide and cyanide poisoning should be considered if there is a history of fire in an enclosed space. Clinically this presents as weakness, nausea, diarrhoea and vomiting and in extensive exposure, neurological symptoms such as seizures and impaired consciousness.

Electrical burns occur due to electrical current passing through tissues. In high energy electrical injuries, the entry and exit points of the electrical current often hide the injury to the deep tissue, particularly muscle, nerves and blood vessels. Rhabdomyolysis, myocardial damage and multiorgan failure can follow. High voltage electrical injuries including lightning strikes can also result in direct cardiac effects with children presenting with an arrhythmia or cardiac arrest.

As with any injury, clinicians should be aware of the presentations that suggest NAI and in addition to treating the burn, there should be the appropriate involvement of police and social services if there are concerns raised about the history and presentation.

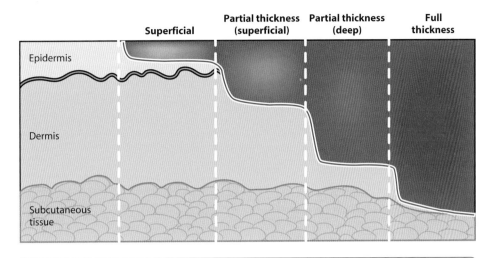

Depth	Superficial – limited to epidermis	Partial thickness (superficial)	Partial thickness (deep)	Full thickness
Possible cause	Sunburn, minor scald	Scald	Scald, brief contact with flame	Significant flame contact
Appearance	Dry and erythematous	Moist, erythematous, blistered	Moist with white slough, erythematous, mottled	Dry, charred, white
Pain sensation	Painful	Painful	Painless	Painless
Healing	Rapid – 1 week	1–3 weeks	3–4 weeks – often requires grafting	Needs skin grafting to heal

Fig. 9.3 Diagram showing features found in burns to the skin (Image use with permission Illustrated Textbook of Paediatrics. Ed. Lissauer T, Carroll W. 5th edition. Chapter 7. Anderson M, Elsevier Ltd.)

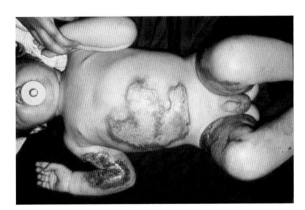

Fig. 9.4 Full thickness burn in 3-month-old boy following exposure to boiling liquid.

Investigations

- full blood count
- biochemistry to guide fluid therapy
- creatine kinase and troponin—if electrical burns
- chest x-ray—if chest trauma or inhalation burns are suspected
- blood gases
- carbon monoxide levels
- ECG—if electrical burns looking for features of myocardial injury

Treatment and management

First aid management requires the removal of all clothing that is wet, burnt or, in the case of chemical burns, potentially contaminated with the causative agent. The burn areas should then be cooled under running tap water for 20 minutes and

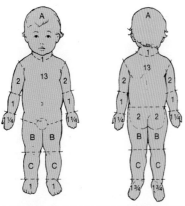

RELATIVE PERCENTAGES OF AREAS AFFECTED BY GROWTH

AREA	BIRTH	AGE 1 YR	AGE 5 YR
A = ½ of head	9½	8½	6½
B = ½ of one thigh	2¾	3¼	4
C = ½ of one leg	2½	2½	2¾

A

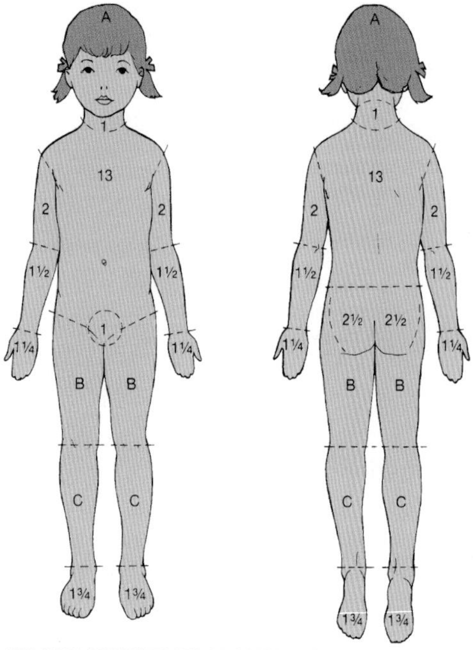

RELATIVE PERCENTAGES OF AREAS AFFECTED BY GROWTH

AREA	AGE 10 YR	AGE 15 YR	ADULT
A = ½ of head	5½	4½	3½
B = ½ of one thigh	4½	4½	4¾
C = ½ of one leg	3	3¼	3½

B

Fig. 9.5 Lund-Browder chart used to estimate extent of burns in children. (A) Birth to 5 years. (B) Older children (Image use with permission and adapted from Saunders Comprehensive Review for the NCLEX-RX Examination Ed. Silvestri LA 2011 Elsevier Inc. Originally from Perry S et al Maternal child nursing care. 4th edition. 2010 St Louis: Mosby.)

those resulting from contact with caustic chemical agents need irrigation with copious amounts of water or saline.

Where inhalation burns are suspected, oxygen should be commenced, involvement of anaesthetic colleagues sought and a plan made for intubation.

PRACTICE POINT—fluid resuscitation for patients with extensive burns

- should be started when burns are greater than 10% of total body surface area
- volume for first 24 hours = **% burn x weight (kg) x 3**
- use Hartmann's solution (also known as Ringer's Lactate)
- half of volume given over first 8 hours; remainder over the following 16 hours

---

Major burns result in a significant amount of fluid loss from the burn itself and so IV resuscitation fluids should be started as outlined in Practice Point box.

Adequate analgesia is crucial and, for those with extensive burns, opiates such as intranasal or intravenous fentanyl are recommended. Ketamine may be needed to provide procedural sedation to facilitate full examination and debridement.

The choice of a suitable dressing is important in effective management of burns and should be discussed with a tertiary burns centre. Dressings need to be nonadherent and have an absorptive component especially for deep dermal and full thickness burns.

Potential complications

Burns may become infected and when extensive, the infection can produce a toxic shock or burns sepsis syndrome. The most common causative organisms are *Staphylococcus aureus* and Group A Streptococci.

With deep and extensive burns there is the long-term complication of scarring, strictures and contractures and such patients will need multiple operations and extensive rehabilitation. Many of the children can have significant psychological trauma as a result of a burn injury and are at increased risk for posttraumatic stress disorder.

Limb-threatening injuries

Upper extremity trauma can cause simple fingertip lesions or more complex injuries involving multiple tissue structures whilst lower extremity injuries will include pelvic and long bone fractures and crush injuries. The range of such injuries is extensive, but some important features are described here.

CLINICAL SCENARIO

A 14-month-old girl presented to the emergency department with her mother and grandmother. They reported that she had fallen into a bath of scalding hot water after her mother had left her in the bathroom to answer the front doorbell. She had been playing with her 4-year-old brother and when her mother responded to the screams, she found her 'standing in 6 inches of hot water, wearing just her nappy'.

Examination identified obvious partial thickness burns covering about 64% of her trunk, legs and arms. The only parts of her body that were spared were her face, neck, chest and tip of her left shoulder.

Immediate management required IV fluids for resuscitation, IV opioid analgesia and sedation. Episodic hypotension indicated a need for inotropic support and she was therefore intubated, ventilated and transferred to PICU.

Safeguarding concerns were raised but it was recognised that the distribution of the burns was consistent with the story of a child falling into a bath, possibly aided by an older sibling, rather than the expected distribution of 'buttocks and thighs' if she had been placed seated in a bath or 'socks' distribution if placed in a standing position. The safeguarding team, however, ensured that this aspect was considered and investigated. The brother was not considered 'at-risk' although he was taken home to his grandmother's house.

Discussions were had with the mother at a later date about basic safety issues to ensure her young children were not left unattended in such situations along with a review of the family's hot water arrangements that allowed extremely hot water to be produced. The rental property was old, the hot water system had not been serviced for many years and the bath did not have thermostatic mixer valves. Social services were involved in supporting the mother and her children to find new accommodation. The landlord was prosecuted.

Vascular injuries

Vascular interruption should be suspected in any significant limb injury and a pulse assessment should be undertaken on a regular basis following presentation. Critical compromise can be recognised if there are cold peripheries with discolouration, prolonged capillary refill time or absent pulses.

Compartment injuries

Compartment syndrome is a surgical emergency and refers to swelling within a fascial compartment, resulting in tissue hypoperfusion. It is seen with fractures, limb muscle contusion, haemorrhage from vascular injury or extravasation injury from excess fluid administrated. Treatment requires urgent surgical review with a view to fasciotomy.

Neurological injuries

Fractures, and particularly dislocations, can cause significant neurologic injury and need prompt recognition and treatment. Assessment of nerve function typically requires a cooperative patient which can be difficult in those with multiple injuries. Progression of neurologic findings is indicative of continued nerve compression and needs intervention.

Open fractures

An open fracture describes a broken bone breaching the skin, and prompt management is needed to minimise complications such as infections. Intravenous antibiotics should be given early along with antitetanus toxoid if there is any doubt regarding full immunity.

Common poisonings

The most common causes of poisoning in younger children are due to household substances, such as cleaning products, cosmetics and pharmaceuticals.

Nonpharmaceuticals and household products

This group includes caustics, antiseptics and disinfectants, and unintentional exposure generally does not result in significant morbidity due to the low concentrations and the small quantities usually ingested.

A caustic substance causes damage on contact and significant injury is caused by substances with pH <3 or >11. The extent of the injury is also determined by other factors such as duration of contact, concentration, volume, or the presence of food in the stomach.

Predictors of injury following swallowing are drooling, haematemesis, hoarse voice and stridor. An urgent upper endoscopy should be performed within the first the 12 hours after ingestion as this will allow appropriate treatment for those with severe injury and the safe discharge of those with minimal evidence of mucosal damage.

Hydrogen peroxide is available as a 3% solution for household use (hair bleaching) and as a 30% solution for industrial use. Following ingestion, a child may present with abdominal pain, hematemesis and rapid mental status deterioration due to oxygen embolisation. Patients with evidence of air in the heart should be placed flat with their head down (Trendelenburg position) to prevent gas from blocking the right ventricular outflow.

Laundry detergent pods are single capsules with concentrated detergent within a water-soluble membrane that dissolves on contact with moisture. They are small, colourful and attractive to children. Ingestion results in gastrointestinal upset and possible CNS depression but activated charcoal is ineffective. Treatment is mainly supportive with airway protection and observation until patients return to baseline mental status.

Moth repellents contain naphthalene and paradichlorobenzene and unintentional ingestion usually causes non-life-threatening toxicity. Haemolysis and methemoglobinemia may occur following acute exposure to naphthalene and methylene blue may be appropriate if this is symptomatic.

Pharmaceuticals

Paracetamol (acetaminophen) overdose is defined as one that occurs over an 8-hour period, and doses over 150 mg/kg are considered capable of causing toxicity. The serum paracetamol concentration for the acute ingestion should be plotted on the Rumack-Matthew nomogram to determine whether N-acetylcysteine antidote therapy is needed. Serum paracetamol concentrations above 150 μg/ml at 4-hours post-ingestion are considered toxic

N-acetylcysteine has a rapid action and is effective in both preventing and treating hepatotoxicity. Monitoring for potential liver toxicity can be undertaken with serial AST and ALT measurements. Where the patient has ingested a dose of paracetamol greater than 150 mg/kg, then commencing N-acetylcysteine treatment is appropriate if the results would not be available until more than 8 hours from the time of the ingestion.

Salicylates produce nausea, vomiting and tachypnoea after an acute ingestion that is followed by tinnitus, lethargy and altered mental status. Respiratory alkalosis develops early after ingestion whilst metabolic acidosis is usually a late finding in acute toxicity. Serum salicylate concentrations are key in guiding therapy. Management requires activated charcoal, fluid replacement and urine alkalinisation via intravenous sodium bicarbonate infusion with the aim of producing a urine pH 7.5–8.0

Nonsteroidal antiinflammatory drugs taken in overdose produced nausea, vomiting and abdominal pain. With a moderate to severe overdose, tinnitus, drowsiness, seizures and acute kidney injury develop. Those patients with ibuprofen ingestions over 400 mg/kg require active management, and activated charcoal should be considered in massive overdoses.

Antihistamines are commonly found in cold and cough preparations and children are at increased risk of toxicity, especially with diphenhydramine. Overdose may result in an anticholinergic effect of tachycardia, drowsiness, hallucinations and urinary retention. An ECG may show a widened QRS complex especially in a large overdose. Management is mainly supportive although decontamination with activated charcoal is reasonable. Benzodiazepines can be given for agitation, hallucination and seizures whilst IV sodium bicarbonate can be given if there is a widened QRS complex.

Advice to parents on unintentional injuries and their prevention

Although the term 'accidents' is commonly used, it creates the impression that such injuries are unavoidable. Further assessment of injuries in children presenting to emergency departments reveals that many are preventable by forethought and changes in behaviour of both patient and parent. Invariably, medical contact usually occurs after the injury has occurred but the attendance is still an opportunity to offer advice that may avoid future injury.

Paediatricians have important roles to play in identifying children at risk of injuries, educating patients and carers about ways in which injuries may be avoided and ensuring that the carers have an understanding of an appropriate responses to any injuries. The paediatrician should also act as an advocate for prevention of injury at local and national levels.

Head injuries and fractures

These can occur from various types of play and do differ somewhat depending on age. Falls in younger children are common and many may be unavoidable, but some may be from a high window where window locks would have provided protection. Head injuries in older children and adolescents are well recognised and the increasing acceptance of helmets for cyclists and clearer guidance for those occurring during sports, particularly if there is obvious concussion, will minimise potential for long-term problems. Many of the major sporting bodies provide clear information on the management of player concussion.

Falls

Advice on how to reduce the fall risk in the house would focus on ensuring that small children are appropriately

PRACTICE POINT—Guidance on concussion in sport

If player displays recognised 'red flag' symptoms
- loss of consciousness
- significant headache
- confusion
- seizure
- focal neurological symptoms
  Response
- player removed from play
- health care professional review within 24 hours
- 14 days of rest
- health care professional review before starting training
- slow gradual return to play

supervised, using window locks and fitting gates across stairwells. Very young children can be trapped in poorly constructed beds which can lead to limb fractures and even strangulation on rare occasions. If children present with fractures caused in this way, then it is important to explore whether beds are appropriate for the age and size child and properly assembled. The potential cause of a nonaccidental injury should always be considered. Children who are involved in sports and recreational activities should be advised to wear appropriate protective gear such as knee and elbow pads and helmets.

Foreign body aspiration or ingestion

The ingestion or aspiration of a foreign body is a particular issue for young children who have narrow airways. Certain food items, such as grapes and nuts, can completely obstruct the upper airway or be inhaled into the trachea and obstruct airflow. Ensuring that any young child does not have open access to such foods is advisable.

Small toys, batteries and magnets may cause significant problems when swallowed although most parents are unaware of the potential impact of such ingestion. Disc batteries can be highly corrosive when lodged against mucosal tissue and erosions can occur within a couple of hours; therefore, removal must occur as soon as possible. The ingestion of multiple small and powerful magnets may lead to perforation if they attract each other and trap bowel mucosa.

Poisoning

Medicines and household cleaning products can appear attractive to children and it is therefore important that these are placed out of reach of children. Clearly any child who has ingested, inhaled or come into contact with dangerous medicines or toxic products should be reviewed and the above advice reinforced at that attendance.

Burns

The impact of burns in children can be devastating and all hot liquids should be made inaccessible to children by keeping them away from the edges of counters and tables and ensuring handles to pans and kettles are not within easy reach. The impact of house fires can be devastating and it is now well recognised that all homes should be equipped with smoke detectors which are tested once a month.

Drowning

Drowning happens quickly and quietly even in a few inches of water in a bath and children should therefore always be supervised by a responsible adult. Distractions occur easily and the supervising individual should avoid reading, talking on the phone and being under the influence of alcohol or drugs. The importance of learning to swim is well recognised and most children attend swimming classes through school. Every encouragement should be given to ensure that all know the basics of swimming and cardiopulmonary resuscitation.

Road traffic impact

No matter how short the trip, all children who are under 12 years should be backseat passengers and wearing a seat belt. They should not be seated in the front seat as most cars now have airbags, and, if discharged, the force of expansion can kill a young child. Road awareness campaigns are well established in many schools and have helped reduce injuries to pedestrians.

IMPORTANT CLINICAL POINTS

Trauma
- falling blood pressure indicates decompensating shock
- pain assessment and appropriate analgesia are high priority

Drowning
- hypothermia is common and rewarming should occur at a controlled rate
- medical cause should be sought for competent swimmers

Life-threatening haemorrhage
- hypotension is a late sign
- fluid resuscitation to rapidly replace circulating volume to age-appropriate level
- blood products are preferred over crystalloids after initial bolus infusion

Head injuries
- consider nonaccidental injury as a cause in under 2-year age group
- fluids should be restricted to 70% of normal maintenance

Cervical spine injuries
- neck must be immobilised in the neutral position and movement minimised
- a defined sensory level is most important clinical sign

Burns and scalds
- fluids to be started for burns greater than 10% of total body surface area
- Hartmann's solution should be used

Poisoning—caustic substance
- patients present with drooling, hoarse voice, stridor and haematemesis if mucosal damage

Poisoning—paracetamol
- doses over 150 mg/kg are considered toxic
- N-acetylcysteine has a rapid action
- N-acetylcysteine is effective in both preventing and treating hepatotoxicity
- N-acetylcysteine treatment is appropriate if results delayed

Poisoning—salicylates
- respiratory alkalosis develops
- manage with activated charcoal, fluid replacement and urine alkalinisation

Further reading

Head injury: assessment and early management. NICE Clinical guideline [CG176]. Published January 2014. Updated September 2019. https://www.nice.org.uk/guidance/cg176

Poisoning, emergency treatment BNF treatment summary. https://bnfc.nice.org.uk/treatment-summary/poisoning-emergency-treatment.html Accessed January 2022

Unintentional injuries: prevention strategies for under 15s. Public health guideline [PH29]. Published November 2010. https://www.nice.org.uk/guidance/ph29

Chapter | 10 |

Fluids and electrolyte management

Lucy Cliffe, Andrew Lunn

After reading this chapter you should:
- be able to assess, diagnose and manage fluid and electrolyte disturbances
- be able to assess, diagnose and manage disorders of acid-base balance (included elsewhere)

An understanding of fluid and electrolyte requirements in children and young people is of major clinical importance. Patients who are well may need little intervention with their fluid requirements, but an assessment should always be made of their fluid status and reassurance obtained that the normal expected intake and output is appropriate for their age. Patients who are unwell will usually require a detailed review of fluid balance and close monitoring of electrolyte levels. Dehydration and severe electrolyte disturbance need careful management as there is a significant risk of complications if not appropriately addressed. The proposed management of fluids in paediatric practice has to take into account the body changes present in the growing child and the differing impact of any pathological process on differing ages.

Fluid requirements

All children admitted to an inpatient unit should have their fluid status assessed and their requirements and mode of fluid administration determined. The term 'maintenance fluids' is used to describe the volume of daily fluid required to replace the insensible losses (from breathing, perspiration and in the stool) and allow excretion of the excess solute load (urea, creatinine, electrolytes etc.) in a volume of urine that is of an osmolarity similar to plasma.

The standard rates of fluid administration are well established in clinical practice and are calculated from the weight of the patient using the Holliday-Segar formula in the following way (Table 10.1):

Table 10.1 The Holliday-Segar formula for maintenance fluid replacement

Weight	Proposed fluid volume
1–10 kg of weight	100 mls/kg/day
11–20 kg of weight	50 mls/kg/day
each kg over 20 kg	20 mls/kg/day

PRACTICE POINT—Calculation of maintenance fluid requirements

A 23 kg child will require:
- 100 mls/kg for the first 10 kg = 1000 mls
- 50 mls/kg for the second 10 kg = 500 mls
- 20 mls/kg for all additional kgs = 60 mls
- Total = 1560 ml
- Hourly rate = 65 ml/hr

Young adult males rarely need more than 2500 mls and young adult females more than 2000 mls of maintenance fluids in a 24-hour period.

The basis for the Holliday-Segar formula is a proposed correlation between energy requirements and the associated fluid requirements in healthy, growing children. Children who are unwell and admitted to hospital are more likely to be catabolic, inactive and have altered organ function, and there are concerns that the standard formula shown above may overestimate the actual fluid requirements of the ill child. Although the Holliday-Segar formula should be used in the first instance when fluids are required, the potential for overhydration should be borne in mind during ongoing review.

If the weight of the patient is above the 91st centile then it may be advisable to use the body surface area value to calculate IV fluid requirements. In these situations, intravenous maintenance fluid requirements should be given using an estimate of insensible loss of 400 ml/m^2/24 hours plus urine output.

There is little strong evidence for the fluid requirements in a newborn child, but NICE guidelines recommend the following volumes for babies who are given formula feeds (Table 10.2).

While most children will tolerate standard fluid requirements, some acutely ill children with inappropriately increased antidiuretic hormone secretion (SIADH) may benefit from their maintenance fluid requirement being restricted to two-thirds of the normal recommended volume. These children include those with:

- pulmonary disorders (e.g. pneumonia, bronchiolitis)
- CNS disorders (e.g. brain injury and infections, CNS tumours)

Appropriate intravenous fluid

If intravenous fluids are necessary, then isotonic solutions should be used in almost all circumstances to avoid iatrogenic hyponatraemia. There is currently little evidence to recommend a particular strength of glucose. Hypotonic fluids—0.18% and 0.45% sodium chloride with added glucose—should NOT be used as routine maintenance fluids in otherwise healthy children.

A commonly used standard solution for maintenance fluids is 0.9% sodium chloride with 5% dextrose, with or without added potassium. The use of 0.9% sodium chloride solutions will provide more than the required sodium maintenance for most children but, in a well child with normal renal function, this additional sodium will be excreted. In the example given, the 23 kg child given their fluid requirements as 0.9% saline would receive over 10 mmol/kg of sodium in the 24 hours (Table 10.3).

Neonates (0–28 days of life) may have higher glucose requirements and lower sodium requirements, particularly in the first week of life, than these standard fluid preparations provide. Caution and senior supervision is required in prescribing intravenous fluids in this age group.

Ongoing losses

Ongoing losses should be assessed every four hours and the fluids chosen as replacement should reflect the electrolyte composition of the fluid being lost. In most circumstances this will be sodium chloride 0.9% with or without the addition of potassium.

Monitoring

Hyponatraemia can develop within a short timescale, and a robust monitoring regime is essential. Weight should be measured, if possible, prior to commencing fluid therapy and daily thereafter whilst fluid balance, including oral intake and ongoing losses, should be recorded and the balance calculated. Plasma sodium, potassium, urea, creatinine and glucose should be measured at baseline and at least once a day in any child receiving intravenous fluids with further electrolyte measurements every four to six hours if an abnormal reading is found.

Glucose monitoring is particularly important as plasma levels may rise during treatment with glucose containing solutions. Analysis of the urine chemistry may be

Table 10.2 Maintenance fluid amounts for a newborn baby	
Day 1	50–60 ml/kg/day
Day 2	70–80 ml/kg/day
Day 3	80–100 ml/kg/day
Day 4	100–120 ml/kg/day
Days 5–28	120–150 ml/kg/day

Table 10.3 Composition of commonly used fluids						
Fluid type	Osmolality mOsmol/l	Tonicity	Sodium (mmol/l)	Chloride (mmol/l)	Potassium (mmol/l)	Glucose (gm/l)
0.9% saline	308	Isotonic	154	154	0	0
0.45% NaCl with 5% dextrose with 20 mmol/l K+	432	Hypotonic	77	77	20	50
Hartmann's solution	278	Isotonic	131	111	5	0
Plasma-Lyte	294	Isotonic	140	98	5	0
5% glucose	278	Hypotonic	0	0	0	50

Table 10.4 Assessment of hydration status. Items in capitals are recognised RED FLAG findings.

	No clinically detectable dehydration (< 3% weight loss)	Clinical dehydration (3%–10% weight loss)	Clinical shock (>10% weight loss)
Symptoms	appears well	APPEARS TO BE UNWELL OR DETERIORATING	
	alert and responsive	IRRITABLE AND LETHARGIC	decreased level of consciousness
	normal urine output	reduced urine output	
	skin colour unchanged	skin colour changed	pale or mottled skin
	warm extremities	warm extremities	cold extremities
Signs	eyes not sunken	SUNKEN EYES	
	moist mucous membranes	dry mucous membranes	
	normal heart rate	TACHYCARDIA	tachycardia
	normal breathing pattern	TACHYPNOEA	tachypnoea
	normal peripheral pulses	normal peripheral pulses	weak peripheral pulses
	normal capillary refill time	normal capillary refill time	prolonged capillary refill time
	normal skin turgor	REDUCED SKIN TURGOR	
	normal blood pressure	normal blood pressure	hypotension

Table 10.5 Fluid requirement in response to assessed dehydration

	No clinically detectable dehydration (< 3% weight loss)	Clinical dehydration (3%–10% weight loss)	Clinical shock (>10% weight loss)
Action	Oral rehydration solutions (ORS) given following maintenance phase	repletion—ORS at 50–100 ml/kg over 4 hours plus ongoing losses maintenance—required amounts plus ongoing losses	repletion—emergency IV fluids at 20 ml/kg isotonic solution.

useful in a small number of patients with high-risk conditions or when the cause behind an abnormal sodium result is unclear. Fluid balance and the ongoing need for intravenous fluids along with the details of the fluid prescription should be reviewed twice daily.

Assessment of hydration status

The clinical assessment of hydration is difficult and often inaccurate. In children who are dehydrated the accepted gold standard of assessment is a calculation of an acute weight loss but this is often not possible due to lack of accurate pre-illness weight. A weight should, however, be recorded at presentation and compared to any subsequent weight measurements (Table 10.4).

Prolonged capillary refill time, abnormal skin turgor, dry mucous membranes and absent tears have been shown to be the best individual examination measures. If two out of four of these parameters are present the child has a high chance of being more than 5% dehydrated.

Management of dehydration
Oral rehydration therapy

Gastroenteritis is one of the major causes of morbidity and mortality in children worldwide, and in those under 5 years of age, death is the more likely outcome. There has, however, been a decline in mortality over the last few decades due to the introduction and availability of oral rehydration solutions (ORS).

Management of children with significant diarrhoea is usually divided into two phases for management:
- **repletion phase**—any calculated fluid deficit is replaced over 2–3 hours with frequent, small amounts of the oral rehydration solution. Ongoing fluid losses are added to the calculated requirement.

- **maintenance phase**—continued use of rehydration solutions until child able to reestablish normal feeding pattern. Ongoing fluid losses are added to the calculated requirement.

The fluid deficit from dehydration needs to be calculated and introduced to the rehydration management plan (Table 10.5).

PRACTICE POINT—Fluid deficit

Fluid deficit in ml = % dehydration x weight (kg) x 10

This estimate is calculated from the child's weight and the clinically assessed degree of dehydration.

PRACTICE POINT—Calculation of fluid deficit

A 23 kg child is assessed as moderately dehydrated at an estimated 5% dehydrated. 23 kg is equivalent to 23 litres and if he is 5% dehydrated, then his deficit is 5% of 23 litres:

$$5/100 \times 23 \times 1000 = 1150 \text{ mls}$$

The deficit is usually replaced over 24 hours and so should be added to the total daily maintenance volume before determining the hourly rate:

One day maintenance (1560 ml) plus 5% deficit (1150 ml) = 2710 ml over 24 hours = 112 mls/hr

---

If the fluid deficit is to be replaced over a longer period, as in hypernatraemic dehydration, then the deficit has to be added to twice the daily maintenance and divide by 48 hours. It will also be important to also add any ongoing losses. In these situations, very close monitoring and accurate fluid balance checks are vital.

Resuscitation

If signs of circulatory collapse are present (prolonged capillary refill time, tachycardia or hypotension), then immediate resuscitation of intravascular volume must occur. This should take place through intravenous or intraosseous access lines, and an initial bolus of 20 ml/kg of isotonic 0.9% sodium chloride should be used. Reassessment of volume status and consideration of the cause of circulatory collapse is crucial.

More details are presented in Chapter 8 Emergency medicine.

Risk of acute kidney injury

Certain children and young people are particularly at risk of developing acute kidney injury from dehydration if any of the following are present or likely:
- young age
- hypovolaemia or hypotension
- chronic kidney disease/transplant
- oliguria (urine output less than 0.5 ml/kg/hr)
- sepsis
- a deteriorating paediatric Early Warning Score

Serum creatinine must be checked against any known baseline values for that patient, and if it is 1.5 times or more above that baseline then the risk of acute kidney injury is high. An estimated GFR (eGFR) of less than 90 ml/min per 1.73 m^2 would also indicate that a patient may be at risk of developing acute kidney injury.

Electrolyte disturbance

Hyponatraemia

Hyponatraemia is defined as a plasma sodium of less than 135 mmol/l and severe hyponatraemia when the plasma sodium falls below 130 mmol/l. It is a common electrolyte abnormality in hospitalised children, and the most common cause is the result of an expanded extracellular fluid volume rather than by sodium depletion—the child with severe gastroenteritis who then receives hypotonic fluid replacement is then likely to develop hyponatraemic dehydration. Consequently, it is important to assess the fluid volume status of a child in order to understand the cause of the hyponatraemia and the required management. A major consequence of hyponatraemia is an influx of water into the intracellular space resulting in cellular swelling.

Causes of hyponatraemia

- iatrogenic
  - intravenous fluid administration (hypotonic solutions)
  - diuretic medication
  - diluted formula feeds (including factitious illness)
  - desmopressin use
- SIADH
  - CNS infections
  - head injury

- bronchiolitis, pneumonia
- surgery
- extrarenal sodium losses
  - gastroenteritis
  - skin (sweating, burns)
  - third space losses
- renal sodium losses
  - polyuric phase of acute tubular necrosis
  - interstitial nephritis
  - cerebral salt wasting
  - absence of aldosterone or lack of effect
- other
  - glucocorticoid deficiency
  - hypothyroidism
  - nephrotic syndrome
  - diabetic ketoacidosis
  - psychogenic polydipsia

Clinical presentation

The symptoms and signs of severe hyponatraemia are predominantly neurological and the result of cerebral oedema and include:
- headache
- nausea, vomiting
- lethargy or irritability
- hyporeflexia
- confusion and disorientation
- seizures
- decreased conscious state

Hyponatraemic encephalopathy is a serious complication and children are particularly susceptible to developing neurological complications. This is due to the reduced space for brain swelling in the skull and impaired ability of the paediatric brain to adapt to hyponatraemia.

Investigations

The serum osmolality (paired with urinary osmolality) taken before fluid replacement can be diagnostically helpful particularly in suspected SIADH when a concentrated urine (high urine osmolality) is seen with a relatively low plasma osmolality (Table 10.6).

Treatment and management

All children with confirmed hyponatraemia should have two hourly neurological observations until the plasma sodium level returns to normal.

The child with normal or increased volume status

The maintenance fluids should be restricted to 50% of requirements to slowly remove the increased body water, and 0.9% sodium chloride with added dextrose should be used if IV fluids are necessary. Hypotonic solutions must not be given.

The child with moderate dehydration and serum sodium 130–135 mmol/l

The child should be offered oral or nasogastric rehydration to provide both a maintenance and a deficit amount. If nasogastric rehydration is not possible or it results in a too rapid rise in sodium, then intravenous 0.9% sodium chloride with 5% dextrose should be used.

The child with severe dehydration or dehydration with serum sodium less than 130 mmol/l

Intravenous fluids are necessary and 0.9% sodium chloride with 5% dextrose would be the appropriate choice of fluids until the child can take enteral feeds. The calculated amount will again include maintenance plus deficit. Close monitoring and recording of both fluid intake and output along with daily weighing are all important.

Acute hyponatraemic encephalopathy is a medical emergency

Intravenous fluids are necessary and 0.9% sodium chloride with 5% dextrose would be appropriate. The ideal rate of correction of a low serum sodium depends on the presence and severity of symptoms. Correction that is too rapid (greater than 8 mmol/l of sodium per 24 hr) can

Table 10.6 Examples of changes in plasma and urine osmolality in various conditions					
	Normal (after 12 hr fluid restriction)	Central diabetes insipidus	SIADH	Decreased plasma sodium	Increased plasma sodium
Plasma osmolality (mOsmol/kg)	275–295	305	260	265	325
Urine osmolality (mOsmol/kg)	> 850	110	650	90	690

result in cerebral demyelination with risk of severe and lasting brain injury. This is especially a risk if hyponatraemia has been present for more than 5 days and is then rapidly corrected.

The hyponatraemic child with seizures or CNS depression

Such a child requires prompt resuscitation and intravenous anticonvulsants as clinically indicated. Hyponatraemic seizures often respond poorly to conventional anticonvulsants and sodium correction should not be delayed. The sodium should be raised until it reaches 125 mmol/l or until seizures stop using intravenous hypertonic sodium chloride solution over 15–30 minutes.

Potential alternative causes for seizures (fever, meningitis, hypoglycaemia) should be sought and addressed. After the seizures have resolved the total increase in sodium, including the rise following the bolus, should not exceed 8 mmol/l per 24 hours. Electrolytes should be measured hourly until the patient is stable, then every 4–6 hours until the serum sodium is normal and the child is off intravenous fluids.

Hypernatraemia

Hypernatraemia is defined as a serum sodium greater than 145 mmol/l; however, it is usually acted on once sodium is over 150 mmol/l.

Causes of hypernatraemia include:
- water and sodium loss
  - gastroenteritis
  - burns
  - diabetes mellitus
- water deficit
  - diabetes insipidus (nephrogenic or central)
  - increased insensible losses—preterm, phototherapy
  - inadequate intake—failure to establish breastfeeding
- excessive sodium intake
  - inappropriately prepared infant formula
  - salt poisoning
  - hypertonic intravenous fluids
  - hyperaldosteronism

Clinical presentation

Most children with hypernatraemia are clinically dehydrated since there is a shift of water from the intracellular to extracellular space and initially infants and children can be less symptomatic. Clinical features of hypernatraemia include:
- 'doughy' feel to the skin.
- irritability
- weakness, lethargy

The degree of dehydration should be assessed from the clinical features and a fluid deficit calculated. If there is no sign of dehydration in the setting of hypernatraemia, it is important to consider causes related to excessive salt intake from infused fluids, medications given or salt poisoning which may be intentional or accidental.

Treatment and management

An understanding of the likely cause of the dehydration will direct the subsequent management of the hypernatraemia.

For hypernatraemic dehydration with serum sodium greater than 150 mmol/l

Any proposed correction of this degree of hypernatraemia should avoid rapid changes as this may cause cerebral oedema, convulsion and death. The deficit can be corrected over 48 hours with the aim of a fall in serum sodium concentration of less than 0.5 mmol/L per hour. If the plasma sodium is over 170 mmol/l then even greater caution is required and a slower correction of the deficit over 72 hours would be more appropriate.

The route of administration of the replacement fluid can be by a nasogastric tube using oral rehydration solution or with IV fluids using 0.9% sodium chloride with 5% dextrose although the concentration of sodium in the administered fluid may need to be adjusted at a later stage according to the clinical response and underlying cause. Close monitoring is required with repeat electrolytes undertaken every 4 hours until stable.

Hypernatraemic dehydration with excessive weight loss in breastfed babies will require specific additional management to support mothers with newborn feeding.

Hypokalaemia

Hypokalaemia is defined as a potassium level below 3.4 mmol/l but symptoms tend not to occur until levels go below 3.0 mmol/l. As potassium falls, there is a net movement from the intracellular spaces into the extracellular spaces and therefore the serum levels will underestimate total body stores.

Causes

The common causes of hypokalaemia are:
- gastrointestinal losses due to protracted diarrhoea or vomiting
- iatrogenic—diuretic therapy, salbutamol, amphotericin
- diabetic ketoacidosis and its treatment
- sepsis

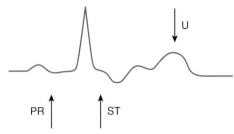

Fig. 10.1 ECG changes in hypokalaemia. Prolonged PR interval, ST depression, inverted T waves, U wave evident.

- renal tubular defects
  It is also a manifestation of:
- hypomagnesaemia
- Cushing syndrome
- hyperaldosteronism
- Bartter syndrome

Clinical presentation

Clinical signs tend to become apparent when potassium level falls below 2.5 mmol/l and recognised features include:
- muscle weakness and cramps
- characteristic ECG abnormalities (Figure 10.1) include:
  - ST segment depression
  - U wave
  - T waves flattened or of low amplitude
  - PR interval prolonged

Treatment and management

When potassium fall below 2.5 mmol/l, patients should have continuous cardiac monitoring and attempts made to identify and treat the underlying condition. Options for treatment depend on the state of the child and ability to tolerate oral fluids.

Oral supplementation

Supplementation, in the form of potassium chloride, to a maximum of 2 mmol/kg/day in divided doses is common but more may be required in practice. Unfortunately, most of the standard preparations of potassium are not very palatable and there may be a practical issue in the administration of the medication

Intravenous supplementation of maintenance fluids

Most situations will be managed using preprepared bags of infusion fluid with added potassium and the maximum

concentration via a peripheral vein is usually 40 mmol per litre.

Those patients who are not actively losing potassium through urine, stool or gastric losses will be able to cope with high potassium intakes until the total body stores are replaced and they will suddenly become hyperkalaemic. Such patients need close monitoring.

Hyperkalaemia

True hyperkalaemia is a rare, but life-threatening, emergency. In many incidences, however, the hyperkalaemia may be artefactual (pseudohyperkalaemia), and a repeat of the test may be indicated when high potassium levels are unexpectedly found and the patient is well or ECG changes are not consistent with the potassium level. The causes of a true hyperkalaemia are wide ranging but the clinical priority lies in treating the raised potassium and ensuring the patient remains stable. Once this is achieved, further investigations are required to establish the cause of the hyperkalaemia.

Causes

- pseudohyperkalaemia
  - haemolysed blood sample
  - EDTA contamination of sample (take lithium heparin samples first)
  - significant leucocytosis or thrombocytosis—tumour lysis syndrome
- increased potassium intake
  - sample taken from arm receiving IV fluids containing potassium
  - high potassium load from IV fluids or TPN
  - blood transfusion
- movement of potassium from intracellular to extracellular space
  - cellular injury—rhabdomyolysis, haemolysis, tumour lysis
  - metabolic or respiratory acidosis

- insulin deficiency
- drugs—beta blockers, suxamethonium, digoxin toxicity
- impaired renal excretion of potassium
  - chronic or acute kidney disease
  - dehydration or hypovolaemia
  - aldosterone deficiency
- drugs
  - potassium sparing diuretics—spironolactone, amiloride
  - nonsteroidal antiinflammatory drugs—ibuprofen
  - ACE inhibitors—captopril, enalapril, lisinopril

Clinical presentation

Symptoms are rare but those with potassium levels over 7 mmol/l may experience:

- muscle weakness
- palpitations or syncope secondary to cardiac conduction disturbance
- ECG abnormalities (Figure 10.2) recognised
  - wide complex tachycardia and ventricular fibrillation
  - peaked T waves
  - loss of P waves
  - short QT

Treatment and management

The immediate response to receiving a result indicating hyperkalaemia would be to remove any obvious extraneous source of potassium and any medications that may increase serum potassium levels.

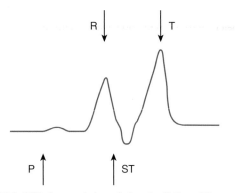

Fig. 10.2 ECG changes in hyperkalaemia. Flattened P wave, flattened R wave, ST depression, peaked T waves.

Moderate hyperkalaemia (potassium over 5.9 mmol/l)

Patients with potassium levels between 5.5 and 7.0 mmol/l are generally asymptomatic but need close monitoring with ECG and repeat levels after a short interval. Discussion with a senior colleague is important as directing the expectant course needs experienced advice.

Severe hyperkalaemia (potassium over 7 mmol/l)

The patient should have a continuous ECG in place and, if characteristic changes to the trace are noted, then intravenous calcium gluconate must be administered promptly. This leads to a rapid increasing ionised calcium and stabilises the cardiac membrane. The effects are, however, short lived and the dose is usually repeated after 5 minutes if the ECG changes are still present. In the interim, other agents such as nebulised salbutamol can be prepared that will move extracellular potassium into the cells. If the potassium level remains high, then sodium bicarbonate, furosemide or an insulin/glucose infusion can be considered following senior discussion. Haemodialysis may be indicated after discussion with colleagues in paediatric nephrology.

Relevant pharmacological agents used

Calcium gluconate—immediate impact on cardiac conduction

Should be given intravenously when significant ECG abnormalities are identified and works by stabilising the cardiac membrane.

Insulin and glucose infusion—10 to 20 minutes to produce an effect

This intervention will move potassium from the plasma into the cells but should only be used if significant ECG changes are noted and the high potassium level is confirmed. The treatment may induce hypoglycaemia and therefore close monitoring of glucose levels is important with supplemental glucose readily available.

Salbutamol—20 to 30 minutes to produce an effect

Can be given via a nebuliser or by slow intravenous infusion over 5 minutes.

Furosemide—60 to 120 minutes to produce an effect

Enhances potassium excretion but may induce hypovolaemia.

Calcium resonium—60 to 120 minutes to produce an effect

Given orally or PR and works by binding to potassium.

IMPORTANT CLINICAL POINTS

Fluid replacement

- oral route should be first choice wherever possible
- intravenous fluids require careful prescribing and close monitoring
- routine IV fluids should be isotonic crystalloids with sodium 131–154 mmol/l
- hypotonic fluids should not be used due to risk of hyponatraemia

Sodium

- Hyponatraemia
  - severe when plasma sodium below 130 mmol/l
  - usually due to expanded extracellular fluid volume and not sodium depletion
- Hypernatraemia
  - significant when serum sodium over 150 mmol/l
  - common cause is inadequate intake in breastfed baby

Potassium

- Hypokalaemia
  - symptoms appear below 3.0 mmol/l
  - ECG—prolonged PR interval, ST depression, flattened T waves, U wave
- Hyperkalaemia
  - ECG—flattened P wave, flattened R wave, ST depression, peaked T waves
  - severe hyperkalaemia (potassium over 7 mmol/l)
  - IV calcium gluconate as has immediate impact on cardiac conduction

CLINICAL SCENARIO

An 8-month-old girl presented with vomiting, diarrhoea and growth retardation. Her mother explained that the vomiting had started some 24 hours previously and the diarrhoea over the preceding 12 hours. There was no obvious blood in the stool. The child had been reviewed by health visitor and GP on numerous occasions with concerns about poor weight gain and a referral to a general clinic had been made.

Apart from the poor weight gain, the child had previously been well following a normal pregnancy and delivery. Her father was a surgical registrar, mother a staff nurse and they had one other healthy boy aged 22 months. No relevant family history.

Examination showed her to be apyrexial, heart rate 110, BP 80/60 and capillary refill of 3 seconds. Her tone was normal but her reflexes were noted to be brisk. No other abnormalities were found on full systems examination.

A provisional diagnosis of viral gastroenteritis with mild dehydration was made and the child was admitted, a nasogastric tube inserted and a rehydration regime commenced. At a review at 24 hours after admission, there had been little improvement although the frequency of diarrhoea stool had reduced. Bloods were requested.

These revealed sodium 182 mmol/l, potassium 3.9 mmol/l, bicarbonate 26 mmol/l, urea 3.9 mmol/l, creatinine 45 μmol/l, glucose 3.9 mmol/l. Repeat samples confirmed these results.

A differential diagnosis at this stage would include gastroenteritis, diabetes insipidus, inappropriately prepared infant formula, salt poisoning or hyperaldosteronism.

Although gastroenteritis was a possible explanation, it was felt that the degree of hypernatraemia was beyond that expected. The volumes of powdered milk used to make the feeds was reviewed and found to be appropriate. Hyperaldosteronism is exceptionally rare in children.

Further investigations were undertaken including urinary sodium. This was found to be markedly elevated and indicated that the child had a greater intake of sodium than required.

Salt poisoning was therefore the presumed diagnosis and an initial discrete discussion was had with social services. Following their involvement, both parents were interviewed and both expressed their shock at this suggestion. The parents were denied access to the child and her blood results returned to normal over the next 48 hours. The sibling of this girl was removed from the parental home and placed in the care of grandparents whilst further safeguarding investigations by social services and police were undertaken.

Further Reading

Intravenous fluids therapy in children. NICE Guideline NG29. December 2015. Updated June 2020. Accessed September 2020. www.nice.org.uk/guidance/ng29

Chapter 11

Safeguarding

Roshan Adappa, Elhindi Elfaki, Colin Powell, Martin Hewitt

After reading this chapter you should be able to:
- recognise the different presentations of abuse
- assess and manage abuse and fabricated illness
- know the emotional and behavioural consequence of abuse and neglect

Safeguarding children is the responsibility of everyone

Parents, wider family members, carers, teachers, health professionals, law enforcement agencies and society at large must have a role in protecting children and young people from physical or emotional harm. It is important to recognise that child abuse occurs in all societies, all cultures, all socioeconomic groups, all ethnic groups and all parental age groups.

Health professionals need to be aware of, and recognise, the features and signs of abuse when they meet children and understand that intervention and taking appropriate actions could prevent potentially catastrophic consequence for the child. Most perpetrators of child abuse are known to the child and are often in a position of authority with the ability to manipulate and coerce the child or young person.

PRACTICE POINT—factors increasing the risk of child abuse

- child disability
- parental mental health problems
- parental alcohol abuse
- parental drug abuse
- domestic violence
- socioeconomic deprivation

Proving that particular injuries are the result of abuse is difficult as usually only the perpetrator and the victim were present at the time of the event. Features that should raise suspicion include:
- age of the child—inconsistent with the explanation of injury
- changing history of events
- unreasonable delay in seeking help
- repeated contact with health care services
- repeated injuries and presentation to emergency department
- suggested mechanism of trauma—"fell off settee onto carpeted floor"
- multiple fractures
- fractures in unusual bones for age
- fractures of different ages
- inappropriate adult reaction including aggression, vagueness, lack of concern
- obvious anxiety or inappropriate reactions of the child
- evidence of neglect or poor growth

The recognised forms of child abuse are:
- physical abuse
- neglect
- emotional abuse
- fabricated and induced illness
- sexual abuse

Physical abuse

Recognising that a particular pattern of physical injury is unusual for the age of the child or that it may be the result of physical abuse is a difficult aspect of paediatric care. The issue is further compounded by the fact that children are prone to falls, accidents and injury and thereby sustain physical injuries that have accidental causes. Types of injury seen in physical abuse are:

- bruises
- fractures
- burns
- head injury

Bruises

Bruising is the most common physical sign of abuse and various factors must be considered when abuse is suspected. These would include:

- age of child
- explanation of cause
- location of bruising
- pattern of bruising

The **age** of the child will dictate mobility; it is unusual for a baby or a nonmobile child to have bruising. Bruising is commonly seen in mobile children especially toddlers who are starting to walk.

The **location** of bruises on the shin, knees and elbows are common in a child who is just starting to walk and are usually on the front of the body. Toddlers are likely to injure their foreheads, nose, chin or the back of their head and hence bruises in these locations are not always suspicious. Unusual areas of bruising that should raise suspicion of abuse are ears, neck, buttocks and back of trunk. Bruises in the upper arm or thigh may represent a forceful grip with small circular 'fingertip' bruises evident. Bruises on sites away from bony prominences (Figure 11.1) are of concern and require further assessment usually with the child in a place of safety.

The **pattern** of bruising can give clues to the mechanism of injury; pinch marks, hand slap marks (Figure 11.2a and 11.2b), belts (Figure 11.3a and 11.3b) and shoes all cause recognisable bruising patterns. Cluster of bruises with petechiae are common in abuse as they suggest a forceful squeeze or sudden impact leading to leakage from small vessels in the skin. Bite marks (Figure 11.4) leave a characteristic circular pattern of bruising on the skin, and although they can be caused by abusing adults, they can also be caused by other children. This distinction may be obvious, but if doubt exists then the opinion of a forensic dentist will help identify specific tooth patterns and differentiate between the bite from an adult or child.

Colour of bruises change over time and the recording of this was previously used to date the injury. Current evidence, however, suggests that such observations and conclusions are not reliable.

Plausible explanations for bruises

- idiopathic thrombocytopenic purpura
- rare causes of low platelets and bleeding—e.g. leukaemia
- coagulation disorders
- congenital dermal melanocytosis in babies

Fractures

Fractures are a common childhood injury but are the second most common physical injury seen in child abuse. X-rays undertaken for other reasons may identify unexplained and healing fractures and thereby raise suspicion of a previous physical injury. Fractures in children under 18 months and, in particular, in those who are not ambulatory should raise suspicion of an abusive cause. The incidence of fractures as a result of abuse reduces as the child grows older.

Multiple rib fractures, particularly those of different ages or posteromedial in position, without a known history of trauma, birth injury or metabolic bone disease

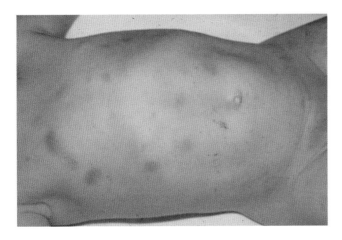

Figure 11.1 Abnormal bruising on anterior surface of chest and abdomen suggesting physical abuse. (Copyright – Dr M Hewitt - used with permission)

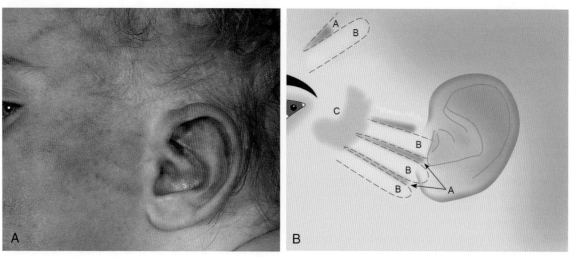

Figure 11.2 A and B. These figures show bruises caused by slap on the face. The ear is bruised. The obvious linear bruises (A) are caused by gap between the fingers allowing capillaries to burst whilst the adjacent paler areas (B) show the impact area of the fingers. The larger bruise (C) is created by the palm of the hand. (Images copyright – Dr M Hewitt - used with permission)

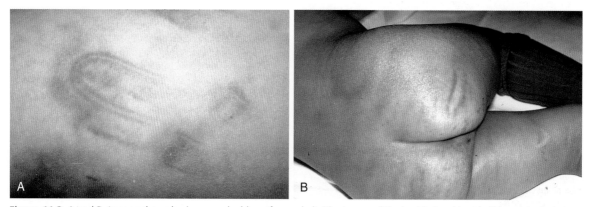

Figure 11.3 A and B. Images shows bruise cause by blows from a belt. The image of the buckle is evident in (A) and the belt pattern in (B). (Copyright – Dr M Hewitt – images used with permission)

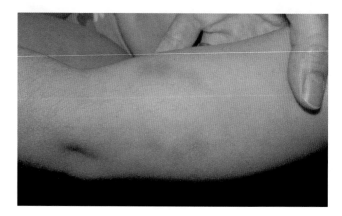

Figure 11.4 This image shows bruise caused by adult bite mark. (Copyright – Dr M Hewitt - used with permission)

should be considered as abusive in origin and a comprehensive assessment undertaken. The presumed mechanism of these rib injuries is that the infant is held tightly around the chest and shaken.

CLINICAL SCENARIO

A 5-month-old boy was brought to the emergency department with a short history of poor feeding, cough and pyrexia. Examination found him to be tachycardic, tachypnoeic with hypoxaemia and localised crackles in left base. He had been born at 34 weeks' gestation and required CPR at birth due to the umbilical cord being around the neck. He had been well since discharge at 3 weeks of age.

A CXR was requested in the emergency department and showed patchy changes in the lower left area. He was given supplemental oxygen and IV fluids and started on IV antibiotics.

The subsequent review of the CXR by the consultant radiologist identified three posterior rib fractures with callus formation. There were no features suggesting an underlying bone disorder.

The question was therefore asked as to whether these identified fractures were the result of the cardiac massage at birth. The radiologist advised that if callus was present on a CXR when the infant was over 3 months of age (and over 3 months since the episode of CPR) then the fractures would not be considered to result from CPR early in the neonatal period. Any fractures induced over 3 months previously would be expected to have healed and be fully remodelled or in a late stage of remodelling without overt callus.

The conclusion was that the fractures were recent and the result of nonaccidental injury. Safeguarding procedures were implemented.

Metaphyseal fractures are also described in abuse and are seen with multiple other injuries in fatal abuse. In the very young, it is thought to be the result of the limb being pulled or twisted, causing the shearing of the metaphysis. Rarer fractures such as scapular fractures or sternal fractures are also highly suspicious of abuse.

Fractures of the long bones such as humerus and femur are common in both accidental and nonaccidental injury. The most common abusive humeral fractures in children aged less than 5 years are spiral or oblique although it is now recognised that some accidents such as falling down stairs could result in spiral fractures. Supracondylar humeral fractures are common in accidental injury

Table 11.1 Features of fractures that are suggestive of abusive trauma

fractures in absence of adequate explanation
multiple fractures
spiral fracture of humerus in under 5 years
oblique fracture of humerus in under 5 years
under 18 months
metaphyseal fractures
spiral fracture of femur in 'nonwalker' (under 15 months)
metaphyseal fractures in young

although a fracture of the humeral shaft in a child less than 18 months is suspicious (Table 11.1).

When abuse is suspected a detailed skeletal survey of the whole body is undertaken and follow-up images at 4 to 6 weeks to reveal newer fractures as they mineralise and calcify.

The dating of fractures is difficult and the confidence in the time of injury will be over weeks rather than days. Even if the initial skeletal survey is normal, a shorter series of follow-up images should be repeated on all children within 11 to 14 days as this may identify fractures which only become visible when healing.

Plausible explanations for causes of fracture

- Preterm babies less than 28 weeks' gestation at birth or babies with a birthweight less than 1500 gm are at risk of osteopenia and therefore an increased risk of fractures. The most common abnormality seen is fractures to the ribs and are usually an incidental finding on a chest x-ray. Long bones are rarely involved.
- Osteogenesis imperfecta is described in more detail in Chapter 29 Musculoskeletal system.
- Vitamin D deficiency and rickets, scurvy and osteomyelitis can cause metaphyseal changes but rarely cause fractures.
- Children with severe disability have a higher risk of fractures due bone demineralisation from prolonged immobility. Unfortunately, this group of children and young people is also at an increased risk of physical abuse and attempting to clarify the cause of any fracture can be difficult.

Burns

Burns can be caused by:
- contact with hot surfaces—hot radiators or an iron
- immersion of limbs in hot water (Figure 11.5)—produces a glove or stocking distribution

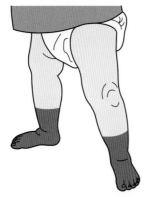

Figure 11.5 Diagram showing 'stocking distribution' of burns in both legs when forced immersion in hot water (Image used with permission from Illustrated Textbook of Paediatrics. Lissauer T, Carroll, W. 5th Ed. 2017. Elsevier Ltd.)

- cigarette burns (Figure 11.6)—produce deep, circular craters with discrete margins

Plausible explanations for causes of skin lesions

- skin infection such as impetigo, staphylococcal scalded skin syndrome
- nappy rash
- ringworm skin infection

Head trauma

Physical abuse that causes head trauma has the highest risk of significant morbidity and mortality. Features suggestive of abusive injury have already been presented, but an inconsistency between the severity of the head injury and the explanation given or a history of a sudden collapse in a previously well child should immediately raise concerns.

Skull x-rays are not useful in the investigation of a child presenting with head trauma and they should not be requested. When there is a suspicion of nonaccidental head injury, a CT of the head should be requested and should take place within an hour of the injury. Linear skull fractures are seen in both abusive and nonabusive trauma and often occur after a seemingly short fall whereas the cause of more complex fractures of the skull need to be assessed in context of the history given. There may be associated cervical and spinal injury with any head injury and appropriate imaging should be considered.

Retinal haemorrhages can be the result of violent shaking and are often associated with head injury and consequently an early ophthalmology assessment is important.

CLINICAL SCENARIO

A 15-month-old boy was brought to ED by both his parents at about 22:00 hrs. They described that he had tried to climb a bunk bed ladder and had fallen backward and hit his head on the bedroom floor. He became drowsy after the fall. There were no relevant features in the past history and he was described as usually very active child.

Examination showed a reduced conscious level and a large haematoma on the left parietal area. There were no other bruises identified.

An urgent CT of head showed a complex, left-sided skull fracture and subdural haematoma and the child was promptly referred to the neurosurgical team for intervention. A subsequent skeletal survey showed no other abnormalities.

The paediatric team felt that the described cause was not consistent with the severity of the findings and the concerns were shared with the parents. The need for further investigations was outlined and parents refused permission for the skeletal survey. Clotting was normal and ophthalmology review reported no abnormalities. A senior surgeon at the hospital made contact with the paediatric consultant to say that he knew the family socially and reassured the team that the parents were 'well balanced' and would not harm their child.

The social worker and paediatric consultant again met with the parents and pointed out that the skeletal survey was part of normal and expected safeguarding practice and that if they refused permission for this to take place then an urgent court order would be requested. After consideration, the parents agreed to the radiological investigation; this was reported as normal.

The child remained in hospital and the parents were only allowed supervised access.

Some two days later, the mother confided in nursing staff that both parents had attended a party at a friend's house and left the young child in the care of their 11-year-old daughter. The daughter had taken the young boy onto the top bunk to play and he had fallen from that height. The story was confirmed by the 11-year-old daughter.

The safeguarding MDT accepted the updated description of events but decided that both children should be placed on the 'at-risk' register and so allow ongoing social work access. The phone call from the consultant surgeon was reported to the medical director of the hospital who reprimanded the senior surgeon for the inappropriate intervention and poor understanding of safeguarding issues.

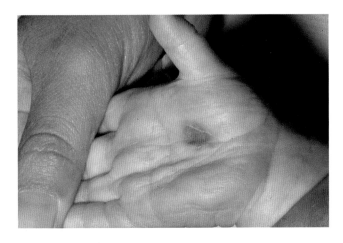

Figure 11.6 Cigarette burn (Copyright – Dr M Hewitt - used with permission)

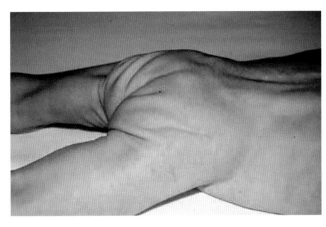

Figure 11.7 Wasting of the buttocks suggesting inadequate nutrition due to parental neglect (Copyright – Dr M Hewitt - used with permission)

Neglect and emotional abuse

Neglect is a form of child abuse where in the normal needs of the child are not met by the carers. This takes the form of poor nutrition (Figure 11.7), lack of hygiene, failure to address medical needs, educational neglect, lack of supervision and awareness of safety and emotional abuse. This could be the result of the parent or carer having significant mental, physical or other social issues resulting in them being unable to care for the child or meet the expected parental responsibilities. Parental use of drugs and alcohol, poverty and social isolation are also contributing factors.

If poor growth is observed in an infant and neglect is considered to be a likely cause then a period of admission to a hospital ward with the exclusion of parents from participating in feeding may be required. A prompt return towards the expected growth trajectory would be observed and is supporting evidence for parental neglect (Figure 11.8).

Emotional abuse and emotional deprivation are a part of neglect where the child experiences ridicule, denigration, aggression, intimidation and rejection in a nonphysical but hostile environment. Emotional abuse and neglect are common but they can be very difficult to recognise or prove particularly if these are the only forms of abuse experienced by the child. Unfortunately, many children who experience neglect also experience physical and emotional abuse.

Some of the identifiable features of neglect and emotional abuse are age related.

Infants and toddlers can display a passive or muted interaction with mother or carer and be withdrawn with poor attachment behaviour.

Toddlers may have episodes of anxiety and fearfulness that may evolve into aggression and resistant behaviour whilst others become apathetic and withdrawn. These young children often show cognitive delay and language delay.

School-aged children who are subjected to emotional abuse or neglect may become aggressive,

113

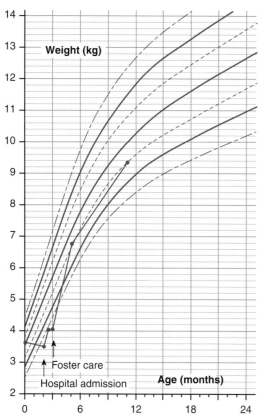

Figure 11.8 Growth chart demonstrating growth retardation that then corrects during a period of hospital admission suggesting neglect through inadequate feeding

disruptive and have friendship difficulties and poor social interactions. They may have poor academic performance, delinquent tendencies and have significant mental health issues such as depression and suicidal tendencies.

Perplexing presentation and fabricated or induced illness (FII)

Perplexing presentation is a situation where the signs and symptoms in a child cannot be explained by, or fit into, any known medical condition. One of the possible explanations is that the symptoms are either exaggerated or invented by the parents or carers that then raises questions regarding their motivation.

The child might need admission to allow the observation of the suggested signs and symptoms. The parents or carers

should be informed that the symptoms and signs do not fit into an obvious medical condition and hence in such situations there is a need to ensure that there are no child protection issues. This may be a difficult discussion and should be undertaken by a senior member of the paediatric team.

The term fabricated or induced illness replaces terminology such as Munchausen by proxy, and is used when a parent or carer gives an exaggerated or false history of symptoms or is suspected of inducing the symptoms. In this situation, the child is at risk of harm as they may be exposed to injury or unnecessary investigations and treatment.

The child is in danger of significant harm when symptoms are suspected of being induced by smothering, overdosing of medications or the administration of noxious substances or poisons. In such situations, it is important to admit the child to a place of safety for a period of observation and the parent or carer denied access. Such actions will require the involvement of social services and police. If no symptoms or signs are observed during the period of admission then the likelihood is that the symptoms were induced by the carers.

CLINICAL SCENARIO

An 8-year-old girl was referred for outpatient review by her GP with a potential diagnosis of seizures. The family had recently moved to the area and the mother reported that the child had been investigated at a hospital near their previous residence. Mother described episodes of collapse during the day when her daughter became unresponsive with her arms and legs shaking wildly. The episodes lasted about 10 minutes and required buccal midazolam that had been provided by the previous hospital. The episodes occurred roughly twice a week. The daughter was described as 'sleepy' after the episodes and she had no memory of the events.

Mum said she had tried to video the episodes but was never able to find her phone when needed and she had never called an ambulance for the events as she herself had epilepsy and was confident in their management. There were no other witnesses to events and none had been seen by staff at the school. The girl had missed a significant number of days from her previous school. Father was well and worked away from home. There was a 6-year-old brother.

Examination showed no abnormalities.

Following the consultation, contact was made with the previous hospital to obtain the results of investigations and it was discovered that the child had not been brought for the planned EEG and ambulatory EEG appointments but had had normal blood tests for electrolytes, calcium and magnesium. The buccal midazolam had been provided from the emergency department following one attendance on the understanding that the child was to be seen in outpatients.

CLINICAL SCENARIO—CONT'D

Contact was made with the current school and the head teacher reported that the mother was highly protective and overindulgent with her daughter but was noted to be dismissive and unsympathetic towards the younger brother.

The child was not brought for the newly requested EEGs.

The reported events raised concern and were discussed with members of the Safeguarding MDT. It was felt that the story could be true but that there were a sufficient number of points to suspect that the events may be fabricated by the mother.

A meeting was arranged and the concerns presented to the mother who initially denied that the events were fabricated. In view of the uncertainty, both children were removed from the family home and placed in the care of paternal grandparents whilst further investigations were undertaken. Mother later recanted and stated that the child did not have seizures. It was not possible to define the motives behind these actions.

Sexual abuse

Sexual abuse is difficult to identify and address but the consequences are devastating and have a long-term effect on the child or young person. More often the abuser in known to the child and is a family member or friend or knows the child in a professional capacity. Stranger abuser is much less common but with increased access to the internet and social media among children, there is an increase in the chances of a young person being groomed by strangers.

Presentation

Disclosure at an early age by the victim does occur, but in later adult life many victims recount being threatened by the perpetrator or fearful of any consequences should they report the assaults. Consequently, disclosure at an early age often does not occur and even when it does occur, many victims report that they are not believed by responsible adults. The identity of children abused sexually may also be discovered while investigations are conducted on child pornography.

Inappropriate behaviour and actions such as long periods away from home, overnight absences from home, reports of visits to distant towns and locations, episodes of profound intoxication from drugs or alcohol or seemingly expensive gifts from unknown friends should alert health care professionals of a likely abusive environment. In some situations, the presence of 'relatives' who are unwilling to allow private conversations with the patient would suggest coercive and controlling behaviour.

Emotional or behavioural issues and difficulty in school or in forming relationships have all been recognised in children who have been sexually abused. Soiling, secondary enuresis, sexualised behaviour in younger children or self-harm in young people are more common in those who have been abused.

Vaginal or rectal bleeding or discharge, the identification of a sexually transmitted disease or the revelation of an unexpected pregnancy in a young girl should also raise suspicions of sexual abuse and therefore require further assessment.

When a disclosure or suspicion of sexual abuse occurs, it is important that immediate referral is made to a clinician experienced in assessing child or teenage victims. Clinicians have a professional responsibility to involve social services and police.

Dedicated units have now been established across the UK that are staffed by members of the sexual abuse team and where police and social services can take individuals for assessment. A detailed history is recorded, including sketches and photographs and a report written by the medical examiner detailing the findings. The social services and police will investigate further the circumstances and the individuals involved but it is vital that the young person is placed in a protective environment as a priority.

Assessment of a child where abuse is suspected

Early identification of child abuse is important and the consequent safety of the child in question, along with the safety of any other children in the family who may not be in attendance, should be the prime consideration. The actual place of safety for at-risk children will be decided following discussion between health and social services team members but it is usually as an in-patient on a paediatric ward until investigations are completed. In rare situations, a child or young person may be placed with a known, safe relative or in foster care.

Children who present with suspicious injuries should be assessed as soon as possible after presentation and the assessment should be carried out by a paediatrician trained in child protection or by junior doctors supported by such a clinician. Consent must be obtained for the examination, investigation or the taking of photographs and this must be provided by those with parental responsibility—mother, registered father or court-directed adult. More information on consent is in Chapter 32 Ethics and Law. If consent is refused then a court order should be obtained.

A suitable designated place for assessment should be identified that must be free from interruption. Examination of young people should be undertaken in the presence of chaperone.

An accurate and well-documented history and examination supported by appropriate investigations, drawings and photographs should be recorded and any forensic evidence collected by those experienced in the process. The history should be taken from the individuals caring for the child before any injury, from witnesses to any event and from the child depending on their age and understanding. Older children should be allowed to discuss the events in private without the possibility of coercion. Variations and changes in the histories from the same individual or from others must be recorded in timed entries to the medical notes as these will become important in future safeguarding and legal presentations.

Further information about the child and the family may be obtained from the child protection registers which can be accessed by the duty social worker. This register is maintained by social services departments throughout the whole of the UK and contains background details of individuals who are considered vulnerable or who are receiving support from social services.

Information on the register will be released to known members of the Safeguarding MDT on a 'need to know' basis and can reveal if the child or other members of the family are considered to be 'at risk' and if there were records of domestic violence. The family structure could also be shared and would be important in identifying the appropriate responsible adult.

PRACTICE POINT—assessment of a child where abuse is suspected

- follow the local procedures and policies
- discuss with senior paediatrician at an early stage
- admit the child to a place of safety
- consider safety of other children in the family
- inform safeguarding nurse
- check the child protection register via the duty social worker
- obtain written consent to undertake assessment
- child or young person can refuse examination and this should be respected
- avoid repeated examination of a child or young person
- produce clear written statement and include an opinion of causation of findings

Investigations may be indicated and these would include:
- full blood count—excludes thrombocytopenia as a cause of bruising
- clotting studies—if bruising or bleeding
- liver transaminases, amylase, lipase levels—if abdominal injury suspected
- toxicology screen—if drug overdose or poisoning suspected

- skeletal survey
- ophthalmology review—if indicated
- cranial imaging—if indicated

Once the police, social services and medical teams have completed their interviews and examinations, a formal MDT meeting is arranged as soon as possible and the reports from all the involved professionals are discussed. Parents or carers are usually invited to contribute to the discussion regarding the finding.

The MDT will make a decision on future plans for the child and any siblings. The outcome may be that the child is returned to the family without any further intervention needed, that the child is placed on an at-risk register but social services offer support for the family or that the child is placed into foster care and legal proceedings are taken to remove the child from the high-risk situation.

Organisation of child protection services

In most areas in the UK, the child safeguarding services are the responsibility of the local authority and administered through the social services department. A duty social worker is always available and can be contacted by any professional or members of the public to discuss concerns about the welfare of children and young people.

When safeguarding issues are identified, a review of each child and their family circumstances will be undertaken by members of the multidisciplinary team—social services, health services, education, police and legal services. A convened MDT will make decisions on how best to protect the child and, where possible, to achieve this through keeping the child within the family setting.

If it is felt that the child should be removed from the family, the allocated social workers will then prepare evidence to present to a judge sitting in the Family Courts. These judges are specially trained in family law and they will ensure that the interests and welfare of the child remain paramount. The children are represented by their own lawyer and hearings are held in private with only those who are involved attending.

Legal proceedings may take place some months or years later and the value of clear contemporaneous notes made by paediatric staff cannot be overemphasised.

Long-term effects of abuse

Long-term effects of abuse are devastating on the child's development and affect both physical and emotional development. It is recognised that abuse and neglect increase the risks of growth failure, behavioural problems including sexualised behaviour, difficulties in forming and maintaining friendships, school underachievement, truancy and pregnancy. Mental health problems including depression, eating disorders and suicidal ideation are also common.

Some individuals who were the victim of abuse go on to be perpetrators of abuse.

IMPORTANT CLINICAL POINTS—safeguarding

General
- safeguarding children is the responsibility of everyone
- are recognised factors that increase risk of child abuse

Physical abuse
- bruises
  - consider age, explanation given, location and pattern
  - dating of bruises by colour is not reliable
- fractures
  - suspicious if child not ambulatory
  - skeletal survey necessary with follow up CXR
- burns
  - pattern important
- head trauma
  - more complex fractures of skull associated with abuse
  - retinal haemorrhages are associated due to shaking insult

Neglect
- poor nutrition, lack of hygiene, failure to address medical needs

Fabricated or induced illness
- exaggerated or false history of symptoms
- lack of corroboration

Sexual abuse
- possible explanation for inappropriate behaviour
- refer to clinician experienced in assessing victims

Further reading

Child protection evidence RCPCH. https://www.rcpch.ac.uk/key-topics/child-protection/evidence-reviews

Systematic review on Fractures RCPCH. Published September 2020. https://www.rcpch.ac.uk/sites/default/files/2020-10/Chapter%20Fractures_Update_280920.pdf.

Chapter | 12 |

Infectious diseases

Lucy Cliffe, Gillian Body, Khuen Foong Ng, Srini Bandi

After reading this chapter you should:
- be able to assess, diagnose and manage infections acquired in the UK and overseas

Infections acquired in the UK

Infections present at all ages, in any organs and can cause mild or life-threatening illness. They can present with symptoms that are nonspecific, particularly in younger infants, where it can be difficult to distinguish between viral and bacterial infection. Clinical presentation may be the direct result of the causative infection or the sequelae of that infection. The management, therefore, should aim to address the presenting clinical problem of the patient, identify the responsible organism and anticipate the possible consequences of that infection.

Bacterial Infections

Bacterial Septicaemia

Sepsis is caused by the immune response of the body to an infecting organism—usually bacterial—although it can be caused by viral or fungal infections. The normal body response to sepsis leads to inappropriate vasodilatation of vessels, increased vascular permeability, white cell proliferation and abnormal cell signalling. If left untreated, it can develop into septic shock, with a significant morbidity and mortality from multiorgan failure.

Children with an isolated bacteraemia will usually present with a pyrexia of unknown focus along with nonspecific malaise. Those with meningococcal disease will often develop a rash that may initially be morbilliform before rapidly becoming petechial and purpuric. Signs of severe sepsis may develop rapidly and include:
- hypotension and shock with cool or mottled extremities
- weak pulse; delayed capillary refill
- confusion
- rigors

The most common organisms are *Staphylococcus aureus* including methicillin-resistant strains (MRSA), *Streptococcus pneumoniae, Streptococcus pyogenes* and *Escherichia coli*. Children who have asplenia are at risk of overwhelming infection from encapsulated bacteria including pneumococcus, meningococcus, H. influenzae and salmonella.

Investigations

It is important to obtain full blood count, C- reactive protein, blood cultures (obtained prior to starting antibiotics), renal function tests, liver function tests, clotting studies, glucose and lactate.

Treatment and management

Bacterial sepsis requires prompt treatment with urgent resuscitation. Antibiotics must be administered as soon as possible and certainly within one hour from attending the clinical area as delays beyond this time period will lead to a significant increase in mortality. Patients are likely to need significant fluid volumes, blood products and intensive care (with ventilatory support) if in septic shock. The monitoring of patients once admitted should follow a structured approach using a Paediatric Early Warning System (PEWS) to identify any potential deterioration.

If subsequent culture results isolate a specific organism, then a full investigation should be undertaken to identify the source including unusual sites such as mastoid area, sinuses, bones and heart. Secondary seeding of distant sites may cause infections such as septic arthritis, meningitis and endocarditis.

Potential complications

These include:
- high mortality rate
- hypoxic seizures and brain injury leading to disability
- extremity loss (limbs, ears, nose tips) from initial coagulopathy and poor perfusions
- adrenal haemorrhage (Waterhouse-Friderichsen syndrome)

Bacterial meningitis

Meningitis is a medical emergency and any children or young person with symptoms and signs suggestive of the diagnosis need immediate treatment. The recognised findings are fever, headache, photophobia, confusion and nuchal rigidity. In younger children, symptoms can be nonspecific with irritability, reduced conscious level, poor feeding and apnoea.

Signs of raised intracranial pressure include a bulging fontanelle, hypertension with bradycardia, papilloedema, abnormal posturing and localised neurological signs and these indicate the need for an urgent response.

The most common organisms are identified in children are:
- *Streptococcus pneumoniae*
- *Neisseria meningitidis*

Immunisation programmes in many countries have seen a marked reduction in meningitis caused by *Haemophilus influenzae type b* (Hib) and pneumococcal disease.

The common organisms in those under 3 months of age are:
- *Escherichia coli*
- *Group B streptococcus*
- *Listeria monocytogenes*

Those patients with an identified CSF leak (basal skull fractures, those with indwelling shunts or cochlear implants) are at risk of pneumococcal meningitis (Table 12.1).

Investigations

The diagnosis is made by CSF microscopy and culture (Table 12.1) and there should be a low threshold for performing a lumbar puncture particularly in the younger age group where there is a lack of localising signs. The procedure would not be needed if the classical meningococcal rash and signs of sepsis were present, and there are also clinical situations where a lumbar puncture would be contraindicated. Microscopy of CSF fluid would usually show bacteria, although these may not be evident if there was partial treatment with antibiotics. In this situation, subsequent CSF culture may be negative and PCR may offer further information. Full blood count, CRP, blood culture, coagulation screen, glucose, electrolytes and liver function tests are necessary initial investigations. Should it be necessary to delay the lumbar puncture for imaging, then antibiotics must be given after the blood culture is obtained.

> **PRACTICE POINT—lumbar puncture would be contraindicated if**
>
> - signs of raised intracranial pressure
> - GCS less than 9 or acute deterioration in GCS
> - shocked patient
> - suspected meningococcal septicaemia with spreading petechial rash
> - within 30 minutes of a seizure
> - following focal seizures and a persistent focal neurology
> - severe coagulopathies

Treatment and management

Patients with a possible meningitis need prompt treatment with IV antibiotics and the current UK guideline advises ceftriaxone for those over 3 months whilst those under this age should have cefotaxime plus amoxicillin or ampicillin to cover a potential Listeria infection. The administration of intravenous dexamethasone is advised if:
- purulent CSF
- high CSF white count (greater than 1000/microlitre)

Table 12.1 CSF findings in meningitis						
	Appearance	WCC	PMN	Lymph	Protein g/l	Glucose mmol/l
Normal	Clear	0–5 10⁶/l	0–2 10⁶/l	0–5 10⁶/l	0.15–0.45	2.2–4.4
Bacterial	Cloudy	>500	90%	Low initially	Raised	<2.2
Viral	Clear	<1000	Rise later	raised	<1	Normal
Tubercular	Fibrin web	100–500	Normal	raised	0.1–0.5	low

- bacteria on gram stain
- high protein count (greater than 1gm/litre)

The administration of fluids and the monitoring of electrolytes are important and require frequent review and those with features suggestive of raised intracranial pressure will need a fluid-restricted plan. The syndrome of inappropriate secretion of antidiuretic hormone (SIADH) is a recognised complication and can make fluid management challenging.

Many children will make a full recovery but some may develop deafness, seizures, neurodevelopmental disability and hydrocephalus. Sadly, some may die. A follow-up review should be made and a hearing assessment requested within 4 weeks of discharge.

Pneumococcal infections

Streptococcus pneumoniae is a capsulated, gram-positive diplococcus and multiple serotypes exist. Carriage in school-age children is up to 60% and even higher during winter months.

Overwhelming pneumococcal infection can occur in those with:

- functional or anatomical asplenia
- B-cell and complement deficiency
- immunosuppression
- cochlear implants
- base of skull fracture

There is an increased risk of disease with intercurrent viral respiratory infection such as influenza, parainfluenza, human metapneumovirus, respiratory syncytial virus or adenovirus, with peaks during winter months. There are few contraindications to vaccination with the conjugate vaccine and its introduction has led to a significant reduction on incidence of invasive disease.

Pneumococcus causes four main clinical problems:

- pneumonia (see Chapter 17 Respiratory)
- meningitis
- bacteraemia
- otitis media (see Chapter 18 ENT and Hearing)

Invasive disease usually follows a bacteraemia, but occasionally local spread can occur. Invasive pneumococcus and acute meningitis are both notifiable diseases.

Meningococcal disease

There are 12 capsular serotypes and the commonest serotype in the UK is type B (up to 80%), with C, W135 and Y the source of less common disease. Asymptomatic carriage is between 5% to 11% in adults and up to 25% in adolescents. This figure increases dramatically in outbreaks, particularly in crowded close contact environments such as university accommodation or residential schools. Spread is by close contact with infected respiratory secretions.

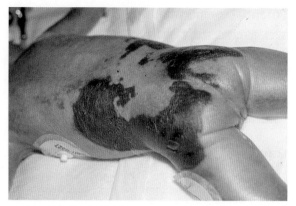

Fig. 12.1 Clinical appearance of meningococcal disease in 2-year-old girl.

Certain travel destinations are considered a high-risk source for meningococcal disease and include Mecca for the Hajj pilgrimage and sub-Saharan Africa. Vaccination against Serotypes A, B, C, W and Y is given in the UK immunisation schedule.

Meningococcal disease typically presents with meningitis, septicaemia (Figure 12.1) or both although other sites can lead to myocarditis, endocarditis, arthritis, pneumonia and chronic meningococcaemia. Meningitis and septicaemia are discussed above.

Streptococcal disease

Streptococci are divided into those which produce in vitro haemolysis (alpha, beta or gamma) and Lancefield groups. The organism produces tissue damaging factors such as streptolysins, hyaluronidase, DNase and exotoxin. Activated cytokines lead to shock, organ failure and death and are responsible for many of the manifestations of severe invasive streptococcal disease. Group A streptococcus is the most significant pathogen and is a normal inhabitant of the nasopharynx. Incidence is highest in school-age individuals, in winter and in areas of crowding and close contact but asymptomatic carriage of streptococci is common as it tends to colonise throat and skin (Table 12.2).

Streptococci produce disease by local invasion, toxin production and nonsuppurative sequelae. The commonest presentations are pharyngitis, skin infections and scarlet fever.

Pharyngitis is a common condition and fever and sore throat may be caused by both bacterial and viral infections. Those with a streptococcal pharyngitis will usually present with:

- acute sore throat and tonsillar exudates
- fever
- cervical lymphadenitis

These findings can also be seen in Epstein-Barr virus which can lead to difficulties in diagnosis. Local spread of

Table 12.2 **Clinical conditions caused by Streptococci**		
Classification	**Example**	**Commonly associated diseases**
Group A (beta haemolytic)	*S. pyogenes*	pharyngitis, tonsillitis, wound and skin infections, septicaemia, scarlet fever, pneumonia, rheumatic fever, glomerulonephritis, necrotising fasciitis
Group B (beta haemolytic)	*S. agalactiae*	sepsis, postpartum or neonatal sepsis, meningitis, skin infections, endocarditis, septic arthritis, UTIs
Group C, G (beta haemolytic)	*S. equi* and *S. canis*	pharyngitis, pneumonia, cellulitis, pyoderma, erysipelas, impetigo, wound infections, puerperal sepsis, neonatal sepsis, endocarditis, septic arthritis
Viridans (alpha or gamma)	many including *S. anginosus*	endocarditis, bacteraemia, meningitis, localized infection, abscesses

streptococcus may lead to sinusitis, mastoiditis or pharyngeal and peritonsillar abscesses. However, a throat swab that is positive for streptococcus may simply reflect carriage rather than invasive disease.

Scarlet fever occurs secondary to toxin production and usually presents with pharyngitis followed, within 48 hours, by a rash which starts in the groin, neck and axillae and spreads over the trunk before fading after 3–4 days. On close inspection, the rash has small papules and is often described as 'sandpaper-like' and is the result of a delayed skin reaction to the exotoxin. Circumoral pallor, a white coated 'strawberry tongue' and desquamation of palms and fingers are all common findings. On clinical grounds, the condition may be indistinguishable from Kawasaki disease but a shorter duration of pyrexia and the lack of mucous membrane involvement will be more suggestive of streptococcal infection.

Investigations

Streptolysin O is produced by Group A streptococci and antibody titres (ASOT) can be measured in blood but this does not help with diagnosis of acute infection. It is only some weeks later when a rise of greater than twofold between samples taken in the acute phase (week 1) are compared with those taken in the convalescent phase (weeks 2–4) that is considered diagnostic of recent infection. Confirmation of a current infection will come from blood culture or tissue samples of infected sites.

Treatment and management

Management of acute pharyngitis is usually conservative and antibiotics are not given as most infections are due to a viral cause. Children with a proven streptococcal pharyngitis or with classical scarlet fever are treated with phenoxymethylpenicillin or clarithromycin. Treatment

of pregnant women is aimed at preventing early Group B streptococcal disease (GBS) but has no effect on late GBS morbidity and mortality.

Potential complications

These can be suppurative or nonsuppurative in nature. Suppurative complications include otitis media, tonsillar abscess, pneumonia, meningitis, cerebral abscess, endocarditis and osteomyelitis. Nonsuppurative complications are delayed effects and immunologically mediated and include acute rheumatic fever and poststreptococcal glomerulonephritis.

Staphylococcal infections

Staphylococcus aureus is a gram-positive aerobic organism and its marked pathogenicity is due to its virulence, potential toxin production and its ability to develop antibiotic resistance.

Transmission is usually by hand-to-hand contact or nasal discharge. Neonates are particularly susceptible due to the umbilical stump, thin epidermis and poor defences. Handwashing is the most effective preventative measure whilst topical antibiotics (mupirocin) and topical washes can be used to decrease carriage rates.

Common sites of infections include blood, skin, bones, joints and heart whilst less common sites are lung and meninges. Exotoxin production is responsible for staphylococcal scalded skin syndrome (Figure 12.2), toxic shock syndrome and acute gastroenteritis.

Septic arthritis presents with a hot, swollen joint with restricted movement and decreased function. It is unusual to have infection in more than one joint, so multiple joint involvement should suggest a reactive or inflammatory arthritis. Direct sampling from the joint is necessary to confirm diagnosis and guide antibiotic treatment.

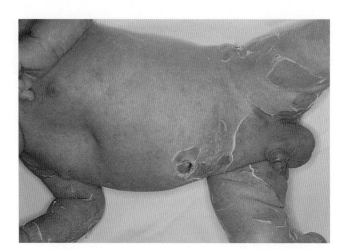

Fig. 12.2 Clinical appearance of staphylococcal scalded skin. Note sheets of lifted epidermis with curled edges (Image use with permission from Clinical Dermatology. Habif TP. 5th edition. Chapter 9. Elsevier Inc)

Osteomyelitis usually presents with localised bony pain, tenderness and redness over the affected area. Initial plain films may be normal and a periosteal reaction may only become evident at a later stage and so MRI usually provides more immediate information.

A preseptal orbital cellulitis presents with pain, redness and swelling of the eyelid and anterior soft tissues. An ophthalmology opinion would be important to exclude a more deep-seated infection which may produce restricted eye movements or severe proptosis. MRI should be performed if any doubt about orbital involvement.

Endocarditis is presented in Chapter 16 Cardiology.

CLINICAL SCENARIO

A 5-year-old girl was admitted with a 2 day history of fever, malaise and vomiting. She was previously well. No other family members had a febrile illness. On admission, her temperature was 38.3°C, BP 110/65 and GCS was 13. There was no obvious rash. Photophobia and neck stiffness were confirmed.

A clinical diagnosis of meningitis was made and a full infection screen was undertaken including lumbar puncture. She was started on intravenous antibiotics. Initial CSF results showed raised white cell and protein values and low glucose compared with plasma glucose. CSF culture results became available at 12 hours and showed *E. coli* and *S. millerii*.

The microbiology team was clear that this was not a contaminant and advised more detailed investigations to identify a possible route of entry for the organisms. Repeat examination noted a 'sacral pit'.

Further investigations were undertaken to identify possible entry sites including ENT review for potential sinus defects and MRI of spine and sacrum. The MRI identified a dermal sinus—a type of spinal dysraphism. She was referred to colleagues in paediatric neurosurgery for surgical correction.

Pertussis

Bordetella pertussis and *Bordetella parapertussis* are gram-negative bacilli that remove the cilia in the major airways. It is this loss of the 'ciliary escalator' and the dependence on coughing to clear the airway which accounts for the symptoms and protracted nature of the illness.

A mild prodrome of fever, coryza, and occasional cough occurs early in the clinical picture but progresses to the paroxysmal cough followed by a whoop or a vomit whilst infants may also present with apnoea. The cough may persist for up to 10 weeks and is typically worse at night. Illness caused by *Bordetella parapertussis* is usually less severe than that of *Bordetella pertussis*.

Alternative diagnoses and differing features

In younger infants, bronchiolitis may initially be mistaken for whooping cough although the coughs are very different in each. In older children, a viral (adenovirus) or bacterial pneumonia can produce similar symptoms whilst inhalation of a foreign body, thoracic lymphadenopathy and poorly controlled asthma with nighttime cough should be considered.

Investigations

Diagnosis is made by culture from a nasal swab and although this is the gold standard investigation, it is typically not reported in time to be clinically useful. A marked lymphocytosis may support the clinical diagnosis and is known to be an independent predictor of fatality from the infection. PCR and serological testing may be used although IgG to Bordetella may simply indicate either a past infection or vaccination.

Treatment and management

This is primarily supportive as an infant may become exhausted and fail to maintain respiratory effort or adequate oral intake. Antibiotics will only decrease infectivity and not reduce the duration of the paroxysmal phase of the disease.

Potential complications

These include subconjunctival haemorrhage, pneumonia, pneumothorax, seizures and alkalosis secondary to tussive vomiting. In overwhelming infection with extensive symptoms, there is the potential for hypoxic brain injury and death.

Important sequelae

Pertussis is part of the routine vaccination schedule and now offers an acellular vaccine produced from fragmented organisms. There are few contraindications. Due to concerns raised in the 1970s about a possible link between cellular vaccines and neurodevelopmental problems, the parents of children with an emerging neurological condition are still advised to consider a delay to immunisation until the neurological problem has been fully investigated. Immunisation in pregnancy has been introduced recently due to a number of outbreaks with the aim of increasing maternal IgG and placental transfer.

Lyme disease

Ticks transfer the causative organism of Lyme disease, *Borrelia burgdorferi*, when they bite the host. The prompt removal of the tick reduces the risk of transmission of the bacteria although removal of the embedded tick requires a specific technique to ensure all parts of the insect are removed. Infected ticks are found throughout the UK and high-risk areas include wooded areas in Scotland, New Forest and the Lake District.

Children and young people present with:
- fever, fatigue, lymphadenopathy
- muscle aches, migratory arthralgia
- unexplained cranial nerve palsies
- cognitive impairment—memory problems and difficulty concentrating

Erythema migrans, often at the site of a tick bite (Figure 12.3), is the pathognomonic rash of Lyme disease and, if identified, no further investigations are needed. It can appear between 1 to 4 weeks after a tick bite and can last for several weeks.

Investigations

There is no gold standard diagnostic test to confirm Lyme disease although serological testing may be recommended by the local microbiology team.

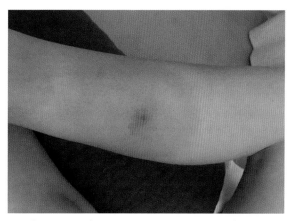

Fig. 12.3 Erythema marginatum seen in Lyme disease.

Treatment and management

The choice of antibiotic depends on the age of the child and clinical features but either oral doxycycline or amoxicillin are recommended as the first-line treatment. If CNS disease identified then the patient should receive intravenous ceftriaxone. There is a potential for long-term problem with chronic arthritis in infected individuals.

Pharmacological agents used

Doxycycline causes staining and dental hypoplasia in growing teeth and should only be given to children over the age of 12 years.

Tuberculosis

Mycobacterium tuberculosis (TB) is spread from person to person through the air and primarily affects the lungs leading to pulmonary TB. Most infected individuals remain asymptomatic although most have a latent infection which becomes active within the first two years after exposure.

The individual with latent TB is usually detected by contact tracing from a known infected individual. Those with pulmonary TB will present with:
- malaise
- cough
- loss of appetite
- weight loss

Examination of the chest may show signs of parenchymal (reduced breath sounds, crackles) and pleural (effusion) involvement. Extrapulmonary TB could include any system and the symptoms at presentation would vary. TB meningitis is one such site and individuals would have the same symptoms and signs of someone with bacterial meningitis.

Investigations

A range of investigations are used to clarify the possible diagnosis of TB.

Mantoux test is an indirect assessment to show immunity against Mycobacterium TB but it does not differentiate between active and latent TB and a negative test does not rule out the active disease. The test site on the skin needs a follow-up examination to interpret the response.

Interferon Gamma Release Assay (IGRA) has the advantage that there is no need for the child to return for the review of the test but, again, does not differentiate between active and latent TB. The assay is less accurate in those under 2 years of age and hence Mantoux is preferred in this group. The test is also useful in the assessment in patients who had previously received a BCG immunisation.

Chest radiograph will show hilar or mediastinal lymphadenopathy along with a peripheral focus that are indicative of active infection whilst other radiological findings include patchy consolidation, pleural effusion, nodular infiltration and less commonly cavitating lesions and miliary dissemination.

Early morning sputum samples and gastric aspirates can be obtained and stained for acid fast bacilli before being cultured. A positive culture is only seen in around 30% to 40% and can take up to 40 days to be available and so would not be helpful in the early stages of management.

GeneXpert MTBRIF® is a PCR-based assay which gives information within a few hours on positive samples. It can also detect the main genetic mutation for rifampicin resistance.

Diagnosis of latent TB infection is based on a positive Mantoux or IGRA in an asymptomatic child with a normal CXR. The diagnosis of pulmonary TB usually comes from clinical suspicion and hilar lymphadenopathy on the chest radiograph whilst a diagnosis of extrapulmonary TB requires a high index of suspicion and investigations tailored according to the site. CNS infection will require neuroimaging and CSF analysis.

Treatment and management

An asymptomatic child with a positive Mantoux and a normal CXR would receive a 12-week course of isoniazid and rifampicin.

A symptomatic child or one who has an abnormal CXR should be assumed to have active TB and further investigations are warranted. It is imperative that all the diagnostic samples are collected before starting TB treatment although treatment can start before culture results are available. The standard TB regime is for a total 6 months (26 weeks) with four drugs for the first 2 months (isoniazid, rifampicin, pyrazinamide, ethambutol) followed by 4 months of isoniazid and rifampicin.

TB meningitis requires a 12 month course with 2 months of quadruple therapy and 10 months of isoniazid and rifampicin. Steroids should be added in CNS TB and pericardial TB.

Relevant pharmacological agents used

Isoniazid—may cause hepatoxicity, peripheral neuritis or Stevens Johnson Syndrome.
Rifampicin—may cause hepatoxicity, turns urine and all body fluids red (must inform patient), induces liver enzymes and can increase metabolism of oestrogens and anticoagulants.
Pyrazinamide—good meningeal penetration
Ethambutol—can affect visual acuity which corrects if drug stopped

Non tuberculous mycobacterium

Atypical mycobacterial disease is the result of infection from mycobacteria other than *Mycobacterium tuberculosis* or *Mycobacterium leprae*. The most common type seen in well children would be *Mycobacterium avium* which may lead to a cervical lymphadenitis (Figure 12.4). The patient

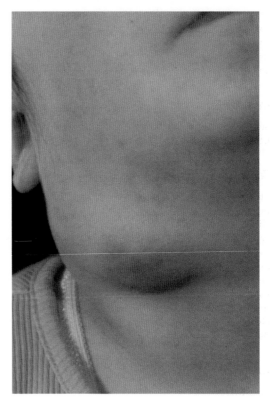

Fig. 12.4 Classical appearance of atypical mycobacteria in a 9-year-old girl.

is usually well and presents with an erythematous cervical mass which is usually nonpainful. Surgical excision alone usually leads to full resolution.

Viral Infections

Rotavirus

Rotavirus is an important cause of acute diarrhoeal illness in children. Since the introduction of an oral, attenuated rotavirus vaccine in the UK national immunisation schedule, the incidence of rotavirus gastroenteritis has fallen dramatically. The infection is easily transmissible through the faecal oral route and in England and Wales is seasonal, occurring mostly in winter and early spring. Groups at high risk for rotavirus infection are unimmunised children, persons caring for patients with rotavirus gastroenteritis and immunocompromised hosts.

Symptoms of gastroenteritis are usually present and include fever, vomiting, abdominal pain and watery diarrhoea without blood.

Alternative diagnoses

Other causes of acute diarrhoea and vomiting need to be considered. Bacterial and parasitic infection tend to affect children above 2 years old, those with animal contact and returning travellers. Presence of blood and mucus in the stool and high fever are more indicative of bacterial gastroenteritis.

Investigations

Stool PCR and ELISA for rotavirus antigen assays are diagnostic of an acute infection.

Treatment and management

Management of rotavirus gastroenteritis is mainly supportive and, in particular, patients should be assessed clinically to determine their hydration status. Fluid management by enteral method (either orally or via nasogastric tube) with oral rehydration salt solution is preferred but intravenous fluid therapy may be required if the enteral route is not tolerated. It is important to prevent spread of pathogens by the applying strict infection control measures including hand washing, nonsharing of towels and isolation until 48 hours after the last episode of diarrhoea or vomiting.

Enterovirus and parechovirus

Enterovirus and parechovirus infections have diverse clinical manifestations and can affect different organ systems. They are particularly severe in neonates and immunocompromised children.

Enteroviruses include:
- Polioviruses
- Coxsackieviruses—Group A and Group B
- Echoviruses
- Other enteroviruses

Parechoviruses share many clinical characteristics with enteroviruses. Transmission of all types is usually via the faecal–oral route. This section relates to nonpolio enterovirus and parechovirus infection.

There is variable incubation period after the acute infection and virus can be shed in respiratory droplets for up to 3 weeks and in faeces for up to 8 weeks.

Children may present with skin manifestations including:
- **Hand, foot and mouth disease**
  - vesiculobullous rashes on the lateral borders of hands and feet (Figure 12.5)
  - oral lesions such as vesicles and ulcers
- **Herpangina**
  - fever
  - odynophagia
  - enanthem of tonsillar fauces and soft palate

The patient may develop central nervous system involvement such as encephalitis and meningitis and certain enteroviruses can also produce acute flaccid paralysis and cranial nerves deficit. Brainstem encephalitis due to enterovirus A71 infection has high fatality rate. It may infect the respiratory system leading to upper respiratory infection, bronchiolitis, pneumonia and pleurodynia.

Severe infection is seen in neonates as a result of perinatal acquisition of the virus from mother or postnatal transmission. There can be wide variation in

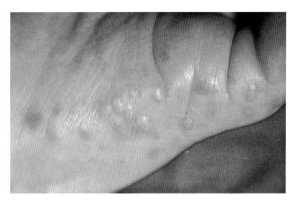

Fig. 12.5 Clinical appearance of hand, foot and mouth disease. Vesiculobullous rashes on the lateral borders of hand

presentation from nonspecific symptoms through to meningitis, sepsis, multiorgan failure, disseminated intravascular coagulopathy, myocarditis, fulminant hepatitis and encephalitis.

Alternative diagnoses

- Herpes simplex virus infection
  - in herpetic gingivostomatitis, the vesicular lesions are usually in the anterior part of the oropharynx and bleed easily; in herpangina, the vesicles are located in the posterior pharynx and do not usually bleed
- Kawasaki disease
- serious bacterial infection including meningitis, sepsis and toxic shock syndrome
- other respiratory viral illness, EBV and CMV infections
- group A streptococcal tonsillopharyngitis and scarlet fever

Investigations

In self-limiting infection, clinical diagnosis alone is sufficient. However, in the event of severe infection, samples should be obtained from different sites for viral culture and PCR.

Treatment and management

Treatment is mainly supportive as there are no proven benefits, even in severe disease, of using antiviral drug or intravenous immunoglobulin.

Human herpes virus

There are currently eight known human herpesviruses and all have double-stranded DNA:
- Herpes simplex virus 1 & 2
- Varicella-zoster virus (VZV)
- Cytomegalovirus
- Epstein Barr virus
- Human herpesvirus 6, 7 and 8

After primary infection, the herpesviruses enter a dormant state and, after certain stimuli, infection may occur by reactivation.

Herpes simplex virus (HSV)

There are two major types of Herpes simplex virus (HSV-1 and HSV-2) and the incubation period for primary infection is 1–26 days. Severe and disseminated disease occurs mostly in immunocompromised children and neonates. Children with HSV encephalitis tend to have poor outcome.

Primary infection is usually asymptomatic although when clinically evident, it is more severe and associated with fever and malaise along with eruption of vesicles on an erythematous base. Recurrent infection occurs by the reactivation of latent virus in ganglion neurons.

Herpetic gingivostomatitis is commonly seen in children aged 1–6 years old, and the vesicular lesions are usually in the anterior part of the oropharynx and often progress to extensive, painful ulceration with bleeding. It is associated with high fever, cervical adenopathy and dehydration as oral intake is painful.

Herpetic whitlow describes painful, erythematous skin lesions with vesicles on the distal fingertips. Eczema herpeticum describes clustered vesicles in eczematous areas of individuals with atopic dermatitis whilst recurrent herpes labialis describes 'cold sores' or 'fever blisters' on the border of the lips. Adolescents may present with genital herpes characterised by vesicular or ulcerative skin lesions.

Investigations

Diagnosis of HSV infection is usually made by sampling an active lesion or affected site and testing it for the presence of the virus by PCR, viral culture or immunofluorescence. Serological tests have limited value.

Treatment and management

Parenteral aciclovir is the drug of choice in severe HSV disease especially in immunocompromised patients and neonates or when associated with disseminated disease (encephalitis) or visceral complications (hepatitis).

Complications

Recognised sequelae include:
- encephalitis (typically affect temporal lobe) (Figure 12.6)
- aseptic meningitis
- transverse myelitis
- Bell's palsy

At least two thirds of children who survived HSV encephalitis develop long-term neurodevelopmental sequelae. Involvement of the eye may lead to keratitis, conjunctivitis, chorioretinitis, corneal scarring and ultimately loss of vision.

Varicella-zoster virus (VZV)

Varicella-zoster virus is a type of human herpesvirus which causes chickenpox in primary infection and shingles when there is reactivation of endogenous latent virus in the sensory nerve ganglia. The diagnosis is usually made clinically

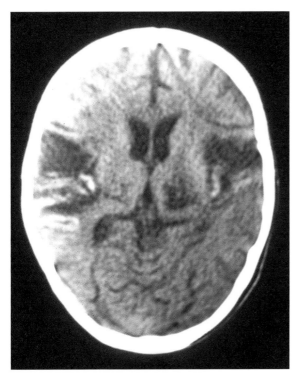

Fig. 12.6 CT scan of 2-year-old child presenting with seizures. Bitemporal lesions suggest herpes encephalitis that was confirmed by CSF culture.

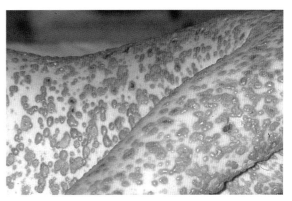

Fig. 12.7 Severe chickenpox in 7-year-old boy with immunodeficiency. Shows lesions at different stages of evolution – obvious new, tense vesicles and older scabbed lesions

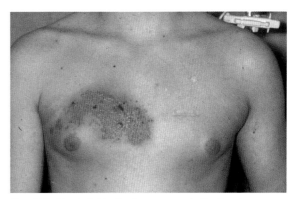

Fig. 12.8 Classical shingles (herpes zoster) affecting dermatomes T2 and T3. Note horizontal scar on left which relates to a previously placed venous access device and suggests that the patient may have been immunocompromised.

and, if indicated, treatment is with aciclovir. It is important to know the period of incubation and infectivity to understand the need of any post-exposure prophylaxis.

VZV is highly infectious and it spreads by airborne droplets from nasopharyngeal secretions and from fluid of fresh skin vesicles. VZV can only be spread from an individual with shingles by direct contact and not by nasal droplets.

The child with chickenpox infection will have a 24-hour prodrome of fever and malaise followed by appearance of skin lesions in crops, first appearing on the head and trunk before spreading to extremities. Mucosal sites can also be affected. The skin rash starts as a macule which then becomes papular and progresses to a fluid-filled vesicle on an erythematous base and before finally crusting. The lesions are at differing stages of development (Figure 12.7).

Pruritus may be intense and scratching may lead to secondary bacterial infection. The key diagnostic clues are a systemic illness and crops of lesions in different stages present at the same time in close proximity.

VZV establishes latency in the posterior root of sensory ganglia and, when immunosurveillance declines due to advanced age or immunosuppression, the virus may reactivate, causing shingles (Figure 12.8). These lesions are characterised by crops of vesicles in different stages of development limited to 1–3 sensory dermatomes. Pruritus and pain may be severe and persistent.

Treatment and management

The treatment of chickenpox in immunocompetent children is supportive with antipyretics and antihistamine to treat pruritus. Aspirin must be avoided as there is a concern that this may precipitate hepatic encephalopathy (Reye's syndrome). Immunocompromised individuals of any age tend to have severe disease and therefore require antiviral therapy.

Children with chickenpox or shingles on exposed areas should be excluded from school until all lesions are scabbed.

The mainstay of VZV prevention is active immunisation with live attenuated vaccine but its use in the UK is limited to healthcare workers, laboratory staff and contacts of immunocompromised patients.

PRACTICE POINT—varicella zoster virus—postexposure management

VZIG postexposure prophylaxis is preferably given within 10 days after exposure and is indicated for
- infants whose mothers develop chickenpox within the period of 7 days before and 7 days after delivery
- VZV antibody-negative infants exposed to chickenpox or herpes zoster (other than in the mother) who are in the first 7 days of life
- VZV antibody-negative infants exposed to chickenpox or herpes zoster (other than in the mother) who still require intensive or prolonged high-level care especially those born before 28 weeks, those weighing below 1 kg at birth and those aged above 60 days old
- Immunocompromised contacts should receive prophylactic acyclovir or valaciclovir from day 7 to day 14 after exposure (not immediately after exposure)

Potential complications of VZV infection include pneumonia, encephalitis, acute cerebellar ataxia—may develop some weeks after primary infection and congenital varicella syndrome (if mother develops chickenpox in first 28 weeks of pregnancy).

Cytomegalovirus (CMV)

CMV causes a wide range of illness in children and young people but in immunocompetent individuals is usually a self-limiting condition. Most individuals are exposed to CMV, and the majority develop antibodies by the time they reach later adulthood. CMV infection is of particular concern, however, for the newborn or immunocompromised patient where it can lead to significant morbidity and mortality.

Spread of the virus is by:
- close contact—young children; nursery
- during pregnancy and childbirth
- sexual transmission
- blood transfusions—common before donated blood was screened

Immunocompetent individuals usually have no symptoms or mild features of infection but those with more severe disease will present with lethargy, prolonged fever, myositis, tonsillitis and cervical lymphadenopathy.

Babies with congenital CMV demonstrate the following features:

- small for gestational age
- jaundice and hepatosplenomegaly
- petechiae from thrombocytopenia
- microcephaly
- sensory hearing deficit
- chorioretinitis

Immunocompromised children and adolescents are at significant risk of developing serious CMV disease. The infection may result from reactivation of previous infections or from any transplanted organ and may lead to significant morbidity and mortality.

Investigations

In the newborn child, infection is confirmed by culture or PCR testing of urine for CMV. IgG serology is unhelpful as it usually reflects maternal status.

In children and adolescents, CMV infection is confirmed from detecting CMV IgM whilst urine and saliva cultures or PCR of blood may be positive in the early phases of the illness. The heterophile antibody test is negative (in contrast to EBV). Full blood count will show mild anaemia and absolute lymphocytosis.

Treatment and management

Most immunocompetent patients with symptomatic CMV infection will have a complete recovery over a period of days to weeks and antiviral therapy is not usually indicated. Children with congenital CMV should be offered hearing, vision and developmental surveillance for the first years of life. Those who are immunocompromised may be treated with ganciclovir although senior discussion should be undertaken before prescribing as treatment may induce a leucopenia.

Epstein Barr virus (EBV)

EBV is the main organism causing infectious mononucleosis and, in common with human herpesviruses, has a DNA core and persists for life without symptoms in nearly all adults.

The clinical picture of infectious mononucleosis includes:
- malaise, headache, fever
- tonsillitis with an obvious exudate
- cervical lymph node enlargement (Figure 12.9)
- palatal petechiae
- mild hepatitis
- splenomegaly
- chronic fatigue persisting for months in some

The clinical history and examination, along with the presence of atypical lymphocytes on a blood film, often raise the possibility of acute leukaemia.

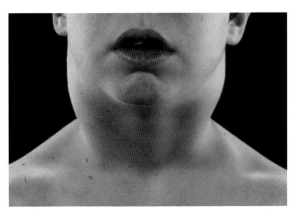

Fig. 12.9 Cervical lymphadenopathy in 12-year-old boy with EBV infection.

Associations

EBV is recognised as a potential aetiological factor in the development of B- and T-cell lymphomas, Hodgkin lymphoma and nasopharyngeal carcinomas.

Investigations

A full blood count usually demonstrates a lymphocytosis along with atypical lymphocytes. Further examination of the peripheral film and assessment of cell markers on the peripheral lymphocytes may be needed to exclude a leukaemic process.

Treatment and management

Support with antipyretics and fluids is appropriate and most symptoms will resolve over a few weeks.

Respiratory viruses

Respiratory viruses can cause both upper and lower respiratory tract infections with similar symptoms and signs. Common respiratory viruses encountered in infants and children in the UK include *Rhinovirus, Respiratory Syncytial Virus, Coronavirus, Human Metapneumovirus, Parainfluenza virus, Adenovirus, Influenza virus* and *Bocavirus*.

Influenza

Influenza is a highly infectious virus that causes seasonal epidemics during the winter. It is spread by respiratory secretions from infected persons and transmitted by aerosols, droplets or direct contact. Incubation period is between 1–3 days. Influenza viruses are classified into three distinct types; A, B and C with Influenza type A and B being responsible for most clinical episodes. Influenza viruses undergo constant antigenic drift over sequential seasons and so can lead to an influenza pandemic.

Influenza causes coryzal symptoms of nasal discharge, sneezing and sore throat along with systemic symptoms of fever, myalgia, anorexia, fatigue and gastrointestinal upset. Signs of a complicated influenza are the result of lower respiratory tract infection. *S. pneumoniae* and *S. aureus* are the most common causative bacteria for secondary bacterial pneumonia. Streptococcal A infection is another secondary infection that is associated with influenza and can cause localised infections or invasive disease and septicaemia.

Investigations

Nasopharyngeal aspirate (NPA) or throat swab will identify the virus by PCR.

Treatment and management

Supportive treatment with antipyretics and oral fluids is given for mild symptoms whilst those with complicated influenza or those at-risk for serious infection, may benefit from treatment with antivirals such as oseltamivir and zanamivir and antibiotics to cover secondary bacterial infection.

Pharmacological agents used

Oseltamivir and **zanamivir** are neuraminidase inhibitors that reduce viral replication and are most effective if started within a few hours of onset of symptoms. NICE guideline recommends use in at-risk patients following contact with infection.

Respiratory Syncytial Virus (RSV)

RSV in infants causes an inflammation of the small airways, producing mucus and airway narrowing. The child develops the clinical picture of bronchiolitis and presents with a cough, breathlessness, difficulty in breathing and reduced feeding. Clinical assessment identifies:
- tachypnoea
- nasal flaring, head bobbing, tracheal tug
- subcostal, intercostal and sternal recession
- bilateral fine crepitations
- wheeze

There may be reduced oxygen saturations in air and the clinical impact is recognised to peak around the fourth day of illness.

Investigations

NPA or throat swab taken should be taken for viral PCR but chest x-ray and bloods are not routinely required.

Treatment and management

Treatment is supportive and can be undertaken at home for those with mild disease but hospital admission is required if oxygen saturations are falling below 92% or if feeding is less than 50% of requirements (individual units will also have their own admission policies). Supplementary oxygen can be administered by nasal cannula, head-box or high flow systems. Feeding options include reducing feed frequency, nasogastric tube feeding or intravenous fluids. Occasionally respiratory support with noninvasive or invasive ventilation is required for apnoea, respiratory failure or bacterial lower respiratory tract infection.

Patients at risk of severe complications from infection are offered prophylactic palivizumab which provides passive immunity against RSV. It is given as an IM injection each month for 5 months during the RSV season and is administered to those who were:
- under 9 months with chronic lung disease
- under 6 months with significant acyanotic congenital heart disease
- under 1 year and on long-term ventilation
- under 24 months with Severe Combined Immunodeficiency Syndrome

SARS-CoV-2 (COVID-19)

The pandemic caused by SARS-CoV-2 has had a devastating impact on mortality and morbidity for millions of people. COVID-19 in children is usually mild but a small number present with a Paediatric Inflammatory Multisystem Syndrome Temporally associated with SARS-CoV-2 (PIMS-TS). This is a new disease in humans and guidelines are being updated to reflect the current best evidence.

Children with COVID-19 will present with symptoms similar to many common respiratory infections including fever, cough, coryza, headache, myalgia, diarrhoea and anosmia. Gastrointestinal symptoms are common in the early stages of the illness and can occur in the absence of respiratory symptoms.

PIMS-TS is now recognised and affected children present with persistent fever, hypotensive shock, rash, conjunctivitis, mucous membrane involvement, swelling of the extremities and lymphadenopathy. This condition is associated with increased inflammation affecting multiple organs, predominantly cardiac, leading to left ventricular failure and coronary artery dilatation. A differential for PIMS-TS would include Kawasaki disease, toxic shock syndrome, viral and bacterial sepsis and haemophagocytosis lymphohistiocytosis.

Investigations

Diagnosis is achieved by detection of SARS-CoV-2 RNA in the respiratory sample or saliva by PCR method. Previous infection is determined by the presence of SARS-CoV-2 immunoglobulin IgG. Chest radiograph should be undertaken in patients who continue to require oxygen or respiratory support by day 3 of admission or in acute deterioration. Investigations for patients manifesting PIMS-TS clinical features should be directed by up-to-date guidance.

Treatment and management

This includes early supportive care with antipyretics, respiratory support, bronchodilators and fluid management. Children with acute respiratory presentation and severe or critical COVID-19 may benefit from dexamethasone.

Potential complications

Children tend to have milder course of COVID-19 disease compared with adults but some may develop multiorgan failure.

Important sequelae

'Long COVID' describes long-term sequelae as a result of COVID-19 with persistent symptoms including fever, fatigue, diarrhoea and arthralgia lasting more than 4 weeks. Some children and young people have been identified as suffering from 'long COVID'.

Hepatitis B (HBV)

HBV is endemic in countries in sub-Saharan Africa and in some Asian countries. It is mainly transmitted by the mother to the child during pregnancy and birth but other routes of transmission would include:
- exposure to infected blood or body fluids
- sexual intercourse
- intravenous drug use
- medical, surgical and dental procedures
- tattooing

HBV is highly infectious and the incubation period can vary from 60 to 150 days. Hepatitis B can present with both acute and chronic infection and both phases will produce elevated liver function. Symptoms of acute HBV include fever, flu-like illness, abdominal pain, jaundice and vomiting.

Investigations

Liver enzymes will be elevated during acute and chronic disease. The stage of HBV infection can be assessed by the reviewing:

the **HBV DNA load**

the **antigen levels**:
- HBeAg—early antigen—reflects viral replication and high infectivity

- HBsAg—surface antigen—indicative of current or past infection
- HbcAg—core antigen—an intracellular antigen expressed in infected hepatocytes. It is not detectable in serum

  and anti-B antibody levels:
- anti-HBeAb, anti-HBsAb, anti-HBcAb

The detection of IgM anti-HBc is usually seen as an indication of acute HBV infection. HBsAg usually appears about 4 weeks after the initial viral infection and any patient with detectable HBsAg should be considered as infected and potentially infectious. The presence of antigen and antibody through the illness are shown (Figure 12.10).

PCR is used to detect HBV DNA in blood samples and is therefore able to quantify the viral load in the host. Levels of HBV DNA can persist into the chronic phase, indicating there is an ongoing viral presence that is controlled by the host immune system.

Treatment and management

Courses of antiviral agents are given with the aim of eliminating HBV from the host. When successful, this reduces or stops further progression of fibrosis and thereby cirrhosis and the future risk of liver cancer.

There is a safe and effective vaccine available and its introduction has led to a reduction in the incidence of chronic HBV in children. The vaccination is part of the immunisation schedule in the UK and all babies are offered the vaccine at 8, 12 and 16 weeks of age as a component of the 6 in 1 vaccine.

Hepatitis C (HCV)

HCV can cause a chronic infection of the liver and both acute and chronic infection can be asymptomatic with normal liver function until 10–20 years after infection. Mothers with high viral loads of hepatitis C carry an increased risk of transmitting the virus to the baby. Vertical transmission is almost always confined to women who have detectable HCV RNA. The mode of delivery does not affect risk of transmission and the current recommendation is that women with HCV without coinfection with HIV, can be advised to breastfeed.

> **PRACTICE POINT—Hepatitis C screen of 'at risk' groups**
>
> Children and young people in the following groups should be tested:
> - infants born to mothers with acute or chronic HCV
> - father with chronic HCV
> - IV drug use (in either parent)
> - unexplained hepatitis (acute or chronic)
> - IV drug use or needle stick injuries
> - sexual intercourse with those at risk of blood-borne infection

Most children and adolescents are identified through screening programmes of at-risk family contacts rather than having specific illness.

Investigations

The diagnosis of perinatal transmission is confused by passive transfer of maternal antibody which can then be present for up to 13 months and occasionally 18 months after birth. Consequently, HCV antibody testing is of limited value in those under 12 months although the infant is considered infected if HCV RNA is detected on two or more occasions.

In older children, the presence of anti-HCV antibody is suggestive of HCV infection although it can persist even after the infection has cleared. Chronic infection is confirmed if the HCV PCR is positive after 6 months.

Treatment and management

There is no vaccine available to prevent infection and hence early diagnosis and management is the key. Those

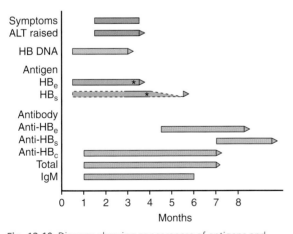

Fig. 12.10 Diagram showing appearances of antigens and antibodies in HBV infection. (Bars with arrow heads show findings that may persist into the phase of chronic infection. Bars with stars indicate findings may not always persist into chronic infection).

with acute problems are treated symptomatically with analgesia and fluids whilst those with chronic HCV infection are treated using direct-acting antiviral drugs. These drugs are highly effective and cure more than 90% of the treated individuals.

Patients are monitored regularly on treatment and blood tests are undertaken at the end of treatment to ensure negative HCV PCR and antibody results. A second blood test is done 12 to 24 weeks after the treatment is stopped to confirm cure.

Human Immunodeficiency Virus (HIV)

HIV infection is a retroviral infection and children acquire the infection mainly through vertical transmission during the peripartum period. Prompt diagnosis and treatment with Highly Active Antiretroviral Treatment (HAART) has resulted in near normal life expectancies for people with HIV.

Some of the more common signs and symptoms include:

- growth retardation
- opportunistic infections—Pneumocystis jirovecii pneumonia
- recurrent bacterial infections
- candidiasis
- chronic diarrhoea
- neuro-developmental delay—due to HIV crossing the blood–brain barrier directly

---

PRACTICE POINT—HIV testing

Children and young people should be tested in the following:

- where the mother has HIV or may have died of an HIV-associated condition
- those born to mothers known to have HIV in pregnancy
- those newly arrived in the UK from high-prevalence areas
- signs and symptoms suspicious of an HIV infection
- those being screened for immunodeficiency

Investigations

Testing a child for HIV requires full informed consent from the appropriate parent or guardian.

If the child is under 18 months of age and vertical transmission is suspected, then HIV PCR should be performed at birth, 6 weeks and 3 months. If the child is over 18 months of age then an HIV 1+2 antibody testing for seroconversion should be performed.

Treatment and management

HAART aims to:

- reduce the circulating viral load
- increase the child's CD4 cell count
- promote normal growth and development
- prevent immune system damage

Neonatal postexposure prophylaxis with zidovudine monotherapy should be commenced as soon as possible after birth. Breastfeeding is not advised and formula feeding should be offered to all infants born to HIV-infected mothers.

Fungal infections

Minor fungal infections such as candida or tinea (ringworm) of the skin or scalp are relatively common. Invasive fungal infections are uncommon and usually only occur in patients in intensive care settings with indwelling catheters or children who are immunocompromised by disease or treatment.

Candida albicans

Candida species is a recognised commensal in some individuals and can colonise the oral cavity, GI tract, skin and genital membranes.

Skin infection occurs in moist sites such as the groin, axillae or skin creases and in infants, candida can cause nappy rash with erythematous areas and satellite lesions. Oropharyngeal infection causes white plaques on the buccal mucosa, tongue and palate which cannot be scraped off and may cause pain, discomfort and reduced oral feeding. Persistent oral candidiasis should raise the possibility of immune deficiency including HIV.

Investigations

Candida infection is predominately a clinical diagnosis but swabs can be obtained for fungal culture.

Treatment and management

Oral candidiasis is treated with oral antifungals, usually either miconazole gel or nystatin solution. Treatment should be continued for 48 hours after symptoms resolve. Nappy rash is treated with topical nystatin cream.

Aspergillus

The most common Aspergillus species—*Aspergillus fumigatus*—spreads by airborne transmission to penetrate the lower respiratory tract. It is an environmental mould found in many settings, including building sites. An immunologically competent host would usually eliminate the spores although in some it can cause allergic hypersensitivity, whilst in the immunocompromised patient it will lead to invasive disease.

There should be a high index of suspicion of invasive disease in at-risk patients presenting with persistent fever.

Investigations

Sputum culture has a low sensitivity and a negative test does not exclude infection. Galactomannan is a circulating antigen that is detectable 5–8 days before any clinical signs and therefore can be assayed if Aspergillus suspected. Skin prick testing or specific IgE (RAST) to Aspergillus can be assessed to support clinical suspicion.

Treatment and management

If infection is suspected then antifungals such as amphotericin should be started following microbiology advice.

Pharmacological agents used

Amphotericin is given intravenously for systemic fungal disease but it is potentially nephrotoxic and requires the monitoring of renal function.
AmBisome® is a liposomal preparation of amphotericin which reduces the risk of nephrotoxicity.
Trizoles—voriconazole, posaconazole—may cause prolongation of QT interval
Echinocandins—micafungin, caspofungin—can be given for invasive Aspergillus

Infections acquired overseas

Travellers' diarrhoea

A returning traveller with diarrhoea should always be evaluated for infectious diseases especially when it is associated with fever. Indications for investigations and antimicrobial treatment depend on host factors, severity of disease and specific pathogens. The incubation period is variable but is usually up to 2 weeks. The aetiologies can be divided into bacteria, viruses and parasites.

Table 12.3 Recognised infectious agents causing 'travellers' diarrhoea'

Bacteria	*Escherichia coli*
	Campylobacter jejuni
	Salmonella
	Shigella
	Clostridioides difficile
	Vibrio parahaemolyticus and *Vibrio cholerae*
	Yersinia enterocolitica
Virus	*Rotavirus*
	Norovirus
	Adenovirus
Parasite	*Giardia lamblia*
	Cryptosporidium parvum and *hominis*
	Microsporidia
	Entamoeba histolytica

Patients usually present with fever, malaise, abdominal pain, nausea, vomiting and profuse watery diarrhoea with or without blood and mucus. The duration of the illness can last more than a month.

Investigations

Patients with mild symptoms may not need investigations. Those with fever and bloody stools, severe nonintestinal symptoms, prolonged diarrhoea of more that 7 days and those who are immunocompromised will need further investigation.

Treatment and management

The main goal of treatment is the prevention of dehydration with either enteral or intravenous fluid therapy. Antimicrobial treatment is generally not required. Certain conditions will also indicate the need for antibiotics and these would include:

* *Clostridioides difficile* gives pseudomembranous enterocolitis
* cholera
* giardiasis
* amoebiasis

Malaria

Symptoms of malaria can be nonspecific and there should be high index of suspicion with early assessment especially when the child has recently travelled to endemic malarial area. Rapidly progressive disease, with high risk of mortality and morbidity, is commonly associated with falciparum malaria.

Imported disease is usually from endemic areas including South Asia, Africa, Central and South America and Oceania. About 75% of infections in the UK are caused by Plasmodium falciparum which has an incubation period between 6 days and 6 months although patients with malaria infection due to other species may present more than 12 months after return from endemic area.

Symptoms include fever and excessive sweating, myalgia, headache, somnolence and vomiting.

Patients suspected to have malaria should be assessed as a medical emergency as the condition can be rapidly progressive. Physical signs commonly found in children are hepatomegaly and splenomegaly whilst cerebral malaria caused by *Plasmodium falciparum* leads to reduced consciousness, seizures, decorticate or decerebrate posturing.

Investigations

Microscopy of thick and thin smear samples is diagnostic although a rapid diagnostic test for malarial antigen can be employed at the same time as smear samples. The percentage of cells with parasitic inclusions should be determined after the infection has been confirmed whilst three negative samples over 24–48 hours are required to exclude malaria.

Treatment and management

Children who travel to malarial endemic area should receive antimalarial prophylaxis. Those who are diagnosed with malaria should be treated using local protocols and following microbiological advice. *Plasmodium falciparum* in most parts of the world is resistant to chloroquine and mefloquine and these should not be used. The treatment of choice for severe or complicated malaria in adults and children is intravenous artesunate. Primaquine is used to ensure the eradication of the hepatic stage of *Plasmodium vivax* and *ovale* as otherwise relapse is possible. Any patient who requires primaquine must be tested for G6PD deficiency prior to commencement.

Typhoid fever/enteric fever

Typhoid fever is endemic in South Asia, South East Asia, Middle East, Africa, South and Central America. It is a severe systemic illness classically caused by *Salmonella enterica* serotype Typhi (formerly known as *Salmonella typhi*). Illness from *Salmonella enterica* serotype Paratyphi A, B and C (previously known as *Salmonella paratyphi*) leads to a similar but milder clinical syndrome called paratyphoid fever.

Both typhoid and paratyphoid fevers are collectively known as enteric fever. Transmission is through ingestion of contaminated water or food. Asymptomatic carriers are a recognised reservoir for the organisms and play an important role as vehicles of transmission.

Individuals with typhoid fever follow a recognised pattern of disease evolution:
- first week—a rising fever and a relative bradycardia
- second week—abdominal pain, diarrhoea and rose spots
- third week—hepatosplenomegaly, intestinal bleeding, perforation due to ileocecal necrosis

Investigations

Diagnosis will usually come from the culture of blood, stool and bone marrow aspirate; although the latter is the most sensitive test, it is rarely required.

Treatment and management

There is increasing antibiotic resistance to *Salmonella enterica* serotype Typhi especially in the Middle East, South Asia and South East Asia. If there is strong suspicion of enteric fever, then empirical treatment with parenteral antibiotics should be started following local guidelines (ceftriaxone, cefotaxime, meropenem). Dexamethasone may be considered in patients with severe systemic illness (delirium, obtundation, stupor, coma or shock).

Prevention of the disease comes from food and water safety and hygiene when travelling to typhoid endemic area and immunisation for children prior to travel. The available vaccines are:
- Ty21a live attenuated oral vaccine
- intramuscular injection of Vi capsular polysaccharide vaccine

Potential complications

Recognised sequelae include intestinal perforation, meningitis, encephalomyelitis, pneumonia, haemolytic uraemic syndrome and hepatitis. Relapse can occur some 2–3 weeks after the resolution of the fever and may be associated with incorrect antibiotic choice or inadequate duration of therapy. Chronic carriage is defined as excretion of the organism in stool for more than 12 months after the acute infection.

Kawasaki disease

Kawasaki disease is a systemic vasculitis predominately affecting the coronary arteries. The precise aetiology remains unknown however it is suspected that an infectious agent may trigger an abnormal immunological response in genetically susceptible children. It is an important differential in presentations of fever of unknown origin.

Clinical presentation

The majority of children are under 5 years of age with the peak age incidence 18-24 months. There are usually no localising signs to suggest an infective cause. The diagnostic features are outline in adjacent box.

PRACTICE POINT—Kawasaki disease: diagnostic features

- fever persisting for 5 or more days
plus four or more of:
- early in presentation
  - erythema of palms or soles
  - non-pitting oedema
- later presentation
  - desquamation of fingers or toes
  - polymorphous rash
  - bilateral nonsuppurative conjunctival injection/conjunctivitis
  - lips and oral mucosal changes
    - red cracked lips
    - strawberry tongue
  - cervical lymphadenopathy

Alternative diagnoses

Streptococcal infection, including scarlet fever, is the main differential for the constellation of symptoms and signs of Kawasaki disease.

Investigations

There is no diagnostic test for Kawasaki disease. Diagnosis is made on clinical grounds with investigations undertaken to exclude other causes such as infection. An echocardiogram should be undertaken at diagnosis with coronary artery diameter and any dilatation or aneurysms commented on specifically. A normal echocardiogram does not exclude the diagnosis

Treatment and management

The aim of treatment is to reduce the occurrence of coronary artery aneurysms. Immunoglobulin is a blood product of pooled antibodies which is given as an intravenous infusion. The efficacy of immunoglobulin treatment is associated with use early in the disease process with limited efficacy after 10 days of symptoms. Aspirin is started at anti-inflammatory doses during the acute phase of illness and then reduced to anti-platelet doses once fever and inflammation have resolved. It is then continued until any aneurysms have resolved. Corticosteroids may have a role in treatment of cases refractory to immunoglobulins where ongoing fever and inflammation and coronary artery changes persist.

Potential complications

Coronary artery dilatation and aneurysms are a significant risk in Kawasaki disease and can occur in 15–25% of untreated cases and the risk of an acute cardiac event is increased. Other cardiac complications include pericardial effusion, pericarditis, myocarditis, coronary artery stenosis and myocardial infarction.

IMPORTANT CLINICAL POINTS

Bacterial disease
- Neisseria meningitides
  - notifiable disease
  - public health staff will advise on contact tracing and prophylaxis
- Streptococcus
  - notifiable disease—invasive group A
- Pertussis
  - notifiable disease
  - lymphocytosis common
- Lyme disease

- high-risk areas for infected ticks are wooded areas in Scotland, New Forest, Lake District

Tuberculosis investigations
- Mantoux test does not differentiate between active and latent TB
- IGRA test does not differentiate between active and latent TB
- early morning gastric aspirates cultured over weeks and positive culture in 30% to 40%
  - PCR-based assay gives information within few hours on positive samples

IMPORTANT CLINICAL POINTS—CONT'D

Viral disease
- Herpes simplex virus
  - HSV-1 is usually transmitted in saliva
  - HSV-2 is usually transmitted in genital secretions
- Varicella zoster
  - spreads by airborne droplets
  - incubation period is 10–21 days
  - infectivity starts 2 days before onset of rash and until all lesions crusted
- EBV
  - lymphocytosis along with atypical lymphocytes
  - may clinically mimic acute leukaemia
- Covid
  - may produce multiorgan failure (PIMS-TS) with coronary artery dilatation and aneurysm

- Hepatitis B
  - incubation period between 60 to 150 days
  - in UK national immunisation programme
- Hepatitis C
  - incubation period for postnatal infection is 6–12 weeks

Overseas infections
- malaria
  - incubation period between weeks and months.
  - notifiable disease
- typhoid fever/enteric fever
  - incubation period is 5–21 days.
  - notifiable disease

Further reading

Fever in under 5s: assessment and initial management. NICE guideline [NG143]. Published: November 2019. https://www.nice.org.uk/guidance/ng143

Sepsis: recognition, diagnosis and early management. NICE guideline [NG51]. Updated September 2017.

Meningitis (bacterial) and meningococcal septicaemia in under 16s: recognition, diagnosis and management. NICE Clinical guideline [CG102]. Updated February 2015. https://www.nice.org.uk/guidance/cg102

Pesch MH, et al.: Congenital cytomegalovirus Infection, *BMJ* 373:n1212, 2021.

Coronavirus – COVID 19 NICE. https://www.nice.org.uk/covid-19.

Chapter 13

Infection control

Ruth Radcliffe, Lucy Cliffe, Gillian Body

After reading this chapter you should:
- be able to follow the UK national guidelines on notification of communicable diseases
- know the principles of infection control
- be able to advise on immunisation in children with certain medical conditions
- know about the appropriate use of antimicrobials
- know the current infection control strategies for local, epidemic and pandemic infections

Notification of communicable diseases

Public health services in the UK provide a nationwide system of identifying and managing infectious diseases within the community. The aim is to detect possible outbreaks of disease and epidemics as early and as rapidly as is possible. It is recognised, however, that underreporting is widespread. Registered medical practitioners have a statutory duty to refer a patient to Public Health officials if they are considered to have one of the conditions listed on the UK schedule of Notifiable Disease. Additionally, if the patient is thought to be infected in a way that may cause significant harm to others, then the doctor must notify the local health protection team. Laboratories must also report to the Public Health Service if they isolate any of the listed causative organisms.

The list is updated periodically and does change with local disease outbreaks or worldwide health threats. In 2020 there were 33 infectious diseases which required notification.

Table 13.1 Infectious diseases which require notification to Public Health Services (This list shows examples and is not exhaustive)

Description	Examples
those preventable by routine vaccines	mumps, measles, rubella, diphtheria, whooping cough
those which spread quickly and for which a 'source' may be identifiable	food poisoning, haemolytic uraemic syndrome, Legionnaires' disease
those from overseas	malaria, viral haemorrhagic fever, enteric fever
those which spread through populations and can be carried asymptomatically	tuberculosis, meningococcal septicaemia, SARS, COVID-19
other common paediatric conditions	acute encephalitis, acute meningitis, invasive Group A streptococcal disease, scarlet fever

Infection control

Knowledge of common infections in children, their routes of transmission, incubation periods and methods to prevent transmission is important and timely clinical diagnosis or suspicion of an infection is the first step in infection control. Microbiological samples should then be sent promptly for confirmation.

Modes of transmission

Droplet

Droplets may be generated from the respiratory tract during coughing, sneezing, talking or singing. If droplets from an infected person come into contact with the mucous membranes or surface of the eye of a recipient, they can transmit infection. These droplets remain in the air for a short period of time and travel up to two metres, so physical distancing helps limit transmission.

Airborne

Aerosols are smaller than droplets and can remain in the air for longer and, therefore, potentially transmit infection by mucous membrane contact or inhalation. Aerosol-generating procedures are therefore high risk for spreading infection.

Contact

Contact transmission may be direct or indirect. Infectious agents can be inadvertently passed directly from an infected person to a recipient who may then transfer the organism to the mucous membranes of their mouth, nose or eyes. Indirect contact transmission takes place when a recipient has contact with an object, such as furniture or equipment that an infected person may have contaminated by coughing or sneezing. Correct hand hygiene is, therefore, important in controlling the spread of disease.

Infectious period

The time period during which an infected person can transmit infection to someone else varies depending on the pathogen and person.

Standard precautions

Standard precautions are work practices that are required to achieve a basic level of infection prevention and control and are recommended for the treatment and care of all patients. These precautions include hand hygiene with soap and water or alcohol gel, glove use and a 'bare below the elbow' policy for staff to allow effective hand-washing. The World Health Organisation promotes the principle of the 'Five Moments of Hand Hygiene' when hands should be washed:

- before touching a patient
- before a clean or aseptic procedure
- after exposure to body fluids
- after touching a patient
- after touching the patient's surroundings

Transmission-based precautions are recommended for patients known or suspected to be infected or colonised with infectious agents that can spread and may not be contained by standard precautions alone. Patients who require transmission-based precautions should be isolated in individual side rooms.

Personal protective equipment refers to a variety of barriers which must be used alone or in combination, to protect mucous membranes, airways, skin and clothing from contact with infectious agents and includes apron or gown, gloves and surgical mask. For procedures in patients with highly infectious disease which may generate an aerosol then protective eyewear, face shields or an FFP3 respirator should be considered. Local workplace infection control policies for general procedures and specific infections should be followed.

Contact tracing is an important part of limiting the spread of some infectious diseases. An assessment should be made regarding the risk of transmission of infection to any contacts in the household, at work, during social events and normal daily activity. For some infections such as meningococcal disease, antibiotic prophylaxis would be offered to significant contacts.

Frontline health staff should be up to date with immunisations and be aware of their own immunity to protect themselves from vaccine preventable infectious diseases. This would include MMR, BCG, Hepatitis B, Influenza and Varicella vaccinations.

Immunisation

Routine immunisation

Vaccination has made a massive positive impact on the global health burden, frequently quoted as being only second to that of the provision of clean water and sanitation. The UK childhood immunisation schedule provides protection against a range of conditions and a standard schedule is in place.

The immunisation programme is designed to protect the very young from dangerous diseases whilst ongoing boosters offer continuing coverage. The ages chosen for immunisation balances the risk of the disease against the ability to respond to the vaccine (Table 13.1). The schedule may change at short notice and the most up-to-date listing is found on the UK government website.

Premature infants should be vaccinated at their chronological age and not at the corrected age. Those born extremely prematurely are at risk of apnoea after vaccination and should be monitored for 48–72 hrs following vaccination.

Complications of vaccination

Adverse events following immunisation relates to any event occurring around the time of immunisation but

Table 13.2 UK Immunisation schedule (as of September 2020)	
Age Due	**Vaccines Given**
8 weeks	diphtheria, tetanus, pertussis, polio, Haemophilus influenza type b (Hib), hepatitis B (6-in-1) meningococcal group B* rotavirus—oral vaccine
12 weeks	diphtheria, tetanus, pertussis, polio, Hib, hepatitis B rotavirus (oral vaccine) pneumococcal conjugate vaccine
16 weeks	diphtheria, tetanus, pertussis, polio, Hib and hepatitis B meningococcal group B*
1 year	Hib and meningococcal group C pneumococcal conjugate vaccine measles, mumps and rubella meningococcal group B*
2 years to 16 years (annually; to be phased in)	influenza (live attenuated nasal vaccine)
3 years 4 months or soon after	diphtheria, tetanus, pertussis, polio measles, mumps and rubella
12–13 years (girls and boys)	human papillomavirus–two doses
14 years	tetanus diphtheria and polio meningococcal groups A, C, W, Y

*Conjugate MenB has been shown to increase risk of fever when given with other vaccines, and this is the one time when prophylactic paracetamol is recommended during the standard immunisation schedule.

which may or may not be caused by the vaccine. This is a deliberately vague definition which aims to encourage the reporting of such events.

Vaccine-induced events include both local and systemic reactions. Common local responses include pain, redness and swelling and, even if severe, do not contraindicate further doses of the vaccine. Systemic reactions include fever, malaise, headache and myalgia and the timing of these can vary depending on the vaccine given. Fever can start within hours of tetanus-containing vaccine but 7–10 days after measles-containing vaccine, and these fevers may be complicated by febrile convulsions. Systemic reactions do not contraindicate further doses of the vaccine.

Contraindications to vaccinations

Practically all children and young people can be safely vaccinated with all the vaccines in the schedule. The main contraindication recorded in the UK 'Green Book' include:
- anaphylactic reaction to a previous dose—extremely rare
- immunosuppressed children—should not receive live vaccines although if the child only has antibody deficiency, then live vaccines are safe

Senior advice should be sought whenever there is doubt about administration of the vaccine and this is preferable to delaying the vaccination. The details of specific contraindications to each immunisation can be found in *Immunisation against Infectious Disease* ('The Green Book') published by the UK Government which should be checked prior to the administration of any vaccine.

There are many spurious or unfounded reasons for avoiding vaccination and these should be sensitively challenged. An example of one such spurious reason is 'children with egg allergy should not be given the MMR vaccine'. MMR is completely safe for those with proven egg allergy and the vaccination can be given in the GP surgery with standard precautions.

Specific issues to be clarified with each patient include:
- if any confirmed anaphylactic reaction to a previous dose of the vaccine
- presence of primary or secondary immunodeficiency
- close contact with another individual with immunodeficiency

Vaccination in pregnancy

In 2012 there was an increase in notifications of pertussis in the UK and a temporary programme was introduced to vaccinate pregnant women against pertussis between 16 and 32 weeks. As the mother's immunity to pertussis would have waned, it allowed boosted antibodies to be passed from mother to baby. This gave protection to the baby until the primary immunisations begin. Pregnant mothers are offered annual influenza immunisation to protect both the mother and, via passive immunity, the baby.

Vaccination of children with unknown or incomplete immunisation status

Children who are not immunised or have an uncertain vaccination status and are born in the UK should be reviewed and every effort made to administer any outstanding doses. Children arriving from abroad who do not have a reliable history of immunisation should be assumed to be unimmunised and a full course of required immunisations should be arranged. A more detailed algorithm to aid decisions is available on the Public Health England website (see Further reading).

Immunising the immunocompromised child

Children with clinical conditions where vaccinations are contraindicated

There are some clinical situations where it is not safe to administer a vaccine to a child. This would include children with significant T cell suppression where a live vaccine strain may cause disease.

PRACTICE POINT—live vaccines in current UK routine childhood programme

- measles, mumps and rubella
- rotavirus
- influenza (live attenuated nasal vaccine)
- BCG

Children with clinical conditions may need extra vaccinations

Certain immune deficiencies leave some children at risk of specific infections and they may therefore require extra vaccines. Those with asplenia and complement deficiency are at increased the risk of infection by encapsulated bacteria. These patients should receive additional protection against Meningococcus A, C, W, Y and B, Pneumococcus and Haemophilus influenza type b. Some children may not respond well to their vaccines, and extra vaccinations to these three may be advised depending on tested antibody results.

When future immunosuppression can be predicted, vaccines may be given in advance to reduce the risk of infection once the child becomes immunosuppressed. An example of such practice is the administration of chickenpox vaccine to those due to receive a renal transplant. In general, all immunosuppressed children should receive an annual influenza vaccine, unless critically immunosuppressed.

Children who have received a bone marrow transplant should be considered for a revaccination schedule which usually commences at least 12 months after BMT and 6 months off immunosuppression.

Children where some vaccinations may not be effective

Children with significant T cell or B cell immunosuppression may not be able to mount an immune response to vaccination, so it cannot be relied upon to prevent infection. In the event of their exposure to certain illnesses such as varicella or measles, it may be appropriate to offer prophylaxis in the form of immunoglobulin or antimicrobials.

Children where family members to be vaccinated

All family members of children with moderate to severe immune suppression should receive an annual influenza vaccine. Those with significant T-cell abnormalities should avoid contact with people receiving the live intranasal vaccine for 7 days. Family members of those with severe immune suppression should be vaccinated against measles, mumps and rubella, if they have not already received a full course of this vaccine.

Antimicrobial use

Antimicrobial resistance is a global public health issue driven by the overuse of antimicrobials and inappropriate prescribing. The increase in resistance is making antimicrobial agents less effective and contributing to infections that are difficult to treat. The number of infections due to organisms resistant to multiple antibiotics is growing but the number of new antimicrobials in development is extremely limited. Antibiotic stewardship is an approach to promote judicious use of antimicrobials to preserve their future effectiveness.

Antibacterial drug choice

A number of factors should be considered when selecting the most appropriate antibacterial agent to use.

PRACTICE POINT—principles of good antibiotic stewardship

- do not start antibiotics without clinical evidence of bacterial infection
- if there is suspicion of bacterial infection, use local guidelines to start prompt, effective antibiotic treatment
- document clinical indication, duration, route and dose on the medicines chart and in the medical notes of the patient
- obtain cultures—knowing the infecting organism can lead to narrowing of broad-spectrum therapy, changing therapy to effectively treat resistant pathogens and stopping antibiotics when cultures suggest an infection is unlikely
- prescribe single-dose antibiotics for surgical prophylaxis if antibiotics have been shown to be effective
- review the clinical diagnosis and the continuing need for antibiotics by 48 hours from the first antibiotic dose and make a clear plan of action

---

Patient-related factors include age, weight, immune status, renal and hepatic function, other medications taken including oral contraception and route of administration. The availability of suitable formulations such as syrups instead of tablets and palatability of these will affect the adherence to treatment and this should influence prescribing decisions.

Suspected or known organism-related factors include site and severity of the infection and antibacterial susceptibility will also influence antibiotic choice.

Prescription dosing should be checked against those listed in the British National Formulary for Children (BNFc) and local prescribing guidance should also be consulted as these recognise local prevalence and resistance.

Infection control for epidemic and pandemic infections

Epidemics and pandemics are rare but the effects can be devastating in both their direct effect on the health of individuals or in their indirect effects on mental health, economic impact and national and international tensions. All of these issues have been clearly demonstrated by the recent COVID pandemic.

The World Health Organisation has presented a strategy document in the face of the COVID pandemic and outlined a structured plan of action to epidemics and pandemic infections. They advise:

- ensuring that the population is aware of the importance of limiting disease transmission through handwashing, avoiding hand contact with mucous membranes and physical distancing
- identifying infected individuals as early as possible and ensure they quarantine themselves
- establishing a mechanism of contact tracing from infected individuals
- promoting social distancing and nonessential contact and minimising domestic and international travel
- establish adequate health care facilities for those who become seriously ill with the infection
- establishing robust and effective public health measures
- supporting development of safe and effective vaccines
- clearing national leadership and communication

Further Reading

Immunisation against infectious disease (The Green Book) Public Health England. Published: September 2013. Last updated: November 202. https://www.gov.uk/government/collections/immunisation-against-infectious-disease-the-green-book

Vaccination of individuals with uncertain or incomplete immunisation status Public Health England. Published September 2013. Updated December 2019. https://www.gov.uk/government/publications/vaccination-of-individuals-with-uncertain-or-incomplete-immunisation-status

Chapter | 14 |

Allergy

Nicola Jay, Eleanor Minshall, Sibil Sonmez-Ajtai

> After reading this chapter you should be able to:
> • to assess, diagnose and manage allergies

Allergic conditions can present in a wide variety of ways from mild episodic rashes through to dramatic, rapid-onset, life-threatening illness. Many symptoms are common to those seen in other conditions and consequently the true aetiology can be missed and inappropriate diagnoses and management plans provided. Similarly, an incorrect allocation of an allergic cause to some of the problems presented in children can impact on their lifestyle. Although many atopic conditions can be managed by the general paediatric team, those with multisystem atopy, IgE food allergy or drug allergy require the advice and input of colleagues in a specialist allergy service.

Allergic reactions and anaphylaxis

Every year many children attend for unscheduled care at their primary care centre or local emergency department due to acute symptoms suggestive of allergy. The responses will vary from mild rhinitis or conjunctivitis or cardiorespiratory collapse due to an anaphylactic reaction.

Clinical presentation

Features of an allergic reaction include:
• urticaria
• peri-orbital oedema
• oral mucosal irritation
• vomiting
• diarrhoea
  The child with acute anaphylaxis will have stridor due to laryngeal oedema, respiratory distress with wheeze or acute circulatory collapse. Children or young people presenting in this way require urgent action.

Treatment and management

The immediate response to a child with acute anaphylaxis is the administration of intramuscular adrenaline. This administration must not be delayed whilst attempting to secure intravenous access or other hierarchical manoeuvres on the ABC pathway. A second dose of IM adrenaline can be given after 5 minutes if the patient has shown little or no evidence of clinical improvement. The airway should be maintained, supplemental oxygen given and intravenous crystalloid fluids provided in the knowledge that the adrenaline is administered. Any potential colloids which might be causative to anaphylaxis should be stopped. Chlorpheniramine and hydrocortisone should also be administered either IM or as a very slow IV dose. The anaphylaxis algorithm 2021 produced by the Resuscitation Council (UK) summarises the management plan (Figure 14.1).

Investigations

There are no investigations required during an episode of acute anaphylaxis although a blood sample taken after the child is stable may reveal an elevated tryptase (produced by mast cells) level. This would indicate that the presenting problem was due to an allergic reaction rather than any other cause of the acute collapse. If the history implicates a potential allergen, then a specific IgE can be requested.

Relevant pharmacological agents used

Nonsedative antihistamines should be used in the acute situation to ensure that sedation does not confuse the

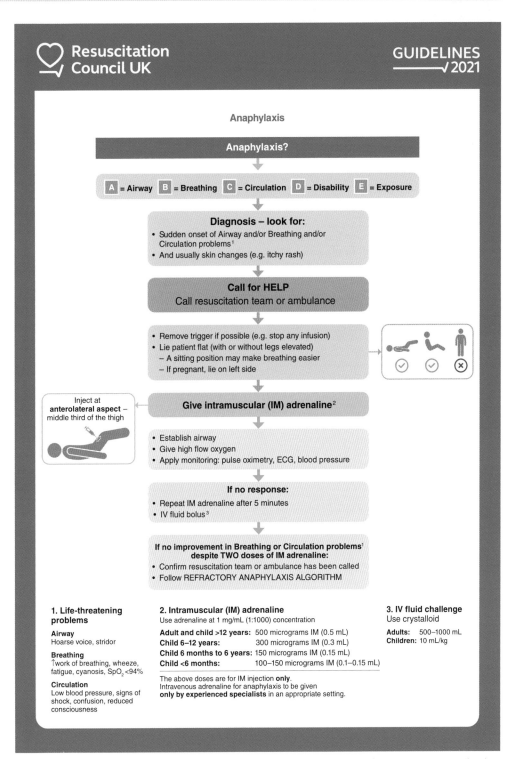

Fig. 14.1 Anaphylaxis Guideline 2021 (Reproduced with the kind permission of Resuscitation Council UK).

acute management. Similarly, when prescribed as part of a take home allergy plan, nonsedating antihistamines, such as cetirizine, are most commonly used due to their duration of action.

Adrenaline will relieve bronchospasm and support central blood pressure by vasoconstriction and therefore requires prompt administration. Adrenaline auto-injectors allow patients and carers to administer doses quickly and easily if necessary and are produced in two dose strengths—150 mcg and 300 mcg. It is important to explain the correct administration technique to the patient and family (Table 14.1).

Important sequelae

After the episode of the allergic reaction has been managed, it is important that a plan is put in place to ensure the child or young person remains safe in the future. A period of observation may be necessary, particularly if anaphylaxis was the presenting problem, and the current NICE guidelines advises a 12-hour period for those under 16 years. Clearly an attempt must be made at identifying the trigger so that appropriate avoidance advice can be given and an 'allergy plan' put in place. Templates for such plans are available online. The details of the reaction must be recorded in GP and hospital notes and a medical alert added to electronic records. A referral to a clinician with expertise in allergy management should be made if there is a concern regarding IgE-mediated food allergy, drug allergy or acute bronchospasm secondary to aeroallergen exposure.

Food allergy

Food allergy is common and affects up to 8% of infants in the UK. Many of the symptoms are nonspecific, leading to the diagnosis being overlooked or dismissed. There is, however, an increasing number of children being wrongly diagnosed with food allergy, probably due to a greater public awareness of allergies. The most important diagnostic tool for food allergy is a focused clinical history which enquires about:
- family and personal history of atopy
- relevant signs and symptoms
- how signs and symptoms related to the food ingested in terms of onset
- details of previous management of the condition

Table 14.1 Doses of 1:1000 adrenaline used in acute anaphylaxis

Dose	Age
Under 6 years	150 micrograms
6 to 12 years	300 micrograms
Over 12 years	500 micrograms

Table 14.2 IgE versus non-IgE mediated food allergies in children

	IgE-mediated food allergies	Nonallergic (non-IgE) food hypersensitivity
Typical signs and symptoms	urticarial rash; itchy red skin; swollen lips and eyes; itchy mouth and throat; vomiting; anaphylaxis	gastroesophageal reflux; vomiting; diarrhoea or constipation; blood or mucous in stools; eczema; poor weight gain
Onset of symptoms in relation to food ingestion	within minutes (up to 1 hour)	several hours or days (usually 4–72 hours)
Duration of symptoms following onset	few hours	several days
Frequency of symptoms	Episodic but each time the food ingested	chronic (since usually caused by a food consumed very frequently)
Common foods leading to allergy	egg milk peanuts other common foods: soya, tree nuts, sesame, fish, shellfish, wheat	milk soya wheat
Age of onset	1–4 years but can develop later	within the first year

It will also consider the need for, and interpretation of, any investigations.

In general, non-IgE mediated food allergies carry a more favourable prognosis with resolution common and likely to occur before 3–5 years of age in most children. In those with IgE-mediated food allergy, the prognosis differs depending on the allergenic food (Table 14.2). The majority of children with milk and egg allergy will experience full resolution over time whilst those with nut, fish and seafood allergies usually have lifelong problems.

There is a distinction in management between allergic reactions and nonallergic hypersensitivity reactions to food as demonstrated by the difference between cow's milk protein allergy and lactose intolerance. There is also a difference between IgE and non-IgE mediated food allergy in diagnosis, management and prognosis.

Contrary to earlier beliefs, it is now known that a prior episode of ingestion is not required in order to develop allergic sensitisation. Defective skin and gut barriers combined with altered microbiome (caused by caesarean birth, inappropriate use of antibiotics, antacids) are thought to play a big role in food allergy pathogenesis, alongside genetic factors such as a family history of atopy.

Clinical presentation

Children with adverse reactions to food can present with a wide and varied range of symptoms including:
- cutaneous rashes
- eczema
- vomiting
- diarrhoea
- poor weight gain
- mucosal sensitivity
- acute anaphylaxis

Investigations

Supportive allergy investigations are available for the confirmation or exclusion of IgE-mediated food allergy, including skin prick tests, specific IgE tests and oral food challenge tests. These tests are not appropriate for the investigation of non-IgE mediated food allergy, where the only investigative tool is exclusion diet followed by reintroduction to prove causality between suspect food and clinical symptoms.

Skin prick testing or specific IgE testing should be directed at suspected trigger foods and not for foods which the patient is consuming on regular basis without consistent symptoms after each and every ingestion.

Interpretation of a positive skin prick test (Figure 14.2) or specific IgE test must be undertaken with caution in children with coexisting atopic disease such as eczema, asthma, allergic rhinoconjunctivitis and eosinophilic gut

---

PRACTICE POINT—performing skin prick testing

- explain procedure to child and carers
- ensure no antihistamines in last 72 hours (ideally 5 days)
- ensure medications and equipment to treat allergic reaction available
- use volar aspect of the forearm and ensure skin appears normal
- mark skin with the initial letter of the allergen being tested
- mark skin for controls—POS + (histamine) and NEG— (normal saline)
- apply drop of extract and push lancet gently through drop
- use separate lancet for each drop
- read at 15 minutes after positive completed
- measure the longest extent of the wheal (excluding the flare) in millimetres
- wheal diameter of 3 mm or larger is considered positive
- IgE-mediated allergy to the test allergen is more likely with large wheal
- size of wheal cannot not predict severity of future allergic reactions

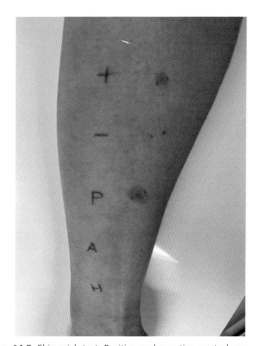

Fig. 14.2 Skin prick test. Positive and negative controls are visible along with the test for reaction to peanut, almond, hazelnut showing a reaction to peanut. The results should be interpreted in conjunction with the history.

CLINICAL SCENARIO

A 7-month-old infant with severe early-onset eczema was being fed by her mother. During the meal the infant developed perioral urticaria which quickly progressed to generalised urticaria, lip swelling, coughing and breathing difficulties. The infant then went limp and floppy and her mother called an ambulance. The meal consisted of a homemade puree of chicken and vegetables made with a stock cube. The infant previously tolerated this same meal the week before. On arrival at hospital, the infant was resuscitated with adrenaline, had intravenous fluids and antihistamines and was observed overnight. Her parents were told not to give her the meal again or any of the constituents and to carry their adrenaline auto-injectors and antihistamines at all times. Appropriate training and management plans were given prior to discharge and bloods taken for specific IgEs to chicken, carrot, onion and celery.

The infant was seen in clinic 2 weeks later and her eczema remained florid. Her specific IgEs to chicken, carrot, onion and celery were all negative and prick-to-prick testing to the puree was also negative. Further history taking revealed that her mother had been eating scrambled egg whilst feeding the infant and had cross-contaminated the puree when checking to ensure the puree was of the correct temperature. The infant had a 12 mm wheal to egg.

Common allergens in infancy are egg, dairy, wheat, nuts, sesame, fish and soya, and it is important to take a detailed allergen-focused history in any child with a history of anaphylaxis asking about potential exposure to these major allergens in particular. Anaphylaxis to trace exposure is uncommon but it is essential that the allergen responsible is identified as soon as possible and appropriate avoidance advice given.

disorders such as eosinophilic oesophagitis. Such atopic individuals often have positive test results to common foods and this does not always translate to clinical allergy.

Negative skin prick test or specific IgE tests make IgE-mediated food allergy unlikely, but if the history is suggestive, they cannot exclude it completely. In these children, a diagnostic oral food challenge may be required, to confirm or rule out allergy. This test carries a risk of an allergic reaction and must be performed in hospital under the supervision of staff who are trained in the recognition and management of allergic reactions and with immediate access to full resuscitation equipment.

High values in both the skin prick test (in mm) and specific IgE test (in kAU/L) increase the probability of food allergy, but they cannot predict the severity of future allergic reactions. The predictors of the severity of food allergy reactions are identified from the focused history and include:
- history of previous anaphylaxis
- coexistent atopic disease especially with asthma
- IgE-mediated allergies to multiple foods

- risk of exposure to the trigger food, depending on family diet, lifestyle, environment (e.g. home versus school versus holidays away from home)

There is often no need to perform all the tests (skin prick testing, specific IgE testing and oral food challenge) to reach the diagnosis of IgE-mediated food allergy. Following a focused history, the first-line test would usually be skin prick testing or specific IgE testing, depending on availability. Certain patient-specific conditions such as extensive eczema on the usual skin prick testing sites will also direct which specific test is the most appropriate. Systemic antihistamine must be excluded in the previous 72 hours prior to skin prick testing as they will reduce the intensity of any allergic response. The diagnosis does not need to be confirmed by oral food challenge, if the focused history is convincing and the supportive skin prick testing or specific IgE testing tests are positive.

PRACTICE POINT—undertaking a food challenge test

- explain procedure to child and carers
- ensure no antihistamines in last 72 hours (ideally 5 days)
- record vital signs—PEFR for those with asthma
- ensure medications and equipment to treat allergic reaction available
- portion challenge food into small to large portions
- starting with smallest portion administer 20–30 minutes apart
- aim for an age-appropriate full portion of the food
- ensure no signs or symptoms of allergic reaction before giving next portion
- if signs or symptoms of reaction, omit next portion and give oral antihistamine
- observe for 1–2 hours if full amount consumed and no problems
- observe for at least 2 hours if oral antihistamine alone given
- observe at least 6–8 hours if anaphylaxis
- outcome communicated to GP and carers (school with permission)
- provide up-to-date written allergy management plan

The oral food challenge tests can be performed for different reasons, including:
- to confirm or rule out allergy where initial management has not been able to confirm or refute the diagnosis of food allergy
- to assess whether the child has developed tolerance and outgrown their food allergy
- to reconfirm the diagnosis and educate the patient in the recognition and management of a food allergic reaction

Treatment and management

All children with IgE-mediated food allergies need strict avoidance of the offending allergenic foods, including education on reading food labels. It is important to involve a dietitian who will offer advice on alternative safe foods to replace those to be avoided. Education of the recognition and emergency management of allergic reactions, including adrenaline auto injector training and the provision of emergency medications and written allergy management plans is crucial for patient, parent, school and anyone with a supervisory role for the child.

Not all children with food allergy will require an adrenaline auto injector provision, but all children with food allergy must have allergy management plans in place (see BSACI allergy plans link).

It is essential to emphasise the adrenaline auto injector must be available to the patient at all times and should never be left at home, even if there is no intention to eat when the child is out. Schools and nurseries must keep at least one adrenaline auto injector for the child, and there is UK legislation which allows schools to purchase an injector for any child with a diagnosis of food allergy. Such children must be in possession of a written allergy plan with signed consent from their parents in case of anaphylaxis.

At some stage in the care of a child, it may be considered important to assess whether the allergic reaction has resolved. The history may reveal an absence of reactions in the last 6–12 months and this, combined with significant reduction in skin prick testing measurements or a reduction in specific IgE levels, suggests that an oral food challenge is appropriate.

Dietician assessment and input must be available at each consultation to all patients, particularly young children, those with milk allergy and multiple food allergies and families who need support and ideas of safe nutritious foods and recipes.

Children with non-IgE mediated food allergy may start a programme of food reintroduction if there had been no reactions to the foods in the preceding 6 months and there was a general improvement in eczema and gut symptoms. In infants with mild to moderate non-IgE cow's milk allergy, this is generally undertaken via the 'milk ladder' and directed by their dietitian.

A delay in the introduction of allergenic foods into the weaning diet of infants increases the risk of food allergy in high-risk infants (those with family history of atopy and early onset eczema). Weaning should be initiated between 4–6 months of age (but no earlier than 17 weeks). Although there is no clear evidence that breastfeeding reduces the risk of food allergy, it has proven benefits and so, whenever possible, exclusive breastfeeding should be encouraged and should be continued alongside weaning to a solid diet. The introduction of peanut butter and egg into the weaning diet as early as possible reduces the risk of peanut and egg allergy.

Acute and chronic urticaria
Clinical presentation

Both wheals and angioedema are recognised features of urticaria.

Wheals affect the upper skin surfaces and are more commonly known as 'hives' or a 'nettle sting rash'. They are red, raised, itchy swellings generally between 2 to 10 mm in diameter with a pale centre. In the vast majority of individuals, these lesions are transient with the skin returning to normal within 20 to 30 minutes, although occasionally they persist for up to 24 hours.

Angioedema describes swelling of the deeper skin structures which can be painful and usually involves the periorbital area and mucosal surfaces of the mouth and airways. These swellings usually last for 24–48 hours but rarely can persist for several days and can leave areas of hyperpigmentation (Table 14.3).

Investigations

In acute urticaria, wheals and angioedema are transient and, by definition, persist for less than 6 weeks. Viral infections are a frequently reported cause in over 40% of affected children, but as the condition is self-limiting, no diagnostic investigations are necessary. Only children with suspected IgE-mediated food or drug allergy require further testing.

In chronic urticaria, lesions may occur daily with symptoms lasting longer than 6 weeks. Although rarely life-threatening, chronic urticaria may lead to misery, embarrassment and significant school absence. Chronic urticaria is classified into two main groups, spontaneous and inducible urticaria. While chronic urticaria is not thought of as an atopic disorder, a history of atopy or other allergic conditions is present in up to 40% of this population (Table 14.4).

Treatment and management

Acute urticaria requires the use of an appropriate dose of nonsedating antihistamines such as cetirizine or loratadine.

For most children with chronic urticaria, symptomatic treatment with antihistamines will be the mainstay of treatment, and parents should be reassured that this condition regresses with time. Although food allergy is a common concern voiced by families, an IgE-mediated food allergy is rarely the cause of chronic spontaneous urticaria.

Table 14.3 **Swellings in the absence of rashes**

Diagnosis	Description of lesions	Clinical information
Hereditary angioedema	angioedema of: face throat extremities	often family history of angioedema starts in first to second decade of life swelling not itchy can be life threatening
Drug-induced angioedema	angioedema	associated with: NSAIDS codeine ACE inhibitors may occur weeks to months after starting the drugs

Table 14.4 **Recommended classification of chronic urticaria**

Description	Type	Examples of triggers
Chronic spontaneous urticaria (CSU)	spontaneous appearance of wheals, angioedema or both for longer than 6 weeks due to known or unknown cause	stress; drugs (nonsteroidal antiinflammatory drugs, codeine, angiotensin inhibitors); infections
Chronic inducible urticaria (CIU)	aquagenic	contact with hot or cold water
	cholinergic/exercise	emotion; physical exertion
	cold	swimming in cold water; cold wind
	delayed pressure	sitting; lying; tight clothing
	dermatographism	minor trauma; heat; hot bath/shower
	solar	sunshine
	vibratory	use of vibrating tools

In chronic urticaria, symptom diaries may be useful in trying to determine a causative trigger and objectively monitoring severity and frequency of symptoms. If triggers are found, then avoidance advice would be key. Since approximately one third of children with cold-induced urticaria will exhibit features suggestive of anaphylaxis, then prescription of an appropriate adrenaline auto injector and training in its use may be necessary. Most children with physical urticaria outgrow their symptoms within 2 to 3 years.

Management of chronic urticaria involves avoidance strategies when an obvious precipitant is identified, and this may be possible with the recording of symptoms in a diary. Standard doses of non sedating antihistamines, such as cetirizine or loratadine, may be offered if the symptoms are troublesome and, on occasions, a short course of corticosteroids for severe exacerbations. Once symptoms are controlled, it is recommended that the child stays on daily treatment for 3 to 6 months, but a referral to an allergy specialist should be considered if the above plan is not adequate.

Relevant pharmacological agents used

Cetirizine and **loratadine** are nonsedating antihistamines and block histamine H_1 receptors. They are generally well tolerated but should be used with caution in children with epilepsy as they can precipitate seizure activity.

Asthma and allergy

Asthma is defined by clinical symptoms, response to anti-asthma medication and abnormal physiological tests. Allergic sensitisation in the early years of life, below the age of five years and particularly less than aged one, is associated with the persistence of an asthma diagnosis into the teenage years.

There is little concrete evidence that perennial allergen avoidance in most children is effective in improving asthma control and reducing the need for medication. Seasonal allergies often cause exacerbations and this may be by having poorly controlled allergic rhinitis which extends into the lower airways or due to allergens such as grass pollen causing immediate hypersensitivity reactions within the lungs.

Moulds such as Cladosporium, Aspergillus and Alternaria can be particularly problematic acting synergistically with house dust mite to compound the effect of both. Alternaria allergy is associated with severe exacerbations of asthma, particularly during thunderstorms.

Clinical presentation

Children with an acute asthma attack will present with the classical features of breathlessness, feeling of a 'tight' chest and cough. Examination reveals tachypnoea, intercostal recession, chest indrawing and a 'tracheal tug'. Many allergens have a seasonal influence on the timing of the presentation:
- winter—house dust mite
- spring—tree pollen (birch, oak, willow, moulds)
- summer—grass and weed pollen
- autumn—weed pollen and house dust mite
- all year—animals (dogs, cats, rabbits, horses), moulds

Investigations

Evidence of exacerbating factors such as aeroallergen sensitisation must be sought as identification of the offending antigen is helpful in management. Specific IgE or skin prick tests may contribute to understanding the aetiology of the problem.

Management of allergic aspect of asthma

Allergen avoidance is important and attempted with steps such as:
- **house dust mite**—minimising exposure at night time with hypoallergenic bedding and mattress covers and ensuring that the room is cool with air being able to circulate around the bed can improve symptoms. The presence of soft toys in bed should be minimised and they should be washed or frozen to remove house dust mite allergens.
- **pollens**—ensuring that the bedding is not dried outside during the offending pollen season, keeping bedroom windows closed and reducing allergens by washing of hair and using nasal douching prior to sleep. Other measures in the daytime include the placing of petroleum jelly at the nasal entrance and avoiding playing on freshly mown grass or under trees.
- **moulds**—avoiding areas around compost heaps and any fallen leaves may be helpful. Indoor moulds are much less likely to cause respiratory exacerbations unless they are present in significant amounts.

- **pets**—it may be appropriate to restrict pets to specific areas of the house, but if symptoms are severe, then removing the animal from the home may be necessary.

Allergic rhinoconjunctivitis

Rhinitis describes the condition when symptoms of inflammation are limited to the nasal mucosa but can also be rhinoconjunctivitis when the conjunctivae are also involved and rhinosinusitis when the sinus linings are involved. It can be described as allergic, nonallergic or infective rhinitis.

Clinical presentation

Patients with allergic rhinitis will present with clear bilateral nasal discharge, nasal itch, congestion and sneezing. Symptoms are triggered by exposure to suspected allergens and usually respond to oral antihistamine and regular use of nasal corticosteroid spray. Symptoms may be seasonal or perennial, intermittent or persistent or mild or severe.

Common allergens:
- house dust mite (carpets, bedding, duvets, pillows, soft furnishings, stuffed toys)
- tree pollen in spring
- grass pollen in summer
- weed pollen in late summer/autumn
- animal dander (cats, dogs, horses, rabbits)
- mould
- air pollution, tobacco smoke and strong perfumes

  Examination can reveal:
- red watery puffy eyes
- 'allergic salute' (the palm of the hand swept upward over the nose)
- horizontal nasal crease across dorsum of nose (a result of the allergic salute)
- mouth breathing

Investigations

Skin prick tests to specific inhalant allergens should be performed and have a high negative predictive value making allergic rhinoconjunctivitis unlikely if negative. Serum specific IgE to specific inhalant allergens should be performed if skin prick tests are not possible or when the skin prick tests together with the clinical history give equivocal results. Further laboratory investigations are usually unnecessary.

Treatment and management

Treatment includes avoiding known allergens where possible. Pharmacological support includes oral antihistamines, nasal steroid spray and finally leukotrienes such as montelukast. Immunotherapy is a treatment that may be appropriate for a selected group of patients with severe allergic rhinitis.

Relevant pharmacological agents used

Montelukast is a leukotriene receptor antagonist and is commonly used in treatment of allergic disorders. The recognised side effects include diarrhoea, fever and skin reactions. There have been recent concerns over psychological effects and the drug should be withheld if there is a history of depression. The patient and families need to be warned about the risk of night terrors and mental health problems (particularly anxiety and suicidal ideation).

Important sequelae

- rhinitis significantly reduces quality of life and interferes with school attendance and performance
- both allergic and nonallergic rhinitis are risk factors for the development of asthma
- rhinitis impairs asthma control and increases its costs
- sleep problems leading to effects on concentration, mood and behaviour

Drug allergy

Adverse drug reactions, including any undesired effects that appear during a course of treatment, should be considered as potential drug allergies. The majority of these are predictable from the known effects of the drug whilst a minority are unpredictable.

Surprisingly, atopy is not a risk factor for IgE-mediated drug allergy, but it may predispose to more serious reactions. As many as 10% of parents report their child to be allergic to a drug, with beta-lactams being the most frequently suspected. There are, however, many published studies which have confirmed the low incidence of true drug allergy by formal challenge testing, and this is particularly notable for supposed antibiotic allergy where less than 4% of individuals are truly allergic. The second most common reported allergy is to NSAID.

Clinical presentation

When a child is thought to have undergone an allergic drug response, it is important that a full history is obtained, documenting signs and symptoms as well as temporal relationship to administration of the drug in question. Where a potential antibiotic reaction has occurred, it is important to record the reason for the prescription as infections such as beta-haemolytic streptococcus can independently cause urticaria whilst cross-reactivity

between EBV and amoxicillin causes a morbilliform rash. The most common reason for children being given the diagnosis of 'penicillin allergy' is the result of an exanthem caused by a virus infection being inappropriately treated.

Drug hypersensitivity reactions are categorised into immediate (within one hour of drug administration) and delayed (being more than one hour after drug administration) (Table 14.5).

The active ingredient is only part of a drug with many other ingredients making up the whole compound. Consequently, it is important to record the brand name of the medication so that the extra components of the drug formulation can be considered.

Investigation

During a potential reaction to a drug, it may be useful to obtain blood for:
- tryptase
- LFT—delayed reactions may cause increase in transaminases
- U&E—acute kidney injury may occur
- FBC—delayed reactions may cause eosinophilia, leukopenia and thrombocytopenia
- specific IgE to the drug concerned

Treatment and management

Any acute allergic response must be manged appropriately with an ABC approach:
- IM adrenaline if cardiac compromise
- removal of the trigger
- antihistamines and corticosteroids
- the drug in question should be avoided with the allergy status documented on the hospital and primary care record. If the drug is difficult to avoid or an acceptable alternative needed, then it is important to refer to an allergy specialist where skin prick testing and, if appropriate, intradermal testing can be undertaken.

Table 14.5 **Recognised features seen in drug reactions**		
Allergic response	**Symptoms**	**Nomenclature**
Immediate	swollen mucosa; erythematous skin; bronchospasm; hypotension	probably IgE mediated
Delayed	morbilliform rash; fixed drug eruption; Steven-Johnson syndrome; toxic epidermal necrolysis	

The majority of children who are said to be allergic to beta-lactam antibiotics are not. However, it is important to ensure that relabelling of beta-lactam allergy status is done in a safe way. In children who have a history of mild exanthem to beta-lactams more than one hour after administration of a dose of the antibiotic, it is advisable to give a test dose of the antibiotic under medical supervision. No allergy testing is needed. A 'test dose' involves the administration of 10% of the total standard dose followed 20 minutes later by the remainder of that dose. If tolerated then the rest of the course of the antibiotics can be given as an inpatient or outpatient as required.

There is no evidence that IgE-mediated drug allergy has an inherited predisposition. There is a possibility, however, that non-IgE mediated drug allergy can be associated with human leucocyte antigen (HLA) types or other genetic abnormalities.

IMPORTANT CLINICAL POINTS acute anaphylaxis

Acute anaphylaxis
- presents with laryngeal oedema, respiratory distress, wheeze or circulatory collapse
- requires immediate administration IM adrenaline
- elevated tryptase, produced by mast cells, would indicate allergic reaction food allergy

Food allergy
- allergy focussed clinical history is crucial
- allergy tests aid diagnosis and monitor IgE-mediated allergies
- non-IgE allergy can only be assessed by exclusion and reintroduction acute and chronic urticaria

Acute and chronic urticaria
- angioedema usually involves periorbital area and mucosa of mouth and airways

- only children with suspected IgE-mediated allergy require further testing
- symptom diaries may be useful in trying to determine a causative trigger allergic rhinoconjunctivitis

Allergic rhinoconjunctivitis
- skin prick tests to specific inhalant allergens have a high negative predictive value drug allergy

Drug allergy
- beta-lactams most common reported
- NSAID is second most common reported
- atopy is not a risk factor for IgE-mediated drug allergy
- atopy may predispose to more serious reactions
- active ingredient is only part of a drug and other ingredients may cause reaction

---

Further reading

Erlewyn-Lajeunesse M, Weir T, Brown L et al. The EATERS method for the diagnosis of food allergies Erlewyn-Lajeunesse M, Weir T, Brown L et al. *Arch Dis Child Edu Prac.* 2019; 104:286–291.

Allergy UK (charity). https://www.allergyuk.org/health-professionals/resources.

British Society for Allergy and Clinical Immunology (BSACI). Allergy templates and plans. https://www.bsaci.org/professional-resources/resources/paediatric-allergy-action-plans/

Food allergy in under 19s: assessment and diagnosis. NICE Clinical guideline [CG116]. Published date: February 2011. https://www.nice.org.uk/guidance/cg116

Chapter | 15 |

Immunology

Nafsika Sismanoglou, Ruth Radcliffe, Lucy Cliffe

After reading this chapter you should:
- primary and secondary immunodeficiency
- understand the presentation and management of autoimmune disorders

The impact of an infection depends on many factors including those of the host, those of the infecting organism and those of the environment including access to medical care. Recurrent infection is seen frequently in paediatric practice and there is often a need to assess whether this is a result of deficiencies within the individual.

Common causes for recurrent infection include:
- disruption in physical barrier of the host—cystic fibrosis, skin trauma, foreign bodies
- structural anomalies and dysfunction—CSF leaks, swallow dysfunction
- host immunodeficiency

Systemic immunodeficiency can present in many ways with some being overwhelming and catastrophic whilst others are indolent and subtle. Immunodeficiency diseases can be grouped by the underlying aetiology:
- primary immunodeficiencies
  - antibody immunodeficiencies
  - T-cell and combined immunodeficiencies
  - phagocytic disorders
- secondary immunodeficiency
  - treatment related
- immunodeficiencies as part of a syndrome

Primary immunodeficiencies

Primary abnormalities of the immune system can have significant and devastating consequences for a child or young person, and certain features of an illness raise the prospect of an underlying immunodeficiency. These infections include those which are Serious, Persistent, Unusual and Recurrent (SPUR). Those presenting with recurrent infections should be assessed for underlying primary immunodeficiency when two or more of the following signs are present:

PRACTICE POINT—consider immunodeficiency if:

- four or more ear infections in a year
- two or more severe sinus infections in a year
- two or more months of antibiotic treatment with little effect
- two or more pneumonias per year
- insufficient weight gain or growth delay
- recurrent deep skin or organ abscesses
- persistent mouth thrush or fungal skin infection
- need for iv antibiotics to clear infections
- two or more deep-seated infections
- family history of primary immunodeficiency

Other important indicators can be found in the family history, especially early infant deaths, other individuals affected by immunodeficiency, history of autoimmunity and malignancy.

Antibody immunodeficiencies

Children with these conditions are unable to produce protective antibodies, and this can be evident from birth or manifest later in life. There may be a deficiency in the level of one or more of the immunoglobulin classes, the IgG subclasses or in the response to polysaccharide antigens, and there are some children who present with combinations of all these abnormalities. In those children where the genetic defect has been identified, the mutation usually affects genes that regulate the B-cell development or the immunoglobulin genes themselves.

Conditions include
- X-linked agammaglobulinaemia
- common variable immunodeficiency disorder
- selective IgA deficiency
- specific antibody deficiency (SPAD)
- transient hypoglobulinaemia of infancy (THI)
- secondary antibody deficiencies

Clinical presentation

Patients with antibody deficiencies typically present with:
- recurrent sinopulmonary infections (otitis media, sinusitis, bronchopneumonia)
- chronic diarrhoea with *Giardia lamblia* infection
- skin infections are also common
  Viral infections are normally cleared as T cell function is usually intact.

Investigations

Initial assessment will include leucocyte count, lymphocyte subsets, immunoglobulin levels and functional antibodies to tetanus, *Haemophilus influenzae type b*, pneumococcal serotypes. HIV serology would also be important.

Treatment and management

In general, the aim of managing patients with a humoral deficiency, is to support growth and development and prevent organ damage, especially bronchiectasis. This is achieved by treating comorbidities, treating infections with antibiotics and ensuring appropriate immunisations, if indicated. In more severe or recurrent infections, prolonged prophylactic antibiotics would be appropriate and immunoglobulin replacement therapy may be necessary.

X-linked agammaglobulinaemia

X-linked agammaglobulinaemia (XLA) is caused by abnormal development of B cells and presents with near absence of these cells. It is caused by a mutation in Bruton's Tyrosine Kinase (BTK) gene although this is a spontaneous mutation in about 60% of the children.

Clinical presentation

XLA usually presents after the first 4–6 months of life, following the decline in maternal IgG. Half of children become symptomatic in the first year of life and 95% by the

age of 5 years. XLA is only seen in boys although autosomal recessive agammaglobulinemia has the same clinical picture as XLA and affects both boys and girls. Patients with XLA are also found to be more frequently affected by sensorineural hearing loss and eczema and have a higher risk of malignancy compared to the unaffected population.

Susceptibility to infections is the common presentation, especially chronic sinopulmonary infections from encapsulated pyogenic bacteria. Gastroenteritis with chronic diarrhoea from salmonella and campylobacter are also seen.

Investigations

The laboratory findings include hypogammaglobulinaemia or agammaglobulinaemia, an absence, or significant reduction, of B cells and a deficient response to immunisations. There is usually an absence of the BTK protein and the diagnosis is confirmed with genetic studies.

Treatment and management

Timely diagnosis and initiation of immunoglobulin replacement is paramount in reducing the burden of infection. General supportive care with appropriate inactivated vaccines and antibiotics for acute infections is the basis of ongoing care.

CLINICAL SCENARIO

An 18-month-old boy was referred to the General Paediatric team with concerns regarding recurrent ear infections. The family reported at least 10 courses of antibiotics over the previous year, with recurrent ear discharge and tympanic membrane perforations. He had one hospital admission for chest infection which was treated with oral antibiotics and oxygen. He was fully vaccinated for his age and was the first child of healthy unrelated parents.

On examination, he did not appear dysmorphic and he had atrophic tonsils.

Initial investigations revealed normal full blood count with normal lymphocyte and neutrophil count; however, his lymphocytes subsets showed slightly elevated CD3 T cells, normal numbers NK cells and absent CD19 B cells. He had a panhypoglobulinaemia with IgG <0.5 g/l (lower normal for age 3.7 g/l), IgA and IgM undetectable. His vaccination responses to tetanus, H. influenza b and pneumococcal serotypes were very low.

The child was commenced on prophylactic antibiotics and immunoglobulin replacement with presumed diagnosis of X-linked agammaglobulinaemia. Genetic testing confirmed the diagnosis.

Common variable immunodeficiency disorder (CVID)

A heterogeneous group of conditions with a significant decrease in IgG and at least in one of the IgM or IgA classes. Diagnosis in those under 4 years is difficult to establish as the picture can be indistinguishable from Transient Hypoglobulinaemia of Infancy in this age group. Children have susceptibility to infections of the sinopulmonary tract, skin and gastrointestinal tract whilst some patients develop a coeliac-like enteropathy with villous atrophy. Patients with CVID have increased risk to develop malignancies, especially lymphomas and stomach cancers.

Treatment and management

General supportive and monitoring measures for infection prevention and treatment with immunoglobulin replacement.

Selective IgA deficiency

This is the most common primary immunodeficiency and presents with an isolated deficiency of IgA with normal levels of the other immunoglobulin subclasses. Due to physiological delay in the onset of IgA production, the diagnosis can only be made with confidence after the sixth year of life when IgA levels become stable. The T cell–mediated immunity is intact in most of the patients.

Clinical presentation

Most patients are asymptomatic and the low IgA is incidental finding, often in the process of coeliac screening.

Treatment and management

There is no need for specific treatment for asymptomatic children but some patients may need prophylactic antibiotics if they experience recurrent infections. A proportion of children will develop Common Variable Immunodeficiency Disorder and therefore long-term follow up maybe appropriate.

Specific antibody deficiency (SPAD)

A condition that is identified when there is inadequate response to polysaccharide antigens in a patient with normal immunoglobulin levels, IgG subclasses and responses to protein antigens. In young children, an inadequate response to polysaccharide stimuli is physiological and improves with age as the immune system matures. Recurrent or severe rhinosinusitis and bronchopulmonary infections due to *Streptococcus pneumoniae*, *Haemophilus influenzae* and others are the main findings at presentation.

Transient hypogammaglobulinemia of infancy (THI)

IgG is actively transported across the placenta and the term newborn infant is protected by the maternal IgG for the first few months of life. These antibodies break down and are undetectable from 6–9 months. As the child's own immunoglobulin production starts slowly, there is a physiological nadir at around 4–6 months of age and during this period, the bacterial infection risk increases. Eventually immunoglobulin levels increase and IgM is the first major class to reach adult levels, followed by IgG and then IgA during puberty. THI is common and has an incidence of around 1 in 100 births. It is a clinical diagnosis usually given retrospectively in a child with:
- persistently low immunoglobulin levels
- no evidence of other primary immunodeficiency
- normalisation of immunoglobulin levels by 2 years
  Prophylactic antibiotics may be required, and immunoglobulin replacement is reserved for children presenting with significant infections.

Secondary antibody deficiencies

Low levels of immunoglobulins can be the result of other, nonimmune conditions. These may need to be considered and excluded in some children presenting with recurrent infections. The conditions include:
- excessive protein losses (nephrotic syndrome, inflammatory bowel disease, extensive burns)
- medication—carbamazepine, phenytoin, valproic acid, corticosteroids
- chronic infections—HIV, congenital CMV, rubella, EBV
- malignancies—lymphoma

Combined immunodeficiencies

This is a diverse group of conditions leading to a spectrum of severity in presentations, ranging from increased susceptibility to opportunistic infections from the first months of life through to less severe infections in later childhood. Those with the condition are also at risk of autoimmune disease and malignant disease. Examples of these conditions include:

Severe combined immunodeficiency (SCID)

Maternal antibodies passed through the placenta and offer some protection initially, but as levels fall, infections develop and the infant usually presents within the first 6 months of life with:
- persistent mucocutaneous candidiasis
- opportunistic and viral infections

- chronic diarrhoea
- growth retardation
- lack a thymic shadow on CXR
- absent peripheral lymphoid tissue
- lymphopenia

Symptomatic vaccine-strain rotavirus infection is common in babies who are later diagnosed with SCID.

Management

Infection prevention measures must be started with some urgency if a diagnosis of SCID is considered. Placing the baby in protective isolation and commencing prophylactic antimicrobial agents are paramount. Pneumocystis prophylaxis and antifungal medication are used in all patients whilst passive immunity is offered with immunoglobulin replacement therapy. Urgent referral to regional bone marrow transplant centre is required.

All live vaccines are contraindicated and the inactivated vaccines are unlikely to be effective but safe to give. Household contacts need to be up to date with all the inactivated immunisations and live vaccinations are strictly avoided in all close contacts.

Caution is required if blood, platelet or plasma transfusions are needed. Only CMV negative and leucodepleted irradiated products can be used. Haemopoietic stem cell transplantation is curative although it has an associated morbidity and risk of mortality.

From September 2021, a pilot newborn screening program for SCID will be introduced into UK clinical practice. The dried blood spot will be used to measure small circular DNA pieces (TRECs) formed during T cell development. Absent or very low TRECs suggest a SCID-like condition and appropriate measures would need to be instigated until the diagnosis is confirmed.

Combined immunodeficiencies

A heterogenous group of very rare conditions which present with SCID-like infections and a predisposition to malignant and autoimmune disease. A variety of syndromes are also associated with combined immunodeficiency and these include Wiskott-Aldrich syndrome, ataxia telangiectasia and chromosome 22q11.2 deletion (Di George syndrome, velo-cardio-facial syndrome).

Combined immunodeficiencies with syndromic features

Wiskott-Aldrich syndrome is X-linked recessive and presents with bleeding of varying severity due to thrombocytopenia, eczema and combined immunodeficiency with sinopulmonary and skin infections. Investigations demonstrate low platelets, T cell lymphocytopenia with normal IgG and low IgM values. Treatment is initially supportive but stem cell transplant can be curative. Children should have irradiated and CMV negative transfusions.

Ataxia telangiectasia is autosomal recessive and usually presents with progressive neurological features, particularly ataxia. Telangiectases can be seen in the bulbar conjunctiva and skin. There may be a history of recurrent infections particularly sinopulmonary infections. Immunological investigations commonly show lymphopenia, reduced IgA levels and raised alpha-fetoprotein. The treatment is supportive with some patients requiring prophylactic antibiotics or immunoglobulin replacement therapy

Chromosome 22q11.2 deletion (Di George syndrome, Velo-Cardio-Facial Syndrome) leads to a variable T cell lymphopenia due to the absence of a thymus. In complete Di George syndrome, the immune deficiency is comparable to that of SCID and can be managed with thymic transplantation. Treatment of milder presentations of immunodeficiency is supportive. Other aspects of management are to be found in Chapter 25 Endocrinology and Chapter 27 Neurodevelopmental Medicine.

Complement deficiencies

These are rare inherited disorders where the child is at risk of encapsulated bacterial infections and may also develop some types of autoimmune disease such as SLE. Those patients with an increased susceptibility to infections are managed with antimicrobials and additional vaccinations.

Abnormalities of neutrophil function

Congenital neutropenia

A neutropenia of less than 0.5×10^9/l that persists for over 3 months is diagnostic of congenital neutropenia if other causes for secondary neutropenia have been excluded. The infections present early, in the first year of life, affecting skin, GI mucosa and respiratory tract. Examples of the various types of congenital neutropenia include:

Severe congenital neutropenia (SCN)

Presentation of SCN is with severe pyogenic infections, usually within the first few months of life along with severe neutropenia, mild anaemia and hypergammaglobulinaemia. The prognosis, however, has improved significantly following the introduction of G-CSF therapy. SCN predisposes to myelodysplastic syndrome and acute myeloid leukaemia.

Cyclical neutropenia

In this condition, the neutropenia lasts for 3 to 6 days, every 21 days and the affected child usually presents in the first year of life with recurrent infections, fever, recurrent malaise and stomatitis. Bacterial causes may not always be identified. Cyclical neutropenia is not associated with increased risk of blood dyscrasias.

Schwachman-Diamond syndrome (SDS)

The condition is inherited as an autosomal recessive disorder that affects both the number and the movement of neutrophils into inflammatory sites. Presentation includes:

- diarrhoea and growth retardation
- bone marrow failure—intermittent neutropenia, anaemia, thrombocytopenia
- steatorrhea due to exocrine pancreatic insufficiency

Full blood count, bone marrow aspirate and faecal elastase would support the diagnosis and genetic testing would identify the specific gene defects. Supportive measures and G-CSF significantly reduces the infection burden whilst a bone marrow transplant may be considered in children who are severely affected. Pancreatic enzyme replacement and fat-soluble vitamin supplementation are usually required.

Chronic granulomatous disease (CGD)

CGD results from defects in phagocytes, and in those with a positive family history the condition invariably follows an X-linked pattern of inheritance. It usually presents in early childhood, before the age of five years with a susceptibility to bacterial and fungal infections, growth retardation and impaired wound healing. It should be considered and excluded in young children who present with inflammatory bowel disease. The affected individuals have normal responses to virus infections. Neutrophil function testing (currently DHR assay is preferred) is undertaken and those with a positive result require specific genetic test to confirm the diagnosis. Current treatment includes lifestyle advice on how to avoid fungal spores and antibiotic and antifungal prophylaxis and this has led to a marked improvement in prognosis. Bone marrow transplantation may be considered and is curative and has high success rates.

Autoimmune disorders

These conditions have a common aetiology and develop when the immune system of the individual is directed at host tissue. The target of the immune attack is usually very specific but the consequences of the tissue injury will be widespread. Coeliac disease, diabetes mellitus type 1 and Addison disease are all examples of autoimmune disease with specific tissue destruction and a systemic impact. Autoimmune conditions have identifiable abnormalities of the immune response to host antigens and the process includes abnormalities of T- and B-cell function (Table 15.1).

Some examples of these conditions are presented here and more details can be found in their related systems chapter.

Autoinflammatory disorders

There are some conditions which are similar to auto-immune disorders and demonstrate an increased host inflammatory response to host tissue, but the abnormal pathological process has not been identified. Fever is a common symptom of these conditions and they can be difficult to diagnose as they may mimic infectious or malignant disease when first seen. Periodic fever syndromes exemplify this group of conditions in the paediatric age group.

Periodic Fever syndromes

These are a group of conditions with recurring episodes of fever and inflammation. They have similar associated symptoms but differ in their pattern of inheritance, duration and frequency of episodes. The inherited diseases

Table 15.1 **Some recognised conditions with autoimmune aetiology**	
rheumatic fever	inflammatory bowel disease
dermatomyositis	juvenile arthritis
systemic lupus erythematosus	reactive arthritis
vitiligo	rheumatoid arthritis
Addison disease	acute disseminated encephalomyelitis (ADEM)
autoimmune thyroiditis	Guillain-Barre
diabetes mellitus type 1	multiple sclerosis
Graves disease	myasthenia gravis
autoimmune hepatitis	Sydenham's chorea
coeliac disease	lupus nephritis

usually present early in childhood, and Familial Mediter-ranean fever (FMF) demonstrates the range of features seen at presentation.

Clinical presentation

Children and young people with FMF present with a history of fevers of 2 to 3 days duration which recur over months or years and other causes such as infections and malignancy are excluded. The fever is described as high grade and of rapid onset. Other multisystem symptoms are associated including conjunctivitis, rash and mono or polyarthritis. There is absence of infective symptoms such as coryza and cough and children are usually well in between fever episodes.

Alternative diagnoses and differing features

- relapsing fever—caused by Borrelia species and is spread by tics or lice. Patients have very high temperatures of acute onset and often have associated rigors

- cyclical neutropenia—fever is episodic and often associated with mucosal ulcers
- tuberculosis
- systemic juvenile idiopathic arthritis—fevers with macular rash and arthritis

Investigations

Acute phase reactants (ESR, CRP) are elevated but other investigations undertaken to exclude more common causes of fever are negative. Genetic analysis can be undertaken to support clinical suspicion of inherited autoinflammatory disease.

Treatment and management

This should be guided by colleagues with experience of autoinflammatory disorders. Colchicine is used in FMF with good effect although the mechanism of action is uncertain whilst corticosteroids, such as prednisolone, at the onset of a fever episode can be effective.

IMPORTANT CLINICAL POINTS

General
- there are recognised features suggestive of underlying immunodeficiency

Antibody deficiency
- present with sinopulmonary infections, chronic diarrhoea, skin infections
- treat with immunoglobulin replacement

Severe combined immunodeficiency
- presents with a wide range of bacterial, viral and fungal infections

- is an immunological emergency at presentation
- all live vaccines are contraindicated

Abnormalities of neutrophil function
- congenital neutropenia if neutropenia of <0.5 x 10^9/l for over 3 months
- cyclical neutropenia—neutropenia lasting for 3 to 6 days every 21 days
- chronic granulomatous disease—usually X-linked if positive family history

Further reading

Wekell P, Hertting O, Holmgren D, et al. Fifteen-minute consultation: Recognising primary immune deficiencies in children. *Archives of Disease in Childhood - Education and Practice.* 2019; 104: 235–243.

Chapter | 16 |

Cardiology

Robert Tulloh

After reading this chapter you should:
- understand investigation of cardiac diseases, e.g. ECG, echocardiograms, cardiac catheterisation and their appropriate selection in diagnosis and management
- know the various presentations of congenital heart problems and to be able to assess, diagnose and manage
- be able to assess, diagnose and manage murmurs, chest pain, palpitations, cardiac arrhythmias and syncope
- be able to assess, diagnose and manage heart failure, myocarditis, pericardial disease and cardiomyopathy
- be able to assess, diagnose and manage pulmonary hypertension and make appropriate referrals
- be able to assess, diagnose and manage infective endocarditis
- know the cardiac complications of other system disorders
- know the indications and common side effects of drugs used to treat common cardiac conditions including duct dependent cyanosis, heart failure and arrhythmias

Many conditions will impact on cardiac function in children and although specific diseases of the heart are less common, they are a regular feature in the clinical practice of paediatricians.

Investigations

Chest radiograph

A plain radiograph can provide information on cardiac shape and size, appearances of main vessels and any change in pulmonary perfusion. Many of the classical appearances of congenital heart disease are now rarely seen on radiographs as echocardiography has superseded the plain film as the most appropriate initial investigation.

Furthermore, treatments will often be undertaken before classical radiological features develop. It is, however, important to understand the contributions that the various cardiac structures make to the radiological appearance (Figure 16.1).

Electrocardiogram

A 12 lead ECG is a basic investigation and will reveal rate, rhythm, wave interval and axis (table 16.1). It has the added issue in paediatric practice in that it changes in appearance depending on the age of the child (Figure 16.2). The ECG of a newborn baby will reflect right ventricular dominance up to the age of 6 months.

Ambulatory ECG monitoring

Useful for patients who may have episodic arrhythmias who have a 3 lead ECG attached to a recording device for one or more days. Abnormal rhythms, however, can still be difficult to record even with this close monitoring. Alternatives are now available such as rhythm cards, digital watches or smartphone ECG recordings.

Echocardiography

Echocardiography is a skilled technique which gives real-time information about cardiac structure and blood flow. The AKP exam will not expect candidates to be able to interpret echocardiographic images.

Cardiac catheterisation

Catheterisation will allow the insertion of specific devices which may close defects or dilate strictures. The inserted catheter can also establish pressures and oxygen saturations in each of the four chambers and the major vessels

Table 16.1 Abnormalities of the ECG wave pattern

Wave	Appearance	Implication
P wave (right axis deviation)	prominent (peaked)	right atrial hypertrophy (p pulmonale)
P wave	prolonged m shaped	left atrial hypertrophy (p mitrale)
ST segment (low voltages)	raised	pericarditis or pericardial effusion
QT interval	prolonged	hypocalcaemia
QT interval	shortened	hypercalcaemia
QRS complex	widened	hyperkalaemia
T wave (with U wave)	flattened	hypokalaemia
T wave	peaked	hyperkalaemia
T wave	upright in V1	right ventricular hypertrophy
T wave	downward in V6	left ventricle cardiomyopathy

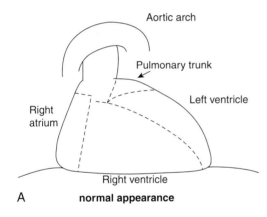

A **normal appearance**

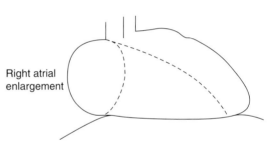

B **right atrial dilation**
The right heart border will bulge into the areas of the hilar region and right lung field. In Ebstein's anomaly, the right atrial wall may stretch to the right chest border producing a "wall to wall heart"

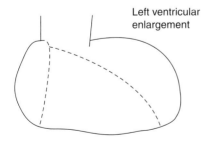

C
left ventricular dilatation/enlargement
prominence and exaggeration of convexity of the left heart border.
lung fields may be plethoric.

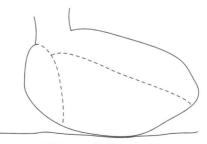

D
Right ventricular enlargement (apex tips up)

right ventricular hypertrophy/ dilation
right ventricle hypertrophies and lifts the cardiac apex.
right ventricular dilation/enlargement produces rounding and elevation of the cardiac apex

Fig. 16.1 Examples of abnormal cardiac contours seen on chest radiographs

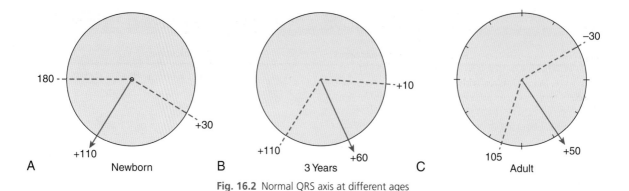

Fig. 16.2 Normal QRS axis at different ages

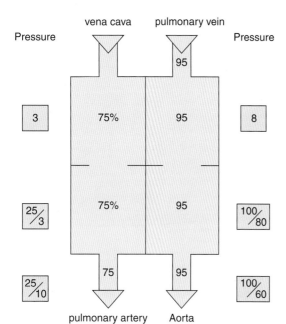

Fig. 16.3 Diagram of the heart showing normal pressure and saturation ranges by chamber

(Figure 16.3). Such information will improve the understanding of the problem and the extend of any abnormalities.

Hyperoxia test

The hyperoxia test is used in newborn babies where there is a concern whether cyanosis is cardiac or noncardiac in origin. The baby is exposed to 100% oxygen for 10 minutes (via intubation or in head box) after which an **arterial blood gas** is taken. If the PaO$_2$ is more than 20 kPa then the cyanosis is not due to congenital heart disease.

Congenital heart disease

Congenital heart disease is identified through antenatal echocardiogram, by the detection of a heart murmur on routine checks and by the acute presentation of a child with cyanosis, heart failure or collapse (table 16.2). Cyanosis is the result of right to left shunting of blood either through defects or connections or through common mixing in the circulation.

Clinical features

Ultrasonography of the fetal heart has become a routine part of the fetal anomaly scan performed in between 18 and 20 weeks' gestation, and approximately 70% of those infants who require surgery in the first 6 months of life are diagnosed in this way. Early diagnosis allows the parents to be counselled appropriately and, depending on the diagnosis, the choice of terminating the pregnancy. The majority, however, continue with the pregnancy and can have their child's management planned antenatally. Those babies with a duct-dependent lesion, which will need treatment within the first few days of life, can be offered delivery at, or close to, a cardiac centre. They will be commenced on prostaglandin at birth in order to prevent them from becoming sick and collapsing.

The most common presentation of more minor congenital heart disease is with a heart murmur although the vast majority of such children will have a normal heart. The murmur is then described as 'innocent' or 'benign'.

Babies with a pathological **left to right shunt** will present **after** the first few days of life, initially with a heart murmur, or at a later date, with signs of heart failure. They never have a murmur on the first day of life, due to the fact that the pulmonary vascular pressures are high, so that there is no 'shunting' until these pressures start to fall. These signs are often detected at the 6 week GP baby check when the baby has faltering growth or may be breathlessness, especially on feeding. Conditions such as ASD, VSD and PDA will present in this way.

Those with a **right to left shunt** can present at any age, but the most critical are those with a duct-dependent cyanotic cardiac lesion where the pulmonary circulation is dependent on a patent ductus arteriosus. They are diagnosed soon after birth when oxygen saturations are found to be less than 94%. Many children with Tetralogy of Fallot are not cyanosed at birth and instead present with a murmur on the first day of life (due to the narrow right ventricular outflow tract).

Children with lesions which result in a **common mixing** of blood within the circulation will present with breathlessness (due to left to right shunt) and cyanosis (due

PRACTICE POINT—some causes of congenital cyanotic heart disease

- Tetralogy of Fallot
- Transposition of the Great Vessels
- Truncus Arteriosus
- Total Anomalous Pulmonary Venous Drainage
- Tricuspid Atresia

Table 16.2 Common congenital heart diseases arranged by physiology

Physiology	Symptoms	Conditions
left to right shunts	breathless or asymptomatic	atrial septal defect ventricular septal defect persistent ductus arteriosus
right to left shunts	cyanosis	tetralogy of Fallot transposition of the great arteries Eisenmenger syndrome
common mixing	breathless; cyanosis	complete atrio-ventricular septal defect complex heart disease
well child with obstruction	asymptomatic	aortic stenosis pulmonary stenosis
sick neonate	collapse	coarctation of the aorta hypoplastic left heart syndrome totally anomalous pulmonary venous connection

Table 16.3 Presentation of left to right shunt in congenital cardiac disease

Defect	Sign	Investigation	Management
Atrial septal defect—secundum	ejection systolic murmur at upper left sternal edge	ECG: partial right bundle branch block CXR: cardiomegaly	ASD closure device inserted in catheter lab age 3 years
Atrial septal defect—primum—now called partial AVSD	ejection systolic murmur at upper left sternal edge apical pansystolic murmur	ECG: superior axis CXR: cardiomegaly	open heart surgery at 3 years to close the defect and repair the leaky left AV valve
Ventricular septal defect	pan-systolic murmur at left lower sternal edge		small defect—closes spontaneously large defect—undergo open heart surgery at 3–6 months
Persistent ductus arteriosus	continuous (machinery) murmur at upper left sternal edge		PDA closure device in catheter lab age 1 year

to right to left shunt) and usually have very complex heart disease.

Children with a mild obstructive cardiac lesion usually present with a heart murmur and are often well and without symptoms. Some babies with severe obstructive cardiac lesions, however, may have a duct-dependent systemic circulation and they will then present in the first few days of life as the duct closes.

Left to right shunt (table 16.3)

Atrial septal defect (secundum)

The majority of children with an isolated secundum ASD will present in infancy with a murmur found on routine examination or when examined because of unconnected chest infection. Classically, it is an ejection systolic murmur at the upper left sternal edge due to the increased flow across the pulmonary valve. It is rare to hear the additional fixed-split of the second heart sound in children.

Investigations

The ECG will show sinus rhythm with evidence of incomplete right bundle branch block and possibly right ventricular hypertrophy. A chest radiograph may show right atrial enlargement, a large heart and pulmonary plethora. The diagnosis is confirmed by echocardiography. This allows measurement of the size and location of the defect and assessment of the degree of right ventricular enlargement.

Treatment and management

For significant ASDs, closure is commonly performed around the age of 3 years using an ASD closure device at cardiac catheterisation which has a very low mortality and an excellent long-term prognosis.

Partial atrio-ventricular septal defect

Previously called atrial septal defect (primum). The child may present in heart failure in infancy if there is significant left to right shunting with left atrio-ventricular valve regurgitation. The ECG shows **superior axis** whilst the radiograph shows cardiomegaly. Correction requires patch closure of the defect and, in all patients, repair of the left AV valve (which leaks because it is not a mitral valve).

Ventricular septal defect

This is the most common congenital heart disease, and those with significant defects, if not detected antenatally, will usually present in the first few weeks of life. The child will have no signs or symptoms on the first day but will gradually develop a murmur and heart failure (if a large defect) over the first week as the pulmonary vascular resistance falls. The classical murmur is a loud pansystolic murmur at the lower left sternal edge. If there is heart failure, this is manifested as breathlessness, faltering growth, poor feeding and cold hands and feet. The defect is often associated with genetic syndromes.

The chest radiograph will show cardiomegaly and pulmonary plethora, the ECG will show bi-ventricular hypertrophy (large total voltage in V3 and V4) and the echocardiogram will establish the definitive diagnosis.

Large defects are closed at 3–4 months of age but, prior to that, the child will need treatment with diuretics and ACE inhibitors. Added calories are introduced to allow the child to put on some weight as cardiopulmonary bypass is undertaken when the child is around 4 kg in weight to achieve the best outcome with the lowest risks.

Those with small muscular VSDs are usually asymptomatic and most do not require any active treatment. The defects tend to become smaller with time and the majority undergo spontaneous closure. Those with a small (restrictive) perimembranous VSD need ongoing monitoring as the aortic valve may become distorted over time.

Persistent ductus arteriosus

These are defined as still being present one month after the baby should have been born and therefore excludes preterm babies who are still within their 'due' dates. They may have no symptoms or may have significant heart failure, and the severity is related to the magnitude of left to right shunting from aorta to pulmonary artery. Their cardinal signs are a systolic or continuous murmur at the upper left sternal edge and the baby may have a collapsing pulse as the blood runs back down the duct in diastole.

The term 'patent ductus arteriosus' refers to preterm babies who are still within their 'due date' and where the duct has not closed. The condition is important in the ventilator dependent preterm infant with lung disease.

Investigations

An infant with a large PDA may have cardiomegaly and pulmonary plethora on a chest radiograph and the ECG will show bi-ventricular hypertrophy (large total voltage in V3 and V4). Small defects will show no abnormalities on these investigations. Echocardiography is used to make the definitive diagnosis.

Table 16.4 Presentation of right to left shunt in congenital cardiac disease		
Defect	**Sign (all are cyanosed)**	**Management**
Tetralogy of Fallot	long harsh systolic murmur at mid left sternal edge	open heart surgery at 6 months
Transposition of the Great Arteries	cyanosis only in most patients may collapse at 2 days old when PDA closes	open heart surgery at 5–7 days (arterial switch operation)
Eisenmenger syndrome	cyanosis only, no murmur tend to be teenagers or older	result of untreated large septal defect pulmonary vasodilator medication

Treatment and management

Large defects may need closure at a young age by catheter device or by lateral thoracotomy surgical operation. The preferred option is to wait until they are over 5 kg and then close them with a device in the catheter laboratory. Until that time, diuretics and added calories can allow the child to put on some weight to reduce the risk of operation.

Right to left shunt (table 16.4)

These present with varying degrees of cyanosis if not detected antenatally.

Tetralogy of Fallot

This condition is most easily understood with four defects (VSD, sub pulmonary stenosis, overriding aorta and, as a result, right ventricular hypertrophy). The sub pulmonary stenosis forces deoxygenated blood from the right ventricle to the left via the septal defect and patients are cyanosed with oxygen saturations below 94%. The condition is usually identified on an antenatal booking scan. The infant will have no symptoms on the first day of life but will have a loud murmur (unlike in VSD) and is unlikely to be cyanosed initially. The obvious cyanosis will gradually develop and increase over the first few months of life and examination reveals a long, harsh murmur at the mid left sternal edge. Many are associated with 22q11 microdeletion. The baby will usually grow well; some infants will develop episodes when they become very blue and then pale before becoming unconscious and limp. This is called a 'spell' and is potentially dangerous as it represents significant reduction in pulmonary blood flow that can be confirmed acutely by absence of their heart murmur (since no blood is crossing the pulmonary valve).

Investigations

The ECG will show sinus rhythm with evidence of right ventricular hypertrophy (upright T wave in lead V1). The

chest radiograph can show pulmonary oligaemia and a boot-shaped cardiac outline—which is the result of right ventricular hypertrophy and hypoplasia of the pulmonary arch (Figure 16.4). The diagnosis is confirmed by echocardiography and allows definition of the precise anatomy.

Treatment and management

Most are repaired at 5–6 months of age, but the children need regular review to ensure they are well and their oxygen saturations remain over 75%. Cardiopulmonary bypass is used ideally when the child is around 6 kg in weight to achieve the best outcome with the lowest risks. Some children have a more complex course and need palliative procedures to increase their pulmonary blood flow until a definitive operation can be performed (such as right ventricular outflow tract stent, PDA stent or arterial shunt). About half of all children will need a pulmonary valve replacement in teenage life, and many adults will have further surgery on their aortic valve.

Transposition of the great arteries

This is the result of the aorta (along with the coronary arteries) arising from the right ventricle and the pulmonary artery from the left ventricle. This is sometimes identified antenatally on the booking scan, allowing the baby to be delivered in a cardiac centre and to start prostaglandin at birth. The infant will have no symptoms on the first day of life and is unlikely to be cyanosed or have a murmur but those who are not identified antenatally will develop cyanosis and acute collapse at 2 days of age when the duct closes. Most have no other pathology, but some will have additional VSD or a coarctation of the aorta.

Investigations

The ECG will show normal sinus rhythm whilst a chest radiograph can show a narrow mediastinum and a cardiac

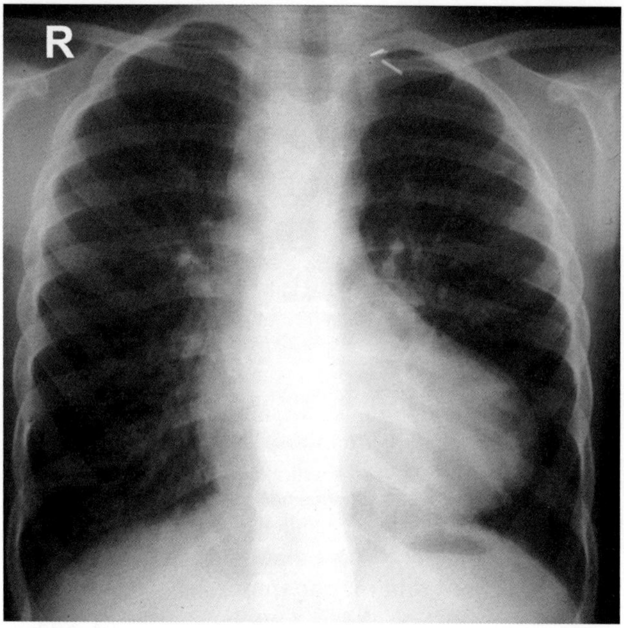

Fig. 16.4 Radiograph of Tetralogy of Fallot showing elevation and rounding of the cardiac apex, creating a 'boot-shaped heart'. There is concavity of the pulmonary trunk region, narrow mediastinum (secondary to overriding aorta) and associated pulmonary oligaemia. A right-sided aortic arch is also present in this image. Surgical clips can be seen as this patient has already had a Blalock-Taussig shunt procedure

Table 16.5 Presentation of common mixing in congenital cardiac disease

Defect	Sign	Management
Complete atrioventricular septal defect	often no murmur very active precordium breathless cyanosis	open heart surgery at 3–6 months
Complex disease with excess pulmonary blood flow, e.g. tricuspid atresia with large VSD	breathless (mostly) cyanosis	pulmonary artery band (to limit pulmonary blood flow and pressure) Glenn shunt at 6 months Fontan at 3 years
Complex disease with reduced pulmonary blood flow, e.g. tricuspid atresia with small VSD	cyanosis breathless (occasionally)	systemic to pulmonary shunt or equivalent (to increase pulmonary blood flow) Glenn shunt at 6 months Fontan at 3 years

contour suggesting right atrial and ventricular enlargement along with pulmonary plethora. The diagnosis is confirmed by echocardiography and allows definition of the precise anatomy.

Treatment and management

If resuscitation is required, then a prostaglandin infusion is effective at reopening the duct, although a quarter of neonates will require a balloon atrial septostomy. An arterial switch operation is then performed, usually on about

day 5–7. The outcome for these children is now excellent with a very low mortality.

Common mixing (table 16.5)

Complete AV septal defect

This congenital abnormality is commonly found in children with Down syndrome. It is characterised by the presence of a common AV valve, a VSD and a defect in the ostium primum part of the atrial septum. Babies usually have cyanosis and, as a result of the excessive pulmonary flow, severe heart failure, feeding difficulties and poor growth. Early management involves medical anti-failure therapy and maximising calorie intake to encourage growth so that definitive surgery can be facilitated.

Well children with obstruction
Pulmonary stenosis

This is a common congenital heart condition and has a very variable presentation. Older infants and children are identified with a murmur, are never cyanosed and are usually completely asymptomatic. Those with a critical pulmonary stenosis will be cyanosed (shunting through PFO or ASD), are very sick and present with a duct-dependent lesion in the neonatal period. The lesion can be part of the more complex abnormalities such as Noonan syndrome. On examination, there is a loud ejection systolic murmur at the upper left sternal edge and if severe enough will have a thrill over the murmur which is generally a guide to the need for intervention.

Investigations

In mild pulmonary stenosis, the ECG may be normal whilst in severe PS there will be evidence of right ventricular hypertrophy (upright T wave in lead V1). In infants with critical pulmonary stenosis, there is generally cardiomegaly with right atrial enlargement secondary to tricuspid regurgitation. The diagnosis is confirmed by echocardiography

Treatment and management

Children with pulmonary stenosis are monitored closely with echocardiography, and when the stenosis becomes significant they are offered balloon dilation via cardiac catheterisation.

Aortic stenosis

Most children are asymptomatic and very rarely breathless and are identified by a murmur at the upper right sternal edge along with a carotid thrill. Some, however, are very sick and present with a duct-dependent lesion in the neonatal period. Supravalvular aortic stenosis is more common in children with Williams syndrome. The first presentation may be with an episode of collapse during exercise, and aortic stenosis is a recognised cause of sudden death in young people.

Investigations

The ECG will show evidence of left ventricular hypertrophy and left ventricular strain with ST depression and

T-wave inversion in the left precordial leads is an important indicator of the need for intervention. The diagnosis is confirmed by echocardiogram.

Treatment and management

Follow up with echocardiography is required until the lesion is severe enough to require treatment by balloon dilation at cardiac catheterisation. However, all children with aortic stenosis will eventually require aortic valve replacement. In general, children with mild aortic stenosis are allowed to take part in all sporting activities, but as the stenosis becomes more severe this may be restricted.

Vascular ring

This is a rare congenital abnormality of the aortic arch with the vessel forming a sling that leads to compression of the trachea or oesophagus and, on occasions, both structures. Children can present with symptoms and signs of airway or oesophageal compression and diagnosis requires a high level of suspicion. Confirmation comes from MRI, bronchoscopy or echocardiography and surgical correction is usually required.

Sick children with obstruction
Coarctation of the aorta

The aortic narrowing can occur at any point along the course of the aorta although it most frequently occurs in the region of the insertion of the ductus arteriosus. The abnormality is usually recognised in utero at the booking scan although some babies will present after birth with collapse and absent femoral pulses. Very rarely, children may present when older with headaches and are found to be hypertensive and examination reveals radio-femoral delay and reduced femoral pulses. An increased incidence is seen in girls with Turner syndrome.

Investigations

In neonates, the chest radiograph will be normal. However, in older children it can demonstrate cardiomegaly due to LVH and rib notching (due to enlarged intercostal arteries). Diagnosis of a coarctation is now almost always confirmed by echocardiography or, in older patients, by CT scan.

Treatment and management

In the neonatal presentation of coarctation, initial management focuses on the medical stabilisation prior to elective surgical repair. Ductal patency is maintained by administration of intravenous infusion of prostaglandin. Surgical repair is undertaken via a left lateral thoracotomy unless the condition is part of a more complex disease. Follow up includes careful palpation of the femoral pulses and measurement of the right arm blood pressure.

Cardiac symptoms and signs

Murmurs

Cardiac murmurs are often discovered during the routine examination of children when they present to their GP or paediatrician with an intercurrent chest infection. Most are benign but it is important to be able to distinguish an innocent murmur from a pathological one.

PRACTICE POINT—hallmarks of innocent murmur

- a**S**ymptomatic
- **S**oft blowing murmur
- **S**ystolic murmur only, not diastolic
- Left **S**ternal edge

On examination
- normal heart sounds with no added sounds
- no parasternal thrill
- no radiation

A venous hum is a continuous noise heard when the child is sitting upright and is created by blood returning through the great veins into the heart. It can be made to disappear by applying gentle pressure over the great veins in the neck.

If there is uncertainty after the clinical examination that the murmur is innocent or if there is any abnormality on ECG or chest radiograph, then a paediatric cardiology opinion is indicated so that a definitive diagnosis can be obtained.

At birth (on the first day of life), many normal babies have a heart murmur. These are due to mild tricuspid regurgitation or increased flow velocity in the newborn pulmonary arteries. The murmur is never due to a closing duct or a septal defect. Those with potential shunts do not have symptoms or murmurs at birth, as the pulmonary vascular resistance is still high. Therefore, conditions such as a ventricular septal defect or ductus arteriosus may only develop signs and symptoms at several days of age when the pulmonary vascular resistance falls.

Chest pain

Chest pain is almost never due to heart disease in children and a proper history and examination will differentiate between the two (table 16.6). An ECG or the measurement of troponin levels rarely identify abnormalities. Noncardiac causes of chest pain:
- gastro-oesophageal reflux
- costochondritis
- asthma
- pericarditis
- anxiety

If, however, there is a strong suspicion of a cardiac cause, then appropriate investigations may be necessary and the value of each will be dictated by the history. Increased suspicion of a cardiac cause would be in the presence of known cardiac disease, syncope or a positive family history of defects.

Table 16.6 **Causes of chest pain**	
Noncardiac	**Cardiac**
sharp in nature	dull or heavy in nature
over the anterior chest wall	in the jaw or down the left arm
when at rest	on exercise
tenderness of costochondral junction	no local tenderness
no other comorbidities	known cardiac disease family history of sudden death

Palpitations, cardiac arrhythmias

Palpitations are a common presentation but single, extra ectopics are unlikely to be the result of a cardiac problem. If there are repeated episodes of palpitation lasting for more than a few seconds, then a cardiac arrhythmia should be considered and further investigations undertaken including 12 lead ECG, 24-hour ECG tape, exercise ECG or portable device recorder.

If the child is thought to have a noncardiac cause of palpitation, then it is worth advising a reduction in coffee, tea, chocolate, cheese and coloured drinks, since these can all cause tachycardia or even precipitate pathological SVT.

Supraventricular tachycardia (SVT)

This is the most common arrhythmia seen in children and the best known example of this phenomenon is

Table 16.7 Abnormalities seen on ECG and their implication

ECG changes	Seen in
prolonged PR interval	hyperkalaemia and myocarditis,
shortened PR interval	Wolff-Parkinson-White syndrome
variable interval	heart block
prolonged QRS complex	Wolff-Parkinson-White syndrome ventricular arrhythmias
prolonged QTc	predispose to collapse and arrhythmias (Normal QTc is less than 0.44 seconds in those older than 1 week)

For those with cardiac compromise, IV adenosine is given whilst preparing for synchronised cardioversion at 1J/kg. The cardioversion should be administered as soon as possible and can be repeated.

Table 16.8 Symptoms suggestive of supraventricular tachycardia

Normal heart rate variation	Suggestive of SVT
occurs on exercise	occurs at rest
no outward signs	pale, dizzy or light headed
no symptoms otherwise	chest discomfort
	terminates with vagal manoeuvres
	family history known cardiac disease

Wolff-Parkinson-White syndrome. About a half of all children with SVT will present in infancy with symptoms ranging from irritability and poor feeding through to presenting in extremis with heart failure. SVT in older children presents with characteristic symptoms with the patient aware of the tachycardia, and they will complain of feeling faint. Certain features in the history will help differentiate SVT from a normal heart rate variation.

Emergency management of acute arrhythmias

A child or young person who presents to the emergency department with an arrhythmia requires an initial assessment of airway, breathing and circulation (ABC). Action may be required if problems are identified and the APLS approach should be followed including the need for ventilation if the child is shocked. Continuous ECG monitoring is important and should be established (table 16.7).

Supraventricular tachycardia (SVT)

Those who are clinically stable should first receive vagal stimulation manoeuvres which, in a young child, include unilateral carotid sinus massage or ice to the face, and in the older child, a Valsalva manoeuvre or unilateral carotid sinus massage. There is **no longer a place for eyeball massage.** If the vagal manoeuvres prove ineffective, adenosine by rapid injection into good vascular access will be needed.

Ventricular tachycardia (VT)

This is a potentially dangerous arrhythmia due to the possibility of it degenerating into ventricular fibrillation. More than three broad complexes in succession will require treatment, and if the patient is not clinically shocked then intravenous administration of amiodarone is an appropriate initial treatment. In the clinically shocked patient, synchronous DC cardioversion under sedation or anaesthesia should be undertaken. It can be the result of hyperkalaemia or poisoning with tricyclic antidepressants.

Further management of cardiac arrhythmias

The advice and involvement of a paediatric cardiologist should be obtained once the emergency management has established a normal sinus rhythm. Treatment of SVT is usually with a beta blocker such as propranolol for young children or atenolol for older ones although some will require more complex therapy with flecainide, sotalol and amiodarone. Older children can be taught the Valsalva manoeuvre or carotid sinus massage to give them some control, but usually after the age of 10 years, these children will be listed for electrophysiological study and ablation of an accessory pathway.

In the management of a child with VT, it is important to consider possible underlying causes which includes previous cardiac surgery and long QT syndrome.

Examples of abnormal ECG rhythms

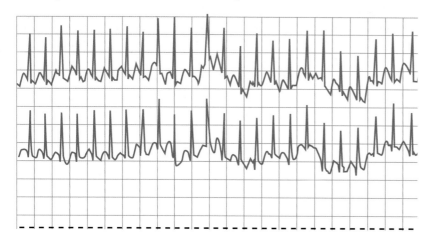

Fig. 16.5 Supraventricular tachycardia. The ECG shows usually narrow QRS complexes and a very fast rate of over 220 bpm (often 250–300 bpm in infants).

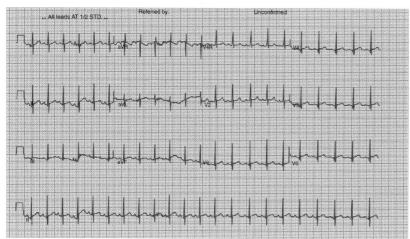

Fig. 16.6 Right ventricular hypertrophy in a 1-year-old boy with pulmonary stenosis. Large R wave in V1, V2 and V3 and upright T wave in V1.

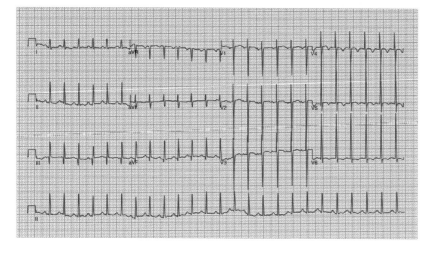

Fig. 16.7 Left ventricular hypertrophy in newborn baby. Left axis deviation (calculated +62°) Large S wave in V1 and V2; Large R waves in V4 and V6. T wave inversion indicates ventricular strain.

Relevant pharmacological agents

Adenosine. Adenosine blocks conduction, primarily at the atrioventricular node, and has a very short half-life of a few seconds. When used, it causes asystole but the heart rate usually recovers rapidly; it is therefore important that full resuscitation facilities are available. Contraindications include heart block, heart failure, long QT syndrome and asthma.

Flecainide. Flecainide is contraindicated if heart failure, haemodynamically significant valvar heart disease or conduction defects are present. Drug levels should be monitored and doses reduced in severe hepatic and renal impairment. Side effects include oedema, dyspnoea, dizziness, fatigue and visual disturbances.

Amiodarone. Amiodarone is contraindicated if bradycardia, thyroid dysfunction and iodine sensitivity are present. Side effects include pulmonary fibrosis, peripheral neuropathy, ataxia, hypothyroidism, hyperthyroidism, corneal micro deposits and hepatotoxicity. Close monitoring of thyroid, pulmonary and liver function tests are required as are regular eye examinations.

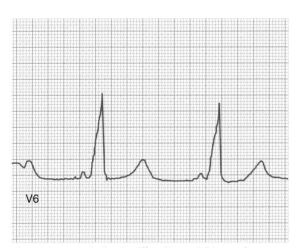

Fig. 16.8 Pre-excitation. Wolff-Parkinson-White syndrome. Short PR interval and pre-excitation delta wave.

Syncope

Transient loss of consciousness is usually due to syncope and is common in adolescents. It is usually benign but rarely is due to life-threatening, cardiac disease.

The causes include:

- neutrally mediated syncope that occurs in response to a range of provocations such as standing up too quickly ('orthostatic intolerance'), the sight of blood or needles and a sudden unexpected pain. There is usually a prodrome of dizziness, abnormality of vision, nausea, sweating or pallor.
- cardiac syncope that may be due to an arrhythmia such as heart block, supraventricular tachycardia, ventricular tachycardia (associated with long QT syndrome) or structural abnormalities (aortic stenosis, hypertrophic cardiomyopathy). This is potentially life threatening if it occurs on exercise. Postural orthostatic tachycardia syndrome (POTS) is **rare** and is not typically associated with syncope or arrhythmia. Features suggestive of a cardiac cause are symptoms on exercise, family history of sudden unexplained death and associated palpitations.

A full assessment must be undertaken if a cardiac cause is suspected and all patients presenting with transient loss of consciousness require a standard 12-lead ECG and assessment of the corrected Q-T interval.

In practice, life-threatening syncope is rare, and consequently investigations beyond a standard ECG are not usually required. If the problem is thought to be due to postural hypotension then the patient is to encouraged drink more water, have added salt in their diet (crisps at breaktime), stand up slowly, sit down quickly if they feel faint and make sure they are in position of safety (not to go climbing without a rope or swim unobserved). Most will be managed successfully and only a few will need added therapy such as a beta blocker, fludrocortisone or other therapies.

Heart failure

In the first week of life, heart failure is more likely to result from left heart obstruction such as coarctation of the aorta. If the obstructive lesion is very severe, then arterial perfusion may be predominantly by right-to-left flow of blood via the arterial duct, so-called duct-dependent systemic circulation.

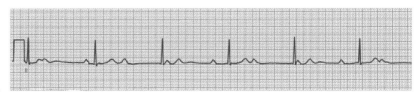

Fig. 16.9 Heart block. Wandering P wave dissociated from QRS complex.

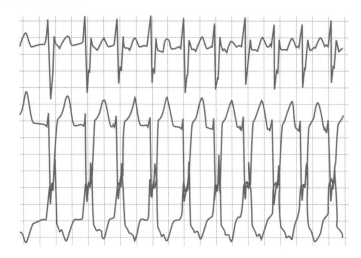

Fig. 16.10 Ventricular tachycardia. Defined as three or more premature ventricular contractions with a rate typically of over 120 bpm. There are wide, bizarre QRS complexes with AV dissociation.

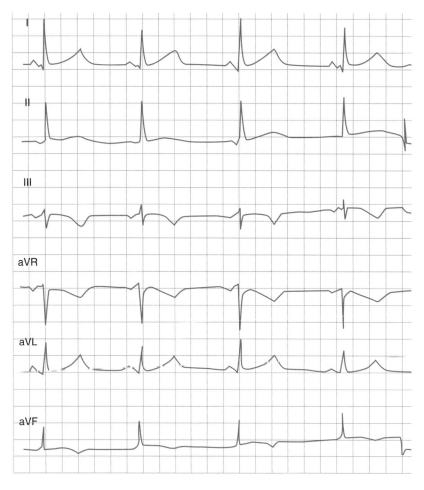

Fig. 16.11 Long QT syndrome. Measured from the start of the P wave to the tail end of the T wave. Normal values after correction for rate (QTc) should be less than 440 msec. QTc from 440–460 msec is considered borderline.

Closure of the duct under these circumstances rapidly leads to severe acidosis, collapse and death unless ductal patency is restored.

After the first week of life, progressive heart failure is most likely due to a left-to-right shunt as the pulmonary vascular resistance falls and the increase in left-to-right shunt and increasing pulmonary blood flow. This causes pulmonary oedema and breathlessness.

Such symptoms of heart failure will increase up to the age of about 3 months but may later subsequently improve as the pulmonary vascular resistance rises in response to the left-to-right shunt. If left untreated, these children will develop Eisenmenger syndrome, which is the result of the irreversibly raised pulmonary vascular resistance resulting from chronically raised pulmonary arterial pressure and flow. The shunt changes direction and becomes right to left leading to cyanosis in the teenager.

Some children will present with heart failure due to poor pump function. This is most likely due to myocarditis or dilated cardiomyopathy. This is classically due to a virus infection occurring a few weeks earlier and the patient will present with varying degrees of heart failure.

Patients will present with breathlessness (particularly on feeding or exertion), sweating, poor feeding and recurrent chest infections. Examination may identify faltering growth, tachypnoea, tachycardia, cardiac murmur, gallop rhythm and hepatomegaly. Features will vary depending upon the age of the child.

Investigations

Chest radiograph will contribute to the understanding of the cardiac problem and may show cardiomegaly and pulmonary plethora or oedema (Figure 16.12).

Clinical Scenario

A 12-yearold girl presented to the emergency department having collapsed at home. She had been well and active at home in the morning but had had an argument with her parents just before the collapse. She had stormed out of the kitchen and slammed the door and then collapsed. Her parents attended very quickly and she recovered fully after about 10 minutes. She had had one previous similar episode when in the garden and had collapsed suddenly after hearing a car back-fire. She did describe frequent episodes of palpitations but had not been formally investigated for these. Her mother added that she herself was one who fainted easily.

On examination she was well and alert but looked slightly pale. Her heart rate was 68 bpm, blood pressure 100/60 and heart sounds were normal.

Initial blood tests showed a normal potassium, calcium and magnesium. An ECG was undertaken and a normal rhythm identified. The QTc interval was found to be 540 ms. A diagnosis of prolonged QT syndrome was made and urgent cardiology opinion sought.

She was advised to avoid competitive sports until further investigations had been undertaken. These would include gene analysis to identify related specific defects. Treatment was started with propranolol beta blocker.

Treatment and management

Standard therapy is with a combination of
- diuretics (typically furosemide and spironolactone/amiloride)
- angiotensin converting enzyme inhibitor (captopril/enalapril/lisinopril)
- beta-blockade (carvedilol)
- anti-platelet medication (aspirin/clopidogrel)
- calorie supplementation (including nasogastric tube feeding if needed)
- possible referral for transplantation opinion if severe or unresolving

Large septal defects between the ventricles are usually closed by the age of 6 months at the latest to ensure the patient does not develop Eisenmenger syndrome. If, however, this does occur then medication is available to palliate the symptoms as surgical intervention would no longer possible.

Relevant pharmacological agents used

Potassium sparing diuretics (amiloride, spironolactone). There is evidence that spironolactone can help the ventricle remodel, so a low dose is often used and often in conjunction with ACE inhibition. It is advised to check the serum electrolytes in heart failure in order to ensure that renal function is not adversely affected. Contraindications include hyperkalaemia and severe renal impairment whilst side effects include dry mouth, jaundice, electrolyte disturbances and gynaecomastia.

Loop diuretics (bumetanide, furosemide). These inhibit the reabsorption of sodium, potassium and chloride in the kidney. Contraindications include hypokalaemia, hyponatraemia, and renal failure. Side effects include

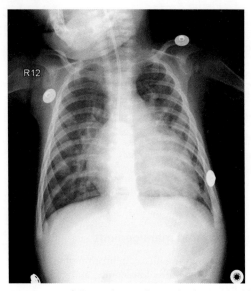

Fig. 16.12 Heart failure. Chest radiograph of 3-week-old girl presenting with tachypnoea, tachycardia, and soft ESM left sternal edge. Image shows mild cardiomegaly with prominent convexity to the left heart margin and pulmonary plethora consistent with a left to right shunt. Large ventricular septal defect shown on echocardiogram.

postural hypotension, hepatic encephalopathy, tinnitus and deafness and consequently meticulous monitoring of electrolytes is required.

Angiotensin-converting enzyme (ACE) inhibitors—(captopril, enalapril, lisinopril) These produce arteriolar and venous dilation and a reduction of aldosterone secretion. Side effects include hypotension, renal impairment, dry cough and bronchospasm.

Beta-adrenoceptor blocking drugs (carvedilol, propranolol, atenolol, sotalol)

These produce vasodilation and reduction in workload of ischaemic myocardium. Contraindicated with heart failure requiring inotropes, heart block, asthma and bradycardia. Side effects include postural hypotension, bradycardia, fatigue and sleep disturbances.

Digoxin. Digoxin decreases the automaticity of sinoatrial node and reduces conductivity within the atrioventricular node. It is contraindicated in heart block, Wolff-Parkinson-White syndrome, ventricular tachycardia and hypertrophic cardiomyopathy.

Other cardiac conditions

Myocarditis

Myocarditis is an inflammatory disorder of the myocardium which is uncommon in children but its potential impact can be significant. Inflammation of the myocardium is usually caused by viral infections such as enterovirus (coxsackie B), adenovirus, parvovirus B19 and EBV.

The children usually present with fever, heart failure and arrhythmias. Chest radiograph will often reveal cardiomegaly (Figure 16.13), and the ECG will show ST and T wave changes indicative of myocardial damage. Troponin levels are usually elevated though not always and cannot be considered a requirement for diagnosis. The echocardiogram will demonstrate a dilated and poorly contracting left ventricle with reduced ejection fraction.

Table 16.9 **Symptoms and signs of carditis**	
Symptoms	**Signs**
shortness of breath	pericardial rub
exercise intolerance	tachycardia
disproportionate tachycardia	apical systolic murmur
fever	basal diastolic murmur
	congestive heart failure

Treatment and management

Management is largely supportive with some patients requiring intensive care and ventilation.

Kawasaki disease

Presentation is usually to general paediatric services and infective cause are usually considered in the first instance. The long-term consequences are cardiac in nature. Further details are presented in Chapter 12 Infectious disease.

Pericardial disease

The commonest pericardial disease is that of pericardial effusion. The causes are many, but include viral infection,

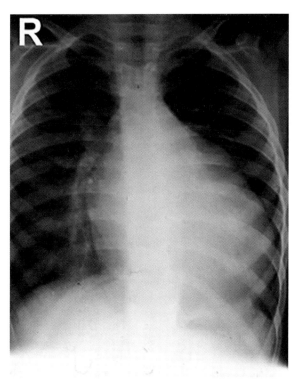

Fig. 16.13 Myocarditis. Chest radiograph of 4-year-old boy presenting with pyrexia, tachycardia, hypotension. Image shows cardiomegaly with globular cardiac configuration, normal pulmonary vascularity but very clearly demarcated cardiac outline; the latter finding can be seen with a poorly contracting heart particularly with pericardial effusion.

streptococcal and staphylococcal infections, Kawasaki disease and after heart surgery (typically at about 2 weeks postoperative).

Many children with a mild effusion can be observed and monitored with echocardiography whilst a large effusion may need to be drained either by percutaneous pericardiocentesis or by a surgical approach.

Rheumatic fever

This is a recognised cause of acquired heart disease in children and young adults. It is an inflammatory disease involving heart, joints and skin and is a complication of Group A streptococcal infection. There is a 2- to 3-week latent period between the infection and the onset of rheumatic fever, and the inflammatory response

involves the myocardium, valves and pericardium leading to fibrotic scarring. The most common valve affected is the mitral valve with the aortic valve being the second.

The criteria for diagnosis of acute rheumatic fever are carditis, polyarthritis, chorea, erythema marginatum and subcutaneous nodules. These are referred to as the Duckett Jones criteria (table 16.10). The presence of two major criteria or one major plus two minor criteria along with evidence of recent group A streptococcal infection indicates a high probability of acute rheumatic fever.

Table 16.10 **Duckett Jones Criteria for Diagnosis of Rheumatic Fever**	
Major Criteria	**Minor Criteria**
carditis	fever
polyarthritis	arthralgia
chorea	first degree heart block
erythema marginatum	elevated acute phase reactants
subcutaneous nodules	

Supporting evidence of streptococcal infection include
- increased ASO titre
- positive throat culture for group A streptococcus
- recent scarlet fever

Arthritis is the most common presentation, and typically the pain is polyarticular, migratory, nondeforming and affecting primarily large joints.

Erythema marginatum presents as a transient rash whilst subcutaneous nodules can be found on the extensor surfaces of the arms and legs as painless, flesh-coloured bumps. Chorea manifests as rapid, uncontrolled movements of the trunk or extremities. This is often the only feature of rheumatic fever to precede the cardiac sequel.

Rheumatic heart disease occurs in 50% of the patients and presents with the clinical features of carditis.

Investigations

- ESR CRP—elevated—are markers of inflammation. Used to monitor disease progress
- ASOT—elevated—often used to determine evidence of active streptococcal infection

- Throat swab—evidence of group A streptococcal infection
- Electrocardiogram—prolonged PR interval indicates first degree heart block

Treatment and management

Primary eradication of group A streptococcal infection from the upper respiratory tract involves treatment with a 10-day course of oral penicillin V. If there are concerns that an oral course will not be completed, it would be better to administer a single intramuscular injection of benzyl penicillin. Prophylactic antibiotics are given to prevent recurrent disease.

Treatment of symptoms includes daily administration of aspirin for 4–6 weeks which will lead to marked improvements in joint manifestations within 24–48 hours. Steroids have shown no enhancement in recovery and have greater risk of side effects.

Important sequelae

These include heart valvular damage (thickened valve leaflets and chordae), atrial fibrillation and embolic complications.

Cardiomyopathy

Cardiomyopathy is a disease of the myocardium and children are often referred following the acute death of an adult relative or due to a positive family history of a cardiomyopathy. It is uncommon in children but can have long lasting effects. There are two main types:
- dilated cardiomyopathy
- hypertrophic cardiomyopathy

Dilated cardiomyopathy

The underlying cause is usually unknown although certain viruses and a genetic predisposition have been implicated. The disease is often identified when a child presents to the emergency department with breathlessness and is found to have acute heart failure. A chest radiograph will show a large heart and an echocardiogram will make the diagnosis.

Management

If an operation is not indicated, then the child is managed with the usual heart failure medication of diuretics, ACE inhibitors, beta blockers and added calories. The outcome is very variable and an often quoted statistic is that one third improve, one third stay impaired and one third need transplantation.

Hypertrophic cardiomyopathy

This can present in the early neonatal period as a consequence of maternal diabetes. The baby will have a high level of insulin and the growth hormone effects of this will lead to a macrosomic baby, with polycythaemia, hypoglycaemia, hypertrophic cardiomyopathy and possible structural heart disease.

Hypertension

Systemic hypertension

Management of this condition falls within renal medicine, and the only cardiac involvement is to exclude the diagnosis of coarctation in children after the neonatal period. Routine cardiac follow up of hypertension is not undertaken unless the child is due renal transplantation where assessment of cardiac function is part of the preoperative assessment. Further details can be found in Chapter 20 Nephro-urology.

Pulmonary hypertension

Pulmonary hypertension is most commonly the result of chronic hypoxic lung disease or from untreated cardiac disease with volume and pressure overload which can occur from any left-to-right shunt. When pulmonary vasculature changes have become severe and pulmonary artery resistance is above systemic, reversal of the shunt from right to left occurs This produces Eisenmenger syndrome (inoperable pulmonary vascular disease) and is usually established by 2 years of age.

Investigations

The ECG demonstrates evidence of right axis deviation and right ventricular hypertrophy whilst the chest radiograph shows cardiomegaly with prominent main and branch pulmonary arteries and pruning of the peripheral vascular markings.

Management

These patients are no longer suitable to undergo any form of cardiac intervention and so the management is with medication or lung or heart and lung transplantation.

Relevant pharmacological agents used

Sildenafil. Promotes relaxation of vascular smooth muscle. It is contraindicated if the patient has sickle-cell disease or recent veno-occlusive disease. Important side effects include altered colour vision, gastritis, reflux oesophagitis, dry mouth and flushing.

Prostanoids—epoprostenol, iloprost, selexipag. Prostanoids produce a vasodilatation but are contraindicated in veno-occlusive disease, arrhythmias, valvar defects and disease of the myocardium. Side effects include systemic hypotension, haemorrhage, and jaw pain.

Nitric oxide. Nitric oxide is a potent and selective pulmonary vasodilator as it is given by inhalation. Side effects include increased risk of haemorrhage and a methaemoglobinaemia.

Infective endocarditis

The presence of congenital heart disease exposes children to the risk of infective endocarditis. This risk is highest when the structural abnormality produces a turbulent jet of blood and is therefore seen in children with a VSD, aortic stenosis and those with prosthetic material inserted at surgery.

Infective endocarditis should be suspected in any child who presents with a sustained fever, malaise, raised ESR, unexplained anaemia or haematuria. The condition may produce infective emboli leading to splinter haemorrhages in nailbed and necrotic skin lesions. neurological signs from cerebral infarction. Although these peripheral stigmata of infective endocarditis are important, their absence does not rule out the diagnosis.

Investigations

If the diagnosis is considered in an unwell patient, then multiple blood cultures should be taken **before** antibiotics are started. Echocardiography may confirm the diagnosis by identifying vegetations of fibrin, platelets and infecting organisms but it can never exclude the condition. Acute-phase reactants are raised and can be used to monitor response to treatment.

Treatment and management

The most common causative organism is alpha-haemolytic streptococcus (*Streptococcus viridans*). The condition is usually treated with high-dose penicillin in combination with an aminoglycoside and both are given intravenously over a period of 6 weeks. The chance of complete eradication of the organism is reduced if there is infected prosthetic material and consequently surgical removal may be required. Repeat echocardiography should be undertaken in all those with new cardiac signs, those with *Staphylococcus aureus* in blood cultures or other signs of infective endocarditis.

Potential complications

The most important factor in prophylaxis against endocarditis is good dental hygiene and brushing of their teeth twice a day should be strongly encouraged in all children with congenital heart disease. Body piercing and tattoos should also be avoided.

Routine antibiotic prophylaxis is no longer recommended in the UK for:
* dental treatment
* procedures involving ear, nose, and throat, bronchi, genitourinary tract and upper and lower gastrointestinal tract

Antibiotic prophylaxis may be required in those with high risk, such as those with prosthetic valves, artificial conduits placed at previous heart surgery when undergoing dental treatment, however trivial, and surgery which is likely to be associated with bacteraemia.

Cardiac complications of other system disorders

There are a variety of conditions which are commonly associated with cardiac disease, especially congenital structural problems (Table 16.11).

Table 16.11 Recognised cardiac conditions with systemic disorders

Disease	Associated condition	Management
Down syndrome	VSD or AVSD pulmonary hypertension	echocardiogram in the first month of life in all patients
Turner syndrome	coarctation or left heart lesions	echocardiogram at diagnosis
Duchenne muscular dystrophy	dilated cardiomyopathy	echocardiogram repeatedly
preterm chronic lung disease	pulmonary hypertension or PDA	echocardiogram at discharge
Williams syndrome	supravalvular aortic stenosis	Echocardiography may need surgery typically at 6 years age.
any genetic condition	congenital structural problems especially VSD	routine cardiac screen in the first 6 weeks of life or when the diagnosis is made
mitochondrial disorders	hypertrophic/dilated cardiomyopathy	echocardiogram and management of heart failure
Marfan syndrome (and other connective tissue disorders)	mitral valve prolapse/regurgitation aortic regurgitation aortic root dilation	screening and monitoring echocardiography

Important Clinical Points

Congenital heart disease
- atrial septal defect (primum) ECG: superior axis

Chest pain
- almost never due to heart disease in children

Cardiac arrhythmias
- ability to interpret ECG and recognition of common ECG patterns is important

Heart failure
- in first week of life likely due to left heart obstruction

- after the first week of life most likely due to a left-to-right shunt

Myocarditis
- children usually present with fever, heart failure and arrhythmias

Rheumatic fever
- defined by the Duckett Jones criteria

Infective endocarditis
- suspect if sustained fever, malaise, raised ESR, unexplained anaemia or haematuria

Further reading

Antimicrobial prophylaxis against infective endocarditis in adults and children undergoing interventional procedures. NICE guidance. Published March 2008; Updated 2016. https://bnfc.nice.org.uk/treatment-summary/antibacterials-use-for-prophylaxis.html

Park's: *The Pediatric Cardiology Handbook: Mobile Medicine Series*, 5th Edition, Elsevier, 2015.
Wernovsky G, et al.: *Anderson's Paediatric Cardiology*, 4th Edition, Elsevier, 2019.

Chapter | **17** |

Respiratory

Alan Smyth, Andrew Prayle, Matthew Hurley, Richard Stewart

After reading this chapter you should be able to assess, diagnose and manage:
- chronic cough
- wheezing illnesses
- lower respiratory tract infection
- cystic fibrosis presentation
- sleep disordered breathing
- life-threatening events including sudden unexpected death in infancy
  and
- select and interpret appropriate respiratory investigations
- understand the indications for long-term ventilation and respiratory support

Respiratory investigations

Blood gases

Values for carbon dioxide and pH do not differ markedly between arterial and venous samples and both will provide important information for clinical care (Table 17.1). Oxygen results from venous and capillary samples reflect values after tissue perfusion and are therefore ignored in clinical practice.

Chest radiograph

Radiological investigation of respiratory disease is commonly used in clinical practice. The posterior-anterior (PA) film is preferable where possible so as to facilitate assessment of cardiac size, although an anterior-posterior (PA) film may be practicable in the acutely ill or small child. Lateral films expose the child to significantly more radiation and rarely add clinically useful information.

Pulse oximetry

The correlation between peripheral saturation measurement and arterial saturation is sufficient for most clinical assessments. Since the technique measures absorbance in haemoglobin, it may provide normal values in anaemic individuals even though the oxygen carrying capacity is significantly reduced and it may also give low saturation values in individuals with poor peripheral perfusion.

Spirometry

Spirometry measures lung volumes, usually during a forced exhalation and inhalation manoeuvre, and the test is usually possible in children over the age of 5 or 6 years (Figure 17.1). In forced manoeuvres such as the Forced Expiratory Volume in 1 second (FEV_1), the increased intrathoracic pressure during forced exhalation is transmitted to the bronchi, acting to decrease the diameter of the lumen and so limiting the rate of flow—this is termed 'dynamic airway narrowing'.

During spirometry, a variety of volumes are measured, and there are recognisable patterns of these (Table 17.2). Reference values allow the spirometry measurements of a child to be compared to the average measurements for their age, sex, height and race and these can be expressed in the form of a percentage predicted or a Z score.

Table 17.1 Responses to changes in plasma oxygen and bicarbonate levels

| abnormality | primary disturbance | EFFECT ON | | base excess | compensatory response |
		pH	pCO2		
respiratory acidosis	↑ pCO2	↓	↑	negative	↑ [HCO3-]
metabolic acidosis	↓ [HCO3-]	↓	N or ↓	negative	↓pCO2
respiratory alkalosis	↓ pCO2	↑	N or ↓	positive	↓[HCO3-]
metabolic alkalosis	↑ [HCO3-]	↑	N or ↑	positive	↑pCO2

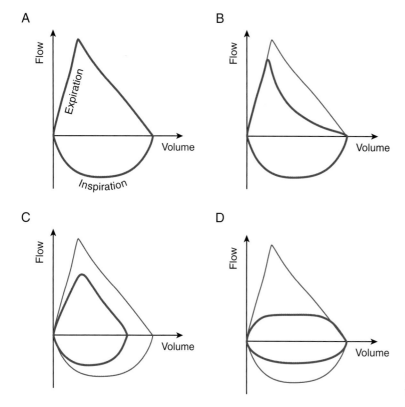

Fig. 17.1 Common patterns of flow volume loops.

A: in a well child, the loop proceeds in a clockwise manner initially with a rapid rise of flow over a small volume, reaching the Peak Expiratory Flow Rate (PEFR). Over the remaining lung volume, the patient expires to the end of vital capacity. The downward reflection of the loop below the zero line, back to the origin, represents the inspiration after the forced expiration.

B: an 'obstructed' loop. Note the concavity of the downward phase of expiration.

C: a 'restrictive' pattern. Note that the volume is decreased—the flow rate may be more normal.

D: extra-thoracic fixed obstruction (e.g. vascular ring around the trachea or mediastinal mass). Note that the peak inspiratory and expiratory flows are both reduced.

Table 17.2 **Patterns of lung volume changes.**			
FEV1	FVC	FEV1/FVC ratio	Interpretation
normal	Normal	Normal	normal
reduced	normal	reduced	obstruction (e.g. asthma, cystic fibrosis)
normal/ reduced	reduced	normal/ increased	restriction (e.g. pulmonary hypoplasia, scoliosis, interstitial lung disease)

Bronchodilator reversibility test

Assesses children and young people (from age of 5 years) for bronchial hyperreactivity by recording spirometry values before and after the administration of a bronchodilator (usually salbutamol). An improvement in FEV1 of 12% or more is regarded as a positive response.

Bronchoprovocation test

The bronchoprovocation test assesses whether a child with initially normal pulmonary function tests may actually produce abnormal results when an inhaled irritant is given. The typical agents used to challenge the airways are methacholine, histamine and adenosine. The concentration of the agent which induces a 20% fall in FEV_1 is recorded and the lower the dose then the greater the degree of airway hyperreactivity. Exercise can also be used as a 'provocation test'. Both these investigations should be undertaken by teams competent in their administration.

Fraction of exhaled nitric oxide (FeNO)

FeNO can be measured in most school-aged children and is an indicator of airways inflammation. It is useful where the history suggests asthma but spirometry is normal or an obstructive pattern is not reversible. Levels of >35 parts per billion are abnormal in children aged 5–18 years.

Bronchoscopy

Bronchoscopy uses either a rigid or flexible bronchoscope and allows direct visualisation of the internal airway structure and allows for microbiological sampling or biopsy. Inhaled foreign may be located and extracted.

Whole body plethysmography (or the 'body box')

This measures thoracic gas volumes, including air that is not directly communicating with the airway opening (such as 'trapped gas' or lung cysts).

Transfer factor of the lung for carbon monoxide (TLCO)

The rate of oxygen diffusion across the alveolar membrane can be assessed by measuring diffusing capacity of carbon monoxide, but the test can only be done in cooperative older children.

Cough

Cough is a reflex which removes mucous and other material from the lungs and is less effective in glottic dysfunction, tracheostomy and neuromuscular weakness.

Cough can be the cardinal feature of both acute, life-threatening and chronic, life-limiting respiratory disease and the causes can be categorised by the age of the child (Table 17.3), the duration of the cough and the character of the cough.

Table 17.3 **Selected causes of cough, grouped by the typical ages at presentation.**		
Infant	Preschool	School age/ adolescent
primary ciliary dyskinesia cystic fibrosis infections (viruses, bacteria, chlamydia, pertussis) congenital malformations (tracheoesophageal fistula)	foreign body infection cystic fibrosis primary ciliary dyskinesia bronchiectasis immunodeficiency asthma passive cigarette smoke aspiration	asthma postnasal drip infection cystic fibrosis primary ciliary dyskinesia immunodeficiency bronchiectasis smoking air pollution tic cough aspiration

The character of the cough can be described as 'wet' or 'dry' with the former suggestive of excessive secretions. In infants and children, a cough associated with sputum production is rarely 'productive' as the sputum is usually swallowed rather than expectorated. A wet cough implies infection and, if chronic, suggests protracted bacterial bronchitis, suppurative lung disease or bronchiectasis. A wet cough might also feature in gastro-oesophageal reflux and aspiration. An acute viral cough can last 3 to 4 weeks whilst the 'postinfectious cough' can last much longer, especially in pertussis.

Protracted bacterial bronchitis

This is the most common cause of a prolonged cough over 4 weeks duration in preschool children. The child usually looks well, has no other clinical signs and has normal growth. It is typically associated with infection by *M. catarrhalis*, *S. pneumoniae* and *H. influenzae* and can be treated effectively with a prolonged (2–4 week) course of an oral antibiotic, such as coamoxiclav. The diagnosis is confirmed by the resolution of symptoms after the trial of therapy. If the cough does not resolve after 4 weeks of antibiotics, then chronic suppurative lung disease or bronchiectasis should be considered.

'Red flags' for cough

A cough should be investigated thoroughly if any of the following are present:
- sudden onset cough after choking
- night sweats
- haemoptysis
- poor weight gain or weight loss
- cough which progressively worsens
- signs of lung disease—clubbing, barrel-shaped chest, Harrison's sulci

Investigations

For a chronic wet cough, a typical approach would involve chest radiographs, bacterial cough swab and viral swabs, a sweat test and an initial immune panel (immunoglobulins, functional antibodies, full blood count and lymphocyte subsets). If primary ciliary dyskinesia is suspected, patients are referred for ciliary studies to a national referral diagnostic centre whilst, if bronchiectasis is suspected, a CT scan should be undertaken. Bronchoscopy may also be indicated.

Treatment and management

Treatment is directed at the underlying cause. There is no role for over-the-counter 'cough medicines' which usually contain opiate-derived compounds to suppress the cough. When a cough is felt to be benign, a watch-and-wait approach is appropriate.

Wheezing disorders

Young children inherently have narrow airways and consequently generate wheeze with only minimal reduction in the diameter of the bronchi and bronchioles. Most wheeze occurs in the expiratory phase as the increased intrathoracic pressure required for expiration will also lead to external pressure on the smaller airways. A biphasic wheeze or a very localised wheeze suggest a fixed area and warrants further consideration (Table 17.4).

Asthma

The key clinical features of asthma are episodic wheeze that is present during exacerbations along with breathlessness and cough. Some patients have interval symptoms, which include breathlessness, cough and wheeze that may be

Table 17.4 Common causes of wheeze

Cause	Examples
infective	mycoplasma pertussis viral induced wheeze—adenovirus, respiratory syncytial virus, human metapneumovirus, parainfluenza, influenza
inflammatory	hypersensitivity pneumonitis irritant inhalation—smoke, illicit drugs sarcoidosis vasculitis
physical compression	foreign body aspiration granulation tissue in airway lymph node enlargement tumour—lymphoma vascular ring, vascular compression tracheo-bronchomalacia bronchogenic or pulmonary cyst
complex pathophysiological	primary ciliary dyskinesia cystic fibrosis bronchiectasis aspiration and gastro-oesophageal reflux disease. hyperventilation.
upper airway	vocal cord palsy vocal fold dysfunction angioedema

exacerbated by exertion, changes in environmental temperatures, damp air, emotion and laughter. Nocturnal cough may also be present. Between attacks many children may be symptom free with normal lung function. Those patients with poorly controlled asthma may have a hyperinflated chest and develop Harrison's sulci (Figure 17.2) which are fixed inward grooves in the chest wall where the diaphragm inserts into the internal surfaces of the ribs.

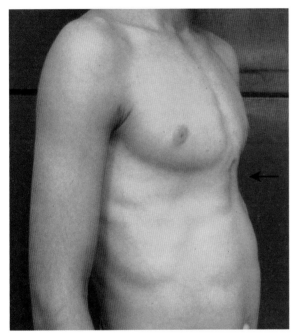

Fig. 17.2 Chest of 11-year-old boy with poorly controlled asthma. Harrison's sulci visible (arrow).

Asthma in the acute setting

An acute asthma attack is associated with breathlessness and a feeling of a 'tight' chest, with a characteristic non-productive cough. Clinical signs include:
- tachypnoea
- intercostal recession
- chest indrawing
- 'tracheal tug'
- prolongation of the expiratory phase of breathing
- wheeze which may be audible without a stethoscope

In more severe asthma, patients use their accessory muscles of respiration. Oxygen saturations are often maintained during an attack and when patients do deteriorate, they are usually hypoxic prior to becoming hypercapnic as the latter finding is a late feature, and indicates a severe, or life-threatening episode (Table 17.5).

Associations

Asthma is often associated with other atopic conditions, in particular hay fever, food allergies and eczema. There is often a strong history of familial atopy.

Wheeze in the under 5-year olds

A current challenge is that many children wheeze in the preschool period and such children are often diagnosed with 'pre-school wheeze' rather than asthma. This can be categorised as either:
- recurrent viral-induced wheeze—evidence of a viral infection with each occurrence of wheeze
- multi trigger wheeze—episodic wheeze after exposure to pollen, moulds or house dust mite

Table 17.5 **Levels of severity of an acute asthma attack**		
Mild-moderate	**Severe**	**Life threatening**
oxygen saturation 92% and above in air PEFR > 50% predicted of best	cannot complete sentences in one breath or too breathless to talk or eat/feed oxygen saturation < 92% in air PEFR < 50% predicted or best	cyanosis silent chest poor respiratory effort fatigue or exhaustion agitation or reduced level of consciousness raised carbon dioxide
under 6 years heart rate < 140/min respiratory rate < 40/min	**under 6 years** heart rate > 140/min respiratory rate > 40/min	
6 years and over heart rate < 125/min respiratory rate < 30/min	**6 years and over** heart rate > 125/min respiratory rate > 30/min	

In reality, many children will move between the two groups and the current NICE guidelines recommend treating them based on observation and clinical judgment along with regular reviews.

Investigations

No single test is diagnostic of asthma, but a history of recurrent wheeze which responds to treatment is useful. Spirometry is the key diagnostic test and can be performed in most children who are 5 years and older. The FEV_1, FEV_1/FVC ratio and the FEF 25–75 are all reduced.

Administration of a bronchodilator (usually salbutamol) should result in an improvement, and an increase in FEV_1 volume of 12% over the baseline is considered reversible airflow obstruction. Peak expiratory flow is highly effort dependent and it alone should not be relied upon.

Exercise challenge tests are useful and spirometry is undertaken before and after exercise. A decrease of 10% of FEV_1 is usually considered diagnostic of exercise-induced asthma.

Treatment and management of chronic asthma

There are several stepwise approaches to increasing asthma treatment but central to all the guidelines is regular review of symptoms and the stepping down of therapy when appropriate. A further key component of treatment is the avoidance of cigarette smoke (Table 17.6).

The major challenge in asthma is adherence to medication and it is well recognised that many patients take only around half their prescribed doses of inhalers. Therefore, rather than automatically 'stepping up' treatment, a careful, sensitive discussion around adherence is often more helpful if patients have frequent exacerbations or loss of control of daily symptoms.

Guidelines for the pharmacological management of asthma are published by NICE, BTS/SIGN and GINA (Global Initiative for Asthma Management and Prevention). There are some differences between these guidelines but all follow a similar approach to management.

Table 17.6 **Pharmacological management of asthma following NICE recommendations**	
Situation	**Therapy**
if infrequent, short-lived wheeze and normal lung function	consider SABA as reliever therapy alone
if asthma-related symptoms 3 times a week or more, or causing waking at night or uncontrolled with a SABA alone	consider low-dose ICS as the first-line maintenance therapy
if uncontrolled on a paediatric low dose of ICS	consider LTRA in addition to the ICS and review the response to treatment in 4 to 8 weeks
if uncontrolled on a low dose of ICS and an LTRA as maintenance therapy	consider stopping the LTRA and starting a LABA in combination with the ICS
if uncontrolled on a paediatric low dose of ICS and a LABA as maintenance therapy	consider changing the ICS and LABA maintenance therapy to a MART regimen with a paediatric low-maintenance ICS dose
if uncontrolled on a paediatric low-maintenance ICS dose with LABA	consider increasing the ICS to a paediatric moderate maintenance dose (either continuing on a MART regimen or changing to a fixed dose of an ICS and a LABA, with a SABA as a reliever therapy)
if asthma is uncontrolled in children and young people (aged 5 to 16) on a paediatric moderate maintenance ICS dose with LABA (either as MART or a fixed-dose regimen)	seek advice from a healthcare professional with expertise in paediatric asthma management
SABA = short acting beta-agonist (e.g. salbutamol); LABA = long-acting beta agonist (e.g. salmeterol or formoterol—unlicensed in under 5s); LTRA = leukotriene receptor antagonist; ICS = inhaled corticosteroid; MART = maintenance and reliver treatment.	

Treatment and management of acute attack

Children and young people with asthma are at risk of acute attacks which may progress rapidly and become life threatening. Presentation requires prompt assessment and administration of high flow oxygen through a tight-fitting mask when the SpO_2 is less than 94% or there is any suggestion of respiratory compromise.

Those with a mild to moderate episode should be given inhaled ß₂-agonist and, if there is a failure of response, inhaled ipratropium bromide should be added via a nebuliser. Oral steroids should be administered at an early stage when possible although their effect will not be immediate.

If reassessment after a short interval reveals a poor response, then an initial single bolus dose of intravenous salbutamol is given followed by intravenous magnesium sulphate if there is a minimal response. Discussions with colleagues from anaesthetics and paediatric intensive care should be undertaken.

CLINICAL SCENARIO

A 15-year-old girl was referred for evaluation of recent onset of cough and wheeze. She had been well previously, had no history of atopy and she was not a smoker. She was, however, a high performing runner but would develop symptoms as soon as he started sprinting on the field. She described an inspiratory stridor, dry cough, tightness of chest and throat. She would stop running and the coughing would cease. She had been on high-dose combination of inhaled steroids and long-acting beta agonists without any benefit.

Her spirometry was entirely normal at baseline; however, after strenuous exercise on treadmill there was marked decrease in inspiratory flow volume. There was associated inspiratory wheeze. Continuous nasolaryngoscopy whilst on treadmill demonstrated severe adduction of laryngeal structures in parallel with severe respiratory distress. Psychological evaluation did not reveal any obvious contributing factors.

A pH study demonstrated frequent gastro-oesophageal reflux and endoscopy indicated that this may be long standing.

A diagnosis was made of exercise-induced laryngeal obstruction secondary to chronic gastro-oesophageal reflux.

Treatment with proton-pump inhibitor was commenced and a referral made to speech therapy with the aim of controlling laryngeal dysfunction. Following this intervention, she had a marked improvement in symptoms and her inhaled medications were withdrawn. She was able to return to high performance running.

Lower respiratory tract infections

A microbiological diagnosis is not made in most children with pneumonia but the organisms likely responsible depend on the age of the child. In older children *Streptococcus pneumoniae* and *Mycoplasma pneumoniae* are commonly implicated with the latter more common in school-age children. In those under 2 years, the commonest bacterial cause of pneumonia is *Streptococcus pneumoniae* which causes around a third of radiologically confirmed pneumonia in this age group. A viral cause is more common in younger children— commonly respiratory syncytial virus (RSV) or human metapneumovirus. Infections caused by group A streptococcus and *Staphylococcus aureus* are more likely to cause necrotising pneumonia and children with these infections are more likely to require intensive care.

Clinical presentation

The physical signs of pneumonia will help make a clinical diagnosis and also assign the degree of severity and guide management. Although some factors differ between infants and young children, the common findings are fever, tachypnoea, respiratory distress, chest pain, abdominal pain and headache. Cough may be absent initially. Wheeze is uncommon in children with pneumonia.

Alternative diagnoses

Many conditions can present in a similar manner to the child with pneumonia but there are often distinguishing features. These include:

- systemic sepsis may be present in infants with pneumonia, and a full infection screen and intravenous antibiotics may be necessary whilst clarity is brought to the diagnosis.
- viral-induced wheeze may produce a low-grade fever, tachypnoea and respiratory distress, in addition to wheezing. Viral wheeze can be distinguished from pneumonia by a history of previous episodes, the presence of coryza and a clinical response to a bronchodilator.
- respiratory difficulty with a cardiac cause due to pulmonary oedema. In older children acute myocarditis may produce biventricular failure.
- metabolic disorders—the child with diabetic ketoacidosis will usually have a sighing, acidotic breathing pattern (Kussmaul) rather than tachypnoea.

Investigations

Pneumonia in children is a clinical diagnosis and invariably a chest radiograph will be undertaken (Figure 17.3a-m). This, however, will not distinguish between bacterial and viral pathogens and is not necessary in children with mild to moderate disease. The terms used to describe clinical appearances include 'consolidation' and 'collapse or atelectasis'. Pure consolidation results in alveolar opacification without volume loss whilst pure collapse results in alveolar opacification and volume loss based on abnormal position of lung fissures and other lung structures. Both can result in loss of normal anatomical landmarks such as diaphragmatic or cardiac outline. Both collapse and consolidation are seen on most radiographs with an infective pathology. Hilar lymphadenopathy is often present (Figure 17.4).

Further investigations are necessary if there is diagnostic uncertainty, an acute deterioration or if complications such as pleural effusion or necrotising pneumonia are suspected. These would include chest radiograph, nasopharyngeal aspirate (in infants), blood cultures (although in most series less than 10% are positive) and acute and convalescent serum for viruses *M. pneumoniae* and *Chlamydia pneumoniae*.

Follow-up chest radiographs are not undertaken routinely but may be useful if there has been a round pneumonia, lobar collapse, persisting symptoms, pleural effusion or necrotising pneumonia detected during the acute phase.

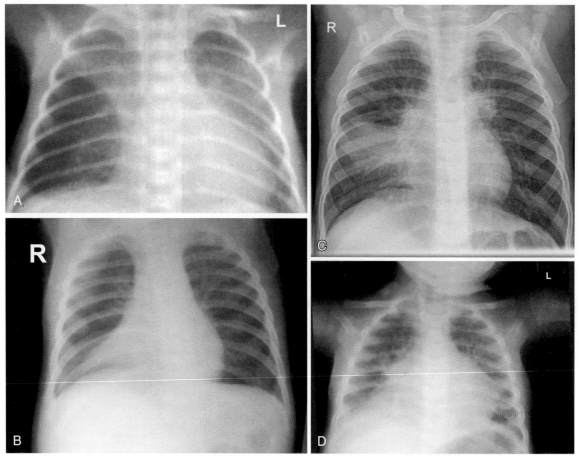

Fig. 17.3 (a) Right upper lobe consolidation with collapse. Opacification in the right upper lobe. Elevated horizontal fissure indicates lobar collapse. Trachea deviated to the right. Additional infective change in left lung field. (b) Right middle lobe consolidation with collapse. Loss of right cardiac border is the key feature in RML consolidation. The horizontal fissure is pulled down indicating collapse. (c) Right middle lobe consolidation without collapse. Loss of right cardiac border due to consolidation. The horizontal fissure remains in position. (d) Right lower lobe collapse. The loss of the line of the right hemidiaphragm by the opacification.

Fig. 17.3 cont'd (e) Right lower lobe consolidation. Right lower lobe consolidation with indistinct diaphragmatic outline but clearly demarcated right heart border. (f) Left upper lobe consolidation. Left upper lobe consolidation affecting mainly the anterior segment of the lobe with some sparing of the apico-posterior segment and lingula. The left heart margin is preserved by virtue of the lingular sparing. (g) Left lower lobe consolidation. Left lower lobe consolidation with opacification obscuring the left hemidiaphragm but with preservation of the left heart border indicating the opacity is behind the heart. (h) Lingular lobe collapse. Lingular consolidation—mid to lower zone air space opacification with cardiac outline lost but diaphragmatic outline preserved.

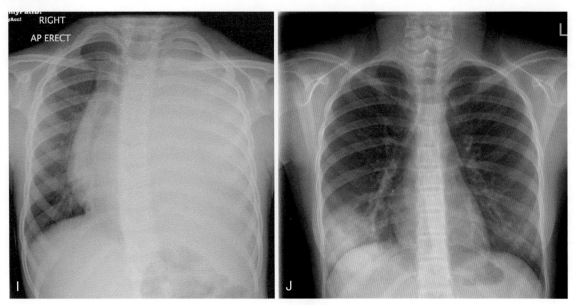

Fig. 17.3 cont'd (i) Left pleural effusion. Diffuse homogeneous opacification of the left hemithorax with cardiac and tracheal shift to the right indicating mass effect. Mild thoracic scoliosis concavity to the left raises the possibility that the effusion may represent an empyema. (j) Round pneumonia. Rounded area of consolidation within the lateral basal aspect of the right lower lobe. Round pneumonias are indicative of Strep pneumoniae infection.

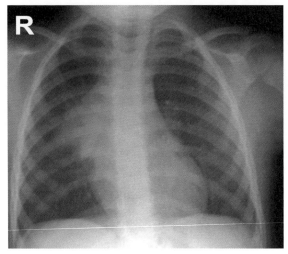

Fig 17.4 Right hilar lymphadenopathy.

Treatment and management

Children in the UK receive the 13 valent pneumococcal conjugate vaccine at 8 weeks, 16 weeks and 1 year. Children with severe pneumonia, those with an oxygen saturation consistently less than 92% and those with an underlying chronic disease should be admitted to hospital. Supplementary oxygen is given to maintain oxygen saturations over 92%, and if there are clinical signs of dehydration then supplementary fluids are needed. Nasogastric tubes partially obstruct the airway and so intravenous fluids are often necessary.

All children with a diagnosis of pneumonia should be given antibiotics, as bacterial and viral causes cannot be distinguished clinically or radiologically. Oral antibiotics are first line provided

- initial oxygen saturation is ≥85%
- the child is not shocked
- there is no underlying chronic illness

First-line oral treatment is amoxicillin but if there is a suspicion of atypical infection then a macrolide should be added. Treatment for 5 days is standard practice although there is some evidence that a 3-day course may be equally effective.

Intravenous coamoxiclav or a cephalosporin can be used but local guidelines, microbiological advice and any positive culture results should guide the decisions.

Important sequelae
Respiratory failure or cardiovascular collapse

Critical care assessment is important at an early stage in a child who is deteriorating. Indications for admission to critical care include difficulty in maintaining an oxygen saturation of over 92% in 60% oxygen, hypercapnia, exhaustion, apnoea and shock.

Pleural effusion and empyema

Small serous effusions are common in childhood pneumonia but when this becomes infected then an empyema occurs. Children may have reduced chest expansion, stony dullness and decreased transmitted vocal fremitus on the involved side with a scoliosis to that side along with tracheal displacement away from the affected side.

Ultrasound and occasionally CT are useful investigations to confirm the diagnosis and plan drainage. Where fever persists and the effusion is of significant size then it should be drained although it is important to consider differentials such as tuberculosis and malignancy.

Intrapleural urokinase administration is of value and is instilled via the chest drain which is then clamped. The drain can be removed when most of the fluid has drained. Early follow up with a chest radiograph is important.

Bronchiectasis

Bronchiectasis describes a condition where the bronchi are dilated and distorted leading to chronic obstructive lung disease. The most commonly identified causes in children are:
- Impaired mucous clearance (cystic fibrosis)
- previous pneumonic infections (pertussis, measles, adenovirus, mycobacteria)
- primary immunodeficiency (HIV, common variable immune deficiency)
- recurrent aspiration
- inhaled foreign body
- primary ciliary dyskinesia

Bronchiolitis obliterans

This is a form of diffuse chronic lung disease with obliteration and constriction of bronchioles. Recognised causes include:
- infection (adenovirus, influenza, measles)
- connective tissue disease
- toxic fume inhalation
- post lung transplantation (part of graft v host disease)

A necrotising pneumonia is suspected where pockets of air are seen within the consolidated lung tissue on chest radiograph and may give a round lesion with a fluid level. The commonest causative organism is *Streptococcus pneumoniae* but methicillin-resistant *Staphylococcus aureus* (MRSA) is also implicated (including strains producing Panton-Valentine leukocidin) as are *Group A streptococci*. Prolonged antibiotic treatment over many weeks is indicated.

Other respiratory conditions

Primary ciliary dyskinesia

Primary ciliary dyskinesia (PCD) is usually autosomal recessive and is characterised by poorly functioning cilia that results in reduced mucociliary clearance and chronic infection. In around half of patients, there is also variable abnormal position of the internal organs such as in Kartagener syndrome which describes dextrocardia with primary ciliary dyskinesia.

A common presentation is prolonged respiratory distress and 'unexplained' oxygen requirement in the neonatal period. In later life, chronic wet cough, reduced lung function and sputum production due to bronchiectasis occurs. Chronic rhinitis and recurrent otitis media and glue ear are frequent. Diagnosis of PCD is by examination of nasal brushings for ciliary function.

CLINICAL SCENARIO

A 13-year-old boy was admitted with a history of cough, wheeze and breathlessness. He had previously been assessed at 4 years of age when restricted growth, a persistent wet cough and wheeze were identified. A definitive diagnosis was not made but he was treated with inhaled beta-agonists, inhaled steroids and then courses of oral steroids. He continued to receive multiple courses of antibiotics but had no hospital admission.

Examination during the current admission showed that his height and weight were below the 3rd centile. He had obvious halitosis, marked clubbing and widespread crepitation on auscultation. A clinical diagnosis of bronchiectasis was made and further investigations were planned. High-resolution CT investigation showed multilobar disease. Sweat test was negative. Sputum culture grew Moraxella catarrhalis and Streptococcus pneumoniae.

He was found to have low immunoglobulins with IgG being very low as was his lymphocyte count. He had a poor antibody response to vaccines.

A diagnosis of common variable immunodeficiency disorder was made and he was referred to the paediatric immunology team. He was commenced on immunoglobulin replacement therapy and made a marked clinical improvement. He continued with regular reviews by both immunology and respiratory teams.

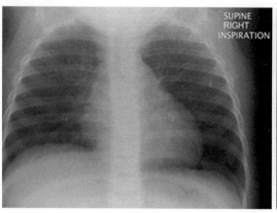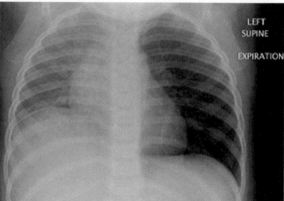

Fig. 17.5 Inhaled foreign body in left lower lobe. Inspiratory and expiratory films showing air trapping as the left lung remains hyperinflated in expiration.

Chronic aspiration

Recurrent entry of food, gastric contents or saliva into the lungs in sufficient quantities to cause respiratory symptoms is termed chronic pulmonary aspiration (CPA). Conditions such as swallowing dysfunction (common in children with neurodisability) and gastro-oesophageal reflux predispose to CPA. The condition should be suspected in children with recurrent pneumonia, chronic cough, stridor and recurrent wheeze. Chronic aspiration results in inflammation, infection, and ultimately bronchiectasis. Treatment is directed at reducing stomach pH (if reflux is demonstrated on an oesophageal pH study) and speech and language therapy advice on reducing aspiration during swallowing. If reflux is severe, a gastrostomy with fundoplication can be considered.

Complication of foreign body inhalation

An inhaled foreign body may obstruct the airway at any level. The site of the obstruction depends on the size and shape of the foreign body and therefore can result in a spectrum of presentations from immediate fatal airway obstruction to chronic respiratory symptoms such as cough, recurrent inflammation and ultimately bronchiectasis of the affected bronchi. Toddlers are usually at greatest risk, though it can affect all ages. Children with neurodisability who have poor swallow are also at increased risk.

After lodgement of a foreign body in a distal airway, mucus and local inflammation will usually result in obstruction of that airway and so reduce the chances of clearing the foreign body by cough. In partial obstruction, air can become trapped in the lung, distal to the obstruction. Diagnosis is sometimes challenging, but a chest radiograph may reveal a radio-opaque foreign body (coins

in the trachea are often rest in a sagittal plane) or chest asymmetry on inspiratory and expiratory films indicating hyperinflation (Figure 17.5). The initial first aid manoeuvres for an inhaled foreign body include back slaps or the Heimlich manoeuvre (for older children) but if this is unsuccessful, then removal through rigid bronchoscopy is then undertaken.

Cystic fibrosis

Cystic fibrosis (CF) is a multisystem disease caused by a mutation of the gene for cystic fibrosis transmembrane conductance regulator (CFTR) that leads to failure of chloride transport at the cell membrane. Gastrointestinal effects include pancreatic malabsorption and faltering growth. In the lung, failure to clear respiratory mucus allows chronic lower airway infection with intermittent exacerbations that leads to lung damage, bronchiectasis and ultimately respiratory failure and death.

Clinical presentation

Since 2007 all babies born in the UK have had a newborn screening test for CF which will identify about 82% of those affected. Around 15% of affected infants will present immediately after birth with 'meconium ileus'—a failure to pass meconium with abdominal distension and bilious vomiting—that requires urgent radiological reduction by contrast enema or surgery. Some children may present at a later stage with symptoms of a chronic wet cough, unexplained growth faltering or evidence of bronchiectasis on a CT scan and these children need prompt investigation with a sweat test. The differential diagnosis at late presentation includes:

- primary ciliary dyskinesia
- immune deficiency (hypoglammaglobulinaemia or common variable immune deficiency)
- postinfectious bronchiectasis (including sequelae of pulmonary culosis)
- bronchiolitis obliterans (which may follow adenovirus pneumonia)
- chronic aspiration
- complication of congenital pulmonary malformation
- complication of foreign body inhalation

Investigations

The newborn screening test initially measures immune reactive trypsin and if this is positive, the same sample is tested for the four most common CF genes. When two genes are identified, the baby is referred to a CF centre and should be seen within 24 hours of the parents being informed.

Those who present with recognised clinical features (chronic wet cough; faltering growth with steatorrhea) will have a sweat test and a sweat chloride of greater than 59 mmol/l confirms the diagnosis. The presence of two gene mutations known to cause CF would also support the diagnosis.

Treatment and management
Nutritional management

Between 80% and 90% of children with CF have pancreatic insufficiency, as identified by a low faecal elastase measurement. They will require pancreatic enzyme replacement therapy (PERT) from the time of diagnosis and specialist dietetic advice is essential. Those infants who require PERT are given a granule formulation (e.g. Creon Micro™) before a feed and this is usually mixed with fruit purée. Many mothers successfully breastfeed their baby with CF.

It is standard practice to prescribe fat-soluble vitamins from diagnosis and to start with vitamin E and vitamin A containing formulations.

Children with CF should be weighed and measured regularly as they require a 20% to 50% greater calorie intake per day than comparable children of the same age. Energy requirements are increased considerably during a pulmonary exacerbation of their condition whilst appetite is often reduced. In some patients, growth failure occurs in spite of adequate PERT and regular dietary advice and further oral calorie supplements may be necessary. If this is unsuccessful then gastrostomy placement and commencing enteral feeds is required.

Airway clearance is a major part of management and specialist physiotherapists will teach percussion and postural drainage which is required once or twice every day. A positive expiratory pressure technique, using a mask or mouthpiece, provides resistance as the child blows out and splints the airway open and aids mucus clearance. Some children will benefit from inhaled treatment with a mucoactive agent, to aid airway clearance. Such agents include dornase alfa, a recombinant enzyme which breaks down viscid DNA from dead cells in the airway, and hypertonic saline (commonly 6% or 7%) that rehydrates airway mucus and induces coughing.

The key to minimising bronchiectasis and optimising respiratory health in CF is the early and effective diagnosis and treatment of airway infection. Children with CF characteristically have different organisms isolated from their respiratory tract as they grow older:

- Infancy: *Staphylococcus aureus*
- Preschool: *Haemophilus influenzae*
- School age: *Pseudomonas aeruginosa*

However, any of these infections can occur at any age and in addition to this, children with CF are vulnerable to highly antibiotic resistant organisms such as nontuberculous mycobacteria (NTM) and *Burkholderia cepacia* complex.

It has been standard practice in the UK to prescribe prophylactic antistaphylococcal antibiotics from diagnosis until 3 years of age. *P. aeruginosa* has the ability to cause chronic, intractable infection in the airways of children with CF, through the formation of biofilms in the airway. When the organism first appears in the CF airway, it can be eradicated with antibiotics. Standard treatment is a combination or an oral antibiotic (e.g. ciprofloxacin) and a nebulised antibiotic (e.g. colistimethate sodium or tobramycin) and prolonged courses of both oral and nebulised therapy are needed (3 weeks to 3 months). It is common for *P. aeruginosa* infection to become established—often after multiple eradication courses over several years and when this occurs, lifelong suppressive therapy with a nebulised antibiotic is necessary. Many organisms are transmissible between patients and strict adherence to infection prevention and control procedures is essential in CF care.

Management of pulmonary exacerbations

Many children with CF will be free of respiratory symptoms but they may develop pulmonary exacerbations which require prompt recognition and treatment. The clinical features of an exacerbation are:
- decreased exercise tolerance
- increased cough
- increased sputum production
- school absence
- decreased appetite

Pulmonary exacerbations require multidisciplinary assessment and antibiotic treatment (guided by the most recent respiratory specimen) and in most cases intravenous antibiotics are required—usually for 2 weeks. Inpatient treatment allows airway clearance to be optimised and nutrition assessment and support to be given. Some children and young people benefit from planned, regular intravenous antibiotics to preempt pulmonary exacerbations and maintain lung function.

Long-term azithromycin, which has both antibiotic and antiinflammatory actions, is used in over half of patients with CF and is indicated for children over 6 years old.

Measurement of lung function

Spirometry is an objective measure to guide the clinician in

- diagnosing a pulmonary exacerbation
- assessing response to treatment
- looking for a year-on-year progression of lung disease

A 10% drop in FEV_1 is in keeping with a pulmonary exacerbation and the average annual decline in FEV_1 should be less than 2%.

Respiratory complications
Allergic bronchopulmonary aspergillosis

Not all lung damage in CF is caused solely by an infectious agent and in some, the patient's immune response is part of the pathogenic process. Aspergillus fumigatus is an environmental fungus which can be found in the airways of children with CF where it can induce a strong, IgE-mediated immune response leading to allergic bronchopulmonary aspergillosis. The diagnosis is confirmed if:

- clinical deterioration is not attributable to another cause
- total IgE >500 IU/mL or a fourfold rise in IgE
- raised aspergillus-specific IgE
- new radiological changes, particularly persistent mucus plugging

Children should receive high dose oral prednisolone for 2–3 weeks combined with an azole antifungal (e.g. posaconazole).

Haemoptysis

Severe bronchiectasis may be associated with hypertrophy of the bronchial arteries leading to haemoptysis. Small haemoptyses are common and often present as blood-streaked sputum. Massive haemoptysis is a medical emergency requiring fluid resuscitation and subsequent bronchial artery embolisation.

Pneumothorax

Occurs when a subpleural bullus bursts into the pleural space, and although uncommon in children with CF it does occur more often as age and lung disease advance. Simple pneumothoraces may be small and managed by aspiration or large and require tube drainage.

End-stage lung disease

Severe bronchiectasis leads to respiratory failure that initially may be characterised by hypoxaemia requiring supplementary oxygen. Respiratory failure can progress to type II respiratory failure (with both hypoxaemia and hypercapnia) and noninvasive ventilation should be introduced. When the FEV_1 falls below 30% predicted there is a 50% chance of death within 2 years and a discussion should take place between the CF team, the young person and the family regarding end-of-life care. For some young people, the right option is good quality palliative care. For others, a referral should be made for transplant assessment although less than five children per year in the UK receive a double lung transplant for CF.

Non respiratory complications
CF liver disease

CFTR is expressed in the intra- and extrahepatic bile ducts and CFTR dysfunction leads to viscid bile, periportal fibrosis and ultimately cirrhosis in some children. Cirrhosis may be accompanied by portal hypertension and oesophageal varices, which may bleed. Risk factors for CF liver disease include pancreatic insufficiency, meconium ileus and prolonged parenteral feeding in infancy. Liver function tests and prothrombin time should be checked at least annually and repeated if abnormal. If the prothrombin time is prolonged then vitamin K should be added. The progress of liver disease is monitored with liver ultrasound every 2 years and where there is evidence of progressive liver disease, the child should be referred to a specialist liver unit, with facilities for liver transplantation.

CF-related diabetes

Failure of the exocrine pancreas is an early feature of CF; however, this may progress to destruction of the endocrine cells. CF-related diabetes is a distinct condition with features of both type 1 and type 2 diabetes. The presentation can be insidious with poor weight gain, and a high index of suspicion is necessary. In the teenage years all children should have an annual oral glucose tolerance test, with additional continuous blood glucose monitoring if the results are equivocal. Children with CF have a high calorie requirement and careful nutritional management is essential to achieve good diabetes control without compromising growth.

CF-related arthritis

CF arthritis can be oligoarticular or a polyarthritis and is frequently flitting in nature. The most important differential diagnosis is hypertrophic pulmonary osteoarthropathy (commonly associated with severe lung disease and finger clubbing) which is characterised radiologically by periosteal reaction. Treatment of lung disease may lead to an improvement in joint symptoms.

Fertility

Infertility in men with CF is almost universal due to congenital bilateral absence of vas deferens. Historically women with CF have found it difficult to conceive but due to improvements in care, many women with CF now have children.

Annual assessment

In a lifelong condition, it is important to review progress each year, to look for complications which may not be evident clinically and to plan care for the year ahead. This annual assessment is a recognised standard of care for all children with CF in the UK and will include:

- review of progress and medications
- full blood count and clotting
- biochemistry for liver and renal function
- vitamin levels
- aspergillus serology
- sputum (induced if necessary) for nontuberculous mycobacteria and other pathogens
- chest radiograph

Other investigations are undertaken when clinically indicated and include:

- oral glucose tolerance test (at secondary school age)
- chest CT scan (where there is concern about progressive bronchiectasis)
- liver ultrasound (if abnormal liver function or to monitor the progress of established liver disease).

Transition to adult care

There are just over 10,000 people in the UK who have CF and over 60% are adults. It is common for young people to experience a decline in their clinical condition during adolescence and so it is critical that the CF team supports the young person, helps them take an increasing amount of responsibility for their treatment and facilitates a smooth transition to adult care. A common approach is for the young person to attend a series of joint adult and paediatric clinics where steadily more of the consultation is with the young person rather than their parents.

CFTR modulator drugs

New drugs have recently become available which treat the underlying defect of CF—the abnormal CFTR protein—although eligibility for treatment depends of the genotype of the individual. These drugs improve spirometry, reduce the number of pulmonary exacerbations and improve nutrition.

Sleep-disordered breathing

Effective sleep is important for optimal neurodevelopment. Sleep may be interrupted by medical conditions, interventions, the environment, or behaviour of the child and those around them. When the child is older, insufficient or inefficient sleep leads to daytime sleepiness with corresponding effects in learning, memory, behaviour and school performance.

Sleep poses particular challenges to the vulnerable child who may present to a wide range of healthcare professionals in primary, secondary and tertiary care.

An understanding of the possible causes for sleep behaviour and disorder (Table 17.7) comes from the clinical history and a careful examination. It is important to clarify the sequence of events before bedtime, those around waking in the night, the appearances and actions of the child when asleep and the reactions when awoken in the morning. Relevant events through the day, particularly sleepiness, will be important.

Table 17.7 Conditions that may result in sleep disordered breathing

Airway and breathing sleep-related disorders	
obstructive sleep apnoea and hypoventilation	
high-risk children	
	Down syndrome
	neuromuscular disease
	craniofacial syndromes
	mucopolysaccharidoses
	achondroplasia
	Prader Willi syndrome
congenital central hypoventilation syndrome	
Nonrespiratory sleep disorders/disorders with daytime sleepiness	
insufficient night sleep	
narcolepsy	
idiopathic CNS hypersomnia	
chronic fatigue syndrome	
delayed sleep phase syndrome	
restless leg syndrome	
non-REM arousal disorders	sleep terror, sleep walking, confusional arousals
sleep–related movement disorders	
REM parasomnias	nightmares, REM movement disorders

Identification of some conditions may be achieved through the measurement of oxygen saturations and blood pressure, calculation of BMI and pharyngeal, tonsillar, neurological and respiratory examinations (Table 17.8; Figure 17.6).

The management of sleep-disordered breathing is directed by the underlying cause. Those patients with an atopic cause for their interrupted sleep may benefit from a medical intervention (antihistamines, nasal steroid, montelukast) whilst those with enlarged adenoids and tonsils may need surgical resection. A small number of patients may require noninvasive ventilation but the majority will be managed with a conservative approach with ongoing monitoring.

Table 17.8 Investigations used for sleep disorders

	Investigation	Information provided
Level 1	oximetry	oxygen saturation and heart rate. Provides ODI reading
Level 2	oxycapnography	oxygen saturation, heart rate, transcutaneous carbon dioxide
Level 3	cardiorespiratory polygraphy (Figure 17.6)	oxygen saturation, ECG, respiratory effort, oronasal flow sensor (occasionally video and carbon dioxide measurements)
Level 4	polysomnography	oxygen saturation, ECG, respiratory effort, oronasal flow sensor (occasionally video and carbon dioxide measurements), encephalography (so that the sleep state may be identified and staged). Provides AHI reading but is labour intensive and expensive
ODI	oxygen desaturation index	number of 4% dips from the baseline per hour and is a proxy for AHI
AHI	apnoea-hypopnoea index	number of episodes of apnoea or hypopnoea per hour

Life-threatening events and sudden infant death

Acute life-threatening events in infancy and sudden infant death are presented together even though they are quite distinct entities. The carer of the child, however, will be concerned that the first may lead to the second and this needs to be acknowledged.

Acute life-threatening event (ALTE)

This is a description of an event that occurs in the first year of life and usually consists of colour change, choking, gagging, apnoea and changes in muscle tone. Such events are most common in the first 3 months of life and the causes include gastro-oesophageal reflux, seizures, respiratory infection, cardiovascular, metabolic and endocrine causes and even physical abuse. The cause cannot be identified in up to 50% of ALTEs.

For children who appear well after the acute event, the term 'brief, resolved, unexplained event' (BRUE) is used. This is defined as a resolved event occurring in an infant that consists of a sudden, brief episode of cyanosis or pallor, absent or irregular breathing, marked change in tone and an altered level of responsiveness. A BRUE is a diagnosis of exclusion.

The appropriate management of the child after a BRUE depends on the outcome of the risk assessment (Table 17.9). A 'high risk' assessment requires investigation and appropriate management whilst a 'low risk' assessment should prompt education and CPR training for the family and might include a period of observation with pulse oximetry and ECG. Further investigation should not be necessary.

Sudden infant death in infancy (SUDI)

The term relates to any death of a child younger than 1 year of age and is applied once all investigations and a post-mortem are unable to find a cause of death. SIDS is more common in babies born prematurely and low-weight infants

SIDS has become increasingly rare since epidemiological studies identified a link to the sleep environment, with the messages of this disseminated through a successful information campaign. The key features of this health promotion message include

- the "Back to Sleep" campaign—placing babies on their back to sleep
- share a room with baby for the first 6 months

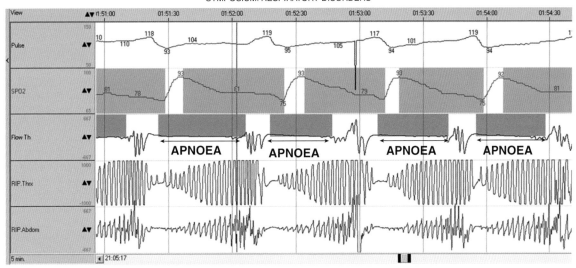

Fig. 17.6 Cardiorespiratory polygraphy in a 10-year-old boy with obstructive sleep apnoea. (Image used with permission from Sleep-disordered breathing in children. Urquhart D et al. Paediatrics and Child Health. 2017.)

Table 17.9 Risk assessment of a BRUE which confers a higher or lower risk of adverse outcomes	
High risk	**Low risk**
younger than 2 months age	older than 60 days
prematurity (< 32 weeks)	gestational age ≥32 weeks and postconceptional age ≥45 weeks
more than one event	
event duration longer than 1 minute	first BRUE and not occurring in clusters
cardiopulmonary resuscitation given and assessed as required by professionals	duration of event <1 minute
	no CPR required by trained medical provider
does not meet all 'low risk' criteria	no concerning historical features
	no concerning physical examination findings

- no exposure to nicotine and cigarette smoke during pregnancy and beyond
- not sharing a sofa or armchair with baby while sleeping
- never co-sleep with the baby if either parent is tired or has consumed alcohol or drugs

Long-term ventilation

Healthy breathing depends upon
- central control (brain and chemoreceptors)
- patent airway (nasopharynx, trachea, bronchi)
- adequate gas exchange (lung parenchyma)
- adequate movement of air (respiratory muscles)

Long-term ventilation (LTV) may be required if any of the above are chronically impaired (Table 17.10). The requirement for such support is often a natural extension from the treatment of sleep-disordered breathing or accompanying prolonged intensive care.

For many children, in particular those with cerebral palsy, impairments of effective breathing are often at multiple levels. In addition to impairments of breathing, many children who require LTV also have a constellation of medical problems and treatment of one may exacerbate other problems and often results in polypharmacy. The LTV multidisciplinary team will include a wide range of health care professionals.

Breathing support is often commenced acutely in a neonatal or paediatric critical care environment but then, at a later date, it becomes clear that LTV will be required. In some circumstances careful consideration is required regarding whether transition to LTV is in the child's best interest. For other children, particularly those with neuromuscular problems, LTV may be planned from the clinic. It is particularly important to consider, and counsel children and their families, whether LTV is 'a bridge' to other treatments such as surgery with the eventual outcome being a good recovery or whether it is 'a destination' and LTV will be required lifelong and occasionally as part of palliative care.

Long-term ventilation consists of a ventilator, humidifier (optional), oxygen (optional), tubing and an interface.

Table 17.10 **Conditions that may indicate a requirement for LTV include:**	
Source of abnormal respiratory control	
impaired central control	brainstem tumour
	central congenital hypoventilation syndrome
	Arnold Chiari malformations
	Prader-Willi syndrome
airway interference	Pierre Robin sequence
	tracheobronchomalacia
	cleft palate
lung parenchymal pathology	cystic fibrosis
	bronchopulmonary dysplasia,
	pulmonary hypoplasia.
neuromuscular disorders	spinal muscular atrophy
	Duchenne muscular dystrophy
	congenital muscular dystrophies
	skeletal dysplasias

Interfaces are the method by which the child is connected to the ventilation circuit and may be invasive (tracheostomy) or noninvasive (face masks, nasal pillows/prongs, oral straw etc.).

The level of long-term ventilation depends upon how critical breathing support is for the well-being of the child and includes:

- Level 1: High—the child is able to breathe unaided during the day but needs to use a ventilator for support; it can be discontinued for up to 24 hours without clinical harm.
- Level 2: Severe—the child requires ventilation at night and would survive accidental disconnection but would be unwell and may require hospital support.
- Level 3: Priority—those with no respiratory drive, are dependent on ventilation at all times and disconnection would be fatal.

Discharge home with support requires a stable airway, a stable oxygen requirement, ventilatory equipment that can be operated by the family or carer at home and nutritional intake adequate to maintain expected growth and development. The opportunities for weaning from support or the need for escalation may then be considered.

Surgical respiratory conditions

Eventration of diaphragm

The condition may be congenital where parts of the diaphragm are replaced by fibroelastic tissue and fail to contribute to the muscular tone or it may be acquired secondary to phrenic nerve injury. As a result, the diaphragm is easily displaced superiorly and the child presents with respiratory symptoms. The chest radiograph shows an elevated (eventrated) hemidiaphragm on a PA film and ultrasound may confirm poor movement of sections of the diaphragm.

Treatment and management

Some children may have minimal symptoms and do not need any intervention whilst others with respiratory symptoms are best managed with a surgical plication of the eventration.

Congenital pulmonary airway malformation (CPAM)

There are three recognised groups of malformations that belong to this clinical description:

- congenital lobar emphysema (Figure 17.17)—hyperinflation of one or more of the pulmonary lobes
- congenital cystic adenomatoid malformations (CCAM) (Figure 17.18)—hamartomas with cystic and solid elements.
- pulmonary sequestrations—mass of lung tissue which lacks normal connections with airways

CCAMs are often detected on an antenatal scan and may be associated with hydrops fetalis. All of the above abnormalities may cause respiratory distress in neonates and infants and large lesions may produce a mediastinal shift. CCAM and sequestrations also being associated with recurrent infection.

Investigations

Chest radiographs show:

- congenital lobar emphysema—hyperinflation of one or more of the pulmonary lobes
- congenital cystic adenomatoid malformations—multicystic, air-filled lesion

Treatment and management

CCAMs diagnosed antenatally are closely monitored as many will resolve or be asymptomatic at birth. If hydrops develops during the pregnancy, thoracoamniotic shunting is indicated and, if respiratory distress occurs, surgical

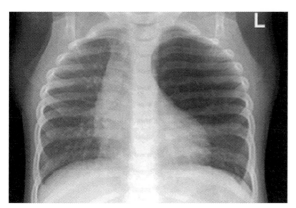

Fig. 17.7 Chest radiograph in newborn child showing congenital lobar emphysema affecting the left upper lobe (commonest lobe to be affected) with mediastinal shift to right.

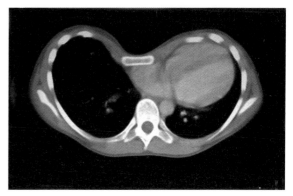

Fig. 17.9 CT chest of 15-year-old boy with marked pectus excavatum. Heart and mediastinum displaced to the left. No clinical compromise in normal activities.

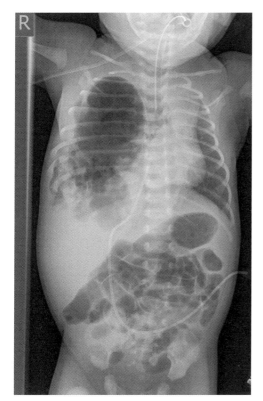

Fig. 17.8 Chest radiograph showing congenital cystic adenomatoid malformations of right lung. Note thin walled cystic areas and some solid elements.

excision is undertaken following delivery. The management of asymptomatic lesions is controversial with some centres recommending excision and others a watch and wait approach. Pulmonary sequestrations and congenital lobar emphysema may be managed conservatively if asymptomatic and resection only performed if complications occur.

Chest wall deformities

These are two major chest wall deformities—pectus excavatum, characterised by sternal depression, and pectus carinatum by sternal protrusion that usually develop in childhood and can progress during adolescence. Both pectus excavatum and pectus carinatum may be associated with Marfan syndrome. Pectus excavatum can displace mediastinal structures and lead to an asymptomatic reduction in pulmonary function whilst pectus carinatum is primarily a cosmetic problem (Figure 17.19).

Treatment and management

Physiotherapy is not beneficial, but in females the deformity may become less apparent with breast development. Pectus excavatum can be surgically corrected by the insertion of a substernal bar or open surgery. Pectus carinatum can be addressed using compression devices which flatten the chest over time, although it is important to introduce this before any pubertal growth spurt occurs when the chest wall tissues are pliant.

Surgical emphysema

Surgical emphysema describes the presence of subcutaneous air present in subcutaneous tissue usually of the chest wall, mediastinum and neck, and palpation of the chest wall reveals obvious crepitations. Causes include postthoracic surgery, severe coughing in asthma, ventilated patients on high pressure settings and penetrating trauma. A chest radiograph will usually reveal the extent of the displaced air (Figure 17.10).

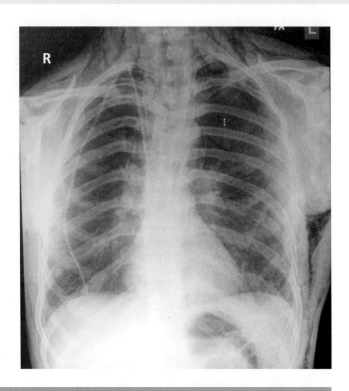

Fig. 17.10 Surgical emphysema. Note the presence of air in the mediastinum, subcutaneous areas round neck and left axilla following left-sided thoracotomy.

IMPORTANT CLINICAL POINTS

Wheezing disorders

- biphasic wheeze or localised wheeze suggests a fixed area of narrowing
- levels of severity of an acute asthma attack need to be formally assessed and recorded
- No single test is diagnostic of asthma
- spirometry shows FEV1, FEV1/FVC ratio and the FEF 25–75 are all reduced
- stepwise management of asthma is required approach

Lower respiratory tract infections

- understanding of radiological changes is important
- bacterial and viral causes cannot be distinguished clinically or radiologically
- commonest bacterial cause in children is *Streptococcus pneumoniae*
- UK immunisation programme includes 13 valent pneumococcal conjugate vaccine
- Recognition of appearances of the chest radiograph changes important

Cystic fibrosis

- part of newborn screening programme which identifies about 82% of those affected

- can present immediately after birth with 'meconium ileus' that requires urgent radiological reduction by contrast enema or surgery
- sweat test with a sweat chloride of greater than 59 mmol/l confirms the diagnosis
- presence of two gene mutations known to cause CF would support the diagnosis
- children with CF characteristically have different organisms isolated from their respiratory tract as they grow older
- the average annual decline in FEV_1 should be less than 2%
- a 10% drop in FEV_1 is in keeping with a pulmonary exacerbation

Sudden infant death

- acute life-threatening event (ALTE) is an event that occurs in a child in the first year of life
- the cause cannot be identified in up to 50% of ALTEs
- risk assessment of a BRUE can confer a higher or lower risk of adverse outcomes

Surgical respiratory conditions

- CCAM are hamartomas with cystic and solid elements
- congenital lobar emphysema results in lobar hyperinflation without solid elements

Further Reading

Asthma: diagnosis, monitoring and chronic asthma management. NICE guideline [NG80]. Published November 2017. Updated March 2021. https://www.nice.org.uk/guidance/ng80

British Guideline on the Management of Asthma BTS/SIGN. Published 2016. https://www.brit-thoracic.org.uk/quality-improvement/guidelines/asthma/

Global Initiative for Asthma Management and Prevention (GINA) Guidelines. Published April 2021. https://ginasthma.org/wp-content/uploads/2020/04/Main-pocket-guide_2020_04_03-final-wms.pdf

Cystic fibrosis: diagnosis and management. NICE [NG78]. Published 2017. http://nice.org.uk/guidance/ng78

Sudden unexpected death in infancy and childhood. RCPCH & RCPath. Published 2016. https://www.rcpath.org/uploads/assets/874ae50e-c754-4933-995a804e0ef728a4/Sudden-unexpected-death-in-infancy-and-childhood-2e.pdf

Urquhart D, Hill EA, Morley A. Sleep-disordered breathing in children. Paediatrics and Child Health. 2017;27:7;328.

Chapter | 18 |

Hearing and ENT

Tawakir Kamani, Roshan Adappa

After reading this chapter you should be able to assess, diagnose and manage
- hearing impairment
- conditions affecting the ears, nose and throat including epistaxis

Hearing Impairment

Paediatric hearing impairment impacts negatively on the speech, language, social, emotional and educational development of a child and should be considered as a cause in any child with speech, learning or behavioural difficulties. Prevention, timely diagnosis and early intervention of hearing loss can prevent further disability in development of linguistic, academic and social skills.

PRACTICE POINT—description of hearing impairment (dBHL)

- mild 26 to 40
- moderate 41 to 70
- severe 71 to 90
- profound more than 90
  dBHL—decibel hearing loss

Hearing Testing

A number of hearing assessments are available for children and the choice of these are dictated by the developmental age of the child.

PRACTICE POINT—hearing assessment by age

- newborn hearing screening
  - automated otoacoustic emission (aAOE)
  - automated auditory brainstem response (aABR)
- 6–18 months
  - visual reinforcement audiometry (VRA)
- 2–5 years old
  - play audiometry
- 5 years–adults
  - pure tone audiometry (PTA)

Newborn Hearing Screening Tests

Newborn hearing screening is a universal programme that aims to identify permanent moderate, severe and profound deafness and hearing impairment in newborn babies. The test can be done on babies up to the age of 3 months.

Early detection and early intervention of hearing problems will lessen the impact of deafness on the child, the child's family and society. All well babies undergo an automated otoacoustic emission test (aOAE). If this is not "passed" after two attempts, then the baby has an automated auditory brainstem response test (aABR). Babies in the neonatal intensive care or at high risk and have both an aOAE and an aABR test.

Acoustic emissions are sounds that are produced by the outer hair cells of the inner ear in response to a noise stimulus and can be measured by placing a small probe in the ear canal. Since the sounds are only produced by normal outer hair cells, their detection correlates highly with normal hearing. The vast majority of hearing impairment is due to damage of these cells and the test therefore provides a sensitive and accurate means of screening for cochlear hearing impairment.

Auditory brainstem response is an electrophysiological response that measures the function of the auditory pathway from the external ear to the brainstem when sounds are presented to the ear. It can determine hearing thresholds allowing targeted treatment depending on the severity of the hearing thresholds.

Visual Reinforcement Audiometry

The test provides a "visual reward" when a child responds correctly by turning their head to sound played from headphones or field speakers on either side of the child and hearing thresholds are determined at different frequencies and amplitudes.

Play Audiometry

This test requires the child to respond to a sound by performing a simple task such as putting a ball in a bucket. This is repeated across different frequencies and at different volumes to determine the hearing thresholds.

Pure Tone Audiometry

The child usually wears headphones and is asked to respond when they hear the sound by pressing a button. The volume and frequency of the sound is adjusted to determine the hearing thresholds.

Tympanometry

The test assesses the status of the middle ear by measuring mobility of the eardrum. It is not a hearing test but an assessment of the compliance of the eardrum.

Types of Hearing Loss

The aetiology of paediatric hearing loss can be classified as congenital or acquired. Congenital hearing loss is present at birth and is due to genetic, prenatal or perinatal factors.

The type of hearing loss depends on where in the auditory pathway the impairment occurs. There are three basic types of hearing loss (Figure 18.1).

Conductive Impairment

Conductive hearing loss occurs when there is impairment of the sound transmission through either the **outer or middle ear** or both. Formal testing demonstrates that the bone conduction thresholds are better than air conduction thresholds. Conductive hearing loss produces losses of up to 50–60 dBHL.

The causes include:
- ear canal obstruction—atresia, wax, foreign body
- perforation of tympanic membrane
- otitis media with effusion
- Down syndrome
- cranio-facial anomalies—Pierre Robin syndrome, cleft palate

Sensorineural Impairment (SNHL)

Sensorineural hearing loss is due to impairment within the **inner ear** or sensory organ (cochlea and associated structures) or the vestibulocochlear nerve (cranial nerve VIII). Formal testing demonstrates that both bone conduction and air conduction thresholds are poor. It can be more severe than conductive impairment and can also be progressive.

The causes include:
- congenital SNHL
  - genetic—syndromic or nonsyndromic
  - infection—congenital infections
  - prematurity
  - hypoxic ischaemic encephalopathy
- acquired SNHL
  - ototoxic drugs—aminoglycosides, furosemide
  - meningoencephalitis
  - head injury
  - neurodegenerative disorders
  - hyperbilirubinemia

The hearing loss in sensorineural impairment is usually profound and usually greater than 90 dBHL. The children need prompt referral to ENT services for a more detailed assessment and consideration of the need for a hearing device. Aminoglycosides classically induce a high-tone hearing loss with a 'ski slope' appearance on the audiogram.

Mixed impairment

Mixed hearing loss occurs when a conductive loss is superimposed on a sensorineural loss. Hearing assessment shows air conduction thresholds to be poorer than bone conduction thresholds, but when the conductive element resolves, the air conduction thresholds revert to bone conduction levels.

Treatment and management

The underlying cause for the loss of hearing will guide the management plan. Most children with conductive loss should be referred to ENT services where they will be managed conservatively or with hearing aids. Full resolution of the problem is likely although some may need surgery. It is important that parents understand the potential effect of the hearing loss on the child's ability to communicate and so accept the importance of wearing hearing aids.

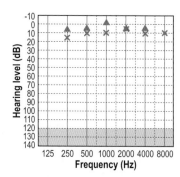

×   Air conduction to left ear

▲   Bone conduction (not masked)

Conductive hearing loss

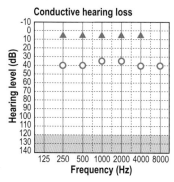

Conductive hearing loss is present if bone conduction thresholds are normal but air conduction thresholds are raised

Bilateral sensorineural hearing loss

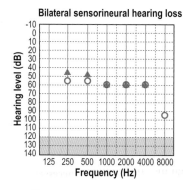

Sensorineural hearing loss exists when the bone conduction and air conduction thresholds are raised

Mixed hearing loss in the right ear

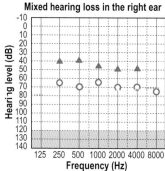

Mixed hearing loss occurs when there is conductive overlay (an additional air-borne gap) on top of an existing sensorineural hearing loss

Fig. 18.1 Pure tone audiograms of normal, conductive, sensorineural and mixed loss.

Any child with identified SNHL should be referred promptly to an ENT service to assess for hearing restoration or rehabilitation. Congenital SNHL needs investigations aimed at identifying the aetiology.

Any child diagnosed with a streptococcal meningitis should have an urgent referral to ENT services as this infection leads to time-critical ossification of the cochlea and any delay will reduce the benefit of cochlear implantation.

Involvement of the multidisciplinary team for children with hearing difficulties will utilise the different skills of the audiologist, parent, ENT specialist and speech and language therapist with later involvement of the teacher once options for preschool and schooling are discussed.

Conditions Affecting Ears, Nose or Throat

Otitis Media

Otitis Media with Effusion

This diagnosis describes an accumulation of fluid behind an intact tympanic membrane in the absence of symptoms and signs of an acute infection. Commonly referred to as 'glue ear', it is the most common cause of hearing difficulties in childhood and is more common between the ages of 2–7 years. On examination, the eardrum looks dull with loss of its light reflex and a fluid level or bubbles may be observed.

Treatment and management

Intervention in a child with **otitis media and an effusion** is indicated if there is hearing loss of 25–30 dBHL in the better hearing ear on two occasions, 3 months apart. Most problems resolve over this time although they do require follow up to ensure the hearing returns to normal. If there is no improvement in the hearing then hearing aids or the insertion of grommets will be considered and, in some, adenoidectomy may be of benefit.

Acute Otitis Media

Acute otitis media (OM) is a common infection in childhood and presents with ear pain, fever and irritability but in younger children the infection may lead to pulling of the ear or banging of the head. Purulent otorrhoea may occur following perforation and otoscopy may be difficult if the external canal is full of pus. The diagnosis is made by direct observation when a red bulging tympanic membrane is seen along with loss of normal light reflex and an effusion behind the membrane.

Bacteria cause the majority of infections in acute OM and the common organisms are:
- Streptococcus pneumoniae
- Haemophilus influenzae
- Moraxella catarrhalis
- Group A streptococcus
- Staphylococcus aureus

Viruses causing acute otitis media are RSV and rhinovirus and therefore symptoms may be seasonal.

Treatment and management

Pain relief with regular paracetamol and ibuprofen is important. Antibiotic management remains controversial as spontaneous recovery occurs in 80% of children and they do not alter outcomes with regards to risk of complication (perforation or mastoiditis). Amoxicillin may be considered in those under 1 year if the child has a high temperature or fails to improve in 2–3 days. Antihistaminic and decongestants are not effective. Risk of serious complications such as mastoiditis and meningitis are recognised but rare consequences for acute OM.

Epistaxis

Epistaxis is common in children and usually the result of local trauma. Little's area describes a venous plexus on the nasal septum and is the most common origin of the bleed. If there are recurrent nose bleeds with bruising or family history of bleeding disorders, then alternative diagnoses should be considered and would include:
- coagulation disorders
- leukaemia
- foreign body
- hypertension

Pressure on the nose below the nasal bone will usually stop the bleeding, but if this fails and the bleeding is profuse then nasal packing or cauterisation may be necessary.

Tonsillar Hypertrophy

This is a common finding in children and usually causes minimal problems. Tonsillar tissue increases in size during the first 6–7 years of life before gradually involuting and, by late teenage years, is usually vestigial. If, however, they undergo massive and sustained enlargement, they may lead to clinical problems such as sleep apnoea.

Children with significant tonsillar hypertrophy will usually present with noisy breathing at night with loud snoring that, on occasions, can be heard in other parts of the house. The child may have observed apnoeic episodes that lead to disturbed and interrupted sleep and consequent daytime tiredness. This, in turn, may lead to a deterioration in behaviour and educational attainment. With more extreme and delayed presentation, the child may have developed chronic hyperoxia, pulmonary hypertension and right ventricular hypertrophy. Further details on investigation and management of sleep disorder breathing can be found in Chapter 17 Respiratory.

Pharyngotonsillitis

Pharyngotonsillitis is usually caused by a viral or bacterial infection and therefore peaks in winter months. The most common viral organisms responsible are rhinovirus, adenovirus, influenza, parainfluenza and Epstein-Barr and the most common bacterial agents are streptococcus group A and C. Viral infections usually last 3–5 days with gradual improvement. However, if the symptoms do not improve after 2–3 days, review is needed, and consideration should be given for a bacterial aetiology.

Clinical presentation

Children often present with fever, sore throat, cough and painful swallowing. Examination shows hyperaemic or inflammation in the posterior pharyngeal wall, uvula and tonsils and the latter may have white exudates covering them. It is not possible to distinguish bacterial from viral infection on clinical examination alone.

Investigations

Throat swabs cannot distinguish current streptococcal disease from carriage and are not routinely undertaken in children with tonsillitis. When a child has obvious high fever and exudative tonsils lasting more than 48 hours then a throat swab may help future management.

Treatment and management

The usual practice would be for symptomatic support with antipyretic medication only. Antibiotics are rarely needed and confer minimal advantage in settings with a low incidence of recognised complications. A 10-day course of penicillin would be advisable if symptoms worsen or the child has a past history of rheumatic fever or a chronic illness that impacts on immune function. Recurrent episodes of tonsillitis which impact on school attendance and learning may need an ENT opinion regarding the need for tonsillectomy.

A peritonsillar abscess is an uncommon complication of pharyngotonsillitis where pus collects in between the tonsil and pharyngeal wall muscles. The child will present with increased pharyngeal pain, local swelling, 'hot-potato' voice, odynophagia, otalgia and trismus. The condition can rapidly progress to airway obstruction and requires treatment with surgical drainage and antibiotics.

> **PRACTICE POINT—indications for ENT opinion regarding adenoidectomy**
>
> - obstructive sleep apnoea
> - recurrent otitis media
> - otitis media with effusions and hearing loss

Sinusitis

The maxillary and ethmoid sinuses are present at birth whilst the frontal sinuses do not develop until the end of the first decade of life and therefore can only cause symptoms from that time. The child may develop a purulent nasal discharge, cough, halitosis and facial pain. The causes would include recurrent viral respiratory infections, allergic rhinitis, foreign body or trauma. Important underlying conditions that require consideration are ciliary dyskinesia and cystic fibrosis.

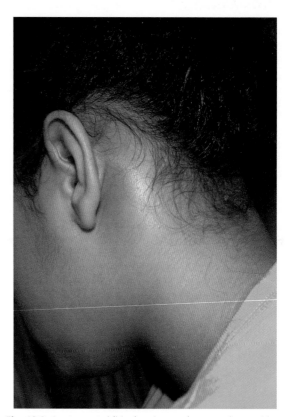

Fig. 18.2 Acute mastoiditis showing erythema and mastoid swelling (Image use with permission from Head, Neck and Orofacial Infections. Ed. Ferneini E and Hupp J. Chapter 19. Eisen MD, Naples. Elsevier Inc.)

Any acute episodes are treated with antibiotics and topical paediatric ephedrine. Acute sinusitis in the young child may cause periorbital cellulitis and this can progress, if untreated, to cavernous sinus thrombosis. The child presents with history of a cold and snotty nose with new onset hyperaemic swelling of the eyelids. It is important that ENT and ophthalmology input is sought urgently and patient commenced on aggressive treatment that includes IV antibiotics, nasal decongestant and intranasal steroid spray. In the event that this does not improve with treatment or progresses, imaging and surgical intervention may be required to drain a periorbital abscess.

Mastoiditis

Acute mastoiditis is rare and is usually caused by infection spreading from the middle ear. Consequently, the responsible organisms are commonly those causing an acute OM. Young children can present with fever, pain in or behind the ear and localised swelling and tenderness over the mastoid bone (Figure 18.2), which displaces the pinna forward and inferiorly. The swelling is tender and may be fluctuant.

Cranial imaging with contrast CT should be considered in the presence of focal neurological signs, reduction in conscious level or prior to a general anaesthetic to drain the mastoid abscess. Treatment requires intravenous antibiotics and an early ENT review to clarify whether mastoidectomy would be indicated.

IMPORTANT CLINICAL POINTS

Hearing impairment

- newborn hearing screening initially uses automated otoacoustic emission test
- conductive impairment due to outer or middle ear problems; gives 50–60 dBHL
- sensorineural impairment due to inner ear problems; gives greater than 90 dBHL

Otitis media with effusion

- glue ear—gives 25–30 dBHL

Acute otitis media

- bacteria cause the majority of infections
- antibiotic management controversial
- spontaneous recovery occurs in 80% of children

Mastoiditis

- CT considered if focal neurological signs or reduction in conscious level

---

Further reading

Sore throat (acute): antimicrobial prescribing. NICE guideline [NG84]. Published January 2018. https://www.nice.org.uk/guidance/ng84

Otitis media (acute): antimicrobial prescribing. NICE guideline [NG91]. Published March 2018. https://www.nice.org.uk/guidance/ng91

Chapter | 19 |

Gastroenterology and hepatology

Lisa Whyte, Rulla al-Araji, David Devadason, Richard Stewart

After reading this chapter you should be able to assess, diagnose and manage:
- conditions presenting with the common symptoms of abdominal disease
- conditions resulting in malabsorption
- diseases and disorders of the pancreas
- diseases and disorders of the liver
- congenital malformations and surgical disorders of the gastrointestinal tract and liver

Gastrointestinal conditions commonly present with the following symptoms:
- abdominal pain
- changes in stool consistency and frequency
- vomiting
- faltering growth
- GI bleeding

Abdominal Pain

Abdominal pain is a common problem in childhood, and a full history and examination is important. Taking a history can be a challenge in younger children as their parents and carers can often interpret vague symptoms such as crying to be caused by abdominal discomfort, when there is little evidence to this as a cause.

Acute abdominal pain

Acute abdominal pain is usually sharp and colicky in nature, and localisation within the abdomen will often suggest the underlying cause (Figure 19.1).

Chronic abdominal pain

Chronic abdominal pain is usually diffuse and dull in nature although some conditions may have acute episodes. The

recognised causes can be divided into organic and nonorganic conditions, and the challenge of identifying the specific diagnosis in children and young people can be difficult.

A diagnosis of functional GI disorders should only be made after organic diseases have been excluded and repeated tests are known to be inappropriate. It can be helpful to raise the idea of a functional disorder at an early stage in the assessments so that patients and carers recognise this as a potential explanation.

Organic causes of chronic abdominal pain

Gastric acid–related conditions

The pain in these related conditions is the result of mucosal erosion although the formation of ulcers is uncommon in children. The children and young people usually present with:
- abdominal pain
- water brash and acid taste in mouth
- vomiting
- epigastric pain that is worse on eating
- melaena stool
- haematemesis
- unexplained anaemia

Treatment and management

The history is often sufficiently clear to warrant a short course of a proton pump inhibitor (PPI) or alginates without the need for more detailed investigations. A follow-up review is advised and, if symptoms do not improve with PPI or if there is evidence of upper GI bleed, then upper GI endoscopy should be considered.

Helicobacter gastritis

Children and young people with a Helicobacter gastritis may develop chronic epigastric pain although many are

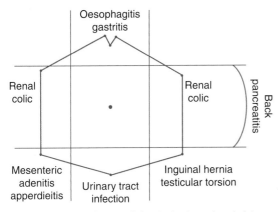

Fig. 19.1 Location of acute abdominal pain and underlying pathology

Table 19.1 **Abdominal pain and associated systemic symptoms**	
Symptom	**Differential diagnosis**
fever, nausea, vomiting, anorexia, diarrhoea	gastroenteritis
tiredness, jaundice	viral hepatitis
cough, shortness of breath	pneumonia or empyema
blood in stool	infection
	necrotising enterocolitis
	inflammatory bowel disease
	intussusception
bilious vomits	small bowel obstruction
urinary frequency, dysuria	urinary tract infection
vaginal discharge	pelvic inflammatory disease

asymptomatic. Some may be identified as part of investigations for iron deficiency anaemia whilst others are identified after adult members of the household are diagnosed with the condition.

Investigations

The older child will be able to perform a urea breath test where radiolabelled carbon in urea is given by mouth. This is then converted to CO_2 and breath analysis will identify the rise in labelled CO_2 after about 20 minutes. The test has a high sensitivity and specificity for Helicobacter. Serology assessing IgG antibodies is less accurate and does not confirm current infection.

Treatment and management

NICE recommend an initial treatment of 1 week with:
- oral omeprazole
- oral amoxicillin
- oral clarithromycin or oral metronidazole

Potential complications

Chronic carriage is possible and transmission and reinfection with 'kissing contacts' and household members is recognised.

CLINICAL SCENARIO

A 14-year-old girl was referred because of shortness of breath on exercise over the preceding 3 years. More direct questioning revealed that she developed a dull central chest pain without radiation and that this was also a significant symptom. There was no associated cough or attendant wheeze. The chest pain also occurred if she undertook heavy lifting. The pain never woke her during the night. Her symptoms did not stop her attending school but she had decided to miss games lesson. Her mother had a specialist referral impending to be assessed for a 'gastric ulcer'.

On examination the patient looked well and her height and weight were both on the 75th centile. Examination showed no adverse findings.

Although the initial problem had been that of shortness of breath on exercise, other aspects of the history suggested she may have significant gastro-oesophageal reflux rather than a primary cardiac or respiratory abnormality.

A pH monitoring study was performed and identified multiple episodes of significant low pH in the oesophagus indicating gastro-oesophageal reflux. A urea breath test was positive.

It is likely that the significant gastro-oesophageal reflux led to chronic aspiration and the respiratory symptoms. The increase in abdominal pressure during exercise would have enhanced the reflux and thereby explain the exacerbation of symptoms on these occasions. The presence of *Helicobacter pylori* also illustrates that two different pathologies can present at the same time and, interestingly, subsequent investigations of the mother revealed she was Helicobacter positive.

Functional causes of chronic abdominal pain

This term describes pain related to the gastrointestinal tract that fits with accepted diagnostic criteria for a nonorganic cause. The common characteristics are:
- central or periumbilical pain
- intermittent pain
- pain worsens with stressors such as exams

Differential diagnosis	Investigation	Findings
pancreatitis	amylase and lipase	elevated
biliary colic	abdominal USS	gall stones
	LFTS	episodic elevation
	amylase and lipase	elevated if pancreatic inflammation
renal colic	abdominal USS	renal calculi
	urea electrolytes	abnormal if obstruction
intussusception	abdominal USS	'target sign' seen
inflammatory bowel disease	faecal calprotectin	elevated with inflammatory changes
	endoscopy—upper and lower	mucosal erythema, loss of vascular pattern, ulcers
	MRE (MR enterography) or ultrasound of small bowel	thickened bowel loops
oesophagitis gastritis peptic ulcer disease	FBC	anaemia
	urea breath test	positive
	stool *H. pylori* antigen	positive
	upper GI endoscopy	inflammatory changes, aphthous ulcers
coeliac disease	coeliac screen	elevated antibodies
	upper GI endoscopy	abnormal histology—flattened villi
constipation	thyroid function	excludes other causes
	coeliac screen	
small bowel obstruction	abdominal x-ray	dilated bowel loops
	contrast study with follow through	abnormal anatomy

Table 19.2 Investigations and findings in acute abdominal pain

- no radiation of pain
- no associated weight loss

Treatment and management

A full and honest explanation of the pathway to this diagnosis is important for the patient and carers. In some situations, the exclusion of serious organic pathology can be sufficient to resolve the current symptoms, but the involvement of colleagues in mental health may be helpful for other patients.

Irritable bowel syndrome (IBS)

The term describes chronic abdominal pain that is cramping in nature and which occurs at least 4 days per month. The pain is often related to defecation and associated with diarrhoea or constipation. Between these episodes, the patient is usually well with good weight gain. Clearly, it is important to exclude other possible causes of such symptoms.

Treatment and management

Treatment options include peppermint oil, probiotics or a FODMAP elimination diet where fermentable sugars are removed from the diet. Behavioural treatments may also be able to support the patient in coping with the problem and many will continue with the problem into adult life.

Abdominal migraine

Young people experience recurrent episodes of intense, incapacitating abdominal pain that lasts over an hour and is associated with nausea, headache and pallor. The episodes can be triggered by stress or fatigue and relieved by rest and sleep. Between episodes the patients are well and lead a full and active life.

Treatment and management

Avoidance of obvious triggers will usually have been tried, but if the episodes are frequent then prophylactic beta blockers may have a role.

Diarrhoea

Diarrhoeal illness is common in children and most episodes reflect a transient infective cause. It can, however, be the presenting problem for more significant conditions and lead to dehydration, electrolyte disturbance, malabsorption and subsequent faltering growth.

Acute diarrhoea

The diarrhoea can be episodic, profuse, explosive and may contain blood or identifiable food particles.

Investigations

The approach is twofold and requires an immediate assessment of potential dehydration and associated biochemical disturbances and a parallel series of investigations to determine the possible underlying cause of the diarrhoea. Investigations are not usually required for acute onset diarrhoea as it is often caused by an infective agent. Blood in the stool is a feature of certain organisms as detailed in Table 19.3.

Treatment and management

Children and young people presenting with acute diarrhoea need to be assessed promptly and an assessment of their cardiovascular stability made. Most young children are only mildly compromised and can be managed with oral rehydration fluids. Profuse, watery diarrhoea, however, can rapidly lead to significant dehydration and the patient may need parenteral fluids to correct any deficit. Details of the management of fluid and electrolyte problems are covered in Chapter 10 Fluids and electrolytes.

Chronic diarrhoea

The episodes of diarrhoea can produce significant amounts of stool which may contain blood or identifiable food particles. The stools may be foul-smelling, greasy and will float in the toilet if they have high fat content usually due to malabsorption.

Investigations

- full blood count and CRP
- electrolytes and urea
- coeliac disease screen
- stool culture (including *Clostridium difficile* and *Giardia lamblia*)

Subsequent blood tests would look for evidence of immunocompromise or autoimmunity.

Specific conditions causing chronic diarrhoea

Children and young people with systemic or local GI disease are likely to have problems with digestion of food and malabsorption of calories and necessary nutrients.

Coeliac disease

Coeliac disease is now recognised as a multiorgan condition with a strong genetic predisposition. Children and young people usually present with gastrointestinal symptoms as the main effect is an immune-mediated, gluten-induced enteropathy that affects small intestine. Gluten is found in wheat, barley and rye and once these are excluded from the diet, a complete recovery takes place.

The close linkage between coeliac disease and specific human leucocyte antigens (HLA-DQ2 and HLA-DQ8) is recognised and most children diagnosed with coeliac

Table 19.3 Common organisms causing acute onset diarrhoea		
Viruses	**Bacteria**	**Parasites**
Rotavirus	Campylobacter jejuni**	Cryptosporidium
Noroviruses	Salmonella**	Giardia lamblia
Adenoviruses	Escherichia coli**	Entamoeba histiolytica
Enteroviruses	Shigella**	
Cytomegalovirus	Yersinia entercolitica**	
Hepatitis A	Clostridium difficile**	
	Listeria monocytogenes	
**Organisms that produce bloody diarrhoea		

Table 19.4 Investigations of stool that will indicate aetiology

Test	Finding	Implications
alpha 1 antitrypsin level	raised	protein losing enteropathy
faecal reducing substances	present	carbohydrate malabsorption
faecal elastase	reduced	pancreatic dysfunction
chymotrypsin	reduced	pancreatic dysfunction
faecal calprotectin	raised	inflammation
fat globules	present	fat malabsorption

Table 19.5 Imaging and endoscopy investigations of stool that will indicate aetiology

Investigation	Information identified
plain abdominal x-ray	abnormalities in bowel gas pattern
abdominal ultrasound	bowel wall thickness and biliary tree structure
contrast study with follow through	congenital or acquired structural malformations
MRI small bowel	small bowel thickness
MRI imaging of the pelvis	perianal disease in IBD
upper GI endoscopy	appearance and biopsies of bowel to first part duodenum
lower GI endoscopy	appearance and biopsies colonic disorders

disease are positive for the two listed HLA types. Iron is absorbed through the ileal mucosa and consequently anaemia is a common finding.

The introduction of gluten into the diet at 6 to 12 months heralds the start of the GI pathological process and the infant develops chronic diarrhoea, abdominal distension, pain and growth retardation. In older children the symptoms may be more subtle but again poor growth along with problems of malabsorption such as diarrhoea, anaemia, vitamin D deficiency and persistent mouth ulcers may suggest the diagnosis. Dermatitis herpetiformis is associated with coeliac disease but is not common in children.

Associations

Coeliac disease has a genetic basis with an autoimmune mechanism of action and is therefore associated with other conditions with a similar underlying pathophysiology. Some units would advocate routine testing for individuals in these groups even if asymptomatic:

- first degree relatives of patients with coeliac disease
- type 1 diabetes
- autoimmune thyroiditis
- selective IgA deficiency
- juvenile idiopathic arthritis
- Down syndrome
- Turner syndrome

Investigations

Specific serological testing is required if coeliac disease is suspected. Prior to blood sampling it is necessary for the child to be exposed to gluten in their diet. This requirement is roughly one slice of bread per day for at least 6 weeks.

The initial coeliac screen includes:

- IgA level (those with IgA deficiency will have a negative IgA-TTG result)
- serum IgA-TTG (IgA antibodies against tissue transglutaminase—high sensitivity and specificity for coeliac disease
- anti-endomysial antibody (EMA—IgA antibodies against intestinal smooth muscle). The test is used to further investigate those patients with a weakly positive TTG-IgA

Previous practice used these blood tests as a screening tool and an elevated result indicated the need for a duodenal biopsy. Current practice, however, is that those with an IgA-TTG greater than 10x upper limit of normal and who are IgA-EMA positive can be recognised as having coeliac disease and a confirmatory biopsy is not necessary.

If these criteria are not met, however, or there is any diagnostic uncertainty, then duodenal biopsy is required. The presence of intraepithelial lymphocytosis and blunting of villi in the tissue sample will confirm the diagnosis.

The assessment of HLA status (DQ2 and DQ8) in the diagnosis can be helpful but should not be used in the initial diagnosis of coeliac disease in nonspecialist settings. The test result may be of value in children who are not having a biopsy, or in those who have limited their gluten ingestion and do not wish to have a gluten challenge.

Treatment and management

Once the diagnosis is established, the patient is advised to remove all gluten products from their diet. The support and advice from an experienced dietitian are important at this stage.

Monitoring of the response to the change in diet is necessary along with review of growth parameters. Children will need to take specific supplements such as calcium or vitamin D if their dietary intake is insufficient.

Once clinical improvement is established, then the patients will be offered annual review where height and weight are plotted, symptoms reviewed and need for bone density assessment considered. Normal growth and development, without GI symptoms, would be expected if gluten continues to be omitted from the diet, but support and reinforcement of gluten avoidance are important particularly through the teenage years.

Inflammatory bowel disease (IBD)

IBD is a chronic relapsing and remitting disease of the gut and includes ulcerative colitis (UC) and Crohn's disease. The diagnosis is made by the combination of clinical features and recognised findings on endoscopy and histology. Crohn's disease is characterised by focal, patchy, transmural and granulomatous inflammation affecting any part of the gastrointestinal tract from mouth to anus and can also have extraintestinal manifestations. Ulcerative colitis involves colonic mucosa and therefore extends from the rectum to the ilio-caecal junction.

The presentation of IBD can vary depending on the area of gut involved and the severity of the disease but typically presents in late childhood or adolescence. The most common symptoms are diarrhoea with or without blood along with episodic abdominal pain. Other presenting features include:
- faltering growth for either height or weight
- delayed puberty
- abdominal mass
- perianal fissures or skin tags
- fever
- lethargy

Some features are less commonly seen in IBD and include:
- erythema nodosum
- uveitis
- arthritis

Investigations

A range of basic investigations is undertaken if there is a suspicion of the diagnosis although normal results do not rule out the diagnosis. Further investigations will be needed to clarify the diagnosis.

- FBC—anaemia is common along with raised white cell and platelet count
- ESR and CRP are usually raised
- albumin levels are often low
- stool occult blood—usually present
- faecal calprotectin reflects disease activity in both UC and Crohn's disease
- small bowel imaging may include contrast studies, ultrasound of small bowel or MRE
- upper and lower GI endoscopy with biopsies define the nature of the condition

Treatment and management

Treatment of IBD based on the site, extent and severity of the disease and paediatric scoring systems have been developed to guide the treatment choices. The drugs used vary, depending on histological diagnosis, but the aim is to achieve steroid-free remission within one year of diagnosis. Patients with Crohn's disease at presentation or with an acute, severe flare will be started on exclusive enteral nutrition to replace all enteral food intake for 6–8 weeks to achieve clinical remission and improve nutrition.

Surgical review and intervention will be required if medical treatment fails to control the disease or if complications such as bleeding, obstruction, perforation or fistulae develop. For Crohn's disease, conservative surgery to relieve obstruction is recommended whilst for ulcerative colitis, a radical pan-proctocolectomy and ileal pouch is preferred. The gastroenterology MDT will always include a paediatric surgeon.

Relevant pharmacological agents used

Corticosteroids will be used in the treatment of an acute flare-up in both UC and Crohn's disease and IV or oral preparations are available. In an acute flare, steroids are usually given over an 8-week reducing course whilst the topical application of prednisolone (by enema or suppository) can be used for short periods (usually up to 2 weeks) for proctitis or left-sided disease.

Aminosalicylates (mesalazine or sulphasalazine) are used to reduce inflammatory pathways in UC, but not Crohn's disease, and work topically on the gut.

Thiopurines (azathioprine or 6-mercaptopurine) reduces the number of cytotoxic T cells and plasma cells and thereby inhibits lymphocyte activity.

Biological therapies act to reduce inflammation and are given parenterally or subcutaneously. Anti-TNF agents will supress inflammatory pathways and so used to achieve and maintain remission. Infliximab is a monoclonal antibody and is highly effective at achieving remission in both UC and Crohn's disease although efficacy can be lost due to antibody-mediated destruction of the drug.

Short bowel syndrome

Short bowel syndrome occurs when a section of small bowel is absent, usually secondary to surgical resection, which then leads to the child being unable to meet nutritional requirements without support. Common causes of short bowel syndrome include:
- necrotising enterocolitis
- malrotation with volvulus
- multiple intestinal atresias
- trauma
  Children have diarrhoea and malabsorption that leads to impaired absorption of calories and nutrients.

Treatment and management

This involves meeting calorific requirements and intensive intestinal rehabilitation with enteral or parenteral support. It is important in infancy as the small bowel, and in particular the terminal ileum, has the capacity for adaptation. Loperamide may help some patients by reducing diarrhoea.

Protein-losing enteropathy

This is a rare condition where children have significant protein loss into the gut. It can be associated with:
- inflammatory bowel disease
- coeliac disease
- giardia
- intestinal lymphangiectasia.
  The intestinal loss will include protein, immunoglobulins and lymphocytes.

  Patients will present with peripheral oedema or dyspnoea due to fluid retention and the diagnosis should be suspected in those with a low albumin without a recognised explanation. Some infants may have diarrhoea and weight loss.

Treatment and management

Assessment of dietary intake is important and introduction of a diet based on medium-chain triglycerides (MCT) which is low in fats and high in protein. MCT fats enter the portal system directly and avoid the gut lymphatic system. Any identified underlying causes will also need treating.

Lactose intolerance

Lactose intolerance may be due to a congenital absence of lactase in the villi of the small bowel or following an inflammatory insult to the same section of bowel.

Patients present with abdominal pain, bloating, flatulence and diarrhoea following the ingestion of milk or milk-containing products. The association between the two events may not be immediately obvious and there may be a long period of discomfort and problems before the diagnosis is made.

Investigations

The hydrogen breath test (Figure 19.2) administers a loading dose of lactose in a drink and then measures the increase in hydrogen in exhaled breath produced from the metabolism of unabsorbed disaccharides by the gut bacteria. The symptoms following the administration of the lactose usually peak at around 60–90 minutes. Younger children may need a jejunal biopsy to assess enzyme activity.

Treatment and management. The avoidance of lactose in the diet will usually lead to symptom improvement.

Constipation

A diagnosis of constipation is based on the observation that the child or young person produces fewer than three complete stools per week of type 3 or 4 on the Bristol Stool Scale. These stools are hard and large although on occasions can be described as 'rabbit droppings'—type 1 stool. The history may also reveal:
- distress before opening bowels
- straining
- blood on the surface of the stool
- overt rectal bleeding
- current or past anal fissures

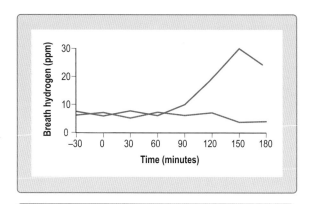

Fig. 19.2 Hydrogen breath test. Normal test (red) with no sugar malabsorption and an abnormal test (blue) when malabsorbed sugars are fermented by colonic bacteria and increase the breath hydrogen

In the older child there may be overflow soiling and the stool may be passed without sensation. Some patients report a poor appetite or the waxing and waning of abdominal pain that improves with passage of a large stool. The child who has faecal impaction will usually be identified from the history and examination.

Examination may identify a grossly distended abdomen with palpable stool but should also include a visual inspection of the lumbosacral spine to exclude spina bifida, perianal area for abnormal positioning and assessment of lower limb neurology. Rectal examination is rarely undertaken in children and, if truly needed, should only be performed by experienced and senior health care professional.

Some findings may indicate an underlying disorder or condition other than idiopathic constipation. These include:
- timing of onset reported from birth or first few weeks of life
- failure to pass meconium or delay of more than 48 hours after term birth
- 'ribbon stools'—suggest Hirschsprung disease
- previously unknown or undiagnosed weakness in legs or locomotor delay
- abdominal distension with vomiting
- faltering growth
- personal, familial and social factors: evidence that raises concerns of safeguarding

Investigations

Investigations are undertaken to exclude other conditions that may present with constipation and, in particular, those with intractable constipation may merit endoscopy and biopsy. Plain abdominal radiographs and ultrasound should not be used to make a diagnosis of constipation.

Table 19.6 Examples of organic causes for constipation

Abnormalities	Conditions
abnormalities of colon and rectum	anal or colonic stenosis anteriorly displaced or ectopic anus
spinal cord abnormalities	meningomyelocele spinal cord tumour
neuropathic gastrointestinal disorders	Hirschsprung disease intestinal neuronal dysplasia
systemic disorders	hypothyroidism hypercalcaemia cerebral palsy
drugs	opiates anticholinergics

Treatment and management

Treatment of impacted faeces in children uses polyethylene glycol in escalating, age-appropriate doses over a one-week period. Stimulant laxatives can cause intense abdominal pains and should therefore be avoided in the initial treatment but may be added if the polyethylene glycol does not lead to disimpaction after 2 weeks. Once the impacted faeces have been cleared then the child must be placed on an ongoing maintenance programme with polyethylene glycol at a lower dose to produce regular soft stools. It is important to maintain treatment for at least 3–6 months to ensure that the bowel tone has improved. Enemas or suppositories are only rarely needed due to potential distress but, if used, should be limited to paediatric preparations.

Education of the child and family by explaining the mechanism of constipation and the principles of management provides the best chance for a successful outcome. Dietary changes on their own are not sufficient to treat idiopathic constipation but should be used alongside medication and toilet training. Ensuring that the young person has a balanced diet which includes an adequate intake of fluid and fibre is important.

Relevant pharmacological agents used

Lactulose is an osmotic laxative and has no significant side effects.

Polyethylene glycol is also an osmotic laxative and is available as a paediatric, unflavoured oral powder which is then mixed with water. The required volume of water may not be tolerated by some children.

Sodium picosulfate, bisacodyl and **senna** are stimulant laxatives and work by increasing intestinal motility. Long-term use may be necessary in some situations and the problem of dependence is not usually evident in children. **Docusate sodium** is both a stimulant and a stool softener.

Encopresis

The term describes the inappropriate passage of stool in inappropriate places and at inappropriate times. Most children with encopresis have a functional cause but it is important to formally exclude neuromuscular or structural abnormalities. Management is usually directed by teams versed in behavioural management.

Vomiting

It is important to differentiate regurgitation, which is the effortless retrograde expulsion of gastric contents, from vomiting, the forceful expulsion of gastric content. Regurgitation usually occurs in babies and younger children and does not

Table 19.7 Common causes of vomiting in children between birth and 5 years

1 and 12 months	1–5 years
any systemic infection	Intussusception
gastroesophageal reflux	gastroesophageal reflux
inborn error of metabolism	toxic ingestion (accidental or fabricated)
pyloric stenosis	
urinary tract infection	

Table 19.8 Common causes of vomiting in those over 5 years

6–12 years	Adolescents
appendicitis	appendicitis
migraine	migraine
cyclical vomiting	alcohol and substance use
pyelonephritis	bulimia nervosa

Table 19.9 Diagnostic clues to causes of vomiting

Symptom	Potential cause
excessive exercise; body image issues	bulimia nervosa
rash; recurring fever	meningitis; systemic infections
abdominal pain	surgical causes—appendicitis; intussusception; hepatitis; gall bladder pathology; renal pathology
diarrhoea	viral—*rotavirus, adenovirus* bacterial—*campylobacter, shigella, salmonella* protozoal—*giardia, cryptosporidium*
headache; dizziness	meningitis; labyrinthitis
bile stained	surgical obstruction
introduction of new food	food allergy
cough	tonsillar enlargement; bronchiolitis; pneumonia; gastroesophageal reflux

have a prodrome whilst children of any age with significant vomiting will usually be pale and retch prior to the vomit.

The cause of vomiting in children and young people is extensive and include both local and systemic conditions. Some diagnoses will affect all age groups and need to be considered in any patient presenting with vomiting. Some symptoms may indicate an underlying cause whilst others are more often seen in individuals of certain ages

Investigations

It is crucial that potential dehydration and electrolyte disturbances are assessed in those presenting with prolonged or excessive vomiting. Diagnostic imaging may also be necessary for some patients and would include:
- abdominal x-ray—if bilious vomiting—abnormal gas pattern; evidence of obstruction
- abdominal ultrasound—gall stones; renal calculi
- swallow contrast study—oesophageal pathology; excludes malrotation
- CT head—excludes raised ICP
- upper GI endoscopy—biopsies for histopathological evidence of GI disorders

Treatment and management

In most clinical situations, the degree of vomiting is usually mild and is often self-limiting. Those patients with dehydration need fluid replacement to cover maintenance,

deficit and ongoing losses whilst those with abnormal electrolytes will need to have the abnormality corrected. Details of fluid and electrolyte management are covered in Chapter 10 Fluids and electrolyte management.

Infant regurgitation

Gastro-oesophageal reflux or 'posseting' is a common condition and should be viewed as a normal physiological process when limited to small amounts of feeds. Peak incidence occurs around 2–4 months and does not usually need any investigation or treatment. There should be no evidence of faltering growth and no other features which suggest a more significant illness.

Gastro-oesophageal disease (GORD)

A small number of babies present with more significant vomiting leading to considerable distress in the baby and parents. Most resolve over time and do not require investigation unless 'red flag' symptoms are reported. These include:
- projectile vomiting
- bile-stained vomit
- haematemesis
- blood in stool

Treatment and management

An initial review of feeding volumes should be undertaken to ensure the baby is not being given inappropriate amounts. Thickening of feeds, anti-regurgitation formulae and upright positioning of the baby after feeds can all be helpful. Some may need proton pump inhibitors if inconsolable crying is a feature. On very rare occasions, some may benefit from a short trial of anti-emetic treatment.

Cyclical vomiting syndrome

The term describes recurrent bouts of intense and unremitting nausea and vomiting separated by many symptom-free weeks and, after evaluation, the symptoms cannot be attributed to another condition. At least two episodes must be recorded in a 6 month period. The cyclical nature of the nausea and vomiting, the duration of the attacks and the possible precipitants for the onset are all helpful for the diagnosis. The median age of onset is between 3.5 and 7 years and a positive family history is not uncommon. The underlying cause is unknown although there seems to be an association with migraine.

Treatment and management

Obvious precipitating events such as stress or fasting should be avoided. The introduction of prophylactic treatment depends on the frequency and intensity of the attacks and antimigraine medications—propranolol, topiramate—can be tried whilst sumatriptan has been used to abort established episodes. Cognitive behavioural therapy may have a place in the management of some children and young people.

Gastrointestinal bleeding

Bleeding from either the upper or lower end of the GI tract is usually obvious although an occult bleeding may be detected during assessment for anaemia. Upper gastrointestinal bleeding is defined as coming from the oesophagus, stomach and duodenum whilst lower gastrointestinal bleeding is from the small bowel and colon.

Recognised causes of upper GI bleeding include:
- vitamin K deficiency—in first few weeks of life
- cows' milk protein allergy—in infants
- Mallory Weiss tear—following prolonged episode of retching in any age
- foreign body ingestion—particularly button batteries
- gastric inflammation—ulceration or stress related
- coagulation disorder
- oesophageal varices—uncommon but can occur in those with liver disease
Recognised causes of lower GI bleeding include:
- anal fissure—usually has associated pain and commonly seen with constipation
- cows' milk protein allergy—in infants

- infectious enterocolitis—*E coli, C difficile, Salmonella, Shigella, Campylobacter*
- intussusception—in young children with episodic, intense colicky pain
- Henoch-Schönlein purpura—with the classic rash on lower limbs and buttocks
- haemolytic uraemic syndrome—usually with associated diarrhoea
- inflammatory bowel disease—usually with diarrhoea and weight loss
- coagulation disorder

Investigations

Initial, and possibly urgent, investigations would include:
- haematology—full blood count; clotting screen; group and cross-match
- biochemistry—electrolytes; liver function tests
Further investigations will be directed by the history and examination but may include:
- abdominal x-ray if NEC or button battery ingestion considered
- contrast studies—to exclude anatomical abnormalities
- Meckel's scan—looking for ectopic gastric mucosa
- endoscopy—direct observation of bleeding point, local treatment and possible biopsy

Treatment and management

The initial assessment and treatment will determine the extent of the bleed and clarify whether episodes are mild or severe. Variceal bleeding is rare but can be profuse and usually occurs in those with a known history of chronic liver disease.

Diseases of the pancreas

Pancreatitis

Children may present acutely with pancreatitis and some even have multiple episodes leading to chronic pancreatitis. Those with recurrent or repeated acute attacks should be referred to specialist teams for further assessment. Underlining causes would include:
- gallstones
- genetic risk—single genes (SPINK1 and PRSS1) with hereditary pancreatitis
- medications—rare—mercaptopurine, L-asparaginase, sulphonamides
- infections—mumps, coxsackie, mycoplasma, toxoplasma, cryptosporidium
- alcohol
Children with chronic pancreatitis present with abdominal pain, vomiting and poor growth. The pain is usually epigastric and classically radiates to the back. There may be

Table 19.10 Management of acute upper GI bleeding

	Mild	Severe	Varices
haemodynamic status	stable	unstable active bleeding	unstable profuse bleeding
investigations	FBC; clotting; cross match; CXR if possibility of foreign body (battery)	FBC; clotting; cross match; CXR if possibility of foreign body (battery)	FBC; clotting; LFTs, cross match
initial response	admit monitor	resuscitate admit monitor	resuscitate octreotide infusion, PPI bolus, IV antibiotics, consider tranexamic acid. rarely Sengstaken tube insertion
surgical intervention	endoscope if progresses	endoscope when stable	endoscope and band/inject if needed
medical intervention	consider PPI (omeprazole) after endoscopy	add PPI (omeprazole) consider Tranexamic acid	octreotide infusion

a history of foul-smelling, greasy stools that are difficult to flush, suggesting fat malabsorption and, with extensive pancreatic fibrosis, some children will develop clinical diabetes.

Investigations

- serum amylase and lipase—usually elevated in acute episodes
- liver function tests—may suggest liver disease or bile duct obstruction
- blood glucose—may elevated in chronic disease
- faecal elastase—low in exocrine pancreatic insufficiency
- fat-soluble vitamins—reduced if malabsorption (ADEK—gives mnemonic of F-AKED)
- ultrasound biliary and pancreatic ducts—to identify obstruction
- MRI abdomen—visualises pancreatic parenchyma
- genetic testing—in those with recurrent episodes

Treatment and management

The initial management of an acute presentation requires administration of appropriate analgesia including opioids if pain is excessive. Enteral feeding is usually omitted in the first instance and intravenous fluids started. With prompt recovery, oral nutrition can be introduced under the guidance of a paediatric dietitian but parenteral nutrition may be required on occasions.

Diseases of the liver

Due to the considerable functional reserves of the liver, disease often remains subclinical until a relatively advanced stage. It is therefore important to be familiar

Table 19.11 Investigations in liver disease in children

Investigation	Indication
liver enzymes	assesses liver cell damage
fractionated bilirubin	identifies conjugated and unconjugated levels
albumin	low level in chronic hepatic—impaired synthesis
viral hepatitis serology	assess potential viral pathology
clotting studies	abnormal if reduction of liver clotting factors
abdominal ultrasound	identify structural pathology

with the 'red flags' of paediatric liver disease, the different age groups affected by these diseases, the initial investigations required and the situations where referral to a specialist liver centre is required.

Many initial investigations are common to most forms of liver disease whilst others are required when specific liver diseases are considered in the differential diagnosis.

Across all presentations, the degree of elevation of liver enzymes must not be relied upon to define severity of disease. Measurement of clotting is most useful and, if a coagulopathy is discovered, then intravenous vitamin K must be given and reassessment performed.

The most common ways that liver disease can present in children and young people are:
- prolonged jaundice in the newborn
- conjugated jaundice in the newborn and infancy
- incidental finding of elevated transaminases
- acute liver disease
- chronic liver disease with portal hypertension and cirrhosis

Prolonged neonatal jaundice

The term describes jaundice lasting for more than 2 weeks in the full-term infant. It is helpful to distinguish between unconjugated (indirect) and conjugated (direct) hyperbilirubinemia in order to define aetiology. A prolonged unconjugated hyperbilirubinemia is usually physiological and related to breastfeeding although it can also be secondary to pathological conditions such as:

- haemolytic diseases (blood group incompatibility or G6PD deficiency)
- congenital hypothyroidism
- urinary infection
- inherited syndromes including Crigler-Najjar or Gilbert syndromes

Crigler-Najjar syndromes (two variants) are autosomal recessive disorders of bilirubin conjugation leading to a very high unconjugated hyperbilirubinemia. There is a high risk of kernicterus.

Gilbert syndrome is an inherited condition of reduced ability to conjugate bilirubin and is usually an incidental finding on bloods taken for other reasons or from the diagnosis being made in other family members. It does not lead to chronic liver disease and no treatment required.

Conjugated jaundice in neonatal period and in infancy

Conjugated hyperbilirubinaemia is seen during the neonatal period and infancy. It is never physiological and should be suspected in all jaundiced infants with light stools and dark urine. The causes are either the result of bile flow obstruction or hepatocellular dysfunction:

- obstructive cholestasis
  - biliary atresia
  - congenital bile duct anomalies (choledochal cysts)
  - Alagille syndrome (intrahepatic cholestasis)
- hepatocellular cholestasis
  - hepatitis (hepatitis A, B, C), herpes
  - alpha-1 antitrypsin deficiency
  - metabolic disorders—fructosemia, tyrosinemia
  - total parenteral nutrition (TPN)–associated

Initial investigations should include
- viral hepatitis serology
- congenital infection serology
- blood and urine culture
- immunoreactive trypsin or sweat test
- alpha-1-antitrypsin levels and phenotype
- galactose-1-phosphate uridyl transferase (GAL-1-PUT)
- clotting studies
- thyroid function tests
- serum cortisol
- fasting ultrasound abdomen

Biliary atresia

Biliary atresia is an important cause of neonatal cholestasis and is the most common cause of the need for liver transplantation in children. It presents in the first weeks of life and is characterised by complete obstruction of the biliary tract. Early detection of this condition significantly improves outcomes, but if it is left untreated, portal hypertension and biliary cirrhosis tend to occur and both can be detected as early as 2 to 3 months of age.

Clinical jaundice along with pale stools (Figure 19.3) and dark urine are suggestive of an obstructive cause.

Investigations

A fasting ultrasound will demonstrate either a contracted or absent gall bladder. HIDA (hepato-iminodiacetic acid) scanning will look for the failure to excrete the isotope into the bowel although the investigation does not have a high sensitivity or specificity. Some liver centres proceed directly to either a liver biopsy or an on-table cholangiogram in order to make an early diagnosis.

Treatment and management

Untreated, biliary atresia leads to progressive liver cirrhosis and death by 2 years of age. Consequently, the above investigations must be completed promptly and referral made to the appropriate liver unit before 6 weeks of age where a hepato-porto-enterostomy (Kasai procedure) will be performed. The operation involves resection of the extrahepatic biliary tree and a small bowel loop anastomosed at the porta hepatis to facilitate biliary drainage.

Alagille syndrome

Alagille syndrome results from a reduction in number and size of the intrahepatic bile ducts and is the most common

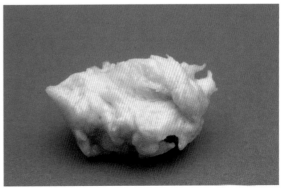

Fig. 19.3 Pale stool seen in conjugated hyperbilirubinaemia

cause of familial progressive intrahepatic cholestasis. The syndrome is diagnosed on the basis of clinical features that include jaundice, pruritis, characteristic facies (broad forehead, deep-set eyes, small, pointed chin), cardiac abnormalities (peripheral pulmonary artery stenosis), vertebral arch defects and corneal defects. Definitive diagnosis is made by liver biopsy and histological examination. Supportive and symptomatic management is required in approximately 50% of children with the condition.

Alpha-1-antitrypsin deficiency

Alpha-1-antitrypsin is a glycoprotein produced in large quantities in the liver to inhibit the neutrophil proteases associated with inflammation. The classical form of the condition that is most closely associated with liver disease is caused by homozygosity for the Z mutation (PiZZ genotype).

The clinical course is variable and may involve neonatal cholestasis, liver dysfunction, liver failure and cirrhosis. Approximately 20% of PiZZ patients develop cholestasis within the first few weeks of life.

Cystic fibrosis

Most patients with cystic fibrosis do not present with liver damage in the early phase of the disease, although hepatic impairment is present in 10% to 30%. Gallstones and micro-gallbladder are the most common biliary abnormalities whilst hepatosplenomegaly and portal hypertension are recognised manifestations of liver disease in older children and adolescents. Further details are in Chapter 17 Respiratory.

Incidental finding of an elevated transaminases

In the older child this is often the mode of presentation of new-onset chronic liver disease when blood tests, as part of a panel investigating an unrelated disease, pick up an elevated transaminase. The underlying cause may well be an intercurrent viral infection but may also be chronic liver conditions such as autoimmune liver disease, Wilson's disease and nonalcoholic fatty liver disease.

Investigations

Essential investigations for the older child with abnormal liver function tests, but not in liver failure, will include those listed in the introduction plus those listed here:

Autoimmune liver disease

Autoimmune hepatitis is a chronic inflammatory liver disease, with an unknown trigger for the autoimmune process. It is classified into subtypes according to the

Table 19.12 Essential investigations in older child with abnormal liver function test

Investigation	Indication
serum caeruloplasmin; serum copper	low levels in Wilson's disease
Immunoglobulins	raised in autoimmune liver disease
autoantibodies screen	positive in autoimmune liver disease
alpha1-antitrypsin levels and phenotype	identifies deficiency and genotype
abdominal ultrasound	assess cirrhosis, fatty liver and portal hypertension

presence of certain auto-antibodies (anti-nuclear; anti-smooth muscle; anti-liver-kidney microsomal antibodies).

Sclerosing cholangitis may have a similar clinical presentation and often accompanies inflammatory bowel disease. Management of both requires the use of immunosuppressants.

Wilson's disease

This is an autosomal recessive condition where copper accumulates in the liver, brain and cornea with hepatic manifestations becoming evident after the first 3 years of life. Patients often have a family history of the condition.

The clinical presentation could be with:
- acute hepatitis with abnormal liver function tests
- liver failure
- cirrhosis with portal hypertension
- gallstones
- Kayser-Fleischer rings in cornea are not evident in younger patients
- neurological symptoms—tremor, dysarthria, behavioural changes

Investigations

Serum ceruloplasmin levels will be low but a liver biopsy is usually required to assess extent of liver toxicity. Genetic assessment will be required and then offered to other family members.

Treatment and management

Patients presenting acutely with symptoms require the administration of copper chelating agents. Thereafter, treatment requires the removal of dietary copper as far as possible. Foods that need to be avoided include chocolate, nuts and shellfish and such restrictions are required throughout life.

Nonalcoholic fatty liver disease (NAFLD)

It is the result of fatty infiltrate of the liver parenchyma and is associated with obesity although many patients are asymptomatic. Raised liver enzyme levels are not sensitive or specific markers for NAFLD but may lead to further useful investigations such as ultrasound. Ultimately the diagnosis is made on histology following biopsy.

Treatment and management

NAFLD is not a benign condition as up to 9% of children with only mildly abnormal LFT can have late-stage fibrosis on liver biopsy. There is no specific treatment for NAFLD apart from weight loss. Affected children are at high risk of developing cirrhosis, type 2 diabetes and cardiovascular disease in adult life.

Acute liver disease

This presentation is usually the result of significant liver cell damage and the usual cause is a viral illness (Hepatitis A, EBV, adenovirus) although a toxic cause also needs to be considered.

The patient will usually present with an acute onset of jaundice, anorexia, vomiting, abdominal pain and pruritis and may develop a rapidly evolving encephalopathy with irritability, confusion, drowsiness and eventually coma. Examination would reveal the obvious icteric appearance and may also identify ascites, hepatomegaly and, if developing late-stage encephalopathy, decerebrate rigidity.

Investigations

Serum transaminases, prothrombin time, INR and ammonia levels may all be markedly prolonged or elevated.

Treatment and management

Management will depend on the underlying aetiology but is likely to require intensive care support. Liver transplantation may be needed for some.

Acute liver failure

Paediatric acute liver failure is a potentially devastating condition, which occurs in previously healthy children of any age and frequently leads to a rapid clinical deterioration. It is associated with a high mortality rate despite optimal medical therapy including emergency liver transplantation.

The main causes of acute liver failure in childhood are:
- viral hepatitis (hepatitis A, B, E; CMV; EBV; adenovirus and enterovirus)
- Wilson's disease
- autoimmune liver disease
- paracetamol overdose
- metabolic diseases
- haemophagocytic syndrome
- Reye syndrome

Reye syndrome is an acute condition resulting in liver toxicity without the appearance of jaundice and occurs in the recovery phase of a viral infection such as influenza or chickenpox. Historically most children had been given aspirin and, as a consequence, the medication now being contraindicated in those under 12 years.

In addition to the clinical features of liver disease, the main abnormality in acute liver failure is abnormal coagulation results. An INR of 1.5 or greater, with evidence of encephalopathy, should indicate acute liver failure and be seen as a medical emergency.

Treatment and management

It is vital that there is early and close liaison with a specialist liver centre and the following supportive measures introduced:
- support with IV Vitamin K and repeat clotting to evaluate
- treat for sepsis and maintain blood sugar levels
- monitor for encephalopathy
- careful fluid balance in an HDU setting
- discuss use of bowel decontamination or lactulose if high ammonia levels
- arrange early transport to a paediatric liver centre

Chronic liver disease

Chronic liver disease, with or without cirrhosis, in children and young people can be the result of a broad group of underlying conditions:
- biliary obstruction—biliary atresia; choledochal cysts; gallstones
- hepatotropic viral infections—hepatitis B, D, C, E
- autoimmune diseases
- metabolic diseases—alpha-1-antitrypsin deficiency; galactosaemia; fructosaemia
- cystic fibrosis; haemochromatosis
- Alagille syndrome
- drugs and toxins—total parenteral nutrition; methotrexate

Children and young people with chronic liver disease are usually known to medical teams and will often develop jaundice and pruritus as liver function deteriorates. Examination will reveal other signs including leukonychia, clubbing, palmar erythema, splenomegaly and undernutrition. They may also develop ascites or encephalopathy whilst the presence of an asterixis ('liver flap') is highly indicative of encephalopathy.

Those with unrecognised liver disease can present with the sequelae of cirrhosis and portal hypertension including upper GI bleeds from varices, splenomegaly or severe malnutrition including deficiency of fat-soluble vitamins.

Treatment and management

Treatment is directed by the underlying aetiology but untreated liver disease that has progressed to cirrhosis and portal hypertension may well require liver transplantation.

Surgical conditions and congenital malformations

Oesophageal stricture

Oesophageal strictures are usually acquired in infancy and the majority present with a history of gastro-oesophageal reflux which has not improved over time. The child will have difficulty swallowing often associated with poor weight gain, pain on swallowing and regurgitation. A previous contrast study meal may have demonstrated a hiatus hernia and lower oesophageal irregularity due to scarring as a result of the acid reflux.

Treatment and management

Upper GI endoscopy will identify the oesophageal stricture and permit dilatation using a bougie or balloon device. All require a fundoplication to control gastrointestinal reflux which, in conjunction with repeated dilations, will allow the stricture to resolve.

Achalasia

Achalasia is an uncommon condition which develops when neuronal cells in the oesophagus degenerate and produces an inability of the lower oesophageal sphincter to relax. This leads to a loss of peristalsis and a dysmotile oesophagus. The child will present with progressive dysphagia and regurgitation which becomes progressively worse over time. A plain x-ray may show a dilated oesophagus with an air-fluid level and a contrast study meal will demonstrate a characteristic narrowing towards the distal oesophagus (Figure 19.4). Oesophageal manometry is diagnostic and demonstrates that the lower oesophageal

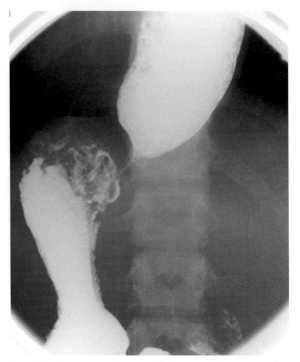

Fig. 19.4 Contrast swallow stud showing narrowing towards the distal oesophagus—'bird's beak' appearance

sphincter fails to relax on swallowing in association with poor oesophageal peristalsis.

Treatment and management

Balloon dilation of the lower oesophagus is effective but has a high recurrence rate and a longitudinal division of the lower oesophageal sphincter (Heller's myotomy) is the preferred treatment.

Hiatus hernia

Most commonly seen in children with developmental motor problems, the condition may present with gastro-oesophageal reflux, growth retardation and haematemesis secondary to oesophagitis. A plain abdominal x-ray may show a retrocardiac mass with or without an air-fluid level.

Treatment and management

Investigation with a contrast meal study, oesophageal pH study and upper GI endoscopy will confirm the diagnosis. Initial medical management is with alginates, H_2 receptor blockers and proton pump inhibitors. Surgical intervention with a fundoplication, usually performed laparoscopically, is indicated when medical management fails.

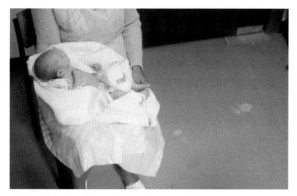

Fig. 19.5 Projectile vomit seen in 6-week-old boy with hypertrophic pyloric stenosis

Infantile hypertrophic pyloric stenosis

The condition is more common in males than females (5:1) and siblings have an increased risk. The infants are usually aged between 2 and 8 weeks with a history of worsening projectile vomiting (Figure 19.5) and growth retardation which may lead to dehydration. A visual inspection of the abdomen may identify peristaltic waves in the left upper quadrant whilst palpation can reveal an olive sized 'tumour' in the right upper quadrant.

Treatment and management

The diagnosis is confirmed by ultrasound which identifies the thickening of the pyloric muscle with consequent narrowing of the pyloric canal giving the 'target sign'. Electrolyte assessment is imperative as the prolonged vomiting of gastric fluid will lead to a **hypochloraemic, hypokalaemic alkalosis**. This must be corrected before the child is taken to theatre where a Ramstedt's pyloromyotomy is undertaken. Infants invariably make a full and uncomplicated recovery with no long-term sequelae.

Ingested foreign body

Many small children will swallow objects and the majority will pass through the GI tract without problems. Some objects, however, need specific management as they can produce significant complications if ignored.

Treatment and management

Batteries, particularly the small button type (Figure 19.6), are small enough to be ingested and can induce mucosal erosion through a local electrochemical reaction. A plain x-ray will

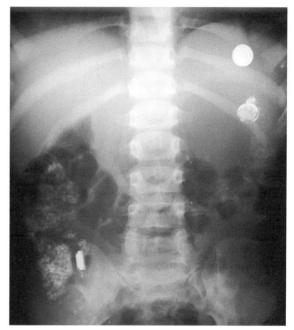

Fig. 19.6 Plain abdominal x-ray of 3-year-old boy who had swallowed button batteries

help to confirm the ingestion if there is any doubt. In most situations, the battery should be removed surgically.

Small magnets can cause significant problems when more than one is swallowed as they may connect and erode through adjacent bowel. Surgical removal is required.

Coins will usually stick in the cricopharyngeal region or at the lower oesophagus and those in the former location may be mobilised with a carbonated drink or may need endoscopic removal. Those at the lower oesophagus will usually pass without problem.

Malrotation and volvulus

Malrotation describes sections of the small bowel which are not correctly located in the abdomen and are not causing problems. They are, however, more prone to twisting in this position and so producing a volvulus. The twisted bowel most commonly develops in children under 1 year of age who then present with bile-stained vomiting. All children with bile-stained vomiting require investigation even if the child has made a full recovery. Some children with malrotation can be shocked at presentation and will need urgent surgical intervention as the potential for ischaemic bowel is high. Plain abdominal x-rays are often unremarkable but an upper GI contrast study will show an abnormal location of the DJ flexure.

Treatment and management

Surgical widening of the mesentery (Ladd's procedure) will place the caecal pole and colon on the left of the abdomen and the small bowel on the right. An appendicectomy may also be performed.

Meckel's diverticulum

This is the embryological remnant of the vitelline duct which connects to the ileum. The majority are asymptomatic but those who do present have features very similar to those of appendicitis with lower abdominal pain although they can also present with lower GI bleeding and intussusception. A technetium isotope scan could be considered if the child is clinically stable but this will only identify the 25% of patients who have gastric mucosa in the lesion. Consequently, the diagnosis can only be confirmed following a surgical exploration.

Intussusception

Typically, the child is between 12 and 24 months old, has **episodic**, severe, cramp-like abdominal pain and fresh blood with mucous ('red currant jelly') in the stool and examination can reveal a mass in the right side of the abdomen. The lead point in intussusception is usually the result of a viral infection producing local lymphadenopathy at the ileo-caecal junction but can be due to a lymphoma or Henoch-Schönlein purpura. A plain abdominal x-ray may identify a soft tissue crescent and exclude bowel perforation whilst an abdominal ultrasound may identify a diagnostic 'target lesion'.

Treatment and management

Following resuscitation with IV fluids and prophylactic antibiotics and providing there is no evidence of perforation, an air enema is undertaken to reduce the intussusception. This is successful in 75% of children, but if it fails then a surgical reduction and possible bowel resection is required.

Hirschsprung disease

This condition mainly affects boys and is due to tonically contracted bowel due to aganglionosis in the bowel segment with some 80% located in the distal colon. Babies may present with delayed passage stool or 'ribbon stool' (Figure 19.7) whilst the older child may have a history of chronic constipation. Some of those with a very late presentation can develop enterocolitis and sepsis and are in extremis at presentation. A rectal examination should be reserved for senior member of the surgical team who will recognise the explosive release of stool.

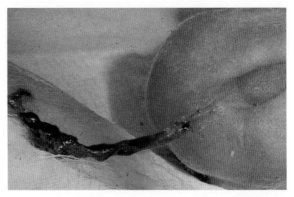

Fig. 19.7 Hirschsprung stool

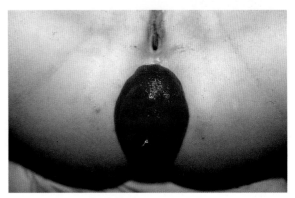

Fig. 19.8 Rectal prolapse

Treatment and management

Confirmation of the diagnosis comes from a rectal biopsy demonstrating aganglionosis. In the neonate, rectal washouts are performed to aid evacuation of the bowel with definitive surgery around 3 months of age. This entails resection of the aganglionic section of bowel with a colo-anal anastomosis. A stoma is only required if rectal washouts fail to decompress the bowel.

Rectal prolapse

Rectal prolapse (Figure 19.8) describes a full thickness of bowel mucosa pushing down and visible through the anus. The child is usually between 3 and 4 years of age and with a history of chronic constipation.

Treatment and management

Manual reduction is usually possible and, with management of the constipation, a full resolution is the expected course.

IMPORTANT CLINICAL POINTS

Abdominal pain
- functional GI disorders should only be diagnosed after organic diseases excluded
- stress ulceration occurs in those in intensive care settings
- *H pylori* is identified by urea breath test
- chronic carriage of *H pylori* is possible and transmission from close contacts occurs

Diarrhoea
- blood in the stool is a feature of certain organisms
- diagnosis of coeliac disease does not always need jejunal biopsy
- most children with coeliac disease are positive for HLA-DQ2 and HLA-DQ8
- coeliac disease is associated with other autoimmune conditions
- patients with acute flare-up of Crohn's disease require exclusive enteral nutrition
- protein losing enteropathy produces low serum albumin and low immunoglobulins

Liver disease
- conjugated hyperbilirubinemia is never physiological
- urgently investigate suspected biliary atresia with ultrasound and HIDA scan
- autoimmune hepatitis is confirmed by identifying certain auto-antibodies

Surgical problems
- infantile hypertrophic pyloric stenosis usually aged between 2 and 8 weeks
- prolonged vomiting of gastric fluid will lead to a hypochloraemic, hypokalaemic alkalosis
- ingested batteries induce mucosal erosion by local electrochemical reaction
- multiple ingested magnets may connect and erode adjacent bowel
- intussusception can be associated with lymphoma or Henoch-Schönlein purpura

Further Reading

Kelly LAM, Whyte LA: Pathophysiology of diarrhoea, *Paediatr Child Health*, 2019.

Campbell C, Slater Y: Approach to the vomiting child, *Paediatr Child Health*, 2018.

Gastro-oesophageal reflux disease in children and young people. NICE Guideline [NG1]. Published January 2015. Updated October 2019. https://www.nice.org.uk/guidance/ng1

Coeliac disease: recognition, assessment and management. NICE guideline [NG20]. Published: 2015. https://www.nice.org.uk/guidance/ng20

Chapter | 20 |

Nephro-urology

Stephen Marks, Ramnath Balasubramanian

After reading this chapter you should be able to assess, diagnose and manage:
- congenital anomalies of the kidney and urinary tract
- acute kidney injury and chronic kidney disease
- urinary tract infections
- renal tubular disorders
- nephritic and nephrotic syndrome
- enuresis

Investigations in renal disease

Proteinuria

Proteinuria above 100 mg/m^2/day reflects abnormal excretion at either the glomerular or tubular level. Children with heavy proteinuria, as seen in nephrotic syndrome, will excrete over 1000 mg/m^2/day of protein.

Glomerular proteinuria will usually produce large protein molecules such as albumin in the urine whereas tubular proteinuria is the result of an inability to reabsorb low molecular weight proteins and is often seen with glycosuria and bicarbonate losses. Small proteins are not detected by standard urinary dipstick testing (Table 20.1).

Haematuria

Microscopic haematuria describes the presence of more than five red cells per mm^3 of urine whilst macroscopic haematuria refers to urine that is visibly discoloured (Table 20.2).

Causes of haematuria include:
- UTI
- malignancy
- renal calculi
- glomerulonephritis
- IgA nephropathy

- Alport syndrome
- clotting abnormalities
- trauma
- haemolytic uraemic syndrome

Urine may be discoloured for reasons other than haematuria and recognition of these potential causes may reduce the need for further assessment.

PRACTICE POINT—causes of discoloured urine

- haemoglobin – haemolysis
- myoglobin – rhabdomyolysis
- food – beetroot, food dyes
- drugs – rifampicin, nitrofurantoin, metronidazole
- metabolic – porphyria
- urates – crystals in neonates

Radiological investigations

Imaging of the renal tract provides significant information to help diagnosis and management, but the interpretation of all radiological imaging relating to the renal tract is the responsibility of the radiologist.

Plain abdominal x-rays—has a limited role in management of renal conditions and their previous role has now been superseded by ultrasonography.

Renal ultrasound—a valuable, noninvasive technique that, in experienced hands, can provide a great detail of information about the structure of kidneys, ureters and bladder.

Micturating cysto-urethrogram (MCUG) investigations (Figure 20.1)—contrast-enhanced images that are produced by introducing radiocontrast material into the bladder through a urinary catheter. The catheter is then removed and abdominal images obtained whilst the child attempts to void urine. Vesico-ureteric reflux, anatomical abnormalities and urethral valves can all be identified by this technique.

Table 20.1 Investigations for a child presenting with proteinuria		
	Investigation	**Rationale for investigation**
urine	urinalysis	haematuria, red cell casts (seen in glomerulonephritis); pyuria
	protein: creatinine ratio (random sample)	quantifies protein output
blood	electrolytes	assess renal function
	urea	assess renal function
	creatinine	assess renal function
	C3 and C4	C3 low post-streptococcal; C3 and C4 low in lupus nephritis
	protein and albumin	low levels supporting protein leak
	lipids	elevated cholesterol and triglycerides with nephrotic syndrome
	ANA	lupus nephritis
	ASOT	raised following streptococcal infection
	hepatitis B and C	assess potential liver disease
imaging	renal ultrasound	parenchymal damage or congenital anomalies

Table 20.2 Investigations for a child presenting with haematuria		
	Investigation	**Rationale for investigation**
urine	urinalysis	red cell casts (seen in glomerulonephritis); pyuria
	culture	identifies urinary tract infection
	urine protein: creatinine ratio (random sample)	quantifies protein output
blood	electrolytes	assess renal function
	urea	assess renal function
	creatinine	assess renal function
	clotting	exclude abnormal clotting
	C3 and C4	C3 low post-streptococcal; C3 and C4 low in lupus nephritis
	protein and albumin	low levels supporting leak
	lipids	elevated cholesterol and triglycerides with nephrotic syndrome
	ANA	usually raised in lupus nephritis
	ASOT	raised following streptococcal infection
microbiology	stool culture	if HUS suspected
imaging	renal ultrasound	parenchymal damage or congenital anomalies

DMSA investigations (Figure 20.2)—radionuclide static scans used to provide information on the distribution of renal parenchymal tissue. The tracer is injected intravenously and the patient is scanned to identify uptake. The scans are able to identify renal agenesis, scarring and dysplastic kidneys and can also identify ectopic renal tissue.

DTPA and MAG3 investigations (Figure 20.3) are radionuclide dynamic scans used to provide information on renal function although the MAG3 scan can also identify some changes in renal parenchymal tissue. The tracer is injected intravenously and the patient is scanned at intervals to record the rate of excretion. The scans can identify delayed excretion of the tracer in each kidney and so assess obstruction to urine flow.

Congenital anomalies of the kidney and urinary tract

Some congenital anomalies of the kidney and urinary tract may be identified antenatally, others are evident at birth whilst some present later. Many syndromic conditions have associated abnormalities of the renal tract.

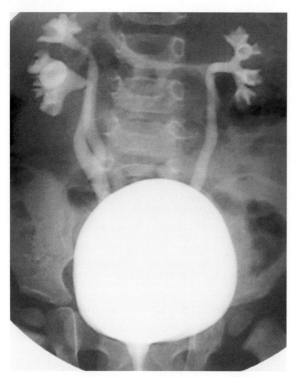

Fig. 20.1 MCUG Image showing bilateral vesico-ureteric reflux and incidental finding of a duplex system on the right side.

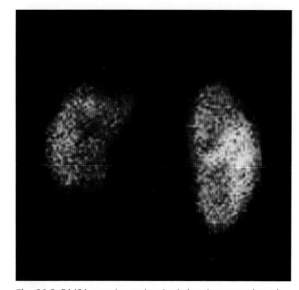

Fig. 20.2 DMSA scan (posterior view) showing parenchymal defects (scaring) of the left kidney.

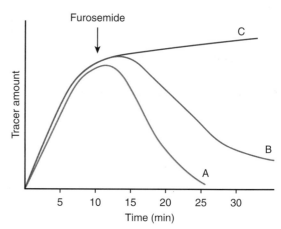

Fig. 20.3 MAG3 scan image showing expected appearances for normal kidney (A), partially obstructed kidney (B) and bladder (C).

Hydronephrosis

Hydronephrosis may be associated with a hydroureter and is usually due to obstruction at the pelviureteric (PUJ) or vesicoureteric junctions. It may also be the result of reflux of urine from the bladder into the ureter and kidneys.

Causes

Table 20.3 **Site of obstruction along the renal tract and possible causes**

Site	Aetiology
renal pelvis	congenital, calculi, tumour, infection
pelviureteric junction	congenital stenosis, calculi, trauma
ureter	megaureter with obstruction, ectopic ureter, ureterocoele, calculi, tumour
bladder	neurogenic bladder, tumours, ectopic ureter
urethra	posterior urethral valve, strictures, phimosis

Treatment and management

Hydronephrosis detected antenatally is usually mild and resolves without intervention although monitoring is undertaken to ensure resolution. Significant hydronephrosis needs investigation with MAG3 or MCUG to ascertain whether the appearances are the result of obstruction or reflux. Children with significant hydronephrosis are likely to need surgical correction.

Pelviureteric junction obstruction

The obstruction is usually identified in antenatal scans and is generally due to congenital stenosis. Mild dilatation does not need extensive investigations and usually resolves whilst most children with significant dilatation will require a pyeloplasty.

Posterior urethral valve

Posterior urethral valves are the most common cause of bladder outlet obstruction in boys. These abnormal valves attach to the urethral wall leading to obstruction and dilatation of the posterior urethra. Over time the bladder detrusor muscle becomes hypertrophied.

Posterior urethral valves are usually suspected when antenatal scans show bilateral hydronephrosis. Severe obstruction may be associated with oligohydramnios which then leads to lethal pulmonary hypoplasia, and most will have some degree of renal dysplasia. Urgent USS and MCUG will identify the obstruction at the bladder outflow.

A urethral catheter should be inserted immediately after birth in those where hydronephrosis is identified antenatally and prophylactic antibiotics administered until investigations are completed. Once the presence of the valves is confirmed they can then be ablated via a cystoscope.

Polycystic kidney disease

Autosomal dominant polycystic kidney disease is the most common inherited renal disease and usually presents in late adolescence or adulthood. Proteinuria and hypertension may develop along with cysts in the liver and pancreas. The screening of asymptomatic family members should be offered as some may have clinically silent disease. End stage renal failure occurs early in the severe type, whereas others may develop failure in later adulthood.

Autosomal recessive polycystic kidney disease can be severe and is identified antenatally with oligohydramnios and pulmonary hypoplasia. These clinical features are consistent with Potter's syndrome and the babies die early in the neonatal period. Those with milder disease can present later with symptoms of progressive deterioration in renal function with polyuria and polydipsia, metabolic acidosis and hypertension. The kidneys are usually enlarged on examination.

The main aim is to control the hypertension and manage the renal failure with some patients needing renal and liver transplantation at a later date.

Acute kidney injury

Acute kidney injury (AKI) describes a sudden loss of kidney function resulting in the retention of nitrogenous wastes and the inability to regulate fluid and electrolyte haemostasis. The conditions that cause AKI are:
- prerenal—hypovolaemia or hypotension
- renal abnormalities—vascular, glomerular, tubular or interstitial
- post renal—congenital or acquired obstruction

Acute kidney injury is identified following the investigations of the conditions presented below. Further investigations will usually be required and can be found under lists for proteinuria and haematuria (table 20.1 and 20.2).

Treatment and management

Prerenal failure is mainly due to hypovolaemia and needs urgent correction with fluid and circulatory support if associated with hypotension.

Primary renal failure results in circulatory overload and retention of fluid and hence fluid boluses are counterproductive. Restriction of fluids with a diuretic challenge may restore urine output, but if oliguria persists, fluid is restricted to that needed to replace insensible loss plus urine output. Nephrotoxic medications should be avoided and all medications with renal excretion need their dose adjusted and, in some situations, levels monitored. Most children will respond to conservative management of fluid balance and a high-calorie, normal protein feed. However, these measures may not be adequate and dialysis will then be required.

Post renal failure needs the relief of the obstruction by bladder catheterisation or nephrostomy and any required surgical correction undertaken at a later date.

Indications for dialysis are:
- the failure of conservative management
- fluid overload resulting in pulmonary oedema
- severe metabolic acidosis
- severe electrolyte imbalance
- hyperkalaemia
- multisystem failure

Long-term follow up is usually required for those patients with AKI as any potential damage can result in hypertension and proteinuria.

Haemolytic uraemic syndrome

One of the main causes of acute kidney injury in children is haemolytic uraemic syndrome (HUS) which is diagnosed by the presence of a microangiopathic haemolytic anaemia, thrombocytopenia and acute kidney injury. HUS is seen most commonly following infection with Shiga toxin-producing *Escherichia coli* although other organisms such as *Streptococcus pneumoniae* have been implicated.

The child usually has usually had a preceding illness with abdominal pain, vomiting and bloody diarrhoea and continues to deteriorate clinically. Hypertension is a common finding on examination. Initial investigations will identify haemolytic anaemia and fragmented red cells, thrombocytopenia and AKI along with a stool culture showing *E. coli O157.H7*. Clotting studies are usually normal in HUS and helps to distinguish it from DIC.

The initial management of children with HUS is supportive, and referral to paediatric nephrology services is advised as renal dialysis may be required. It is also important to notify the local Public Health services as a source of the infection should be investigated.

Chronic kidney disease

Chronic kidney disease (CKD) is the result of a progressive loss of renal function and is diagnosed when the GFR falls below 60 ml/min per 1.73 m^2 for more than 3 months.

The common causes of CKD are:
- congenital—malformations, obstructive uropathy, renal dysplasia, reflux nephropathy
- metabolic—cystinosis, oxalosis, polycystic kidney disease
- glomerulonephritis—focal segmental glomerulosclerosis, congenital nephrotic syndrome, IgA nephropathy

CKD in the earlier stages is mainly asymptomatic but patients with later stage disease present with:
- anorexia and lethargy
- polyuria and polydipsia
- restricted growth
- anaemia
- hypertension

Late features include acidosis, hyperkalaemia, uraemia, left ventricular failure and pulmonary oedema.

Investigations

These are aimed at identifying the underlying cause of the presenting chronic renal failure and excluding any potential causes of acute kidney injury.

Treatment and management

It is not usually possible to reverse the renal damage seen with CKD and hence the aim is to prevent further deterioration of renal function by supportive measures. Ensuring good nutrition, optimal growth, control of hypertension and treatment of anaemia are all required. Any obstructions of the renal tract needs to be relieved and the development of renal osteodystrophy minimised by keeping calcium, phosphate, PTH and alkaline phosphatase within normal range.

Children and young people with CKD are at risk of anaemia and are usually given iron supplements and erythropoietin. They are also at risk of developing metabolic bone disease which is identified by hyperphosphataemia and hypocalcaemia and consequently require phosphate binders, calcium supplements and vitamin D analogues (1-alfacalcidol, 1,25 dihydroxycholecalciferol).

If CKD progress to end-stage kidney disease, renal replacement therapy—renal transplant or dialysis—is required and is usually started when the child or young person becomes symptomatic or the biochemical parameters reach unacceptable levels. A living-donor renal transplant is the preferred option; otherwise, a dialysis programme is offered.

Haemodialysis is undertaken at least three times a week; each session lasts 3–5 hours and the patient and their families usually have to travel some distance to the dialysis centre. The treatment therefore makes significant demands on the patient and their family and both home haemodialysis or peritoneal dialysis have been used to mitigate this disruption. Successful transplant offers a return to near-normal life although immunosuppressive medications are needed for life.

Urinary tract infection

Urinary tract infection (UTI) is one of the most common causes of bacterial infections in childhood and is more common in girls except in early infancy. It can be easily missed as the symptoms are often nonspecific. UTI in the young is known to cause renal scarring leading to long-term morbidity including hypertension and renal impairment, and a child with repeated urinary tract infections may have an underlying renal tract anomaly and needs investigation. Common causative organisms include E. coli, proteus and pseudomonas.

UTI should be suspected in any child presenting with fever and nonspecific symptoms. Recognised added symptoms by age are:
- infants—fever >38°C, irritability, vomiting and, rarely, septicaemia
- preschool children—may complain of abdominal pain, smelly urine and dysuria
- older children—frequency, dysuria, urgency and enuresis

Investigations

The diagnosis may be confirmed when dipstick testing is positive for nitrites or leukocyte esterase along with a mild proteinuria. Formal laboratory testing will identify pyuria and bacteriuria. The method of collection of the sample is important but is challenging in young children, and it is usual to attempt a 'clean catch' in the first instance. If this is unsuccessful, then suprapubic aspiration in those under 1 year or catheter insertion for older children may be needed.

Imaging may be required in some children to identify structural abnormalities, vesico-ureteric reflux or renal scarring, and it is advisable to consult the NICE guidelines for imaging of the various age groups. The guidelines advise different investigations for a child with a first UTI who responds well to treatment within 48 hrs and those with atypical UTIs who are very ill, with a raised creatinine, a failure to respond to antibiotics, a non-E. coli organism or if the child has recurrent UTI.

These can be summarised as follows.

- infants younger than 6 months
  - first UTI only requires a renal USS within 6 weeks and an MCUG if the USS is abnormal
  - atypical UTI requires an USS during acute infection, an MCUG after treatment and DMSA in 4–6 months after infection
- children 6 months–3 years
  - first UTI does not need imaging
  - atypical UTI requires an USS during infection and DMSA at 6 months whilst those with recurrent UTI need a renal USS at 6 weeks after infection and DMSA at 4–6 months
- in children 3 years and over
  - first UTI does not need imaging
  - atypical UTI requires an USS during infection or if a recurrent UTI then USS at 6 weeks followed by DMSA at 4–6 months is required

Treatment and management

- usually treated with oral antibiotics like cefalexin and trimethoprim, but if not tolerated parenteral antibiotics can be given initially
- antibiotic prophylaxis is controversial and is not usually advised

Renal tubular disorders

Renal tubular disorders could affect the proximal and distal tubules, the ascending limb of loop of Henle or the collecting duct.

Renal tubular acidosis (RTA)

RTA develops when the kidneys are unable to acidify the urine and occurs due to loss of either bicarbonate or hydrogen ions. There are three types of RTA:

Distal RTA (type I)

- autosomal dominant and usually mild
- autosomal recessive is usually more severe and associated with deafness

Children will present with faltering growth and renal colic due to the presence of renal stones and nephrocalcinosis. Investigations reveal hypokalaemia and a metabolic acidosis but with a urine pH over 5.5 indicating an inability to acidify the urine.

Proximal RTA (type II) is usually identified as part of a Fanconi syndrome which affects the proximal tubules causing a loss into the urine of bicarbonate, glucose and amino acids. The syndrome is usually the result of cystinosis with the intracellular accumulation of cysteine in kidneys, eyes and thyroid gland. Affected children are usually identified with faltering growth, rickets and a metabolic acidosis.

Hyperkalaemic RTA (Type IV) is due to a reduction in renal excretion of hydrogen and potassium ions and is the result of an inadequate response to aldosterone.

Bartter syndrome

The pathological abnormality in this condition is in the ascending limb of loop of Henle and affects transport of sodium, potassium and chloride ions across the renal cells.

Children commonly present with faltering growth and investigations reveal a hypokalaemic metabolic alkalosis, whilst hyponatremia from sodium loss, hypochloraemia, hypercalciuria and nephrocalcinosis may also be observed. A similar electrolyte picture is seen in children with cystic fibrosis and that is known as pseudo-Bartter syndrome.

Investigation

- plasma electrolytes and renal function
- genetic studies to identify one of associated gene mutations

Treatment and management

Correction of hypovolemia and electrolyte imbalances are the mainstay of treatment. The child will usually require lifelong supplementation of potassium, magnesium or bicarbonate.

Nephrogenic diabetes insipidus

This condition occurs as the result of renal resistance to the effects of antidiuretic hormone (ADH, vasopressin) leading to an increase in water loss through kidneys. The most common form follows an x-linked pattern of inheritance and the patient will present with polyuria and polydipsia with hypernatraemia. Details of management are found in Chapter 25 Endocrinology.

Hypertension

The normal range for blood pressure is determined by age, sex and height of the child or young person and consequently values obtained during examination should be compared to appropriate standardised tables or charts for the above parameters. Hypertension is usually diagnosed if one or the other of systolic and diastolic blood pressure is greater than the 95th percentile for age, sex and height on three or more occasions.

As a consequence of increasing incidence of obesity in childhood, there has been an increase in diagnosis of hypertension in children with a consequent long-term effect of cardiovascular and cerebrovascular disease.

PRACTICE POINT—causes of hypertension in children

- renal parenchymal disease—glomerulonephritis, reflux nephropathy, obstructive uropathy, chronic kidney disease
- renovascular disease—renal artery stenosis, renal artery thrombosis, vasculitis
- cardiovascular—coarctation of aorta
- endocrine—phaeochromocytoma, Cushing syndrome, hyperaldosteronism, congenital adrenal hyperplasia
- malignant disease—nephroblastoma, neuroblastoma, pheochromocytoma
- drug induced—corticosteroids

The problem is usually discovered incidentally in a child without symptoms but can present with headaches, visual disturbance, breathlessness or, if the hypertension is severe, encephalopathy and seizures.

Investigations

Specific investigations include:
- urea and electrolytes—for evidence of impaired renal function
- plasma renin and aldosterone

- urine catecholamines—exclude neuroblastoma and pheochromocytoma
- urine albumin/creatinine ratio—evidence of renal disease
- urine microscopy for red cell casts—evidence of renal disease
- ECG, echocardiogram
- renal USS with doppler of renal vessels

Treatment and management

Treatment depends on the age of the individual, the likely aetiology and the severity of the hypertension. Nonpharmacological interventions such as salt restriction, weight reduction and exercise are as important as medications. The aim of treatment is to reduce the blood pressure of the individual to below the 90th centile.

Pharmacological treatment includes a range of medications with different mechanisms of action and formulations and will be chosen depending on these characteristics.

First-line treatment could be with:
- calcium channel blockers—nifedipine or amlodipine—although these are contraindicated in individuals with diabetes mellitus
- ACE (angiotensin-converting enzyme) inhibitors—captopril—used in patients with chronic kidney disease
- diuretics—furosemide or hydralazine—are useful if features of fluid overload

Hypertensive emergencies are rare in children but can present with seizures, encephalopathy, focal neurological deficit or cardiac failure depending on cause. Urgent intervention is obviously required, but if intracranial pathology is suspected then lowering the blood pressure may lead to adverse consequences. Treatment should be with IV antihypertensives such as sodium nitroprusside or labetalol infusions and undertaken in an intensive care setting. It is important that the pressures are reduced at a slow rate over about 48 hours as rapid falls can produce permanent neurological sequelae such as blindness.

Phaeochromocytoma

Phaeochromocytoma arises from adrenal medulla or sympathetic chain and presents with the classical triad of episodic headache, sweating and tachycardia with 60% to 90% of patients having hypertension. The tumours are removed surgically though adequate preoperative α-adrenergic blockade must be achieved before adding the beta-receptor blockers. This approach will avoid the unopposed α-adrenergic stimulation from the catecholamines that can result in a hypertensive crisis or pulmonary oedema.

Acute glomerulonephritis

Acute glomerulonephritis usually occurs following a systemic infection with streptococcus being the most common causative organism.

Causes

- immune complex mediated glomerulonephritis
  - post infectious
  - Henoch-Schoenlein purpura or IgA vasculitis
  - systemic lupus erythematosus (SLE)
  - IgA nephropathy
  - membranoproliferative glomerulonephritis
- antiglomerular basement membrane antibody-mediated glomerulonephritis (Goodpasture syndrome)
  Children and young people will usually present with an acute onset of haematuria and periorbital or peripheral oedema. Examination will usually reveal hypertension.

Investigations

- listed in Table 20.2
- chest x-ray—to exclude cardiomegaly or pulmonary oedema
- evidence of streptococcal infection—raised ASOT. Levels rise 1 to 3 weeks after streptococcal infection, peaks around 3 to 5 weeks and falls to insignificant levels by about 6 months.
- autoantibody screen—exclude underlying cause
- renal biopsy is rarely required

Treatment and management

The treatment is aimed at addressing hypertension and the acute kidney injury although renal dialysis is rarely needed. Penicillin is given for the streptococcal infection in those with acute glomerulonephritis although it does not change the course of the disease. The overall prognosis is very good with only 1% of children developing chronic kidney disease.

Henoch-Schoenlein purpura

The condition is an IgA-mediated vasculitis and often presents after a preceding upper respiratory tract infection with the classical triad of purpura, abdominal pain and arthritis. The purpuric rash is distributed on buttocks and lower legs though occasionally it can be more generalised. Renal vasculitis is uncommon but may lead to microscopic haematuria and hypertension. The condition resolves without sequelae in most children, but a deterioration in renal function may develop at a later stage and therefore all children should be followed up for at least 6 months with checks for haematuria, proteinuria and hypertension.

IgA Nephropathy

Children may present with:
- recurrent macroscopic haematuria (usually follow a URTI)
- flank pain
- asymptomatic microscopic haematuria with or without proteinuria
- rarely with acute kidney injury and crescentic glomerulonephritis

Investigations

Plasma IgA is increased in some patients but does not correlate with severity or clinical course, but a renal biopsy is usually required and will show IgA deposits in the glomerular mesangium.

Treatment and management

Microscopic haematuria without proteinuria does not usually require further treatment. If the child presents with macroscopic haematuria and proteinuria then immunosuppression with prednisolone or azathioprine may be necessary, although 20% to 25% of patients will progress to chronic kidney disease.

Alport syndrome

This condition results from gene mutation that leads to a defect of type IV collagen and is characterized by kidney disease, hearing loss and eye abnormalities. It is inherited in an x-linked manner in 80% of individuals, and the progressive loss of renal function leads to chronic kidney disease.

Clinical Scenario

A 12-year-old girl presented with a history of tiredness and joint pain over the last few weeks. She had been passing reddish brown ('cola coloured') urine for the past couple of days. There was also reduced urine output over the past 24 hours and a headache.

On examination her BP was 156/80 mmHg. She was pale with a facial rash, peri orbital and pedal oedema and mild ascites.

The differential diagnosis would include causes of macroscopic haematuria such as postinfectious acute glomerulonephritis, nephrotic syndrome, lupus nephritis and IgA nephropathy. While acute postinfectious glomerulonephritis is a common cause of macroscopic haematuria, the presence of a facial rash and pallor would suggest lupus nephritis. The age of the child, gender, history of tiredness and joint pains could also support this diagnosis.

Investigations showed haemolytic anaemia, raised creatinine and positive ANA and double-stranded DNA. Kidney biopsy confirmed the diagnosis and she was started on immunosuppressive therapy.

Nephrotic syndrome

Idiopathic nephrotic syndrome is a characterised by heavy proteinuria, hypoalbuminemia and oedema and is usually associated with hyperlipidaemia. Congenital nephrotic syndrome appears in infancy whilst those presenting later usually have an underlying systemic disorder such as minimal change nephrotic syndrome (MCNS).

MCNS leading to nephrotic syndrome usually presents between the ages of 2–6 years and is more common in boys and Asian children. The condition is often triggered by a viral infection and usually the child will present with an episode of increasing oedema and reduced urine output. Oedema of the periorbital area, ankles and scrotum are usually identified promptly by parents. The child also might have features of hypovolaemia and infection. The loss of proteins includes immunoglobulins and complement therefore results in an increased susceptibility to infections.

Treatment and management

Initial management requires prednisolone at a dose of 60 mg/m^2/day which is given over 4 weeks followed by a reduced dose of 40 mg/m^2/day for another 4 weeks. The subsequent dose reduction is arranged over a further 4-week period, but regular reviews are needed to identify signs of relapse. A no-added-salt diet is also advised.

Potential complications

The child with nephrotic syndrome is immunosuppressed due to the loss of immunoglobulins and complement and the long-term administration of corticosteroids. Infections leading to peritonitis, cellulitis, pneumonia and severe chickenpox are all seen frequently in such children. Many children at presentation may be hypovolaemic and are at risk of thrombotic episodes, and fluid balance needs to be closely monitored.

A renal biopsy is indicated if atypical features such as steroid resistance, macroscopic haematuria, significant hypertension, persistent renal dysfunction and atypical age at onset are identified.

Only a small proportion of children will have a long-term response to treatment of the first episode and most will have relapses and remissions.

Renal calculi

The most common causes are:
- infection—proteus species most common
- metabolic—hypercalciuria most common but hyperoxaluria and cystinuria also responsible

Primary hyperoxaluria is an important genetic cause with almost half of the children developing renal failure by 5 years of age.

Common symptoms at presentations are:
- recurrent flank pain and renal colic
- UTI
- macroscopic haematuria
- dysuria and strangury suggesting bladder stones

Investigations

- plain abdominal x-ray—will show radiopaque calculi but miss small calculi (Figure 20.4)
- renal and bladder USS

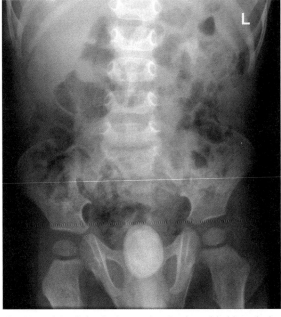

Fig. 20.4 Plain abdominal x-ray showing large bladder calculus

- electrolytes, calcium, phosphate, uric acid, vitamin D level and PTH
- urinalysis to identify raised levels of urate, oxalate and amino acids along with microbiological culture Figure 20.4

Treatment and management

Medical management includes encouraging a high fluid intake, salt restriction, potassium supplements and alkali therapy. Surgical intervention is indicated for debilitating pain and urinary obstruction, and percutaneous nephrostomy may be required as a temporary measure to relieve obstruction. Small calculi may be treated with extracorporeal lithotripsy although it is not effective when the calculi are very hard as seen with cysteine and calcium phosphate calculi. Percutaneous nephrolithotomy is preferred with larger and harder calculi.

Enuresis

Enuresis is voiding of urine due to lack of bladder control in children over 5 years of age and is classified as primary if the child has never been dry and secondary if the bed wetting starts 6 months after the child had previously been dry. The condition is mainly due to maturational delay and an organic cause is only found in less than 5% of affected children.

Nocturnal enuresis is the usual presenting problem and bladder dysfunction should be suspected if diurnal enuresis develops along with frequency and urgency. The condition is usually seen in boys with 10% of 5-year-olds and 5% of 10-year-old boys wetting the bed. Those with daytime wetting are more likely to have a pathological cause compared with those with only nocturnal wetting. Urinary tract infections, constipation and psychological reasons are all recognised causes of eneuresis.

Investigations

Children with nocturnal eneuresis alone do not require investigations whilst those with secondary enuresis or persistent daytime enuresis should have urine examination to rule out a UTI. Primary daytime wetting requires further assessment to exclude anatomical abnormalities such as ectopic ureters in girls.

Treatment and management

Once significant pathology has been excluded, management should consider behavioural modifications such as regular bladder emptying, 'lifting' the children as parents go to bed and walking them to the toilet and motivational approach with 'star charts' for younger children. Enuresis alarms—'bell and pad alarm'—are effective in children who are able to respond and safely go to the toilet in the night although the relapse rate is high on discontinuation.

Pharmacological treatment should be avoided where possible in young children and reserved for those approaching puberty where it is more effective. Oral desmopressin can be prescribed along with fluid restriction and usually leads to control of enuresis. Intranasal desmopressin should not be used for this indication as there is a recognised risk of hyponatraemia. If frequency and urgency accompany daytime incontinence, then anticholinergics such as oxybutynin may help reduce bladder instability.

IMPORTANT CLINICAL POINTS

Acute kidney injury
- prerenal causes are the commonest cause of AKI
- HUS is the most common cause of acquired AKI

Renal tubular acidosis
- present with restricted growth, polyuria, abnormal electrolyte and acid–base balance
- RTA is characterised by metabolic acidosis with normal anion gap

Nephrotic syndrome
- presents with massive proteinuria, hypoalbuminemia and oedema

- minimal change NS responds to steroids
- infection, hypovolemia and thromboembolism are main complications
- FSGS-type progress usually to renal failure

Glomerulonephritis
- postinfectious glomerulonephritis is most common cause
- present with haematuria, hypertension and AKI

Hypertension
- Consult standard tables for age, height and sex

IMPORTANT CLINICAL POINTS—cont'd

Calculi

- main types of calculi are infective and metabolic
- most common metabolic cause is hypercalciuria
- most common infective cause is proteus spp
- high fluid intake, reduced salt intake and alkali therapy are useful but definitive treatment depends on underlying cause

Eneuresis

- daytime wetting more likely to have a pathological cause
- UTI, constipation and psychological reasons can all cause eneuresis

Further Reading

Acute kidney injury: prevention, detection and management. NICE guideline [NG148]. Published December 2019.

Urinary tract infection in under 16s: diagnosis and management. Clinical guideline [CG54]. Published August 2007. Updated October 2018.

Bedwetting in under 19s. NICE Clinical guideline [CG111]. Published October 2010.

Singh C, et al.: Fifteen-minute consultation: the child with systemic arterial hypertension. *Arch Dis Child Educ Pract Ed.* 2017;102:2–7

Chapter | 21 |

Haematology

Subarna Chakravorty

After reading this chapter you should be able to:
- assess, diagnose and manage children with anaemia including bone marrow failure
- understand the risks, benefits and precautions involved in blood transfusion
- assess, diagnose and manage coagulation disorders, hypercoagulable states, purpura and bruising
- assess, diagnose and manage neutropenia

A general principle in all paediatric haematology is the need to refer to age-specific normal ranges. Children with haematological problems can present with a variety of symptoms:
- pallor
- bruising or bleeding
- recurrent infections

Anaemia

Anaemia is defined as a reduction in the haemoglobin concentration below the normal reference ranges for their age and in healthy children, haemoglobin concentrations reach adult levels by approximately 5 years of age. A normal response to anaemia is to increase bone marrow activity that leads to an increase in circulating reticulocytes. These red cells have retained their ribonucleic acid and can be counted separately on standard automated counters and can be recognised on blood films as polychromatic cells.

An understanding of the possible aetiology of anaemia helps during the evaluation of the anaemic patient and the causes can be broadly divided into impaired red cell production, ineffective erythropoiesis and increased red cell destruction (Table 21.1).

Anaemia presents with clinical features such as pallor, fatigue and, in extreme situations, cardiac failure and death. Formal examination would confirm pallor, may detect jaundice suggesting increased red cell haemolysis and identify dysmorphic features indicative of bone marrow failure syndromes.

Investigations

A full blood count, blood film assessment and reticulocyte count will all provide important diagnostic clues in the initial assessment of anaemia. The mean cell volume (MCV) and mean cell haemoglobin (MCH) can help define various aetiological subtypes of anaemia. Other important tests include liver function tests to detect bilirubin levels which may indicate haemolysis, direct antiglobulin test that detects attached antibodies on red cells and haemoglobin electrophoresis to identify abnormal haemoglobin (Figure 21.1)

The reticulocyte count will offer information on the ability of the marrow to respond to a pathological insult (Figure 21.2).

Impaired red cell production
Iron deficiency anaemia

Iron deficiency anaemia is the most frequent cause of anaemia in childhood and is the result of lack of iron in the diet. It may also reflect chronic blood loss, and appropriate investigations to exclude inflammatory bowel disease should be considered. The effects of anaemia are well recognised and include weakness, fatigue, palpitations and collapse. Less common effects of iron deficiency are the epithelial changes seen in the mouth and an attendant drive to eat nonnutritional substances such as soil and clay—pica. Chronic iron deficiency can also impair growth and intellectual development.

Table 21.1 Aetiology of anaemia

Physiological dysfunction	Associated condition
Impaired red cell production	bone marrow failure syndromes (Fanconi anaemia, Diamond Blackfan anaemia) acquired aplastic anaemia transient aplasia due to parvovirus infection bone marrow infiltration with malignancy renal failure leading to reduced erythropoietin haematinic deficiency hypothyroidism chronic inflammation
Ineffective erythropoiesis	thalassaemia sideroblastic anaemia vitamin B_{12} and folic acid deficiency
Increased red cell destruction or loss	congenital haemolytic anaemias haemoglobinopathy autoimmune or alloimmune haemolytic anaemia paroxysmal nocturnal haemoglobinuria (PNH) chronic or acute blood loss

Investigations

An initial full blood count and serum ferritin would likely identify an iron deficiency. It is important to remember, however, that ferritin is also an acute phase reactant and can rise to within the normal range during intercurrent infection. Iron deficiency may be associated with either raised or reduced platelet counts. Poikilocytosis describes the variation in shape of red cells and includes 'target cells' and 'pencil cells' (hypochromic elliptocytes found in iron deficiency).

Treatment and management

Oral iron supplementation and improving the diet are often sufficient. In rare situations where the child is intolerant of oral iron, they may benefit from intravenous iron infusion (Table 21.2).

Relevant pharmacological agents used

All oral ferrous preparations are similar in their efficacy and the choice is usually dictated by palatability and cost. Standard daily doses as listed in the BNFc should lead to an expected rise of the haemoglobin concentration of about 20 g/litre over a 3 to 4 week period, and dosing should continue for a further 3 months to replace iron stores. Term babies are born with adequate iron stores but need to maintain an adequate dietary intake. Iron in breast milk is well absorbed but the iron in artificial or cows' milk is less so, although artificial

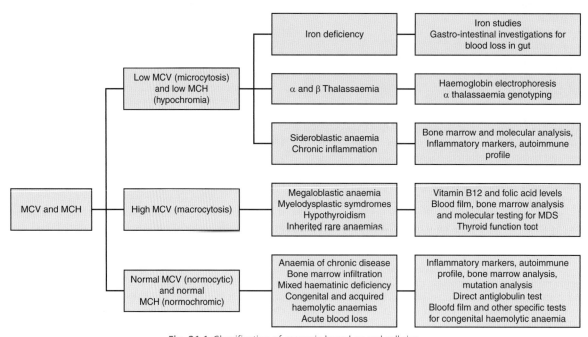

Fig. 21.1 Classification of anaemia based on red cell size.

milks have supplementation. Infants with a poor diet may become anaemic in the second year of life and those with unusual diets may present with anaemia when 3 or 4 years old. Gastrointestinal side effects of oral iron are well recognised and include constipation and production of dark brown or black stools whilst on medication.

Bone marrow failure

Children who present with bone marrow failure may have an underlying congenital cause or may develop the failure due to an inflammatory response, infection or to some environmental insult such as a reaction to medication or chemical exposure. The patient will present with the consequences of the pancytopenia—pallor, exhaustion, severe infection, bruising and petechiae. The causes of the bone marrow failure may be inherited or acquired. Those with inherited bone marrow failure may have dysmorphic features such as skeletal abnormalities, short stature and predisposition to malignancies. A full history will seek information on relevant family history, recent infections and exposure to drugs or potential environmental toxins such as benzene.

Investigations

The full blood count will identify the pancytopenia and a low reticulocyte count will be indicative of the reduced red cell production. Bone marrow aspirate and trephine examination may show a reduced cellularity whilst cytogenetic and molecular testing will look for chromosomal fragility and known genetic mutations which are associated with congenital bone marrow failure syndromes. Tissue typing of siblings is a mandatory consideration at the outset (Table 21.2).

Inherited bone marrow failure syndromes
Fanconi anaemia

Fanconi anaemia is rare but more common in populations with higher rates of consanguinity. It is characterised by increased chromosomal fragility and is caused by mutations in at least 22 genes involved in DNA repair. Clinical severity in Fanconi anaemia is variable, and the age at presentation may vary from infancy to adulthood. Congenital malformations are common presenting features:

- short stature
- absent or hypoplastic thumbs
- absent or hypoplastic radii
- café-au-lait spots
- structural heart defects
- structural kidney defects

Only a small number of children with Fanconi anaemia are identified at an early age and many may first present with bone marrow failure due to myelodysplasia or acute myeloid leukaemia. Children with the condition require lifelong

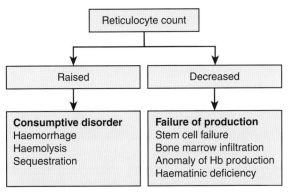

Fig. 21.2 Contribution of reticulocyte count to understanding of response of bone marrow to insult.

Table 21.2 Comparative table of FBC findings in some causes of anaemia in a 3-year-old child				
	Fe deficiency anaemia	Bone marrow failure	Beta thalassaemia	Normal range
Hb	68	68	68	110–140 g/l
MCV	66	87	64	70–86 fl
MCH	22	23	15	23–31 pg
RBC	2.95	3.9	6.8	4.2–6.5 x 10^{12}/l
WCC	4.3	3	6	5.0–12.0 x 10^9/l
Platelets	504	99	354	150–450 x 10^9 /l
Reticulocytes (absolute)	Low/raised or normal	Low	low	50–150 x 10^9/l
Ferritin	low	Normal	high	12–200 µg/l

screening for epithelial tumours, especially in the head and neck, gut and genital areas. Bone marrow transplant improves the aplasia and reduces the risk of myeloid malignancy but not of epithelial malignancies (Table 21.3).

Diamond Blackfan anaemia

This is a congenital erythroid aplasia that is usually identified in infancy. Affected children present with a macrocytic, normochromic anaemia with a low reticulocyte count. Bone marrow aspirate shows an absence of erythroid precursors but normal white cell and platelet precursors. They have congenital malformations of the craniofacial, eye, cardiac and thumb structures and have an increased risk of developing malignancies such as acute myeloid leukaemia, myelodysplastic disease and solid tumours.

Schwachman-Diamond syndrome

This is inherited as an autosomal recessive disorder and is associated with bone marrow failure, exocrine pancreatic insufficiency and skeletal abnormalities that generally present in infancy. The condition often presents in infancy or early childhood with a pancytopenia, short stature and steatorrhea due to exocrine pancreatic dysfunction. Loose, foul-smelling stools and an anaemia should always raise the possibility of this condition.

Acquired bone marrow failure
Aplastic anaemia

Aplastic anaemia is rare and the patient presents with the consequences of a pancytopenia. A bone marrow aspirate and trephine will confirm the absence of the haemopoietic precursor cells and exclude marrow infiltrative conditions. Most presentations of acquired aplastic anaemia are driven by autoimmune aetiologies and therefore many children will not have an identified cause for their disease. However, some drugs (including chloramphenicol, phenylbutazone, sulphonamides, antithyroid drugs and anticancer drugs), chemicals (benzene), viruses (parvovirus, human herpesvirus 6) or antigens have all been implicated.

Treatment and management

Unless treated, children generally succumb to complications associated with bone marrow failure, such as sepsis, bleeding or malignancy, and treatment is aimed at mitigating these complications. Exposure to blood products should be kept to a minimum to prevent development of red cell alloantibodies or HLA-related antibodies that reduce the effectiveness of future transfusions. Bone marrow transplant is recommended in those with available donors at the earliest opportunity. The transplant procedure requires the harvesting of

cells from a donor and infusion into the recipient. The donor is usually a full sibling (matched donor) or an individual from a donor panel (matched unrelated donor—MUD). Severe acquired aplastic anaemia can be cured by bone marrow transplant, and outcomes of unrelated donor transplants are currently almost comparable to those with sibling donors. In the absence of available donors, long-term immunosuppression helps sustain remission.

Haemoglobin disorders
Thalassaemia

Thalassemia occurs as a result of mutations in genes encoding α and β globin proteins (*HBA* and *HBB*, respectively) that make up the tetrameric haemoglobin A molecule. This results in reduced or absent production of the respective proteins required in the haemoglobin chain. Consequently, there is an imbalance between the numbers of α and β globin proteins available and these then combine to produce unstable combinations (Table 21.3).

α-thalassaemia

This condition develops when deletions or mutations occur in the alpha globin genes (four genes in total, two from each parental allele) which then result in reduced production of

Table 21.3 Haemoglobin contribution to various haemoglobinopathies

Status	Haemoglobin
normal adult Hb	HbA (90%); HbA$_2$ (less than 3.5%)
foetal Hb	HbF
alpha-thalassaemia major	HbBarts; HbH
beta-thalassaemia trait	HbA$_2$ (greater than 3.5%) and HbA (90%)
transfusion dependent beta-thalassaemia	variable proportions of transfused HbA; some HbA2; variable proportion of HbF
sickle cell trait	HbS (25%–40%); HbA (50%–60%)
sickle cell disease	HbS (80%–95%); HbF (5%–10%)
HbC disease	HbC (90%–95%); HbF (5%–10%)
HbSC disease	HbS (40%–50%); HbC (40%–50%)

the alpha globin protein. As there are four genes contributing to the total alpha globin content of an individual, deletion of one or two genes (heterozygous state) result in no clinical consequence, as the other two remaining genes upregulate their alpha globin protein production. Deletion of three alpha globin genes causes the clinical syndrome of Haemoglobin (Hb) H disease. Deletion of all four alpha genes is known as α-thalassaemia major or Haemoglobin Barts hydrops fetalis and is incompatible with life as it does not produce any normal haemoglobin to sustain foetal and postnatal life. This type of thalassaemia mainly affects individuals who are of Southeast Asian descent.

Many children with alpha-thalassaemia trait may be asymptomatic or identified by the incidental finding of a microcytic anaemia. Hepatosplenomegaly is not usually present although the spleen may be enlarged on ultrasound assessment. Those with Hb Barts often present in utero with hydrops fetalis and rarely survive beyond the first few weeks of life.

Treatment and management

Treatment depends on the number of deleted alpha globin genes. One or two gene deletion alpha thalassaemia trait does not need any treatment. Three gene deletion state (HbH) can need occasional transfusions during intercurrent illness, pregnancy, puberty or surgery.

HbH

HbH is the haemoglobin formed when three out of four alpha globin genes are deleted, leading to the production of significantly lower amounts of alpha globin, leaving the excess beta globin chains to form beta tetramers (also known as Haemoglobin H). HbH is unstable and leads to ineffective erythropoiesis in marrow. However, due to the production of alpha globin from the single unmutated alpha globin gene, small amounts of HbA ($\alpha_2 \beta_2$) are produced and so patients may not be transfusion dependent.

Hb Barts Hydrops fetalis

If all four alpha globin genes are mutated and no alpha globin is produced at all. This leads to the production of beta globin chains, or other beta-like globin proteins such as gamma globin. These excess gamma globin chains tend to form gamma tetramers (Hb Barts) which are very unstable, leading to ineffective foetal erythropoiesis and severe in utero anaemia and placental disease.

β-thalassaemia

The homozygous beta globin mutation results in underproduction of the beta globin protein that results in the excess alpha globin to form unstable alpha globin tetramers. These structures will denature and precipitate within early red cell precursors in the bone marrow and so lead to ineffective erythropoiesis, severe anaemia and transfusion dependence. There are more than 200 pathological mutations in the beta globin gene which results in β-thalassaemia of variable severity. It is now classified into three subgroups:

- transfusion dependent—homozygous for significant mutation
- transfusion independent
- beta thalassaemia trait—one mutated and one normal beta globin gene

Some individuals have a non-transfusion-independent thalassaemia (previously known as beta thalassaemia intermedia) and are homozygous for mild mutations. They may only require intermittent transfusions during puberty, pregnancy or intercurrent illness. Those with the transfusion-dependent condition may need transfusions as early as 3 months of age and remain transfusion dependent for life, or until they receive curative treatments. The condition is more common in individuals who are of Mediterranean (Greek, Italian and Middle Eastern), Asian or African descent.

Pregnant women who are identified as being at high risk of being a carrier of thalassaemia are offered screening during pregnancy as part of their routine blood tests. The direct assessment of at-risk newborn babies is not undertaken just after birth, as the test is unreliable due to the presence of high amounts of fetal haemoglobin, particularly in preterm infants. Infants must be over 6 months old before the absence or presence of beta-chains can be assessed.

Children with transfusion-dependent β-thalassaemia will be identified from an early age due to a pallor and likely breathlessness on feeding. Anaemia and jaundice are common problems and in the absence of adequate transfusions, the children will develop classical skeletal abnormalities as multiple marrow sites become involved in extramedullary hemopoiesis. Facial deformity is well recognised in under-transfused children as they develop frontal bossing, malar prominence, maxillary overgrowth and dental problems. Other bony sites will also be recruited including spine, skull and pelvis, and many children suffer from bone pain. The changes in the skull give a 'hair on end' appearance on a plain x-ray (Figure 21.3). Bone expansion may lead to some degree of thinning, and the affected individuals are prone to fractures with even slight trauma. Many of these bony changes can be minimised by transfusion regimes particularly if started early in life. Extramedullary haematopoiesis is common in liver and spleen and affected children will often have hepato- and splenomegaly.

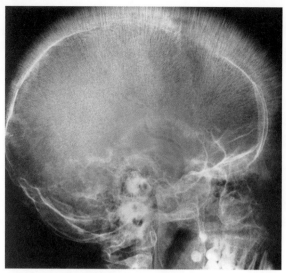

Fig. 21.3 Skull radiograph of 14-year-old boy with β-thalassaemia showing 'hair-on-end' appearance indicating extramedullary hemopoiesis. (Image used with permission from Comprehensive Radiographic Pathology. 7th Ed. Johnson NM; Eisenberg RJ. Ch 9. Elsevier Inc.)

Investigations

A hypochromic, microcytic anaemia is common to both thalassaemia and iron deficiency and consequently most laboratories require ferritin to be assessed in the first instance to exclude iron deficiency. Haemoglobin electrophoresis and genetic testing can then be undertaken to confirm the diagnosis. In children with β thalassaemia, the production of HbF and HbA$_2$ is increased, leading to higher circulating levels of these haemoglobins and can be measured by haemoglobin electrophoresis.

Treatment and management

Treatment of β-thalassaemia major, or transfusion-dependent thalassaemia, includes two to four weekly red cell transfusions to suppress the endogenous ineffective erythropoiesis, allowing children to achieve their full growth and developmental potential. Treatment programmes providing regular transfusions will lead to iron overload in the patient and so all such programmes will also include the administration of iron chelating therapy which may be sufficient to normalise tissue levels of iron. Regular ferritin assessment is an important part of the monitoring process. Bone marrow transplantation from a sibling donor is a curative treatment option. Gene therapy can allow a transfusion-dependent patient to become transfusion independent. This procedure is currently undergoing clinical trials.

Potential complications

Iron has a toxic effect and is deposited in liver, heart, brain and endocrine organs, leading to organ failure. Cardiac iron overload and death from cardiac failure is the commonest outcome in transfusion-dependent patients without chelation. Growth and pubertal failure, endocrinopathy and bone and joint damage are also common in children who are not adequately transfused or chelated. Some children may develop type 1 diabetes mellitus if iron is deposited in pancreatic cells.

Relevant pharmacological agents used

Deferoxamine is a chelating agent which binds to iron and facilitates excretion. It is given as a subcutaneous infusion over 8–12 hours between 3–7 times per week. Oral iron chelators deferasirox and deferiprone are also licensed for use in children and are often the preferred chelators due to their ease of administration.

Increased red cell destruction or loss
Haemolytic anaemia

Patients may present with jaundice and pallor. Examination will reveal icteric sclera and splenomegaly when this is the main site of red cell destruction.

Investigations

The history and examination will offer direction to the appropriate investigations needed, but the initial investigations would include full blood count and film, reticulocyte count, haematinics and liver function tests.

Treatment and management

Treatment include supportive measures such as red cell transfusions, folic acid supplementation and, in selected children, splenectomy. Treatment of autoimmune haemolytic anaemia includes immunosuppression by corticosteroids and supportive measures including folic acid.

Specific haemolytic conditions
Spherocytosis

Hereditary spherocytosis occurs due to mutations in genes encoding red cell cytoskeletal proteins and is mostly inherited in an autosomal dominant manner. Deficiencies in cytoskeletal proteins cause the red cells to adopt a spherical shape leading to premature cell breakdown in the spleen. The condition is characterised by jaundice and splenomegaly with gallstones also being a common finding. Viral infections

Table 21.4 Causes of haemolysis

Intravascular haemolysis	Extravascular haemolysis (haemolysis in reticulo-endothelial cells of the liver and spleen)
paroxysmal nocturnal haemoglobinuria (PNH)	RBC enzyme defects
infections	glucose-6-phosphate dehydrogenase deficiency
C difficile	
meningococcus	
malaria	pyruvate kinase deficiency
burns—due to endothelial damage	membrane defects
	hereditary spherocytosis
drugs	hereditary elliptocytosis
red cell fragmentation	sickle cell disease
haemolytic uraemic syndrome	autoimmune
disseminated intravascular coagulation	malaria
	drugs
mechanical from cardiac valve	
sickle cell disease	

can exacerbate haemolysis, producing an acute haemolytic crisis. Infection with haemotrophic viruses such as parvovirus B19 may result in an aplastic crisis in which the rate of erythropoiesis is reduced, leading to anaemia and reticulocytopaenia. Folate deficiency may also lead to a failure of erythropoiesis but is rare in children with normal diets.

Management consists of appropriate counselling, dietary supplementation with folic acid and occasional red-cell transfusions in the event of significant anaemia especially following in aplastic crisis. Splenectomy is curative and is indicated in patients with significant haemolysis and gallstones although it is advisable to wait until patients are over 6 years of age before surgery is performed. Those who are planned for splenectomy need to have had vaccination against encapsulated bacteria, including pneumococcus and meningococcus prior to surgery. Annual influenza vaccination is recommended and those who have had a splenectomy are advised to remain on penicillin prophylaxis for life.

Autoimmune haemolytic anaemia

In this condition, the anaemia develops due to the presence of autoantibodies that attach to the red cells and lead to extravascular haemolysis and haemoglobinuria (Figure 21.4). The problem may be seen in individuals who already have a diagnosis of systemic lupus erythematosus, scleroderma, juvenile idiopathic arthritis, dermatomyositis or autoimmune hepatitis but can also

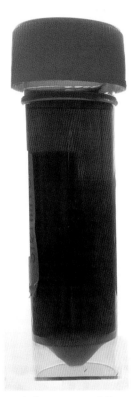

Fig. 21.4 Urine sample from 10-year-old boy with G6PD deficiency who had received rasburicase. The urine is discoloured but translucent.

occur in the absence of other autoimmune conditions. Infection with *Mycoplasma pneumoniae* or Epstein-Barr virus (EBV) can lead to the generation of haemolytic autoantibodies.

Patients with glucose-6-phosphate dehydrogenase (G6PD) deficiency can experience acute haemolysis when given drugs such as rasburicase, dapsone and ciprofloxacin. The condition demonstrates x-linked inheritance.

Paroxysmal nocturnal haemoglobinuria (PNH)

PNH is an acquired disorder leading to intravascular red cell haemolysis although it is very rare in childhood. Patients present with tiredness, jaundice, abdominal pain and nocturnal haemoglobinuria. Low-grade anaemia is evident and is interspersed with acute episodes of intravascular haemolysis occurring at night or during the day resulting in haemoglobinuria. Venous thrombosis and bone marrow aplasia are other known but rare features of PNH.

CLINICAL SCENARIO

A 4-year-old boy was admitted with a 3 day history of lethargy and two episodes of passing dark urine. He had recently seen his GP with dysuria and frequency, and a urine sample was positive to nitrites and protein. He had been started on trimethoprim but had not been able to tolerate the preparation and had therefore been given nitrofurantoin. Both parents were born in Cyprus.

On examination he was well grown, afebrile but pale with mildly icteric sclera. His heart rate was 100 bpm and his BP was 80/60. Examination of the abdomen identified a 1 cm liver and no palpable spleen. The rest of the examination was normal.

Initial blood results showed a haemoglobin of 63 g/l, WCC 18 x 10^9/l, platelets 178 x 10^9/l and a raised reticulocyte count of 600 x 10^9/l (normal 50–150 10^9/l). Bilirubin was 158 μmol/l.

The clinical picture and blood results suggested acute haemolysis. The relevant features in the history were the recent administration of nitrofurantoin and that both parents were from Cyprus. A diagnosis of G6PD deficiency was proposed and confirmed on laboratory assay.

The boy needed a blood transfusion but made a full recovery. Both father and a brother were then tested for G6PD deficiency, as it is an x-linked disorder, and the family were educated on avoidance of foods and drugs that could precipitate a haemolytic episode.

Sickle cell disease

Sickle cell disease (SCD) occurs due to the formation of a functionally pathological β-globin protein. Haemoglobin (Hb)S occurs due to a point mutation in the *HBB* gene and, in conditions of intracellular hypoxia, acidosis or dehydration, tends to polymerise and precipitate within the red cell cytosol as long filaments, damaging the cell membrane and changing the red cell to a crescent or 'sickle' shape. HbS polymerisation is initially reversible and cells can return to the normal biconcave shape. However, some cells become irreversibly 'sickled' and can then become lodged in small capillaries, leading to veno-occlusive disease, tissue ischaemia and further sickling. The tissue ischaemia leads to:

- haemolysis
- severe debilitating pain
- hyposplenism due to splenic ischaemia and infarction
- chronic organ failure

The most frequent disorders which are characterised by sickling are homozygous HbSS, compound heterozygous HbSC or HbS/beta thalassaemia. Sickle cell disease is screened at birth in the UK as part of the newborn screening programme.

Clinical features

Sickle cell diseases are seen most commonly in people of African descent but are also seen in people from the Mediterranean, Middle East and parts of India. The acute painful, vaso-occlusive events (VOE) occur most frequently in bones, lungs and spleen. Large vessel vasculopathy in intracerebral arteries brain may result in acute ischaemic strokes. Chronic dactylitis may lead to digits of variable length. Sequestration 'crises' represent sickling within the spleen or liver and the pooling of blood leading to severe exacerbation of the anaemia. Acute chest syndrome is the most common cause of death. Other features include aplastic crises and priapism. Splenic infarction consequent on sickling leads to a reduction in splenic size and function and increased risk of overwhelming sepsis from encapsulated bacteria.

Investigations

The initial diagnosis is based on haemoglobin electrophoresis which will identify the aberrant haemoglobin (Table 21.3).

PRACTICE POINT—investigations needed for an acute vaso-occlusive episode

- FBC
- reticulocyte count
- U+Es/creatinine
- liver function tests
- tests for evidence of infection

Treatment and management of acute vaso-occlusive episodes

Prompt assessment is required to identify clinical complications such as acute chest syndrome or splenic sequestration and to instigate prompt and appropriate treatment.

Presentation of acute vaso-occlusive episodes

- fever
- significant pain (often bone)
- pallor
- dyspnoea

Presentation of acute chest syndrome

- chest pain
- fever
- cough with or without wheeze
- respiratory distress
- hypoxia
- CXR abnormalities

Presentation of acute sickle sequestration (usually spleen) leading to venous drainage obstruction

- rapid increase in spleen size
- abdominal pain
- symptomatic anaemia
- hypovolaemic shock

Priapism—blockage of venous drainage

- pain
- penile erection

Aplastic crisis—usually caused by infection with Parvovirus B19

- symptomatic anaemia
- not jaundiced
- possible signs of parvovirus B19 infection (fever, red cheeks)
- anaemia
- reduced reticulocytes

PRACTICE POINT—management of acute sickle cell vaso-occlusive episodes

- ensure airway and circulatory stability
- supplemental, high flow oxygen—keep O_2 saturations above 95%
- prompt and adequate analgesia—may require parenteral opiates
- treatment of any infections
- ensure patient is hydrated—encourage oral fluids wherever feasible
- avoid hyperhydration presenting with chest symptoms as that can lead to fluid overload and respiratory failure
- ensure patient is warm—particular attention to peripheries

Treatment and management of chronic problems

Children with sickle cell disease are at high risk of infections with encapsulated bacteria (Pneumococcus, Streptococcus, Haemophilus, Salmonella spp). In addition to the usual childhood vaccinations, additional vaccination with Meningitis ACWY vaccine is recommended for those under one, and the 23-valent polysaccharide pneumococcal vaccine (Pneumovax) is given at age two and five and then yearly thereafter. Annual influenza vaccination is recommended at all ages.

Penicillin prophylaxis, stroke surveillance, additional vaccinations, easy access to hydroxycarbamide and blood transfusions and expert management of surgery and pregnancy are the mainstay of treatment. New drugs addressing the pathophysiology of SCD are currently in development worldwide. Bone marrow transplant is used for children with severe disease and can be curative but is not widely available due to its cost and the lack of suitable donors. Gene therapy is currently under early phase trials and has shown curative promise.

SCD is part of the national newborn screening programme, and children identified with this condition are commenced on penicillin prophylaxis to prevent deaths from encapsulated bacterial sepsis. In countries with good quality publicly funded medical care, most children born with SCD are expected to survive to adulthood. Unfortunately, this is not the case in resource-poor countries, resulting in the death of the majority of SCD children in childhood.

Important sequelae

The consequences of severe vaso-occlusive disease are extensive and potentially life threatening. Stokes, avascular necrosis of bones and retinopathy are all recognised complications of sickle cell disease and all will have major impact on the growth and development of the child.

CLINICAL SCENARIO

A 4-year-old girl presented with cough, fever and generalised abdominal pain for 2 days. She was diagnosed with HbSC sickle cell disease by neonatal screening.

On examination she was clearly in distress, her temp was 38.1°C, heart rate 110 bpm, BP 100/70 and her oxygen saturations were 90% in air. She had a respiratory rate of 40 and extensive crackles were heard at the right base. Examination of her abdomen revealed tenderness over the liver which was enlarged to 2 cm. There was a 3 cm splenomegaly. There was no evidence of guarding of the abdomen.

Initial bloods results showed a haemoglobin of 71 g/l, WCC 22 x 10^9/l with a neutrophilia, platelets 420 x 10^9/l and a raised CRP. A chest x-ray showed right lower lobe consolidation without effusion.

The clinical impression was that she had an acute chest syndrome secondary to a lobar pneumonia but there was a suggestion that she was developing acute sickle sequestration.

She had already been started on high flow oxygen but clearly needed analgesia and was therefore given intranasal opiate with effect. Regular pain relief with appropriate doses of paracetamol, ibuprofen and an oral opiate was initiated. Intravenous access was established and IV antibiotics given. Maintenance fluids only were given intravenously but with frequent reviews to ensure she was not given excessive amounts of fluid. Full blood count was repeated at 4 hours to assess any potential fall in haemoglobin in view of a possible sequestration. She made a full recovery but was in hospital for 8 days.

Transfusion of blood products

Blood products are used in many areas of clinical practice allowing many aspects of patient care and management to be undertaken. Donated whole blood is separated into the constituent cellular (red cells, platelets, white cells) and plasma components (fresh frozen plasma, cryoprecipitate and cryo-supernatant). Several national and international guidelines are in place to ensure appropriate products in the right doses are used.

The transfusion of blood products constitutes one of the most risk-prone aspects of patient care due to the harm caused to the patient if the wrong blood product is given. Hence stringent rules are required whenever the administration of blood products is considered. These rules must be in place before any prescription and administration of blood products is made and the clinician must be aware of their own responsibilities in the decision to administer any such products.

PRACTICE POINT—principles of administration of blood products

- robust indications for administration
- careful identification of patient in need of product
- samples from patient fully labelled with clear identification criteria
- blood products crossed checked with patient ID in laboratory
- blood products collected and cross checked by appropriately trained staff
- blood products checked by trained staff before administration
- patient identity checked by trained staff before administration
- full documentation of blood product details recorded in patient notes
- detailed record of any adverse events

PRACTICE POINT—adverse effects of transfusion

Immediate

- febrile transfusion reaction due to
  - cytokines from white cells present in red cell or platelet transfusion components (rare with leuco-depleted blood products)
- haemolytic transfusion reaction
  - incompatible blood group
- bacterial infection

- volume overload
- air embolus
- transfusion-associated lung injury

Delayed

- haemolytic transfusion reaction
  - red cell antigens other than ABO
- post-transfusion purpura
- pathogen transmission of viruses
- transfusion associated graft versus host disease
- transfusional haemosiderosis (iron deposition with multiple transfusions)

PRACTICE POINT—management of acute transfusion reaction

Reactions to blood products usually start shortly after the start of transfusion
- depending on severity either stop or slow infusion
- send samples to transfusion laboratory for further investigation
- return transfusion bag to laboratory for further assessment
- monitor patient closely for development of anaphylaxis
- in case of acute haemolytic transfusion reaction, patients may develop renal failure
- bacterial infection from infected blood products may result in septic shock—patient will need antibiotics, fluids and close monitoring for complications
- all significant transfusion reactions are reportable in the UK to the 'Serious Hazards of Transfusion' database

Coagulation disorders

Coagulation is the process by which bleeding from vascular injury is stemmed by the formation of a protein mesh containing fibrin strands, platelets and red cells. In the nontraumatic environment, there is a balance between circulating proteins which precipitate coagulation ('procoagulants') and those which remove unwanted clots ('anticoagulants').

The process of clot formation is usually described as a series of reactions involving coagulation factors, cofactors, calcium ions and phospholipids. The endpoint of the coagulation is the generation of thrombin, and this occurs as a result of a large number of enzymatic reactions which are orchestrated by both positive and negative feedback loops. The traditional view of the blood coagulation pathway was a 'cascade' model of reactions in distinct 'intrinsic' and 'extrinsic' pathways. This has now been replaced by a 'cellular model' with three main components of clot formation:

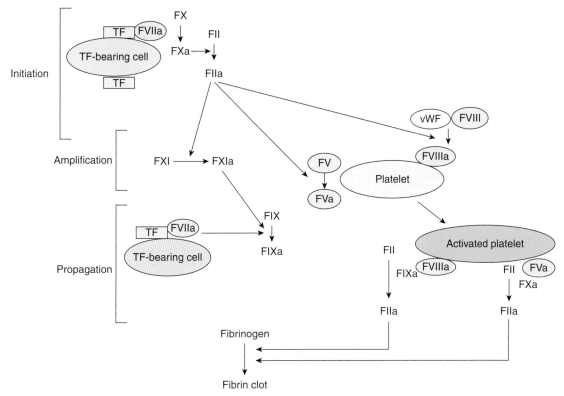

Fig. 21.5 Cell-based coagulation model with an initiation phase triggered by vascular injury and tissue factor (TF) exposure, leading to small amounts of thrombin formation, leading to platelet activation and subsequent amplification and propagation of fibrin (clot) formation. (Image use with permission Illustrated Textbook of Paediatrics. Ed. Lissauer T, Carroll W. 6th edition. Chapter 23. Chakraborthy S Elsevier Ltd.)

- initiation
- amplification
- propagation

The model (Figure 21.5) is based on more recent understanding of the coagulation process. At the same time as the coagulation reaction, there is continuous negative feedback from anticoagulant factors to limit the extent to which the coagulation factors remain activated. This, and enzymatic degradation of thrombin, ensures that hemostasis is maintained at all times. The following factors are produced in the liver—I (fibrinogen), II (prothrombin), VII, IX and X.

Clot formation is balanced by anticoagulation activity which is provided by the naturally occurring Protein C and its cofactor Protein S. This protein is activated by thrombin and, through a negative feedback mechanism, inactivates activated FV and activated FVIII and so limits clot extension. Thrombin also generates plasmin that can lyse fibrin strands and the activation of antithrombin, a naturally occurring anticoagulant protease which results in the inactivation of thrombin and other 'intrinsic pathway' factors.

Investigations

Investigation of bleeding disorders starts with a thorough clinical and family history and an initial coagulation screen comprising prothrombin time (PT) and the activated partial thromboplastin time (aPTT) (Table 21.5).

Prothrombin time

PT is a screening test that measures the ability of blood to coagulate and specifically examines coagulation factors II, V, VII, X, also known as the extrinsic and common pathway factors.

Causes of prolonged PT:
- vitamin K deficiency
- warfarin therapy
- liver disease (reduced production of factors)
- DIC (disseminated intravascular coagulation)—consumption of coagulation factors
- factor II, V, VII, X deficiency
- hyperfibrinogenaemia

Activated partial thromboplastin time

This result reflects the effectiveness of the coagulation factors in the intrinsic and common pathways—namely factors I (fibrinogen), II (prothrombin), V, VIII, IX, X, XI and XII.

The test is used to:
- assess unexplained bruising and bleeding
- diagnose disseminated intravascular coagulation (DIC)
- monitor clotting response to unfractionated heparin (but not low molecular weight heparin LMW)
Causes of prolonged aPTT
- Haemophilia A or B
- von Willibrand Disease
- heparin
- DIC (consumption of coagulation factors)

Thrombin Time

This reflects the effectiveness of the conversion of fibrinogen to fibrin along with platelet effectiveness but is not usually included in the initial coagulation screen.

Causes of prolonged TT:
- heparin (fractionated and LMW)
- liver disease (reduced production of factors)
- dysfibrinogenaemia
- DIC

Fibrinogen levels

The levels indicate a consumptive process and low levels are caused by:
- DIC (consumption of coagulation factors)
- liver disease (reduced production of factors)

D-dimers

These are degradation products of fibrin and are elevated in:
- venous thrombotic disease
- DIC
- liver disease
- renal vein thrombosis
- pulmonary embolus

Relevant pharmacological agents used

Heparin enhances the proteolytic activity of antithrombin against FXa and thrombin by several thousand-fold leading to the reduction of clot formation. Standard (unfractionated) heparin has a rapid onset of action but a short duration of action whilst low molecular weight heparin has longer half-life. Standard heparin may be preferred if the clinical situation anticipates the need for a rapid termination of effect otherwise of protamine sulphate is a specific antidote to heparin and can be used if required.

Warfarin antagonises the effect of vitamin K and takes 48 to 72 hours for full anticoagulant effect to develop. Its use should be avoided in hepatic disease. If major bleed occurs in a patient on warfarin then the drug should be stopped and a dose of IV vitamin K given slowly along with prothrombin complex concentrate or fresh frozen plasma. Such problems should be discussed with a haematologist and the patient monitored with regular INR result.

Bleeding disorders

Gene mutations leading to aberrant procoagulant factors cause haemophilia whilst those leading to abnormal anticoagulant proteins lead to thrombophilia.

The major abnormalities of clotting include:
- Inherited
  - haemophilia A—factor VIII deficiency
  - haemophilia B—factor IX deficiency
  - von Willibrand disease
- Acquired
  - disseminated intravascular coagulation

Haemophilias

Haemophilia is caused by mutations in the genes encoding FVIII (leading to haemophilia A—incidence of 1:5000) and FIX (leading to haemophilia B—incidence of 1:30,000), resulting in reduced or absent production of the necessary protein. Both these genes are located

Table 21.5 Interpretation of results of clotting screen		
	PT normal	**PT prolonged**
aPTT normal	normal clotting screen rare coagulation defects such as FXIII deficiency or dysfibrinogenaemia and 50% patients with von Willebrand disease	vitamin K deficiency warfarin therapy liver disease (reduced production of factors) antiphospholipid antibodies
aPTT prolonged	Haemophilia A or B von Willibrand Disease (50% of individuals) heparin therapy	DIC (consumption of coagulation factors) deficiency of extrinsic factors

on the X chromosome; therefore, males are affected and women are carriers in the heterozygote state. Both conditions result in the reduction of the relevant clotting factor and depending on the exact nature of the mutation, the child is left with little or no protein activity. Both conditions are divided into categories depending upon the extent of factor deficiency compared with a normal value:

- severe: <1%
- moderate: 1%–5%
- mild: >5%

The inability to complete clot formation leads to significant bleeding including joint and muscle bleeds, intracranial haemorrhage and other life-threatening bleeding symptoms. In most children with severe or moderate factor deficiencies, the bleeds are usually spontaneous although mild trauma can lead to a disproportionate and significant bleed.

Investigations

Diagnosis is based on family history and an initial coagulation screen which shows normal PT and prolonged aPTT. Further confirmation is made by genetic studies identifying the specific mutations and so allowing clinical prognostication.

Treatment and management

Severe haemophilia is treated with the appropriate factor concentrates and ideally on a self-administered prophylactic regime from early childhood. Such a regime prevents the development of joint bleeds and other organ bleeds with the resultant long-term pathological changes.

Relevant pharmacological agents used

Recombinant human FVIII and FIX are now the main components used in prophylaxis in children although the costs prevent those in resource-poor health systems to receive these prophylactic concentrates.

New treatment of haemophilias include long-acting recombinant factor concentrates, newer agents that target FX, and activate it directly. Finally, gene therapy in haemophilia B has shown curative outcomes.

Potential complications

Haemophilia treatment is commonly complicated by the development of antibodies against the factor concentrates (also known as inhibitors) which diminishes the expected improvement in clotting and so increases the risks of bleeding.

von Willibrand Disease

Von Willibrand Factor is a circulating protein which attaches platelets to sites of vascular injury and also binds and stabilises FVIII. The disease develops when there is deficient or ineffective factor. The condition is the most common inherited abnormality of bleeding and, as most are autosomal dominant in their inheritance, they are present equally in males and females (although more females are identified due to abnormal menstruation). Acquired von Willibrand Disease can be seen in children presenting with nephroblastoma, non-Hodgkin lymphoma or autoimmune conditions including SLE.

The diagnosis is often missed although it is the most common bleeding disorder. Many individuals have minimal symptoms and are only identified by excessive mucosal bleeding, heavy menstruation or problems postpartum. Surgical procedures can reveal unexpected prolonged bleeding. The severe form, however, can produce easy bruising, cutaneous bleeding and joint and soft tissue bleed.

Investigations

A prolonged aPTT with a normal PT with a suggestive clinical history should lead to screening tests for vWF activity and antigen.

Treatment and management

Most children do not need active treatment if they have the mild form. Advice on avoiding medication such as aspirin and nonsteroidal antiinflammatory drugs which have a direct effect on platelet function should be offered in writing, and any proposed surgical procedure requires prior discussion with colleagues in haematology. Screening of first-degree family members for the condition should be offered. DDAVP administration leads to release of endogenous vWF but assessment of its use should be under the direction of the haematology team.

Disseminated intravascular coagulation (DIC)

The condition occurs in children and young people with a significant intercurrent illness such as overwhelming infection, trauma or malignant disease. The coagulation process is initiated producing excessive fibrin in small vessels along with the concurrent consumption of platelets and clotting factors and a consequent bleeding diathesis.

The range of presenting features is extensive and will vary from prolonged bleeding at sites of venepuncture

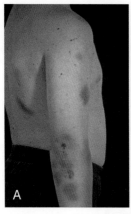 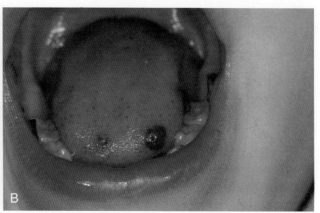

Fig. 21.6a, b Clinical appearance of 7-year-old boy with ITP.

through to purpura and peripheral tissue necrosis. Organ failure due to small vessel thrombosis can affect lung, liver, kidney and central nervous system tissue.

Investigations

- FBC—thrombocytopenia is invariably present
- PT—prolonged—extrinsic and common pathway factor deficiencies
- aPTT—prolonged—intrinsic and common pathway factor deficiencies
- fibrinogen—low consumption
- D-dimer—elevated—increased breakdown of fibrin

Treatment and management

Treatment and management aims to address the underlying cause of the DIC and, in parallel, replace the low levels of clotting factors. Fresh frozen plasma (FFP) provides proteins to encourage both procoagulation and anticoagulation whilst cryoprecipitate also has fibrinogen and clotting factors to correct the low fibrinogen levels. Regular platelet transfusions are also required.

Potential complications

Overwhelming DIC can lead to massive organ failure and death whilst ischaemic and necrotic peripheral lesions may lead to limb amputation.

Thrombophilia

Thrombotic events are rare in children although can be more common in teenage years. An increase in risk of thrombosis is seen in children with indwelling central venous access lines, prolonged periods of immobility or teenage girls taking oral contraceptives. Inherited conditions should be considered in all young people presenting with a thrombotic episode particularly those with a positive family history. Such conditions include:

- protein C deficiency—protein C is a naturally occurring anticoagulant
- protein S deficiency—cofactor to Protein C
- factor V Leiden homozygous

Severe protein S, protein C and antithrombin deficiency present as purpura fulminans in children and require prompt diagnosis and management to avoid life-threatening thrombotic events. Discussion with colleagues in haematology should be undertaken if a condition of increased thrombosis is considered.

Platelet disorders

Acquired thrombocytopenias

Acute immune thrombocytopenia (ITP) is an immune-mediated condition which is described as either allo-immune in neonates or auto-immune in older children.

Children usually present with a short history of purpura and bruising (Figure 21.6a and 21.6b) but are otherwise well, although a recent history of a viral illness or vaccination is not uncommon. Bleeding from mucous membranes and intracranial haemorrhage are both rare, and the previous practice of in-patient observation has been shown to be unnecessary. The diagnosis is one of exclusion by ensuring there are no other adverse findings in the history or examination and that the full blood count shows only thrombocytopenia. Bone marrow examination is not routinely required.

Treatment and management

Treatment is based on the severity of bleeding and should not be based solely on the platelet count as values of 0 or 1 are not unusual. For most children the condition is mild and self-limiting, with some 80% resolving spontaneously within 3 months. Intramuscular injections and nonsteroidal antiinflammatory drugs must be avoided. Active treatment is not required and the child can be managed at home. A repeat full blood count should be obtained after a week to guide the frequency of further counts.

Severe bleeding may occur and includes:

- active bleeding
- GI bleeding—melaena stool, haematemesis—usually in the first week
- uncontrolled epistaxis
- intracranial haemorrhage

Children who meet one of these criteria will need cross-matched blood to be made available and require discussion with a haematologist. Treatment options include:

- intravenous immunoglobulin
- steroids
- platelet transfusion

Chronic ITP is recognised when the thrombocytopenia lasts for longer than 6 months and such children should always be managed by a paediatric haematologist.

Relevant pharmacological agents used

Newer drugs for the treatment of ITP are becoming available and include the thrombopoietin-mimetic drugs eltrombopag and romiplostim.

Kasabach-Merritt phenomenon

Kasabach-Merritt phenomenon describes congenital vascular tumours which often present with bruising due to significant platelet consumption leading to severe thrombocytopenia.

Neutropenia

Neutropenia is identified if the full blood count reveals a neutrophil count of less than $1.0 \times 10^9/l$ whilst 'severe neutropenia' is defined as a neutrophil count less than $0.5 \times 10^9/l$. Children with such low counts are at risk of rapidly progressive, overwhelming, life-threatening bacterial infection. The neutropenia may be part of a pancytopenia or, seen in isolation, as congenital or acquired neutropenia.

Congenital neutropenia

Clinically significant neutropaenia is generally characterised by absolute neutrophil counts of $<0.5 \times 10^9/l$ that persists for over 3 months and is usually associated with recurrent infections in the first year of life affecting skin, GI mucosa and respiratory tract. Severe congenital neutropenia, cyclical neutropenia and Schwachman-Diamond syndrome are all examples of congenital neutropenia and further details on these conditions is presented in Chapter 15 Immunology.

Acquired neutropenia

Transient neutropaenia due to mild viral infections is extremely common. Some children develop antibodies against the neutrophil antigens and consequently have more persistent neutropaenia, but these too mostly resolve within 18 months of diagnosis. Neutropenia can also occur secondary to drugs such as chemotherapy and certain antibiotics.

Congenital neutropenia

Those with inherited neutropenias have severe infections from birth including balanitis, pneumonia, suppurative skin abscesses and other life-threatening infections and often demonstrate poor growth.

Treatment and management

A child with a fever over 38°C requires immediate review by experienced clinical staff and, if neutropenia is likely, intravenous antibiotics must be started following the prompt taking of cultures. The antibiotics chosen are directed by local policy but will be broad spectrum and must cover gram-negative organisms. It is commonly accepted that 'door to needle time' should be less than one hour as any delay in the starting of intravenous antibiotics, even in a well-looking individual, leads to an increased risk of mortality.

Children with chronic neutropaenia may benefit from antimicrobial prophylaxis (for example, azithromycin once daily for 3 days every fortnight). Children with severe congenital neutropaenia are treated with regular GCSF to keep neutrophil counts at safe levels and avoid recurrent infections.

IMPORTANT CLINICAL POINTS

Anaemia

- reticulocyte count reveals how marrow responds to insult
- iron deficiency anaemia may reflect dietary intake or chronic blood loss
- Fanconi anaemia has hypoplastic or absent thumbs and radii
- Schwachman-Diamond syndrome has associated steatorrhea

Thalassaemia

- HbF above 5% after 6 months indicate impaired Hb production
- β-thalassaemia—raised HbF and HBA2

Haemolytic conditions

- spherocytosis—parvovirus B19 may lead to an aplastic crisis

- sickle cell disease can present with vaso-occlusive events and needs active management

Transfusion of blood products

- one of the most risk-prone aspects of patient care

Coagulation disorders

- haemophilia A and haemophilia B are x-linked conditions
- associated with normal PT and prolonged aPTT

von Willebrand disease

- normal PT and prolonged aPTT (in 50% patients) but can have normal aPTT
- most common inherited bleeding disorder
- most inherited are autosomal dominant

Further reading

New HV, Berryman J, Bolton-Maggs PHB, Cantwell C, et al. Guidelines on transfusion for fetuses, neonates and older children, *Br J Haematol*, 2016. https://doi.org/10.1111/bjh.14233.

Helen V. New,; Jennifer Berryman,; Paula H. B,. Bolton–Maggs,; Carol Cantwell, et al. Accessed April 2021.; Neunert CE, Cooper N: Evidence-based management of immune thrombocytopenia: ASH guideline update, *Am Soc Hematology Educ Program* 2018; 2018(1):568–575.

Sickle Cell Disease. Piel FB, Steinberg MH, Rees DC: Sickle Cell Disease, *N Engl J Med* 2017; 376(16):1561–1573.

How I treat children with haemophilia and inhibitors. Young G. How I treat children with haemophilia and inhibitors. *Br J Haematol* 2019; 186(3).

Chapter |22|

Oncology

Madhu Dandapani, Martin Hewitt

After reading this chapter you should be able to assess, diagnose and manage:
- leukaemias and lymphoproliferative disorders
- solid tumours
- understand the associations of specific syndromes with propensity to malignancy
- oncological emergencies

and understand:
- side effects of treatment for malignancy
- risks and benefits of ionising radiation in patient care
- role of bone marrow transplantation and immunosuppressive therapy
- services involved in providing shared care

Although malignant disease in children and young people is relatively uncommon, it remains the major cause of death in the UK of those between 1 and 15 years of age. Like many illnesses, the impact of diagnosis and treatment on the child and family is significant and can have long-term implications for the individual concerned. In the UK, all children with suspected malignant disease are referred to one of 19 Primary Treatment Centres where diagnostic and staging investigations are undertaken, treatment options considered by the multidisciplinary team meeting (MDT) and proposed management discussed with patient and families.

Treatment protocols are complex and evolve over time as further understanding of their efficacy becomes clearer. The AKP exam does not require a detailed knowledge of the chemotherapy or radiotherapy regimens used although a broad understanding of the modalities used and an awareness of some of the common side effects of the drugs and radiotherapy are important.

Leukaemia

Acute lymphoblastic leukaemia (ALL) is much more common than acute myeloid leukaemia (AML) in the paediatric age range and both are seen more frequently than chronic myeloid leukaemia (CML). All can present at any age from infants to teenagers.

ALL and non-Hodgkin Lymphoma (NHL) are overlapping diseases with the distinction based on the major site involved and the cell of origin. A finding of 'extensive bone marrow involvement with lymph node extension' would indicate a diagnosis of leukaemia whilst 'significant lymph node involvement with some marrow disease' would be defined as a lymphoma.

Clinical presentation

Children and young people present with consequences of bone marrow failure—anaemia, white cell abnormalities—initially leucopenia and then leucocytosis—and thrombocytopenia. This leads to:
- pallor
- lethargy
- recurrent infections
- easy bruising and bleeding
- progressive lymphadenopathy
- bone pain
- headache, vomiting—if CNS involvement

On examination, children may demonstrate signs indicative of pancytopenia with pallor, bruising and signs of infection whilst widespread lymphadenopathy is common. A slightly enlarged liver and spleen may be palpable although those with chronic leukaemia may have a

Table 22.1 Interpretation of presenting FBC results in a 3-year-old girl

	RCPCH normal range	Leukaemia— patient 1	Leukaemia— patient 2	Aplastic anaemia
Haemoglobin	110–140 g/l	67	67	67
WCC	5.0–12.0 x 10⁹/l	13	220	0.3
Platelets	150–450 x 10⁹/l	34	34	21
Reticulocytes	50–150 x 10⁹/l	120	120	5
Urate	0.15–0.35 mmol/l	0.21	0.65	0.08

markedly enlarged spleen. Those with CNS disease may have papilloedema and boys can have enlarged and firm testicles indicative of disease infiltration.

Alternative diagnoses

Aplastic anaemia

The underlying pathological process in aplastic anaemia is one of reduced cell division in all three cell lines leading to erythropenia, leukopenia and thrombocytopenia. In leukaemia the process is that of proliferation of immature white cells (blast) which then crowd out the other normal progenitor cells. A bone marrow aspirate is necessary to clarify this distinction (Table 22.1).

Some conditions will lead to changes in appearance or number of the white cells in the peripheral circulation and so mimic the presentation of acute leukaemia, but more detailed investigations will clarify the diagnosis. These would include:

- infectious mononucleosis
- parvovirus B19 infection
- HIV
- pertussis
- autoimmune conditions

Investigations

An initial full blood count will usually raise suspicions of leukaemia with anaemia and thrombocytopenia present to varying degrees. The white cell count may be low or normal in the early stages of disease as the immature blast cells are confined to the bone marrow. Further proliferation of the malignant clone leads to the immature blast cells passing into the circulation and leading to a progressive elevation of the count.

Samples of the malignant cells are obtained by bone marrow aspirate and will identify sheets of blast cells. Further clarification as to the specific cell line (T-cell, B-cell,

myeloid or other) involved will come from immunochemistry on the malignant cells.

Cytogenetics of the leukaemia cells is also undertaken as specific translocations and deletions have been identified which have prognostic implications. Cerebrospinal fluid from a lumbar puncture is examined for the presence of blasts and, if present, indicates CNS disease.

Treatment and management

Intensive chemotherapy is given following the current national trial protocol. For children with ALL, the treatment sequence involves blocks of chemotherapy over the initial months and then maintenance therapy over the following years. Children with AML have blocks of very intensive chemotherapy over a 6- to 8-month period and are rendered profoundly immunosuppressed over this time.

PRACTICE POINT—CNS-directed therapy in acute leukaemia

The direct administration of chemotherapy into the intrathecal space is via a lumbar puncture and, in paediatric practice, this usually occurs under anaesthesia. Clinical errors have occurred whereby an inappropriate chemotherapy agent—usually vincristine—was injected rather than the required intrathecal agent. Death of the patient is the usual outcome of this error.

Following a national review, the current UK practice only allows those who have been specifically trained and whose names appear on the hospital Trust register be involved in any aspect of intrathecal treatment— prescription, transporting or administration.

Clinicians who are not on their Trust register must decline if asked to prescribe, check or administer intrathecal chemotherapy.

Important sequelae

The 5-year survival for good risk acute lymphoblastic leukaemia (female, between 2–10 years, white count under 50 at presentation, no CNS disease and no adverse cytogenetics) is 93%. For AML it is around 70%.

Lymphoproliferative disorders

Non-Hodgkin Lymphoma (NHL)
Clinical presentation

The site of the initial disease in NHL will dictate the presenting features. Children with massive lymphadenopathy in the chest invariably have T-cell (thymic modulated) NHL and will present with:
- dyspnoea (orthostatic in extreme situations)
- pleural effusion
- collapse
- generalised pallor
  Those with abdominal disease will usually have B-cell NHL and will have:
- anorexia
- diarrhoea
- abdominal distention
- ascites
- jaundice (if massive liver involvement)
  Peripheral lymphadenopathy—cervical, axillary or inguinal—may be the first sign of malignancy.

Alternative diagnoses

Other causes of lymphadenopathy would need to be considered and would include:
- malignant diseases (soft tissue sarcomas, thyroid carcinoma)
- infections (Epstein-Barr, Mycobacterium, cat-scratch disease, toxoplasmosis)
- autoimmune conditions (Kawasaki disease, systemic lupus erythematosus)

Associations

Many conditions associated with immunodeficiency lead to an increased risk of developing non-Hodgkin lymphoma and include:
- congenital immunodeficiencies
  - Wiskott-Aldrich syndrome
  - ataxia telangiectasia
  - X-linked lymphoproliferative syndrome
- acquired immunodeficiencies
  - HIV
  - immunosuppressive treatments following solid organ transplants

Investigations

A CXR will be requested for those with respiratory symptoms and shows a mediastinal mass (Figure 22.1). Imaging with CT (Figure 22.2 and Figure 22.3) and MRI is necessary but the exact modality will depend on site of the primary disease. These images will determine the extent of disease and will allow assessment of future response to treatment. Tissue diagnosis is essential for diagnosis and will include histological examination, cytogenetics and immunochemistry which will determine the cell lineage. Lactate dehydrogenase (LDH) is not pathognomonic of lymphoma and can be raised due to any condition which increases white cell activity. Patients are at risk of tumour lysis syndrome and biochemical assessment is necessary before treatment commences and monitored closely through the early stages of chemotherapy.

Treatment and management

Complex protocols are used and the regimens are usually started in the designated UK specialist units before care is transferred to local shared care centres where possible.

Potential complications

Patients with rapidly progressive thoracic disease may develop superior vena caval (SVC) obstruction and airway occlusion (see below). Critical airway compromise may be evident from an inability of the patient to lie flat due to marked dyspnoea. These patients need rapid assessment by a senior anaesthetist and close monitoring in an intensive care setting. Initiation of treatment is required urgently to counter the evolving cardiovascular and respiratory compromise and the tumours usually have rapid response to treatment, shrinking over 24 to 48 hours. Those with abdominal disease can develop rapidly progressive distension from ascites along with peripheral oedema.

Important sequelae

The 5-year survival figures for children with NHL will vary depending on the histological diagnosis. Those with T-cell disease can expect 70% overall response, those with B-cell disease have 90%. Long-term effects are well recognised and will be the result of the chemotherapeutic agents used and the general impact of treatment such as time out of education and impact on family life.

Hodgkin Lymphoma (HL)
Clinical presentation

Hodgkin lymphoma usually presents in teenagers and young adults but has been identified in young children.

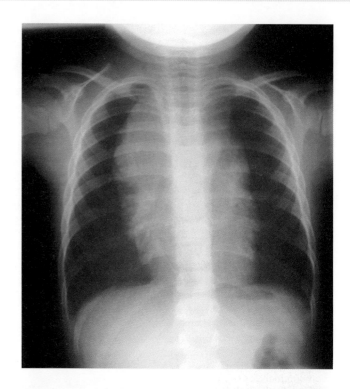

Fig. 22.1 Chest x-ray of 8-year-old presenting with dyspnoea. Mass in upper and middle mediastinum. Biopsy confirmed non-Hodgkin lymphoma.

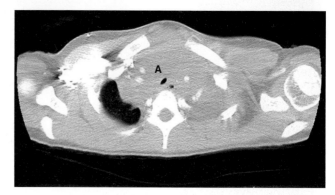

Fig. 22.2 CT upper mediastinum in 9-year-old boy who presented with dyspnoea, orthopnoea and pallor. Upper mediastinal mass shown with critical narrowing of trachea (A)

Patients will present with painless, persistent lymphadenopathy, usually in the cervical or axillary areas, but a large mediastinal mass may produce respiratory symptoms. 'B symptoms' have been identified and their presence leads to more intensive treatment protocols.

PRACTICE POINT—Hodgkin lymphoma—B symptoms

- fever (greater than 38°C)
- weight loss (greater than 10% body weight)
- drenching night sweats

Investigations

A tissue biopsy is needed to confirm diagnosis and exclude other causes of lymphadenopathy. Immunohistochemistry will identify characteristic surface antigens seen in HL.

Imaging has a major role in staging and will include a CT scan (cervical, mediastinal, abdominal and pelvic areas) and positron emission tomography (PET) scan (Figure 22.4). The PET scan will identify sites of active disease in lymph nodes and organs and will be used to monitor treatment response.

Extensive disease is seen in submandibular, cervical, axillary, para-aortic and pelvic lymph nodes. Massive splenomegaly is evident as is liver and bone marrow involvement.

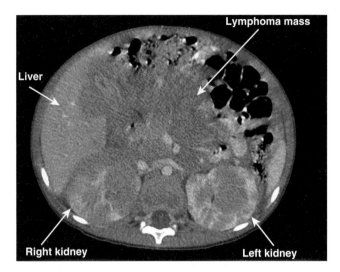

Fig. 22.3 CT of abdomen of 6-year-old child presenting with an abdominal mass. A central mass is evident that has extended into the liver and both kidneys. IV contrast has been given leading to enhancement of abdominal vessels and renal parenchyma.

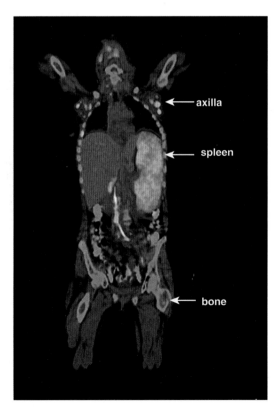

Fig. 22.4 PET scan of 13-year-old girl with Hodgkin lymphoma.

Treatment and management

Although there are differences in the details of management between international protocols, they all use a combination of treatment modalities with systemic chemotherapy and radiotherapy to affected sites. Some patients, however, can omit radiotherapy if they have a sufficiently good response to initial chemotherapy.

Long-term prognosis is dependent upon stage of disease at presentation but is generally very encouraging. Patients with Stage 1 (localised) disease have a UK 5-year survival of over 90% whilst the figure for those with Stage 4 (widely disseminated) disease is around 80%.

Important sequelae

Patients treated for HL during childhood or teenage years are at risk of significant long-term problems. Treatment protocols include an anthracycline which can induce a cardiomyopathy, but current protocols have reduced doses of this agent and therefore minimise this effect.

Radiotherapy to various sites may lead to tissue hypoplasia and an increased risk of malignancy within the radiation field. Further details are presented in the section on radiotherapy.

Central nervous system tumours

Clinical presentation

The presenting symptoms will depend upon the age of the child and the exact site of the lesion, but the most common ones are due to a raised intracranial pressure or from mass effect. They include:

- headaches (often worst when waking up)
- vomiting (usually relieves the headache)
- visual disturbance

Specific neurological signs may indicate the site of the lesion such as those in the posterior fossa (brain stem, fourth ventricle and cerebellum) inducing ataxia.

Very young children with central tumours may have regression of developmental milestones whilst lesions in the cerebral cortex can lead to seizures. Those with hypothalamic or midline lesions can present with endocrinopathies including:

- isolated growth hormone deficiency
- multiple-pituitary hormone deficiency including diabetes insipidus
- growth hormone excess
- gonadotrophin dependent sexual precocity
- pathological pubertal delay

Severe hydrocephalus presents with bradycardia, bradypnea and systolic hypertension, and death can occur from herniation of brain stem if not identified and treated promptly.

The HeadSmart campaign provides age-appropriate cards and online information aimed at increasing awareness of parents and healthcare professionals to the signs and symptoms.

Associations

Syndromes with a higher incidence of CNS malignancy include:

- neurofibromatosis type 1 (NF-1)—gliomas, particularly of optic pathway
- neurofibromatosis type 2 (NF-2)—Schwannomas particularly of auditory nerves
- tuberous sclerosis—develop SEGA (subependymal giant cell tumours).

Investigations

The patient with a suspected CNS tumour may present in extremis and would therefore need an urgent CT scan. This would allow the clinical team to assess the need for neurosurgical intervention to reduce a raised, and potentially critical, intracranial pressure.

MRI scans of the brain and the spine are then required in all patients to delineate the location and extent of the tumour (Figure 22.5). MR spectroscopy can be used to detect chemical composition in some lesions and thereby suggest the tumour type. Histological examination of tissue removed by surgical excision or biopsy is, however, required for diagnosis.

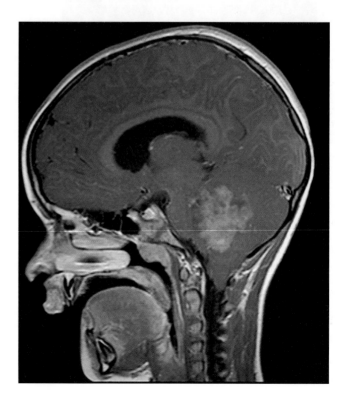

Fig. 22.5 MRI scan of 9-year-old boy showing lesion in the cerebellar lobe. A medulloblastoma was confirmed on biopsy

The common types of tumours include

- glial tumours—includes gliomas which arise from astrocytes
- ependymoma which arise from the cells that line the ventricles (ependymal cells)
- embryonal tumours—includes medulloblastoma in posterior fossa
- craniopharyngioma—involves pituitary
- germ cell tumours—(see later section)
- meningiomas—arises from meninges—extremely rare in children
- secondary metastatic deposits

Treatment and management

Initial management would consider the need for urgent surgical intervention. Relief of raised pressure with the insertion of an external ventricular drain, biopsy or macroscopic excision. The MDT, with the support of the histology results, will then consider the options for further treatment—chemotherapy, radiotherapy, further surgery or a combination of all. Radiotherapy is avoided in those under 3 years of age due to the long-term effect of significant, debilitating impairment on cognitive function, and chemotherapy may be used to defer or avoid the use of radiotherapy. Some low-grade tumours can be treated with chemotherapy alone.

Potential complications

Removal of tumour (and the region of the brain it involves) can cause neurological deficits whilst radiotherapy can cause profound cognitive impairment, endocrinopathies and vasculopathy. Chemotherapy can further compound effects of radiation on fertility and second malignancies.

Solid tumours

Solid tumours outside the central nervous system account for about 35% of all childhood malignant disease in the UK. The range of problems at presentation is wide and the investigation, management and prognosis varied. Those tumours which arise from abdominal tissue produces palpable masses and the location can indicate the most likely tumour type (Figure 22.6).

Neuroblastoma

Clinical presentation

The peak age for presentation is from birth to the age of 5 years although it can occasionally occur in older children.

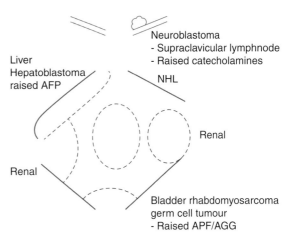

Fig. 22.6 Solid tumours causing abdominal masses and their associated features

The disease can occur anywhere along the sympathetic chain (retro-orbit to pelvis) and consequently the symptoms will vary depending on the site of origin. About two-thirds of children present with an abdominal mass due to an adrenal or parasympathetic primary and they are invariably irritable and miserable. Metastatic disease occurs in two-thirds of patients and involves:
- bone marrow
- left supraclavicular node ('Virchow node')
- skull leading to periorbital bruising (raccoon's eyes).

Alternative diagnoses and differing features

Neuroblastoma can be described as the 'great pretender' as many of its presenting features will mimic other conditions. Persistent pyrexia without a focus, irritability, bone pain, bruising and rash can lead to other diagnoses such as infection or autoimmune conditions. Occasionally patients are referred with safeguarding concerns due to unexplained bruising.

Investigations

- full blood count—evidence of bone marrow infiltration with pancytopenia
- urinary catecholamines (adrenaline, dopamine, HVA, VMA are invariably raised)
- biopsy of primary for histology and cytogenetics
- oncogene assessment—multiple copies of MYC-N confer adverse prognosis
- CT/MRI scan of affected areas (Figure 22.7)
- MIBG radionuclide scan—identifies metastatic disease
Calcification of neuroblastoma tissue and the invasive nature behind the abdominal aorta are characteristic features

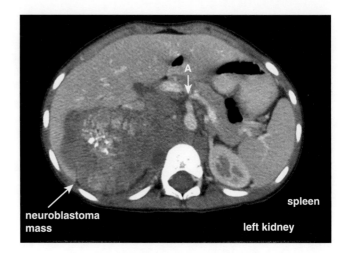

Fig. 22.7 CT of abdomen in 4-year-old boy showing neuroblastoma.

Treatment and management

Treatment is based on the risk factors identified. Patients with very low risk disease (asymptomatic infants) are unlikely to require any treatment as the tumours can spontaneously regress. Chemotherapy and surgery are required for low and intermediate risk patients, but those with a poor prognosis require highly intensive multimodal therapy including high dose chemotherapy, surgery, radiotherapy and immunotherapy. Survival depends on risk group with very low risk patients having a greater than 95% survival whilst the high risk patients have a 5-year survival of around 40%.

Nephroblastoma (Wilms tumour)

Clinical presentation

Classically, the child presents between the ages of 2 and 4 years with an abdominal mass discovered incidentally. Around 10% of children will have haematuria. Examination will identify a flank mass and possibly hypertension.

CLINICAL SCENARIO

A 3-year-old girl presented a with 2-month history of malaise and pallor and 24 hours of being unable to weight bear. She had a good appetite until the last few days. Examination showed that she was pyrexial at 38.4°C, had no obvious rash and, although tachycardic, had no other abnormalities of cardiovascular system. She had an obvious swelling just above the medial left clavicle and obvious lymph nodes in axillae and groin. Examination of the abdomen revealed a firm, left-sided mass about 4 x 4 cm. She was reluctant to move all her limbs.

A differential here would include malignant disease focussed on the abdomen. This would include lymphoma,

neuroblastoma or nephroblastoma. It should also include infectious conditions, particularly osteoarthritis or septic arthritis, although they would not explain the abdominal mass. The presence of a left supraclavicular mass suggests a Virchow node and would be suggestive of metastatic neuroblastoma. The age of the child, the pallor and the reluctance to weight bear would also be consistent with this diagnosis.

Investigations showed pancytopenia indicating marrow infiltrate, urinary catecholamines were elevated suggesting neuroblastoma and initial ultrasound scan and then MRI scan confirm the location and extent of the mass. Biopsy of the mass was needed to confirm the diagnosis and the child started intensive therapy.

Associations

There are recognised clinical syndromes associated with nephroblastoma:

- WAGR (Wilms tumour, aniridia, genital abnormalities, range of intellectual disability)
- Beckwith-Wiedemann syndrome—often detected at birth and is characterised by hemi-hypertrophy, macrosomia, macroglossia, omphalocoele and a cleft on pinna of ear

Both groups of children need regular abdominal ultrasound examination during the first 6 to 8 years of life.

Investigations

Abdominal ultrasound will identify the location and extent of an abdominal mass and will also view the inferior vena cava to identify possible extension of tumour through the renal vein and up to the right atrium. CT/MRI scan of abdomen will identify size and extent of the abdominal mass (Figure 22.8) and CT scan of chest will look for metastatic disease. Biopsy of the abdominal mass is required in most children.

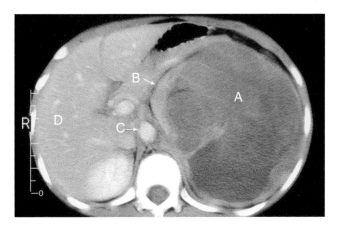

Fig. 22.8 CT scan of large left-sided nephroblastoma (A) in 4-year-old girl IV contrast has been given and highlights residual normal renal tissue (B) at the periphery of the tumour mass (A). Abdominal aorta (C) and liver (D).

Treatment and management

The stage of the disease will dictate the extent of treatment but currently requires initial chemotherapy to reduce the size of the renal tumour before moving to nephrectomy. Further chemotherapy is required after surgery and the duration and intensity of this phase depends on the staging. Radiotherapy may be necessary in some children with high-stage disease or tumour rupture.

Important sequelae

Removal of the affected kidney is standard practice that may lead to hypertension in later life. Radiotherapy to the renal bed or lung tissue may lead to pulmonary fibrosis or hypoplasia and deformity of any muscle or bones included in the radiotherapy field (particularly if given at a young age). Cardiomyopathy could occur due to anthracycline chemotherapy.

Hepatoblastoma
Clinical presentation

The child with a hepatoblastoma usually presents with an asymptomatic, right-sided abdominal mass and is usually under the age of 6 years.

Investigations

The specific investigations of a hepatic mass are:
- abdominal US scan
- MRI scan—identifies the site of the mass and the involved lobes of the liver
- chest x-ray—for evidence of metastases
- alpha-fetoprotein (AFP) is highly suggestive of hepatoblastoma
  - Neonates can have a very high physiological AFP level that falls in the weeks following delivery and nomograms are available to help distinguish this from the pathological levels
- biopsy of mass

Treatment and management

Clarification of disease site and distribution within the lobes of the liver will direct treatment. Single, well-circumscribed lesions within individual lobes can be resected and further treatment with chemotherapy given whilst disseminated disease may need total hepatectomy and liver transplant. The outlook for children with hepatoblastoma has improved dramatically and now over 80% are disease free at 5 years.

Osteosarcoma
Clinical presentation

The peak age for presentation is in the second decade of life (12–16 years), and it is extremely rare in children under 5 years. Most patients present with painful swelling of long bone in the upper or lower limb. The main sites are at the proximal and distal metaphyses of the long bones:
- femur
- tibia
- humerus

Metastatic disease occurs mainly to the lungs but rarely can involve other bones.

Investigations

Patients will usually have plain films of the affected area. These will show an expansile, lytic lesion of the bone shaft, along with periosteal, new bone formation formed as the periosteum is lifted from the normal bone shaft around the lesion (Figure 22.9). MRI scans are undertaken to identify adjacent soft tissue extension and also intramedullary extension. CT of chest is necessary to identify pulmonary metastases. Definitive diagnosis comes from biopsy and in the UK, this must be undertaken at designated supraregional unit.

Areas of sclerosis and ragged border evident.

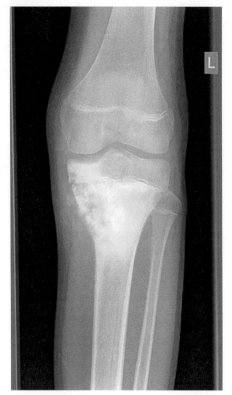

Fig. 22.9 X-ray of left proximal tibia in 15-year-old girl showing osteosarcoma.

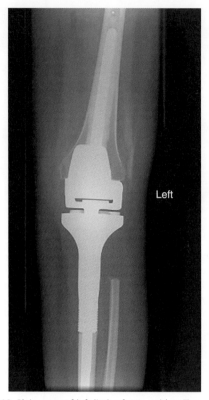

Fig. 22.10 Plain x-ray of left limb of same girl as Figure 22.9 following chemotherapy and insertion of prosthesis

Treatment and management

Chemotherapy is integral to the treatment programme and surgery usually undertaken in the middle of the whole course. The surgical procedures now aim for a limb-sparing approach, and advances in the development of the prostheses have allowed this to happen (Figure 22.10). Replacement joints for knee, hip and shoulder have all ensured the affected limbs can be retained and often with significant residual function. Some patients, however, will need limb amputation. Radiotherapy does not form part of treatment.

Potential complications

The initial problems for the young person after surgery is the impact on motor function. Those with lesions around the hip and knee may have had prosthetic joints inserted which allow good mobility. Those who needed limb amputation will need to master the external prosthesis—although they may go on to compete in high level sports.

Ewing Sarcoma
Clinical presentation

The condition can present between 2 years through to late teenage years and the common sites are:
- axial skeleton
  - skull, spine, scapula, chest wall, pelvis
- appendicular skeleton
  - femur, tibia, fibula

The patient may present with localised pain, swelling or loss of function although the actual location may also lead to other symptoms. Metastatic disease can be detected in lung, bone, lymph nodes and bone marrow.

Investigations

- plain films—show bone destruction, bone expansion and soft tissue extension (Figure 22.11)
- MRI of area—defines disease margins and soft tissue extension
- CT of chest—for pulmonary metastases
- positron emission tomography (PET scan)—identify distant metastases

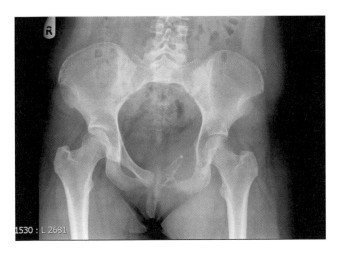

Fig. 22.11 Plain x-ray of pelvis showing lytic lesion arising within the left pubic ramus. Subsequent biopsy confirmed a diagnosis of Ewing sarcoma.

- biopsy—confirms diagnosis
- cytogenetics—demonstrates chromosome 22 translocation

Treatment and management

Treatment involves systemic chemotherapy, surgical resection where possible, and potentially radiation therapy to the primary and metastatic sites. The axial location of many of the presenting tumours makes surgical resection difficult or inappropriate. Proton beam radiotherapy (highly focussed) may be used at difficult anatomical sites to maximise dose intensity and minimise radiation to normal surrounding tissue.

Important sequelae

Surgical resection may impact on mobility whilst local radiotherapy will limit tissue growth and increase the risk of second primary malignancies within the radiation fields. The treatment programmes are intense and patients on this protocol are given prophylactic cotrimoxazole to protect against *Pneumocystis jirovecii*.

Soft tissue sarcomas

This includes a range of tumours arising from mesenchymal tissue with rhabdomyosarcoma being the most common. This tumour can develop in bladder, pelvis or nasopharynx. Investigations will confirm histological subtype and imaging and bone marrow trephine will help define extent. Treatment utilises surgery, chemotherapy and radiotherapy.

Langerhans cell histiocytosis (LCH)

Clinical presentation

Langerhans cell histiocytosis is a condition with a wide range of presenting symptoms and signs—from a life-threatening, multi-system disease through to an 'incidental finding of a single site.'

Widespread multiorgan involvement with systemic symptoms can be seen in children in the first few years of life and such disease is progressive and life threatening. The condition can present in the neonatal period and infancy with skin rashes which can be misdiagnosed as congenital infection or contact dermatitis if in the perineal area (See example image. Dermatology chapters 23. Fig 23.15). Lytic lesions in the bone are the most common clinical finding and consequently children may present initially to orthopaedic teams.

Systemic symptoms are common and children are often investigated for a 'pyrexia of unknown origin.' Presenting features of disease include:
- lymphadenopathy
- gum involvement
- pulmonary involvement
- hepatosplenomegaly
- middle ear (produce persistent discharge)
- pituitary fossa (leading to diabetes insipidus)

Investigations

Histological diagnosis is essential and biopsy of the lesion is essential. Assessment of the extent of disease will come from a skeletal survey looking for single or multiple lytic lesions that are described as having sharp margins.

Treatment and management

Young children with multifocal, multisystem disease require intensive chemotherapy as the condition is progressive and ultimately fatal. Those with isolated bone lesions and who are otherwise well may simply need curettage of the lesion.

Table 22.2 Syndromic conditions associated with increased risk of malignant disease in children and young people

Condition	Inheritance	Features	Associated malignancy
ataxia telangiectasia	autosomal recessive	ataxia, telangiectasia, immunodeficiency	non-Hodgkin lymphoma
Beckwith-Wiedermann	most sporadic uniparental disomy	macrosomia, hemihypertrophy, macroglossia, earlobe crease	nephroblastoma hepatoblastoma
Down syndrome	trisomy 21	Characteristic phenotype, cardiac lesions, Intellectual disability	leukaemia
Fanconi anaemia	autosomal recessive	microcephaly, short stature, developmental delay	leukaemia
Gardener syndrome	autosomal dominant	retinal pigmentation	adenomatous polyposis
Li-Fraumeni	autosomal dominant	early onset malignancy	rhabdomyosarcoma osteosarcoma nephroblastoma
neurofibromatosis type-1	50% sporadic 50% autosomal dominant	cutaneous café-au-lait lesions, neurofibromas, msk abnormalities	glioma—optic nerve
neurofibromatosis type-2	sporadic and autosomal dominant	usually identified from family history	schwannoma meningiomas ependymomas
Rothman-Thompson	autosomal recessive	facial rash, short stature, sparse hair, premature aging	osteosarcoma
tuberous sclerosis	autosomal dominant	Intellectual disability, seizures, facial angiofibromas	sub ependymal giant cell tumours—SEGA
WAGR	spontaneous	Wilms tumour, Aniridia, Genitourinary anomalies, Range of intellectual disability	nephroblastoma
Wiskott-Aldrich syndrome	x-linked recessive	thrombocytopenia, eczema, immunodeficiency	non-Hodgkin lymphoma
X-linked lymphoprolif-erative syndrome	x-linked recessive	early onset lymphoma significant EBV infection	non-Hodgkin lymphoma

Syndromes with propensity to malignancy

(Table 22.2)

Oncological emergencies

Neutropenic fever

Most patients on treatment will be immunocompromised due to the effect of chemotherapy on the bone marrow activity, and in particular, the white cell and neutrophil count will be low. These patients are highly susceptible to invasive infections usually from gut or skin bacteria which can cause septic shock and death. The risk of overwhelming sepsis increases dramatically according to the duration and severity of neutropenia.

> **PRACTICE POINT—Indications for treatment of child with fever and neutropenia**
>
> 1. neutropenia
>   a. neutrophil count below 1.0×10^9/l
>   b. severe neutropenia is count below 0.5×10^9/l
> 2. temperature above 38.5°C or sustained above 38°C over one hour
> 3. possible sepsis on examination (i.e., hypotensive, collapse) even when neutrophil count unknown or normal

Clinical presentation

In those patients receiving blocks of chemotherapy, the period of neutropenia will begin some 7 to 10 days from the **start** of the last block. Patients with a temperature greater than 38°C and a possible low neutrophil count need urgent clinical assessment. Abscess or pus formation **does not** occur in the absence of neutrophils.

Treatment and management

Prompt recognition of the at-risk patient is imperative and the urgent need for intravenous antibiotics is crucial. The current NICE guidelines indicate that systemic antibiotics should be administered within one hour of entry to the clinical area and delays beyond this interval lead to a significant increase in morbidity and mortality. First-line treatment should follow local guidelines and is usually a combination of antibiotics including one effective against pseudomonas. Patients who are at risk of a prolonged period of neutropenia and fever should be started on antifungal therapy following senior discussion.

Tumour lysis syndrome

Clinical presentation

Malignant disease formed by rapidly dividing cells is susceptible to cell lysis when chemotherapy is started, although in some situations the natural turnover of cells may be sufficient to generate biochemical abnormalities even before chemotherapy is introduced. Acute leukaemia, particularly disease presenting with a high white count, and non-Hodgkin lymphoma are the most common forms of malignancy to produce tumour lysis syndrome. It is rarely seen in children with solid tumours.

With cell lysis, the intracellular contents—potassium, phosphate and purines—are released into the circulation. DNA base pairs guanine and adenine (the purines) break down to form urate in the circulation which is then excreted in the urine. The primary biochemical abnormalities are:
- hyperkalaemia
- hyperphosphataemia
- hyperuricaemia

The PTH response to hyperphosphataemia leads to hypocalcaemia. High levels of urate may crystallise in the renal parenchyma and lead to renal insufficiency.

Investigations

It is imperative that frequent and repeated biochemical assessment is undertaken in those patients at risk of tumour lysis once chemotherapy is started. Frequency of testing is usually every 4 to 6 hours in the first few days, and a rising phosphate may be the first indicator of the increased cell breakdown.

Treatment and management

Hyperhydration is required to increase the renal excretion of urates but potassium **must not** be added to the prescribed fluid as impending cell lysis will release extra potassium. Allopurinol is a xanthine oxidase inhibitor and limits the production of urate whilst rasburicase converts urate to allantoin that is then excreted through the liver and stool. Calcium administration to correct asymptomatic hypocalcaemia requires caution as it may lead to calcium phosphate precipitating in renal tissue. Cardiac arrhythmias can occur in the face of hyperkalaemia and hypocalcaemia whilst acute renal failure due to high serum urate may require renal dialysis.

Important sequelae

Tumour lysis syndrome is a clinical issue only during the first few days of treatment and once these abnormalities have resolved then subsequent problems would not be expected.

Superior vena caval obstruction

Patients with rapidly progressive thoracic disease (usually T-cell NHL or Hodgkin lymphoma) may develop superior vena caval obstruction and airway occlusion due to the size and location of the mass. This obstruction leads to venous congestion in the areas drained by the SVC and patients develop:
- generalised facial oedema
- 'slate-grey appearance' to the facial skin
- engorgement of veins on the face and upper chest

Early airway compromise may be evident from an inability to lie flat due to the development of dyspnoea. These patients need rapid assessment by experienced anaesthetists and the urgent commencement of treatment with steroids to reduce the mass.

Radiotherapy

Radiotherapy forms an integral part of the treatment for many solid tumours and is usually combined with chemotherapy and surgery. Preparation and planning of radiation requires relevant imaging of the primary tumour and any potential metastases that would then allow the delineation of the 'radiation fields' and the total dose required. Dosing is dictated by:

- tumour type
- proximity to surrounding normal tissue
- national or international protocol directive

The treatment is usually given once a day over a 10 to 14 day period in a recognised radiotherapy treatment centre. Splints, supports or 'masks' are used to ensure that the patient is located in exactly the same position for each dose administered, and in small children a general anaesthetic may be required.

Radiation therapy can be administered using different techniques. Conventional beam therapy uses a point source and therefore a diverging beam. This does bring the risk of damage to normal adjacent tissue as, for example, irradiation of an orbital rhabdomyosarcoma could damage the pituitary gland. Proton beam therapy uses parallel beams and can be manipulated to irradiate to only a predetermined depth and consequently is useful where sensitive tissue is near to the required field. Implanted radiation devices are available but rarely used in children.

Radiotherapy can have an effect on growing tissue, and its use in children and young people requires careful consideration by the radiotherapist. Treatment to the neck for a thyroid malignancy may lead to hypoplasia of neck tissue which may have cosmetic implications. Abdominal irradiation may limit growth of lower ribs and pelvic irradiation will affect fertility and shape of the pelvic bones. A child with a left-sided nephroblastoma and pulmonary metastatic disease may receive splenic irradiation that will produce a functional asplenism and the need for prophylactic penicillin for life.

The major long-term concern is the potential for a second primary malignancy within the radiation field. Females who received radiotherapy in their teenage years for a mediastinal Hodgkin lymphoma have an increased risk of breast cancer. All current radiotherapy regimes recognise this potential and have adjusted dosing appropriately. This second primary malignancy, however, may not develop for a further 20–30 years.

Radiotherapy is occasionally used in palliative care to control adverse symptoms such as bone pain which are related to tumour progression.

Peripheral stem cell harvest and transplantation

Primarily used in children with leukaemia or lymphoma who have poor-risk disease at presentation or who relapse after multiple courses of chemotherapy. They can be given stem cells harvested from a matched, related donor (allograft) or matched-unrelated donor (MUD). Children with some solid tumours who fail initial treatment may have autografts (stem cells harvested from the patient) and so allow high-dose chemotherapy.

Treatment and management

Patients receiving allografts are usually given myeloablative therapy with very high dose chemotherapy and total body irradiation (TBI). When the chemotherapy is completed, the patient receives the harvested cells and marrow reinfusion is through a central venous catheter. Patients are then cared for in an isolation unit until they develop bone marrow regeneration.

Potential complications

Graft versus host disease (GvHD) occurs when the donated marrow has some degree of 'mismatch' and the transplanted lymphoid cells begin to target host organs. Common sites of GvHD are:

- skin (producing florid rash)
- liver (deranged liver function and clotting problems)
- gut (with consequent diarrhoea and malabsorption)

Immunosuppressive agents are given as part of routine, post-transplant treatment but may need to be adjusted if GvHD develops. Following bone marrow transplant (BMT), there will be some degree of 'graft versus leukaemia' due to mismatching, and such patients have a better survival than those with a 'perfect match.'

Shared care services

The UK has established a system of Principle Treatment Centres (PTC) round the UK to cover the population and each centre then works closely with other paediatric units in the region to establish a 'hub and spoke' service. All children with solid tumours, CNS tumours and leukaemia with adverse clinical features (myeloid features, Down syndrome, high white count) are transferred to the PTC. These children will have the expected investigations to confirm the diagnosis and establish the extent and stage of the disease. A Paediatric Oncology MDT will meet to review the diagnosis and propose a treatment programme that will usually follow national or international treatment programmes or a clinical trial.

The PTC will provide initial counselling for the patient and family, start the agreed chemotherapy regimen, arrange response assessments and provide necessary surgical intervention and radiotherapy.

Agreement is then reached between the PTC and peripheral unit on how best to deliver the required treatment and, if possible, will aim to deliver this close to the family home. The local unit will provide ongoing support for the patient and family including administration of chemotherapy, admissions for neutropenic fever,

transfusions of blood and platelets when necessary and nutritional support. Social and education support can also be provided by the local teams.

Common pharmacological agents used

Details of the treatment programme and the doses used are not required for the AKP exam, but acute and long-term side effects are important and these are listed here (Table 22.3).

Table 22.3 Commonly used chemotherapeutic agents in treatment of malignant disease

Agent	Used in	Acute effects	Long term effects
bleomycin	germ cell tumours	nausea mucositis (Figure 22.12)	lung damage
cisplatin/ carboplatin	osteosarcoma CNS tumours	significant emesis bone marrow suppression ototoxicity—usually high tone loss nephrotoxicity	permanent high tone hearing loss permanent nephrotoxicity

cyclophosphamide/
ifosfamide
	Hodgkin lymphoma
	NHL
	ALL
	Ewing tumour
		significant emesis
		bone marrow suppression
		nephrotoxicity—proximal tubular
		   damage
		mucositis
			Nephrotoxicity—potential problems
			   are the result of a proximal
			   tubular nephropathy similar to
			   Fanconi syndrome infertility

doxorubicin
(anthracycline)
	osteosarcoma
	nephroblastoma
	Hodgkin lymphoma
	NHL
		significant emesis
		bone marrow suppression
		cardiotoxicity—dose-dependent
		mucositis
			cardiomyopathy—repeat cardiac
			   echo every 3–5 years through
			   life

methotrexate	osteosarcoma ALL	hepatotoxicity mucositis	long-term hepatotoxicity
prednisolone	Hodgkin lymphoma NHL	hyperglycaemia weight gain mood disturbance hypertension	avascular necrosis of hip

vincristine	Ewing tumour
	   nephroblastoma
	Hodgkin lymphoma
	NHL
	ALL
		peripheral neuropathy (loss of
		   reflexes, reduced power, ptosis,
		   constipation) during treatment	

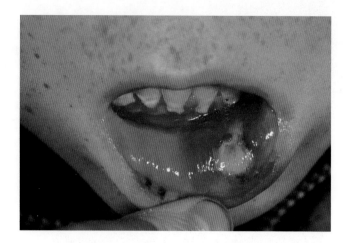

Fig. 22.12 Mucositis as a consequence of chemotherapy.

IMPORTANT CLINICAL POINTS

Leukaemia

- consider diagnosis of acute leukaemia if pancytopenia
- consider diagnosis of acute leukaemia if anaemia and thrombocytopenia with normal white count
- consider Hodgkin lymphoma if B symptoms (fever, weight loss, night sweats)
- both non-Hodgkin and Hodgkin lymphoma can present with a mediastinal mass
- treatment of Hodgkin lymphoma can produce long-term sequelae

CNS tumours

- NF-1 associated with optic nerve gliomas
- NF-2 associated with Schwannomas of auditory nerves
- radiotherapy is avoided in those under 3 years of age

Solid tumours

- consider neuroblastoma in child who is miserable, pyrexial and with unexplained bruising
- nephroblastoma associated with Beckwith-Wiedeman syndrome
- raised AFP with abdominal mass is suggestive of hepatoblastoma

Bone tumours

- bone tumours show expansile, lytic and ragged lesion on plain x-ray
- osteosarcoma commonly at proximal or distal sites of long bone in a teenager
- Ewing sarcoma often midline but can appear at long bone sites

Tumour lysis syndrome

- usually seen with high count leukaemia or non-Hodgkin lymphoma
- major problem at start of chemotherapy
- blood results show raised Potassium, Phosphate, Purines
- hyperphosphataemia is evident before hypocalcaemia
- treated with hyperhydration and rasburicase

Further readings

Davis K, Wilson S: Febrile neutropenia in paediatric oncology, *Paediatr Child Health* 2020;30:93–97.

Madni M, Dandapani M: Genetic syndromes predisposing to paediatric brain tumours, *Paediatr Child Health* 2020;30:98–101.

Chapter | 23 |

Dermatology

Jane Ravenscroft, Jothsana Srinivasan

After reading this chapter you should be able to assess, diagnose and manage:
- atopic eczema
- skin infections
- drug eruptions
- urticaria
- skin manifestations of systemic disorders
- ectodermal dysplasia and epidermolysis bullosa
- birth marks, neurocutaneous lesions

Dermatological disorders in children cover an extensive range of clinical problems and presentations. Primary abnormalities of the skin often have a major impact on a child and their family, and some are known to be incompatible with survival. Cutaneous abnormalities are often clearly visible to all, and their impact on the mental health and educational abilities of the individual are often significant and require active and supportive management. Disorders of many other systems may first become evident through their dermatological manifestation, and the ability to recognise and manage these conditions, either directly or through onward referral to a paediatric dermatology service, is part of the skills of the paediatrician.

Atopic eczema

Atopic eczema is a chronic disease with a huge impact on children and families. The aim of treatment is disease control through the avoidance of trigger factors including irritants, the regular use of emollients and the rapid management of flare ups.

Children present with pruritis associated with a chronic fluctuating rash, often on a background of dry skin and the itch may cause sleep disturbance, irritability and distress. The rash often starts on the face in infants (Figure 23.1), but may be anywhere, and often settles in the knee and elbow flexures after 18–24 months of age (Figure 23.2).

The rash is characterised by erythema and itchy papules or vesicles that may become excoriated and lichenified. Eczema may be aggravated by trigger factors including:
- irritants
- ingested or airborne allergens
- infection (systemic or topical)
- intercurrent illness
- stress

Secondary infection with *Staphylococcus aureus* or *Herpes simplex* virus is a common complication (Figure 23.3).

Associations

Atopic eczema is frequently associated with other atopic conditions in the child or other family members including asthma, hay fever, allergic rhinitis and food allergy (30% of children with severe eczema have immediate reactions to egg, milk and peanut). Severe eczema which is associated with infections and growth retardation may be a feature of immunodeficiency syndromes (Table 23.1).

Alternative diagnoses and differing features

Seborrheic dermatitis can present as a similar rash in the first few months of life but is generally less itchy and favours the scalp and nappy areas. Psoriasis is more common in older children and presents as a bright red, well demarcated, less itchy rash.

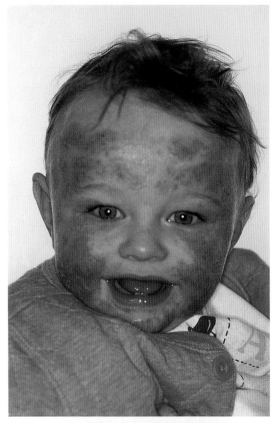

Fig. 23.1 Atopic dermatitis. A 1-year-old boy with severe facial eczema.

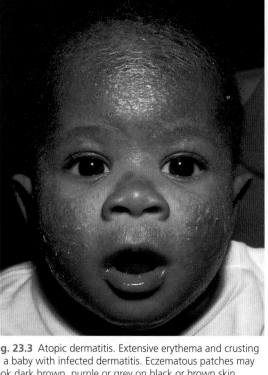

Fig. 23.3 Atopic dermatitis. Extensive erythema and crusting in a baby with infected dermatitis. Eczematous patches may look dark brown, purple or grey on black or brown skin. (Image used with permission from Habif's clinical dermatology: Dinnulos JGH. 7th Edition. Philadelphia. 2021 Elsevier)

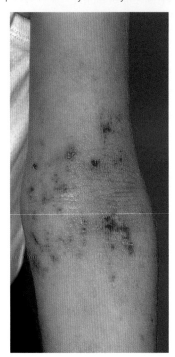

Fig. 23.2 Atopic dermatitis. Left antecubital fossa showing excoriated and infected eczema.

Table 23.1 **Severe eczema associated with immunodeficiency syndromes**		
Syndrome	**Mode of inheritance**	**Features**
Hyper-IgE syndrome	(Two variants— AD and AR	eczema, skin abscesses; eosinophilia; elevated serum IgE
Netherton syndrome	AR	scaly reddish skin; stunted growth; immunodeficiency; high IgE and low to normal IgG
Wiskott-Aldrich syndrome	x linked	eczema; thrombocytopenia; immune deficiency

Table 23.2 Treatment options for management of eczema			
(Reproduced with permission from NICE under Open Content licence)			
	mild eczema	**moderate eczema**	**severe eczema**
Emollients	Yes	yes	yes
topical corticosteroids	mild potency	moderate potency	high potency
steroid example	1% hydrocortisone	clobetasone butyrate	betamethasone
topical calcineurin inhibitors		yes	yes
Bandages		yes	yes
Phototherapy			yes
systemic therapy			yes

Investigations

Atopic eczema is a clinical diagnosis, but investigations may be helpful in specific circumstances. These include:

- bacterial or viral swabs—to exclude super-added infection
- specific serum IgE and skin prick tests—for exacerbating allergens
- patch tests to look for allergic contact dermatitis
- immune deficiency and growth retardation screen

Treatment and management

Assessment at first consultation should include personal and family history of atopic disease, trigger factors, an examination of the whole skin and an assessment of the impact on quality of life. Atopic eczema is a chronic disease with variable severity, and the aim of treatment is to achieve clearance of lesions and then maintain control through regular application of emollients and rapid treatment of flares by parents. General management measures include:

- avoidance of trigger factors
- use of emollients (for washing and daily application to dry skin)
- education of parents to recognise infection
- education of parents to use active treatment on red, inflamed skin

There is a recognised stepwise approach to the pharmacological treatment of eczema which changes with extent of the disease (Table 23.2).

Relevant pharmacological agents used

There are many different types of emollients, and compliance is better if patients are given a choice. The strength of steroids to be used is determined by the severity of disease, age of child and body sites involved. Side effects of prolonged continuous use include skin thinning, systemic absorption and glaucoma. Potent steroids should not generally be used on the face.

Calcineurin inhibitors, such as topical tacrolimus, are useful if eczema is not controlled by safe maintenance doses of topical steroid or the lesions are present at sensitive body sites such as around the eyes.

Systemic treatment using methotrexate, cyclosporin, azathioprine or mycophenolate mofetil have all shown benefit in severe eczema which is unresponsive to other treatments. The first biological treatment for eczema, dupilumab, has been approved for use in the UK.

Bacterial skin infections

Staphylococcal scalded skin syndrome

This is a blistering disorder affecting neonates and infants and is mediated by epidermolytic toxins produced by *Staphylococcus aureus*. The toxin leads to intra-epidermal splitting.

Affected infants usually present with prodromal features such as fever and irritability followed by tender erythematous areas in the flexural areas which quickly progress to other areas. Fragile blisters develop which then desquamate leaving a scalded appearance of skin (Figure 23.4). There is no mucosal involvement. Nikolsky's sign (the sheering of epidermis from dermis upon pressure or the presence of exfoliated epidermis) is typically present. Widespread skin loss in infants can cause temperature instability, fluid and electrolyte imbalance and risk of secondary sepsis.

Investigations

Bacterial swabs from affected sites on the skin may be taken but are often negative as the condition is toxin mediated.

Treatment and management

Prompt initiation of intravenous flucloxacillin is imperative whilst active fluid management is important as fluid

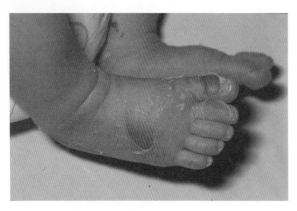

Fig. 23.4 Scalded skin syndrome in 1-month-old child. Note lifting of epidermis and desquamation.

loss and electrolyte imbalance do occur in children with extensive desquamation. Staphylococcal scalded skin syndrome resolves usually in 2–4 weeks without any scarring or pigmentation.

Impetigo

Impetigo is the most common acute bacterial skin infection seen in young children. It is contagious and is usually caused by *Staphylococcus aureus* (rarely *Streptococcus pyogenes*) affecting the epidermal layer of skin.

Non-bullous impetigo is the common form and presents with multiple erythematous papules that coalesce, break down, weep and form crusts. The infection can appear at sites of preexisting skin barrier interruption such as atopic eczema, burns, abrasions or chickenpox. Typically, crusts are golden brown, honey coloured over erythematous base and the usual site is the perioral region. Bullous impetigo can affect intact skin and appears as fragile blisters that deroof leaving a raw erythematous base.

Treatment and management

For localised non-bullous impetigo, treatment with topical antibiotics will be adequate but systemic antibiotics are usually required for widespread involvement. If left untreated, toxic shock syndrome and systemic sepsis can occur.

Cellulitis

Cellulitis is infection of deeper tissues (dermis and subcutaneous tissues) usually caused by streptococci and staphylococci and is invariably preceded by trivial trauma to skin. It usually starts with spreading cutaneous erythema, swelling and pain with systemic features such as fever, malaise and lymphadenopathy and often occurs in the extremities and in the periorbital region.

Treatment and management

Oral antimicrobial therapy is adequate for localised cellulitis but intravenous antibiotics are needed if there is spreading cellulitis or the child is systemically unwell. If left untreated then the infection can progress to localised abscess formation, necrotising fasciitis, systemic sepsis and septic shock. Orbital cellulitis may lead to venous thrombosis if not treated adequately.

Scarlet fever

Scarlet fever is an acute bacterial systemic infection caused by toxin-producing strains of *Group A streptococcus* (GAS), also known as *streptococcus pyogenes*. It is highly contagious and transmission is by aerosol droplets or direct contact with infective secretions.

Dermatological symptoms and signs include widespread maculopapular rash with sandpaper-like texture, strawberry tongue, flushed cheeks with desquamation of peripheries appearing as the rash settles. Fever and lymphadenopathy are also present. Scarlet fever can easily be confused with glandular fever and Kawasaki disease and it is important to assess and investigate a child to exclude these conditions.

Treatment and management

Treatment with oral penicillin for 10 days will suffice for uncomplicated infections and if the child is penicillin allergic, erythromycin or clarithromycin is preferred.

Potential complications

Suppurative complications with abscess formation at different tissue sites may occur. Nonsuppurative complications are delayed effects and immunologically mediated and include acute rheumatic fever and post-streptococcal glomerulonephritis.

Viral skin infections

Systemic viral infections

Generalised viral exanthems are common among children and although many present with nonspecific signs, some have characteristic systemic features with skin involvement.

Infectious mononucleosis (Epstein-Barr virus, glandular fever) presents a generalised morbilliform rash along with fever, sore throat, exudative tonsillitis, lymphadenopathy and palatal purpura. A lymphocytosis is usually seen.

Measles was uncommon until recently when the uptake of the vaccination fell following misinformation. The child develops a widespread morbilliform rash, Kolpik spots in the buccal mucosa, conjunctivitis and fever.

Roseola infantum (HHV-6 infection) presents with an initial fever and malaise. Its importance for clinical practice is that the initial fever settles after a few days just as the rash appears. It is, therefore, a recognised reason why some individuals are diagnosed with 'penicillin allergy' having been started on antibiotics during the febrile period.

Parvovirus produces an erythematous macular rash particularly evident on the face and gives the classical 'slapped cheek' appearance. In children with an existing haemolytic disorder such as spherocytosis, an infection with parvovirus can lead to acute haemolysis whilst immunosuppressed children can develop anaemia from bone marrow suppression.

Varicella zoster (chickenpox) is highly contagious and produces a characteristic pleiomorphic rash. The lesions evolve over time and initially appear maculopapular before changing into vesicles and then scabs. All stages will be evident at the same time at the height of the illness.

Localised viral skin infections

Molluscum contagiosum is one of the common localised cutaneous viral infections seen in children, and there is an increased prevalence in children who are immunocompromised or who have atopic eczema. Transmission occurs by close contact or infected fomites. The lesions appear as flesh coloured dome-shaped, pearly, umbilicated papules (Figure 23.5) over face, chest, body, back and legs and genital areas and are generally asymptomatic. Molluscum lesions clear spontaneously over years and therefore treatment is not routinely required.

Viral warts are common in school age children, particularly in children with eczema as a result of skin barrier dysfunction. Transmission occurs by close contact with affected individuals or indirectly through fomites. They can occur anywhere although hands and feet are commonly affected. Common warts are hard, rough hyperkeratotic papules over hands, around nail beds, toes and on the knees whilst plantar warts are rough, flat lesion with tiny black dot in the centre usually seen on plantar surface of the foot. These latter types of warts are often quite painful. Most warts disappear spontaneously without treatment, but if they are painful and limit function then treatment can be offered. Cryotherapy and topical salicylic acid are widely used. Safeguarding issues should be considered in the underlying aetiology if extensive anogenital warts are seen.

Herpes simplex virus infection (HSV-1 and HSV-2) infections are transmitted by direct contact with cold sores or genital herpes. HSV-1 is primarily associated with

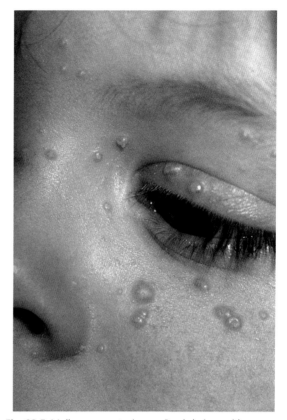

Fig. 23.5 Molluscum contagiosum. Pearly lesions with umbilication.

infections around the mouth, oral cavity and face, and the lesions appear as painful clusters of vesicles that may extend into the gingiva and oral cavity (herpetic gingivostomatitis). HSV-2 lesions predominantly involve the anogenital area.

Children with underlying skin barrier dysfunction such as eczema or burns may develop rapidly disseminating HSV infection known as eczema herpeticum (Figure 23.6). This can be painful and has associated systemic features.

Skin swabs for viral PCR should be sent if the diagnosis is uncertain. Oral antivirals are used to limit the severity of infection and halt progression whilst intravenous antivirals are preferred if the child is systemically unwell.

Fungal skin infections

A number of fungi, moulds and yeast can cause skin infections in children. Most serious fungal infections occur in immunocompromised children where opportunistic

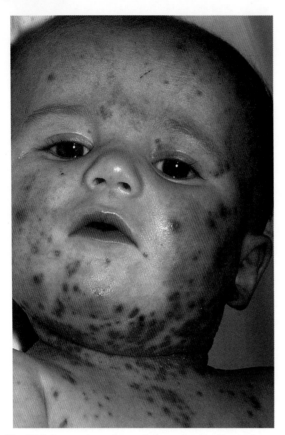

Fig. 23.6 Eczema herpeticum. A 6-month-old with atopic eczema with primary herpes simplex infection.

infection can lead to systemic fungal sepsis. Common superficial fungal infections include:

Tinea (dermatophyte) infections

Tinea capitis can present as a boggy infected scalp swelling (kerion) and often looks like an abscess. Other features include itchy, circular patches of hair loss with dry, scaling skin, broken-off hair shafts and associated cervical lymphadenopathy. **Tinea corporis** (ringworm) appears as annular or ring-shaped lesions with central clearing and peripheral fine scales, redness over trunk, arms or legs. **Tinea pedis** (athlete's foot) presents as redness, scaling and maceration in interdigital areas whilst **Tinea unguium** (onychomycosis) affects the nail bed and nail plate leading to brittle nails, fine white powdery surface and thickening of nail plate.

Fungal scrapings from affected sites are important to establish diagnosis and treatment includes oral antifungal agents such as terbinafine and griseofulvin for scalp and nail infections. For tinea corporis and pedis, topical antifungal agents are suitable.

Candida (yeast) infections

These are common in neonates and young infants and are caused by *Candida albicans* and the common manifestations are oral thrush and napkin dermatitis. Oral thrush typically presents with mucosal involvement with white plaques over tongue, buccal cavity and pharynx that leave a red, raw area underneath when scraped. It can also occur in older children who use recurrent steroid inhalers and recurrent use of antibiotics, as this disturbs oral microbial flora.

Napkin candidiasis describes multiple erythematous, circular 'satellite-like' lesions affecting groin areas and buttock region. Napkin candidiasis is one cause of 'nappy rash.' Other causes include irritant dermatitis from prolonged contact with urine or faeces, atopic dermatitis, infantile seborrheic dermatitis, napkin psoriasis, allergic contact dermatitis, perianal streptococcal infection, scabies and zinc deficiency (acrodermatitis enteropathica). The diagnosis is usually clinical but skin scrapings help to support the diagnosis and treatment includes topical antifungal agents and oral nystatin.

Infestation

Scabies is an extremely itchy, contagious skin infestation caused by a mite (*Sarcoptes scabeii*) and usually affects more than one member of the family. Transmission is through close contact, sharing bedding and towels and is common in crowded living conditions.

Clinical features

- intense pruritus which is particularly worse at night
- excoriated and scratched areas of skin
- linear burrows in the interdigital spaces (Figure 23.7), wrists, and penis
- linear lesions may have a small black dot at the end

Demonstration of mites, burrows and faecal material from skin scrapings is the gold standard method for diagnosis. It is imperative to treat all family members at the same time with 5% permethrin and ensure that the family know the correct application technique. Where permethrin is contraindicated, 0.5% malathion can be used.

Urticaria

Urticaria is a common skin disorder characterised by appearance of intensely itchy, transient wheals on an erythematous base. It can be sometimes be accompanied by angioedema which is swelling of deeper tissues beneath the skin.

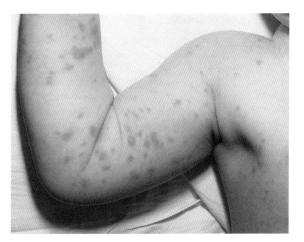

Fig. 23.8 Urticaria. Pink wheals over the upper arm.

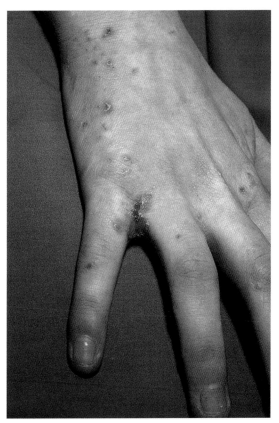

Fig. 23.7 Scabies. Finger web involvement.

Acute urticaria lasts for less than 6 weeks and there is usually an identifiable cause which, in children, is often a viral infection. Other causes include food allergens, drugs and insect sting (bee, wasp) and are often seen in children with an atopic background.

Chronic urticaria describes episodes that last for more than 6 weeks and may be idiopathic or associated with a recognised physical or exogenous stimulus.

Autoimmune urticaria is a form of spontaneous urticaria associated with autoimmune conditions including coeliac disease, type 1 diabetes, hypothyroidism, inflammatory bowel disease, juvenile arthritis and lupus.

Inducible urticaria is a unique subset of chronic urticaria triggered by physical stimulus such as heat, cold, water, pressure, vibration, sun exposure (solar), contact, dermographism and exercise.

Clinical presentation

The lesions appear as pruritic, well-circumscribed, erythematous plaques or wheals with central clearing (Figure 23.8) that are of varying sizes and which may coalesce. Individual lesions last less than 24 hours, but the overall condition can persist with new crops of lesions occurring at fresh sites. Urticaria can be accompanied by angioedema—commonly swelling of lips, tongue, eyes, hands and feet—and in most situations, this resolves without progression to life threatening symptoms although recurrence is common.

Investigations

Investigations are not usually required but, in some children, further testing may be necessary if IgE-mediated food or drug allergy is suspected.

Treatment and management

Treatment of urticaria mainly involves symptomatic relief with the use of antihistamines and avoidance of any known triggers. Second generation antihistamines are the standard first step treatment. For those children with chronic urticaria who are not improving despite antihistamines, a stepwise management approach has been recommended with leukotriene antagonists, H_2 blockers, intermittent short courses of oral steroids and a biologic, omalizumab.

Cutaneous drug eruptions

Cutaneous drug reactions are a common manifestation of adverse drug reactions and the majority of them are of a benign exanthematous pattern. The history and a temporal relationship to the onset of the rash is crucial to diagnosis, and although severe cutaneous reactions are rare, they can constitute a dermatological emergency.

Clinical presentation

Drug reactions may be limited to the skin or may be associated with a severe systemic reaction. The most common cutaneous eruptions are benign and appear as a morbilliform rash although other forms including urticaria, angioedema, erythema multiforme, and bullous eruptions do occur. The initial rash usually appears 3–14 days after exposure and the mucosa is usually spared. Symptoms settle with desquamation over a period of few days after the removal of offending drug.

Severe adverse drug reactions are recognised as a spectrum of mucocutaneous and systemic involvement. Stevens-Johnson syndrome/toxic epidermal necrolysis is the most well recognised presentation with:
- blisters with large areas of skin detachment (positive Nikolsky's sign)
- painful mucus membrane erosions
- atypical target skin lesions
- purpura
- widespread epidermal necrosis

Common culprits are penicillin, high dose cephalosporins, sulphonamides and anticonvulsants (carbamazepine, phenytoin, lamotrigine).

Diagnosis and management

Skin biopsy has a role when the diagnosis is unclear although there are no specific histological features to confirm a drug reaction. Intradermal test for drug allergies is used particularly for penicillin-cephalosporin allergy. Adequate management requires the cessation of offending drug and supportive care. Toxic epidermal necrolysis is an emergency that may require referral to burns unit.

Systemic disorders involving the skin

The skin can give a clue to diagnosis of systemic conditions, and signs may predate other features of systemic disease. Changes may be disease specific and should guide the clinician to look for possible related underlying disease (Table 23.3).

Connective tissue disease

Clinical presentation

Connective tissue disease in children may present as a well-defined entity such as lupus erythematosus or as a mixed picture with features of several connective tissue disorders.

Table 23.3 Systemic disorders commonly associated with characteristic skin manifestations

	systemic disorder	dermatological features
Connective tissue disease and vasculitis	systemic lupus erythematosus discoid lupus erythematosus neonatal lupus erythematosus	butterfly rash; photosensitivity; scarring skin plaques; hair loss
	juvenile dermatomyositis	pale pink rash eyelids; Gottron's papules on the knuckles; photosensitivity
	scleroderma	morphoea
	cutaneous vasculitis	palpable purpura
Endocrine disorders	diabetes	necrobiosis lipoidica; acanthosis nigricans
	thyroid	dry skin; brittle hair
	adrenal	hyperpigmentation
Autoimmune disorders	vitiligo alopecia areata	hypopigmented patches; well-defined bald patches
	coeliac disease	dermatitis herpetiformis
Inflammatory disorders	erythema multiforme	target lesions
	erythema nodosum	red tender nodules on the shins
	Bechet's disease	mouth and genital ulcers
Proliferative disorders	Langerhans cell histiocytosis	greasy papules on scalp, neck, axillae and groins

Lupus erythematosus

This is usually divided into:
- systemic lupus erythematosus
- discoid lupus erythematosus
- neonatal lupus (distinct condition caused by maternal antibodies)

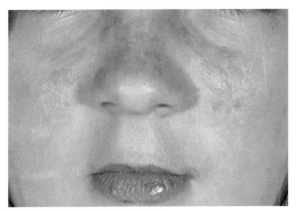

Fig. 23.9 Systemic lupus erythematosus. 9-year-old girl with classical butterfly rash (Copyright - Dr Jane Ravenscroft – reproduced with permission)

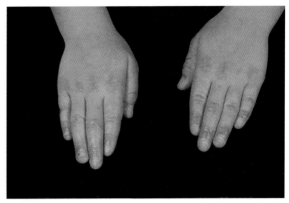

Fig. 23.10 Dermatomyositis. Characteristic distribution of rash over dorsal joint surfaces (Copyright - Dr Jane Ravenscroft – reproduced with permission)

Systemic lupus erythematosus is a systemic disease characterised by multiorgan involvement, most commonly skin, joints and blood vessels. Skin problems may predate other organ involvement and include a butterfly rash over the cheeks and bridge of nose (Figure 23.9), photosensitivity, alopecia and mouth ulcers. Raynaud phenomenon is a common associated finding. All patients should have meticulous sun protection including sun avoidance, hats, sunblock when necessary and, for skin disease alone, potent topical steroids and immunomodulators.

Discoid erythematosus is rare in children and produces red scaly patches most commonly affecting face and scalp. Early diagnosis and treatment with super potent steroids and sunblock helps reduce scarring.

Neonatal lupus occurs in the offspring of mothers with positive Ro/SSa antibodies and occasionally La/SSB antibodies. It presents with:

*   red, scaly eruption on the face and classically around the eyes (raccoon eyes)
*   congenital heart block in the first few weeks of life.

Mother may have a known connective tissue disorder, but many mothers do not have clinical signs and do not know they are carrying the antibodies. It usually resolves within the first year of life. Topical steroids may be used and sun protection is advised.

Juvenile dermatomyositis

Dermatomyositis is an autoimmune disorder, affecting predominantly the skin and muscle. The juvenile type presents with a rash in over 50% of patients. The characteristic features:

*   pale pink rash typically affects the face (often upper eyelids), knuckles (Figure 23.10) and knees

*   rash may first appear after sun exposure (photosensitivity)
*   cutaneous calcinosis
*   diffuse alopecia
*   myositis

Management is with strict sun protection and systemic immunosuppression, usually methotrexate being first line agent.

Scleroderma

Scleroderma comprises a group of diseases which share a common feature of increased collagen deposition in an autoimmune setting. It may take the form of:

*   plaque morphoea—localised round patches of thickened skin, often with purple tinge
*   linear morphoea—linear induration of limbs or scalp
*   pansclerotic morphoea or systemic sclerosis—generalised skin induration

Localised treatment using UVB light therapy or other topical treatment is used for limited involvement whilst more extensive disease requires immunosuppression.

Cutaneous vasculitis

Cutaneous vasculitis is an inflammatory process of blood vessels in the skin, usually presenting as palpable purpura. It may often be isolated to the skin of the lower limbs or may involve other organs as part of a systemic vasculitis. The differential diagnosis of palpable purpura include:

*   cutaneous vasculitis
*   sepsis (meningococcus; DIC)
*   localised pressure, trauma, suction
*   coagulation abnormality
*   other rashes—urticaria, urticarial vasculitis, erythema multiforme

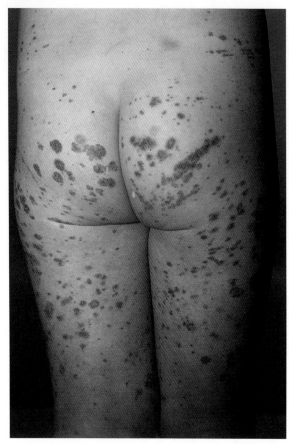

Fig. 23.11 A 6-year-old girl with Henoch-Schonlein purpura showing purpura over buttocks and lower limbs.

Small vessel cutaneous vasculitis usually only affects the skin where palpable purpura is most commonly seen on lower legs, arms and trunk. It can occur at any age although it is more common in those over 12 years. Investigations are aimed at ruling out a systemic condition.

Henoch-Schönlein purpura

Henoch-Schönlein purpura is an immune complex–mediated disease which is IgA mediated and forms part of the classic triad of purpura, abdominal pain and arthritis. The palpable purpura is classically distributed on buttocks and lower legs (Figure 23.11) though occasionally can be more generalised.

Kawasaki disease

An example of a vasculitis affecting larger blood vessels. The child usually presents under the age of 5 years with:
- high fever for over 5 days

- conjunctivitis
- lymphadenopathy
- erythematous rash progressing to acral desquamation

There is a risk of subsequent coronary artery aneurysms at a later stage.

Endocrine disorders

Endocrine disorders in children are uncommon, but many will show skin changes, including:
- Addison disease—hyperpigmentation
- Cushing disease—striae
- Hypopituitism—fair skin and fair hair
- Hypothyroidism—dry skin, brittle hair

Diabetes-related disorders

Necrobiosis lipoidica is a chronic, granulomatous condition which causes characteristic plaques which are waxy textured, yellow or orange and telangiectatic plaques on the shins which are largely asymptomatic. Over 90% of patients with necrobiosis lipoidica have or will develop diabetes mellitus. Treatment is difficult as the condition does not often improve with good diabetic control.

Acanthosis nigricans. This velvety brown hyperpigmentation of the neck and axillae is seen in overweight patients with diabetes or insulin resistance (Figure 23.12).

Autoimmune disorders

Autoimmune disorders may be specific to the skin and include vitiligo which causes hypopigmented patches without systemic involvement. Alopecia areata leads to discrete smooth bald patches on the scalp and sometimes other hair bearing areas. It is often transient, and regrowth occurs without scarring.

Other disorders
Coeliac disease

Dermatitis herpetiformis, which is associated with coeliac disease, is a very itchy, blistering rash affecting the elbows and buttocks and, if problematic, can be treated with dapsone until a gluten=free diet is established. Coeliac disease may also present with generalised hair thinning due to iron deficiency.

Erythema multiforme

This is a hypersensitivity reaction which develops acutely and is characterised by the sudden development of red papules. They can appear anywhere but acral sites, especially hands (Figure 23.13) and arms are commonly affected. Lesions evolve into typical target shapes, and

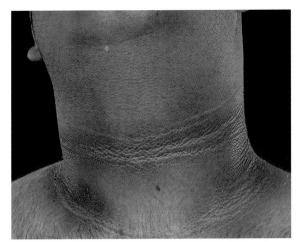

Fig. 23.12 Acanthosis nigrans. Appearance in neck of 15-year-old boy with diabetes mellitus (Copyright - Dr Jane Ravenscroft – reproduced with permission)

prodromal symptoms may include fever, joint pains and myalgia.

In around 90% of children, the lesions are triggered by infections, with *Herpes simplex* being the most common organism. Less than 10% may be attributed to drugs such as nonsteroidal antiinflammatory drugs, penicillins, sulphonamides and anticonvulsants. Erythema multiforme is now seen as a different entity to that of Steven-Johnson syndrome and toxic epidermal cecrosis which are much more commonly triggered by drugs.

Erythema nodosum

Erythema nodosum is clinically characterised by the sudden eruption of several red, tender nodules, typically on the shins (Figure 23.14). It is a reactive process in the skin that may be triggered by a wide range of infections, inflammatory disorders and, less commonly, by medications and malignancy. The commonest causes in children are bacterial infections (group A streptococcal throat infection) and inflammatory bowel disease.

Langerhans cell histiocytosis

Langerhans cell histiocytosis is a rare disease characterised by the clonal proliferation of cells which are phenotypically similar to macrophages. It is described as either a single system disease associated with a generally indolent course and excellent prognosis or multisystem disease which carries significant morbidity and mortality. Single system disease most commonly affects bone, but cutaneous disease usually presents before the age of 4 years with a characteristic rash (Figure 23.15).

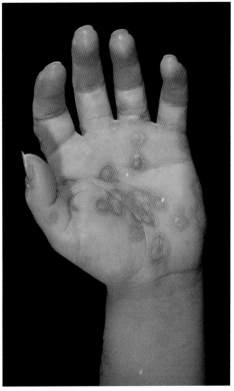

Fig. 23.13 Erythema multiforme. Hands of 12-year-old boy recently given amoxicillin (Copyright - Dr Jane Ravenscroft – reproduced with permission)

Ectodermal dysplasias

Ectodermal dysplasia is a term used to describe a number of different genetic conditions which lead to abnormalities of ectodermal structures:
- hair—absent, sparse or slow growing
- teeth—widely spaced, conical (Figure 23.16) and missing
- nails—dysplastic or absent

Hypohydrotic ectodermal dysplasia is the most common ectodermal dysplasia and the skin is dry and may be scaly. Reduced sweating causes heat intolerance and overheating which can lead to febrile seizures and may even be fatal, especially in early life.

Epidermolysis bullosa

Epidermolysis bullosa is a rare genetic disorder of skin fragility which leads to blister formation of the skin and mucosae following mild mechanical trauma. It should be

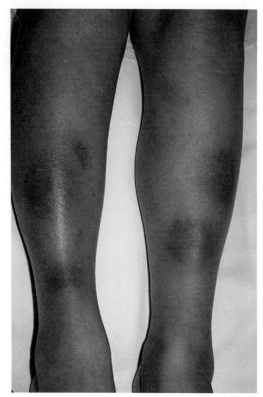

Fig. 23.14 Erythema nodosum. Typical lesions on the shin (Copyright - Dr Jane Ravenscroft – reproduced with permission)

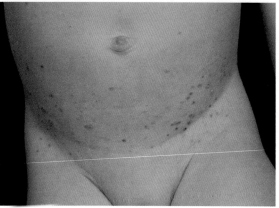

Fig. 23.15 Langerhans cell histiocytosis. Typical rash in 3-month-old child.

suspected in a neonate born with areas of skin loss, and immediate measures should be taken to reduce the risk of further skin damage such as removing wristbands and avoiding tapes. Classification is based on the level of ultra-structural blistering and the deeper the level of the split,

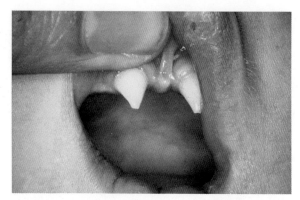

Fig. 23.16 Ectodermal Dysplasia. Conical teeth seen in the condition.

the greater the scarring and deformity. There are three major subtypes of the condition.

Epidermolysis bullosa simplex

Inheritance is autosomal dominant, so there is usually an affected parent. EBS may present with superficial widespread blisters soon after birth or the presentation may be in childhood with blisters without scarring localised to the hands and feet.

Junctional epidermolysis bullosa

Junctional epidermolysis bullosa is an autosomal recessive and the least common type of epidermolysis bullosa. It is characterised by generalised skin and mucosal erosions with wounds tending to form excessive granulations especially around the central face. Nails are dystrophic or absent. Mucosal involvement causes a characteristic hoarse cry.

Dystrophic epidermolysis bullosa

This condition may be is autosomal recessive or dominant. Recessive subtypes are the most severe and may present with large areas of skin loss at birth (Figure 23.17). Blistering and erosions can be extensive and heal with scarring, contractures and mitten deformity of the hands and feet. Dominant dystrophic epidermolysis bullosa is less severe and often localised to areas predisposed to trauma such as knees, elbows and ankles.

Birthmarks

Vascular malformations

Vascular malformations are a group of conditions that arise due to dysfunctional embryogenesis leading to defective vasculature. They are present from birth and

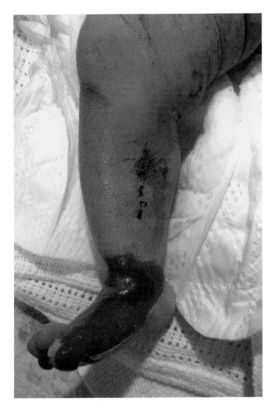

Fig. 23.17 Dominant dystrophic epidermolysis bullosa. Characteristic skin loss on the foot of a newborn child (Copyright - Dr Jane Ravenscroft – reproduced with permission)

persist throughout life and can be classified as capillary, venous, lymphatic and arteriovenous malformations.

Capillary malformations

This description includes salmon patches and stork marks (naevus simplex) and appear as flat pink or red patches with ill-defined borders over the forehead, above eyelids or on the nape of neck. These require no investigation or treatment and rarely come to medical attention.

Port wine stain (also known as naevus flammeus)

These lesions are a subtype of capillary malformations and appear as a large flat pink, purple, red patch with well demarcated borders which can occur anywhere but are often seen over face. Port wine stains do not disappear and they become darker with time and can be associated with lymphatic, venous and arteriovenous malformations. They are seen in Sturge Weber and Klippel Trenaunay

syndromes. Treatment of options include cosmetic camouflage and pulsed dye laser.

Venous malformations

Low flow vascular malformations which appear as bluish-purple, soft, compressible swellings. Spontaneous thrombosis is common due to venous stasis and they then may present as a painful swelling (thrombophlebitis). MRI angiography will ascertain the extent of involvement and treatment includes compression, sclerotherapy or surgery.

Lymphatic malformations

Abnormalities of the lymphatics are usually apparent at birth and present as soft, spongy, nontender fluid-filled masses often around the head and neck. When enlarged they can impinge on nearby structures such as the trachea and oesophagus and cause functional impairment. Treatment includes excision or sclerotherapy depending on the site and extent of the lesion.

Vascular tumours

Infantile haemangiomas

These are the most common benign vascular tumours of infancy and usually clinically inapparent at birth. A superficial lesion is known as a strawberry naevus and appears as a red raised lesion whilst a deeper lesion gives a bluish appearance to the swelling.

They exhibit a unique clinical course that consists of proliferation and then involution. Rapid growth occurs during the first 4–6 weeks and most reach 80% of their maximum size by 3 months. Natural involution or regression takes over from 12 months and continues slowly over 3 to 10 years (Figure 23.18).

Orbital haemangiomas present with proptosis, squint and distortion of eyelid margins. There is the potential for amblyopia and consequently they need prompt assessment and treatment. Life-threatening airway obstruction can occur if sub glottic and supra glottic regions are involved.

Associations

Large and plaque-like cutaneous haemangiomas have a higher association with extra cutaneous abnormalities including cardiac malformations, urogenital anomalies, spinal dysraphism and anogenital abnormalities. Multiple ones (greater than 10 in number) can be associated with hepatic haemangiomas and, in this situation, the initial assessment should aim to identify the possible location of all lesions with cardiac echo, liver ultrasound and cranial imaging.

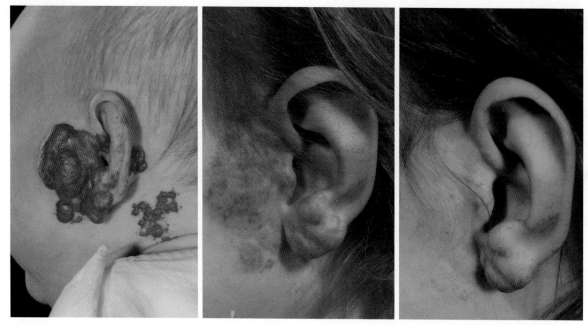

Fig. 23.18 Infantile haemangioma—progress over time. Images of same lesion at 4 months, 28 months and 5 years. Parents elected to not receive any treatment (Copyright - Dr Martin Hewitt – reproduced with permission)

Treatment

Superficial, uncomplicated infantile haemangiomas will usually involute after a year and simply need monitoring to ensure they follow the expected course. For complicated haemangiomas with a risk of functional impairment or cosmetic disfigurement oral propranolol is now the first-line treatment. A full assessment of the child should be undertaken prior to starting propranolol including heart rate, blood pressure and ECG.

Pigmented birthmarks

These birthmarks have a grey or brown colour. Commonly recognised ones include:

Congenital dermal melanocytosis (previously known as Mongolian blue spots) are ill-defined areas of blue, black or slate grey discolouration noted at birth in neonates of Asian or African descent (Figure 23.19). The lumbosacral area is the commonest site though spots can be seen in extremities and face and can be mistaken for bruises in infants.

Café au lait macules are brown, round or oval, well-defined areas of hyperpigmentation of varying sizes. Solitary café au lait macules are common and of no clinical concern whereas the presence of more than five lesions may indicate associated genetic syndromes including:

- neurofibromatosis
- tuberous sclerosis
- ataxia telangiectasia
- McCune-Albright syndrome

CLINICAL SCENARIO

A 3-month-old boy was brought to the emergency department after being found in a collapsed state at home. He was born at term and had no postnatal problems, fed well and had a normal weight gain.

At about 4 weeks of life, his parents had noticed multiple lumps appearing on his face, trunk and arms. Initially small and red, they did not cause distress but they gradually increased in size over the following weeks. Around the same time, he developed coarse sounds in his breathing which gradually increased in volume and was biphasic in nature.

On review in the emergency department resuscitation room, he was pale, responding poorly to stimuli and had obvious biphasic stridor and mark intercostal and sternal recession. Anaesthetic support was called and he was intubated although the intervention proved difficult and fresh blood was noted in the oropharynx after the procedure. Multiple haemangiomas, some up to 2 cm in diameter, were noted across his body.

Dermatology advice was obtained and a diagnosis of infantile haemangiomatosis was made. Imaging identified a lesion in his trachea proximal to the tip of the endotracheal tube, a 4 cm lesion in his liver, a 1 cm lesion in his left kidney and no lesions in the brain or spinal cord. A tracheostomy was performed allowing disconnection from a ventilator.

He was treated with oral propranolol and the lesions gradually involuted. He made a full recovery and the tracheostomy was closed at 15 months.

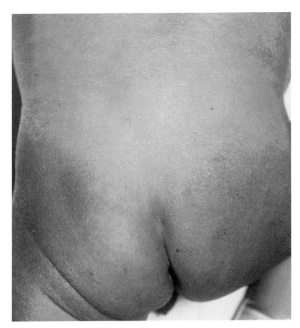

Fig. 23.19 Congenital dermal melanocytosis in a newborn child.

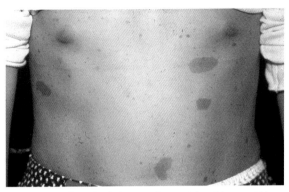

Fig. 23.20 Café au lait lesions on the trunk in a 14-year-old boy with neurofibromatosis type 1.

- Lisch nodules are pigmented iris hamartomas visible on slit lamp examination

Neurocutaneous syndromes

Neurocutaneous syndromes are a group of diverse conditions with a genetic basis presenting with neurological and skin manifestations. The skin and central nervous system share a common embryonic origin, and mutations leading to defective neural crest differentiation are believed to be the underlying basis. Cutaneous manifestations serve as markers to underlying neurological and systemic conditions.

Neurofibromatosis

Clinical presentation

The condition is inherited as an autosomal dominant condition with 100% penetrance by the age of 5 years. The cutaneous manifestations include

- café-au-lait macules that are flat, well-defined, oval brown macules over trunk and extremities (Figure 23.20) and are the first feature of the disease to appear. They increase in number and size in the first decade
- cutaneous neurofibromas are soft pink tumours, over trunk and limbs and many hundreds may develop
- plexiform neurofibroma are diffuse fibroma along trigeminal or cervical nerves which appear in the first 2 years of life
- axillary and inguinal freckling is a characteristic feature of NF-1

Investigations and management

When a diagnosis of NF1 is suspected, children should be referred to Clinical Genetics to confirm a diagnosis and to assess relatives. A multidisciplinary approach involving various professionals is important in management.

Tuberous sclerosis complex

Tuberous sclerosis complex represents a genetic disorder characterised by presence of hamartomas in multiple organs. It is one of the common, single gene disorders transmitted by autosomal dominant inheritance with variable expression. Individuals with the condition may develop classical cutaneous lesions, epilepsy and intellectual disability.

Clinical presentation

Skin manifestations are found in 60% to 90% of patients and classically include

- angiofibromas (previously known as adenoma sebaceum) that usually appear between the ages of 3–10 years. These are firm, discrete, telangiectatic papules over nasolabial furrows, cheeks, chin and often become more extensive around puberty
- periungual fibromas appear after puberty and are smooth flesh-coloured outgrowths emerging from nail folds
- shagreen patches are large, thickened, irregular skin-coloured plaques with orange peel surface and are usually seen in the lumbosacral region (Figure 23.21)
- ash leaf macules (hypomelanotic macules) usually appear in early infancy and are oval hypopigmented macules visible under Wood's lamp examination on the trunk and peripheries (Figure 23.21)

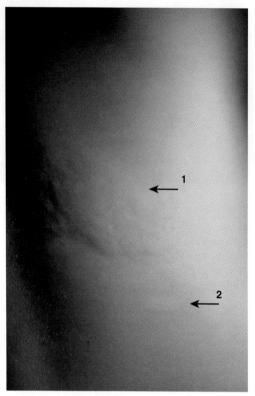

Fig. 23.21 Shagreen patch (arrow 1) and hypopigmented macule (arrow 2) on back in 12-year-old with tuberous sclerosis (Copyright - Dr Jane Ravenscroft – reproduced with permission)

Sturge Weber syndrome

Sturge Weber syndrome is a segmental vascular, neurocutaneous disorder characterised by:

- cutaneous—ipsilateral facial port wine stain in the trigeminal nerve distribution
- neurological—ipsilateral leptomeningeal angiomatosis
- ophthalmic—ipsilateral glaucoma or ocular abnormalities

The facial port wine stain can be treated with a 'pulsed dye' laser but complete clearance is not achievable.

Incontinentia pigmenti

This is an x-linked dominant condition affecting females that is lethal in males. The cutaneous manifestations are classical and diagnostic and evolve over time. They are usually present at birth. The initial lesions are small, grouped blisters on an erythematous base with a **linear distribution** over peripheries and a swirly, patchy pattern which becomes hyperpigmented streaks over time. Management is supportive and the skin lesions require no treatment as the initial blisters heal spontaneously without sequelae.

Ataxia telangiectasia

Ataxia telangiectasia (AT) is a rare, progressive, multisystem neurocutaneous disorder characterised by manifestations secondary to defective DNA repair and neuronal degeneration. The dermatological manifestations include telangiectases over face and bulbar conjunctiva usually appearing around the age of 3 years in sun-exposed areas on the face, eyelids and ears which then spread to neck, hands and feet. Lymphoreticular malignancies occur during childhood and affected individuals have high susceptibility to tissue damage from ionising radiation. There is no specific cure.

IMPORTANT CLINICAL POINTS

Atopic eczema
- presents with rash and pruritus
- associated with other atopic conditions
- first-line treatment is with emollients and topical steroids
- disease control through regular use of emollients, avoidance of irritants and rapid management of flare ups

Skin Infections
- staphylococcal scalded skin syndrome
  - caused by toxins produced by Staphylococcus aureus
  - mucosa is not involved
- scarlet fever
  - toxin producing strains of Group A streptococcus
  - asymptomatic carriage is common
  - is a notifiable disease

- herpes simplex virus
  - HSV-1 primarily around mouth and oral cavity (herpetic gingivostomatitis)
  - HSV-2 predominantly involves the anogenital area

Urticaria
- can be associated with angioedema
- acute urticaria lasts for less than 6 weeks
- identifiable triggers for acute urticaria
- investigations are often not necessary

Cutaneous drug eruptions
- antibiotics are commonest cause
- any drug can be the culprit, and onset can be delayed

Further reading

Atopic eczema in under 12s: Diagnosis and management.
NICE guideline [CG57] Published December 2007. Last update
March 2021.

Chapter | 24 |

Diabetes mellitus

Juliana Chizo Agwu

After reading this chapter you should be able to:
- assess, diagnose and manage diabetes and its complications, including diabetic ketoacidosis
- assess, diagnose and manage hypoglycaemia in the child with diabetes

The diagnosis of diabetes has a significant impact on children, young people and their families. Like all other chronic conditions, it will affect the physical and mental health of the individual and may influence many life choices. All paediatric teams will need skills in the management of patients admitted acutely with the major metabolic abnormalities seen with diabetes whilst the long-term support, advice and monitoring is provided by specialist diabetes teams. Such teams include paediatricians, dieticians, nurse specialists and psychologists and will have experience in the management of biochemical, physical, emotional and behavioural difficulties seen in patients with diabetes.

The most common form of diabetes mellitus in children and young people is type 1 diabetes which is a polygenic disease due to the autoimmune destruction of insulin-producing pancreatic beta cells. Other types of childhood diabetes include type 2 diabetes (the result of multiple gene abnormalities and environmental factors) and monogenic diabetes (due to various single gene defects) Diagnostic criteria are shown in Table 24.1.

Diabetes is a lifelong condition, and those young people who receive their initial care from paediatric teams will need to transfer to adult services at some stage in their teenage years. Such a transition needs careful planning by both paediatric and adult teams, and the patient and their family need to be guided on the process before it occurs. The actual transition should occur at a time of relative stability in the health of the young person and should aim to avoid major events in lifestyle and education such as school exams.

Table 24.1 The recognised diagnostic criteria for diabetes mellitus

Random blood glucose (in the presence of typical symptoms)	greater than 11.1 mmol/l
Fasting plasma glucose	level greater than 7 mmol/l
2-hour post prandial glucose	greater than 11.1 mmol/l
HbA1c	greater than 48 mmol/mol (6.5%)
An abnormal random blood glucose (> 11.1 mmol/l) in the presence of typical symptoms is diagnostic. However, children and young people who are asymptomatic need a second abnormal result on another day to confirm the diagnosis	
Impaired glucose tolerance	
Fasting plasma glucose	greater than 7.0 mmol/l
2-hour post prandial glucose	greater than 7.8 mmol/l and less than 11.1 mmol/l
Impaired fasting glucose	
Fasting plasma glucose	6.1 to 6.9 mmol/l

Type 1 diabetes mellitus

Clinical presentation

Typical symptoms of diabetes are polyuria, polydipsia and polyphagia, weight loss and recurrent infections.

The individual may be relatively well or may present very unwell with diabetic ketoacidosis (DKA) with marked dehydration, shock and a reduced conscious level.

The risk of developing other autoimmune conditions such as hypothyroidism, thyrotoxicosis, coeliac disease, Addison disease and autoimmune liver disease is higher in children with type 1 diabetes when compared to the general population.

Investigations

Children and young people with the clinical features suggestive of diabetes mellitus should be referred on the same day to secondary care for urgent assessment and the initiation of insulin therapy. This is to avoid any delay and risk the child developing DKA.

Investigations in hospital setting include:

- random blood glucose
- blood ketones
- urea and electrolytes—to asses dehydration and electrolyte disturbance
- blood gas—to assess if acidosis
- thyroid function test
- coeliac screen (tissue transglutaminase)
- diabetes related auto antibodies—may aid differentiation of type of diabetes

Treatment and management

Those who are alert, well and not vomiting should be encouraged to take oral fluids. They will also need to start insulin either as multiple daily insulin injections or as a continuous subcutaneous insulin infusion. Both approaches will need the required total daily dose of insulin to be calculated using 0.5–0.75 units/kg/day. Patients will need basal insulin, pre-meal bolus insulin and correction dose prescribed (Table 24.2).

The prescribing of insulin must be undertaken with care and the UK Department of Health and Social Care has identified errors in the prescribing of insulin as 'never events.' It is therefore important that:

- the words 'unit' or 'international units' should not be abbreviated
- specific insulin administration devices should always be used to measure insulin (i.e. insulin syringes and pens)
- insulin should not be withdrawn from an insulin pen or pen refill and then administered using a syringe and needle

The blood glucose targets are:

- on waking: 4–7 mmol/l
- before meals: 4–7 mmol/l
- after meals: 5–9 mmol/litre
- when driving: at least 5 mmol/l

Table 24.2 **Calculation of daily insulin requirements**	
Basal insulin	Between 30% to 50% of total daily dose (TDD) is given as basal insulin using a long-acting insulin analogue (Glargine, Determir or Insulin degludec)
Pre-meal insulin	The pre-meal insulin bolus using rapid-acting insulin analogue (Insulin Aspart, Insulin Lispro, Insulin Glulisine) and is prescribed as insulin:carbohydrate ratio (I:CHO ratio) There are different ways to calculate the I:CHO ratio Some clinicians use the '500 rule' (500/TDD) for children over 5 years and '300 rule' (300/TDD) for those under 5 years. Some hospitals use pre-set I:CHO ratios rather than using either 500 or 300 rules.
Correction dose	This is the amount of **extra** rapid-acting insulin analogue to administer to bring high glucose levels to target To calculate the 'correction' dose: • calculate the child's Insulin Sensitivity Factor (which is how much 1 unit of insulin will reduce their blood glucose in 2–4 hours) by dividing 100 by the total daily dose of insulin (100/TDD). • determine the required fall in glucose level to return the value to the target range • calculate the number of units of insulin which will produce this required fall in glucose level For example, if the calculated Insulin Sensitivity Factor for a particular patient is 4, the measured blood glucose is 11 mmol/l and target blood glucose is between 4–7mmol/l, this indicates that the patient will need to administer an extra 1 unit of insulin to bring their measured blood glucose into the top end of the target range (7 mmol/l). An extra 1.5 units would bring the measured blood glucose towards the lower end of the range (5 mmol/l).

The overall aim is to achieve good glycaemic control without disabling hypoglycaemia or undue emotional distress. An HbA1c of less than 6.5% (48 mmol/mol) and a 'Time in Range' of over 70% is associated with reduced risk of developing long-term vascular complications. Children should monitor their glucose levels at least 4–5 times a day. Some wear continuous glucose monitors (CGM)

PRACTICE POINT—administration of insulin in a young person recently diagnosed with diabetes mellitus type 1

A 14-year-old boy is admitted via his GP and is diagnosed with type 1 diabetes. He is well and weighs 44 Kg.

Total daily dose (TDD) of insulin is calculated as 44 x 0.75 = 33 units

Basal insulin dose = 50% of TDD = 16.5 units

Insulin: Carbohydrate Ratio = 500/TDD = 15.

   Insulin:CHO ratio = 1 unit:15 gm CHO (Some hospitals use a set Insulin:CHO ratios based on age or weight instead of using the '500' rule)

   Correction Dose: Calculate insulin sensitivity (ISF) = 100/TDD = 3.0

Calculating Pre-meal bolus Insulin

If he wishes to consume a meal containing 30 g of carbohydrate and his pre-meal blood glucose is 11 mmol/l, he will calculate the amount of pre-meal insulin needed to address both of these issues separately and bring his glucose level within target blood glucose of 4–7 mmol/l

* **Insulin:CHO ratio**—to accommodate 30 g CHO meal needs 2 units (30/15)
* **Correction dose**—to reduce his BG from 11 mmol/l to 5 mmol/l needs 2 units (2 x 3.0)

   Total Pre-meal insulin dose = 4 units

---

that measure interstitial, rather than blood, glucose levels continuously but displays the readings every 5 minutes.

All children and young people and their families should be taught by dietitians about the need for healthy eating and carbohydrate counting skills at diagnosis. Families should be taught to recognise patterns of high or low blood glucose and how to use the information to adjust insulin dosages to achieve their glycaemic targets.

Fasting blood glucose levels reflect the action of the basal insulin and if patient has a pattern of high fasting blood glucose, then the basal insulin dose will need to be increased to bring the glucose level into target range. The pre-meal blood glucose levels reflect the action of the insulin analogue injected in the preceding meal; for instance, the blood glucose before lunch reflects the action of the pre-breakfast insulin analogue whilst the glucose level before evening meal reflects the action of the pre-lunch insulin analogue and the glucose level before bedtime reflects the action of the pre-evening insulin analogue.

Exercise is essential for all and is to be encouraged and supported, and adjustments to both the insulin dose and the diet will be needed when undertaking planned exercise. Children and young people can be reassured that despite the diagnosis, they may still be able to achieve at the highest levels in sport.

PRACTICE POINT—insulin adjustment

The father of a 7-year-old girl with type 1 diabetes rang for advice as her blood glucose profile has been erratic. She currently takes 6 units of glargine before bed. Her pre-meal insulin: carbohydrate (I: CHO) ratio is 1:10 before breakfast and 1:15 before lunch and evening meal. Her blood glucose profile is shown.

	Blood glucose levels in mmol/l			
Date	Before breakfast	Before lunch	Before evening meal	Before bed
12/11	6.0	2.5	7.1	6.3
13/11	5.7	3.6	4.7	5.6
14/11	5.9	3.4	5.1	6.3
15/11	6.3	3.0	6.3	5.9

Interpretation: Her blood glucose profile shows a pattern of low blood glucose before lunch that suggests she needs less insulin before breakfast. Her Insulin:CHO ratio can be changed to 1:12 to give her less insulin before breakfast.

A specialist multidisciplinary team should manage the ongoing care of patients with diabetes. Patients and their carers should be taught to administer insulin therapy, monitor glucose and blood ketones levels, assess the carbohydrate content of food and use the insulin:carbohydrate ratio to decide the premeal insulin dosage. They should learn how to manage both hypoglycaemia and hyperglycaemia, prevent the development of diabetic ketoacidosis and manage days when other illnesses develop—so-called 'sick days rules.' The young person should be encouraged to wear some form of identification that would alert others to his or her diagnosis if found unwell or acting strangely.

PRACTICE POINT—'Sick Day rules' for individuals with diabetes mellitus

* follow local guidelines given to patient and family by diabetes team
* ensure drinking enough fluids to avoid dehydration
* never stop or omit insulin—though dose may need adjusting
* check blood glucose every 2 hours
* check blood ketones regularly
* administer correction doses of insulin to bring any high blood glucose in target
* if blood glucose and blood ketones are high and the child is vomiting, they need urgent admission to hospital as the child is in DKA

The risk of long-term chronic complications is reduced by improved glycaemic control. Intensive insulin regimens (multiple daily insulin injections or continuous subcutaneous insulin infusion) are superior to conservative regimens (once or twice daily insulin injections) in achieving good glycaemic control.

Potential complications

Acute complications include hypoglycaemia and DKA and the management of these is presented later. Microvascular and macrovascular complications associated with poor glycaemic control include:

- diabetic nephropathy
- diabetic retinopathy
- diabetic neuropathy
- ischemic heart disease, hypertension
- peripheral and cerebrovascular disease

Smoking increases the risk of neuropathy, so young people must be discouraged in taking up the habit. The current UK NICE guideline recommends screening for diabetic nephropathy and retinopathy from the age of 12 years.

Type 2 diabetes mellitus

About 2.2% of all childhood diabetes in the UK is due to type 2 diabetes and the prevalence is increasing due to the rise in childhood obesity. The condition occurs when insulin secretion is inadequate to meet increased demands posed by insulin resistance.

Clinical presentation

Many with type 2 diabetes are asymptomatic at presentation although some will present with the typical symptoms of diabetes. Features which may suggest type 2 diabetes rather than type 1 include:

- family history of type 2 diabetes in close relatives
- being obese at presentation
- being of black or Asian family origin
- evidence of insulin resistance—acanthosis nigricans, polycystic ovarian syndrome, hypertension
  Comorbidities associated with Type 2 diabetes include:
- nonalcoholic fatty liver disease
- sleep apnoea
- polycystic ovarian syndrome
- dyslipidaemia

Treatment and management

The key aspect of management of children and young people with type 2 diabetes is the introduction of intensive lifestyle interventions such as healthy eating and physical activity in order to achieve an appropriate weight. However, compliance with this is limited in many young people and the majority will require the addition of a pharmacological agent to help achieve good glycaemic control.

The only medications currently licensed for use in children and young people with type 2 diabetes are metformin, insulin and liraglutide.

Relevant pharmacological agents used

Metformin improves insulin sensitivity and exerts its glucose-lowering effect by inhibiting hepatic gluconeogenesis and opposing the action of glucagon.

Liraglutide is licensed for children older than 10 years old and is a glucagon-like peptide 1 (GLP-1) receptor agonist and so acts by increasing insulin secretion from the pancreas and reducing glucagon secretion. It also promotes weight loss by delaying gastric emptying and reducing appetite.

Both metformin and liraglutide may also help by reducing appetite.

Monogenic diabetes

Monogenic diabetes accounts for less than 5% of all diabetes and is the result of several identified single gene defects. It should be considered in any child presenting with atypical features of type 1 or type 2 diabetes such as:

- mild stable fasting hyperglycaemia which does not progress
- diabetes presenting in the first 6 months of life
- diabetes associated with extra-pancreatic features such as congenital heart or gastrointestinal defects, CNS malformations
- family history of diabetes which is suggestive of an autosomal dominant inheritance
- atypical features of Type 1 diabetes such as:
  - absence of diabetes-specific auto antibodies
  - low or no insulin requirements and detectable C-peptide more than 5 years after diagnosis
- atypical features of Type 2 diabetes such as:
  - absence of marked obesity, acanthosis nigricans

Types of monogenic diabetes
Neonatal diabetes

Diabetes mellitus presenting in the first 6 months of life is usually due to monogenic diabetes and can be either transient or have resolved by 18 months. Diabetes may recur in adolescence and become permanent. Hyperglycaemia in the neonatal period is usually due to the stress of other illnesses such as sepsis rather than neonatal diabetes. Other rare causes of hyperglycaemia include inborn errors of amino acid metabolism such as methylmalonic aciduria.

The majority of patients with neonatal diabetes mellitus present with intrauterine growth retardation, hyperglycaemia, dehydration and rarely ketoacidosis and some 20% will also present with neurological problems.

Monogenic diabetes in children and adolescents

There are several single gene mutations causing monogenic diabetes in this age group but the two most common mutations are:
- Hepatic Nuclear Factor (HNF1A) MODY. Patients usually present initially with post prandial hyperglycaemia that then develops into frank diabetes mellitus with typical symptoms.
- Glucokinase (GCK) MODY. Patients present with non-progressive mild hyperglycaemia which is usually detected incidentally. It is a benign condition and therefore does not require any treatment or further monitoring.

Investigations

- blood glucose to establish hyperglycaemia
- associated blood tests listed for type 1 diabetes
- molecular genetic testing to identify known gene mutations

Treatment and management

Patients with neonatal diabetes will initially require insulin therapy regardless of cause of the hyperglycaemia although some may later switch to oral sulphonylurea medication.

Patients with a mutation of the HNF-1a gene may be able to control their diabetes by diet in the first instance. However, once they develop frank diabetes, they can then be managed long term with low-dose sulfonylureas to achieve good glycaemic control.

Diabetic ketoacidosis (DKA)

DKA occurs when there is severe insulin deficiency as in children with type 1 diabetes mellitus at presentation or those with established diabetes mellitus following deliberate or inadvertent insulin omission. Identifying the reason for episodes of DKA is important and clues should be sought in the background of the young person that might explain the development of DKA. Recurrent admissions may be a cry for help or an attempt to avoid potentially distressing events at home or school.

DKA can also be due to relative insulin deficiency in conditions where the counterregulatory hormones levels increase in response to the stress such as in sepsis or trauma. This can occur despite the patient taking the usual recommended dose of insulin.

In the presence of typical symptoms, the diagnosis of DKA is based on the following biochemical criteria:
- hyperglycemia (blood glucose greater than 11.1 mmol/l)
- metabolic acidosis defined as venous pH less than 7.3 or bicarbonate below 15 mmol/l
- ketonemia or a moderate to large ketonuria

The classification of the severity of DKA is based on degree of acidosis:
- mild DKA: venous pH less than 7.3 or serum bicarbonate below 15 mmol/l
- moderate DKA: pH less than 7.2 or serum bicarbonate below 10 mmol/l
- severe DKA: pH less than 7.1 or serum bicarbonate below 5 mmol/l

Diabetic ketoacidosis remains the most common cause of death in children and young people with diabetes and is usually the result of clinically apparent cerebral oedema.

Clinical presentation

The clinical signs of diabetic ketoacidosis include:
- dehydration
- tachypnoea and deep sighing respiration (Kussmaul breathing)
- tachycardia
- breath smelling of acetone
- vomiting
- reduced conscious level

Investigations

Measurement of blood glucose, blood ketones, urea and electrolytes and a blood gas must be undertaken with urgency. If clinical features suggestive of infection are present then samples of blood and urine are also sent for culture.

Treatment and management

Children in DKA should be monitored closely in a high dependency care setting with regular assessment of their level of consciousness and Glasgow coma scale. Any assessment at this time should also aim to identify and treat any precipitating event. The goals of therapy include addressing the following issues:

Fluid resuscitation and fluid deficit

The degree of dehydration is based on the severity of the DKA and the advised assessment is:
- mild and moderate DKA: assume 5% dehydration
- severe DKA: assume 10% dehydration

All patients who present with DKA and appear clinically dehydrated require an initial fluid bolus of 10 ml/kg over 30 minutes using 0.9% sodium chloride. A further 10 ml/kg fluid bolus can be given after reassessment in order to improve tissue perfusion. This fluid bolus volume is deducted from the total fluid deficit.

Shock is rare in DKA but can occur especially if there is coexistence of sepsis. Signs of shock in DKA include low volume or weak, thready pulse and hypotension. Children in shock should receive 20 ml/kg fluid bolus of 0.9% normal saline. This bolus is not subtracted from the total fluid deficit.

Maintenance fluids

For the fluid maintenance requirement, use the Holliday-Segar formula with a maximum weight of 75 kg:
• give 100 ml/kg for the first 10 kg of weight
• give 50 ml/kg for the second 10 kg of weight
• give 20 ml/kg for every kg after this
The calculated deficit and maintenance should be replaced over 48 hours using intravenous 0.9% saline plus potassium 40 mmol/l initially (unless patient is anuric) but changing to 5% dextrose saline plus potassium when blood glucose falls below 14 mmol/l. Ongoing urinary losses are not replaced.

Metabolic acidosis

The metabolic acidosis is the result of ketoacidosis and lactic acidosis due to poor tissue perfusion and is corrected by fluid therapy and insulin therapy. It must not be corrected by the administration of intravenous bicarbonate as this increases the risk of cerebral oedema. Capillary or venous blood gas along with urea, electrolytes and creatinine should be measured every 2–4 hours to assess response to fluid management.

Intravenous insulin

Intravenous insulin should be started after the interval of one hour following the start of IV fluid therapy and administered at the rate of 0.05–0.1 units/kg/hour. The blood glucose and blood ketones are monitored hourly to ensure the resolution of the hyperglycaemia and ketosis.

Potential complications

Cerebral oedema

Typical signs include:
• sudden onset headache
• hypertension with bradycardia
• drowsiness
• confusion
• coma
• respiratory arrest and death
Cerebral oedema is unpredictable and occurs in 1% of patients presenting in DKA and typically occurs 2–12 hours after therapy has started. Recognised risk factors for the development of cerebral oedema are:
• severe DKA on presentation as indicated by:
  ○ severe acidosis at presentation.
  ○ severe dehydration
  ○ severe hypocapnia
• use of bicarbonate for correction of acidosis
The role of fluid therapy in the development of cerebral oedema remains controversial. Patients with signs suggestive of cerebral oedema need immediate treatment with either hypertonic saline or mannitol and fluid administration should be reduced to half maintenance until the clinical condition has stabilised. Senior support must be sought immediately.

Other complications

• electrolyte disturbances—hypokalaemia, hypocalcaemia, hypomagnesaemia

---

PRACTICE POINT—calculating fluid requirements in DKA

A 14-year-old girl presents to the emergency department and is assessed to have moderate DKA. She weighs 46 kg and is not on shock. She receives 10 ml/kg bolus over 30 mins.

As she has moderate DKA, she is assumed to be 5% dehydrated. Her weight of 46 kg gives a body fluid volume of 46 litres. Her daily maintenance requirements are calculated using the Holliday-Segar formula.

Her calculated fluid requirements (in mls) are:
Initial bolus given in ED (46 x 10) 460
Deficit from dehydration to be replaced over 48 hours (mls): (46000 x 5/100) 2300
Subtract Initial bolus given in ED from total fluid deficit (2300-460) 1840
Total fluid deficit to be administered =1840
Her daily maintenance: 2020
Total 48-hour fluid maintenance = 4040
Total calculated fluid requirements over 48 hours after fluid bolus subtracted = (1840 + 4040) = 5880
Hourly rate = 5880/48 (mls/hr) 123
Ongoing replacement fluid is 0.9% saline plus potassium 40 mmol/l

- aspiration pneumonia
- neurological pathologies (cerebral venous thrombosis; subarachnoid haemorrhage

Hypoglycaemia

In clinical practice, a level below 3.9 mmol/l is used as the threshold value to initiate treatment and is regarded as an 'alert' value. Some clinicians use 4 mmol/l as the alert threshold to make it easier for families to remember. A level below 3.0 mmol/l reflects a clinically important hypoglycaemia and can lead to impairment of counter regulatory hormones and a lack of awareness of the hypoglycaemia by the individual. Causes of hypoglycaemia include:

- relative excess of insulin following missed meals
- exercise
- mismatch between insulin administered and food consumed

Autonomic symptoms of hypoglycaemia include feeling tremulousness, sweating, palpitations and hunger pangs. Neurologic symptoms include headache, drowsiness, irritation, behaviour changes blurred vision and difficulty concentrating. Symptoms of severe hypoglycaemia include convulsion and coma.

In **mild to moderate hypoglycaemia,** where the individual is able to swallow, immediate oral treatment should be given using a solution containing 10–15 g glucose (3–5 glucose tablets or proprietary products) which can be repeated if the hypoglycaemia persists. If there is any indication of a reduced conscious level, then the oral route should not be used as there is a clear risk of choking and inhalation. In this situation, intramuscular glucagon should be given, if available.

When the symptoms improve or blood glucose levels return to normal, a complex carbohydrate snack (toast or biscuit) should be given to children if they are managed by insulin injections so as to counter the rebound hypoglycaemia, although patients managed by insulin pump therapy do not need complex carbohydrate after treatment of hypoglycaemia. Chocolate or ice cream are not advised for the treatment of hypoglycaemia as they delay stomach emptying and so produce slow glucose absorption.

Severe hypoglycaemia in a young person who is at home should be treated with intramuscular glucagon and, if they are conscious and able to swallow, a concentrated oral glucose solution. Those who are in hospital and have IV access should be given a rapid bolus 10% dextrose infusion (2 ml/kg).

Strategies to reduce hypoglycaemia include:

- regular glucose monitoring
- education on management of exercise and sick days
- good carbohydrate counting skills

New technologies that are reducing the frequency and severity of hypoglycaemia include use of continuous glucose monitors, insulin pump therapy and hybrid closed-loop insulin pumps.

IMPORTANT CLINICAL POINTS

Diabetes mellitus—type 1

- prescribing insulin requires careful consideration and errors are 'never events'
- fasting glucose levels reflect basal insulin action
- pre-meal glucose levels reflect the insulin action of the dose injected at preceding meal
- knowledge of 'sick days rules' important

Diabetes mellitus—type 2

- consider if family history of type 2, obesity, black or Asian family origin
- consider if evidence of insulin resistance— acanthosis nigricans, polycystic ovarian syndrome, hypertension

Monogenic diabetes

- consider if family history of diabetes, condition does not progress or occurs in first 6 months of life

Diabetic ketoacidosis

- cerebral oedema can lead to death in children and young people with diabetes
- assessment of degree of dehydration important
- calculated deficit and maintenance should be replaced over 48 hours using intravenous 0.9% saline plus potassium 40 mmol/l initially
- severe hypoglycaemia in a person at home should be treated with intramuscular glucagon and, if able to swallow, a concentrated oral glucose solution

---

Further reading

Diabetes (Type 1 and Type 2) in Children and Young People: *Diagnosis and Management NICE Guideline NG18*; Published 2015; last 16 December 2020.

Chapter | 25 |

Endocrinology

Kah Yin Loke, Joanna Walker

After reading this chapter you should:
- know the causes and management of pituitary and hypothalamic disorders
- be able to assess, diagnose and manage disorders of the adrenal glands
- be able to assess, diagnose and manage disorders of thyroid and parathyroid glands
- be able to identify endocrine complications of other diseases and refer appropriately

Many complex interactions of normal cellular function are controlled by hormones released by the organs and glands of the endocrine system. Control of electrolytes, both within the cells and circulating in the extracellular spaces, are finely controlled by feedback mechanisms involving hormones. Growth, development and pubertal changes are all under the orchestration of interdependent hormone release which bring about changes evident in everyday paediatric practice. The consequences of untreated endocrine pathology are significant and will have a major impact on the child or young person.

Pituitary and hypothalamic disorders

Anterior pituitary hormone deficiency

Damage to the hypothalamus, pituitary stalk or pituitary gland—congenital or acquired—can cause pituitary hormone deficiencies that can present at any age. The hormones produced (Figure 25.1) by the anterior pituitary are:
- growth hormone
- thyroid stimulating hormone
- luteinising hormone
- follicular stimulating hormone
- adrenocorticotrophic hormone

With expanding knowledge of the genes that direct pituitary development and hormone production, an increasing proportion of pituitary disorders in children can be attributed to specific genetic abnormalities, especially where there is consanguinity or a relevant family history.

Congenital causes increase the likelihood of developing multiple pituitary hormone deficiency (MPHD) and are often linked to other abnormalities of brain development. Examples of these conditions include holoprosencephaly and septo-optic dysplasia with incomplete septum pellucidum, optic nerve hypoplasia and midline abnormalities.

Acquired causes include trauma, post-infection, tumours, surgery and cranial irradiation.

Clinical presentation

Neonates. Craniofacial and pituitary gland development are closely related, so any baby born with midline anomalies such a median cleft palate should be recognised and investigated as they may have holoprosencephaly and be at high risk of evolving MPHD. Most affected babies, however, have no outward signs at birth. Hypoglycaemia and prolonged conjugated jaundice are the most common presenting features. Isolated pituitary hormone deficiencies such as growth hormone deficiency rarely present at this age.

Neonates with suspected hypopituitarism may also display:
- dysmorphic features including subtle craniofacial abnormalities
- roving eye movements and nystagmus due to optic nerve hypoplasia
- nystagmus
- micropenis and maldescended testes (boys)—suggesting gonadotrophin deficiency

Older children. Growth hormone deficiency is the most common axis to be affected, so slow growth is almost always the presenting problem in children over the age of

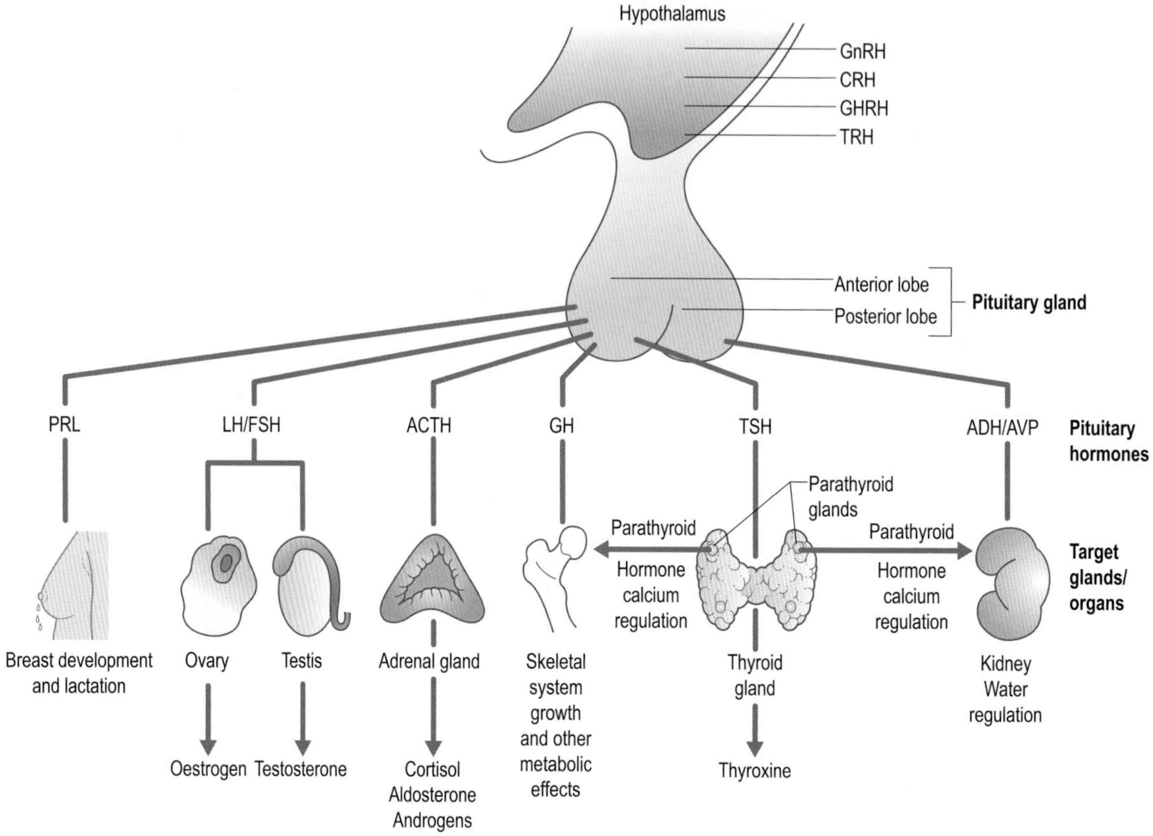

Fig. 25.1 Hormones produced by the pituitary gland and their effects.

(ACTH = adrenocorticotrophin; ADH/AVP = antidiuretic/arginine vasopressin; CRH = corticotrophin-releasing hormone; FSH = follicle stimulating hormone; GH = growth hormone; GHRH = growth hormone-releasing hormone; LH = luteinising hormone; GnRH = gonadotrophin-releasing hormone; PRL = prolactin; TRH = thyrotrophin-releasing hormone; TSH = thyroid stimulating hormone)

2 years when the predominantly nutrition-driven phase of growth is completing. Other symptoms suggestive of pituitary hormone deficiency include:

- tiredness and malaise
- muscle weakness
- headache
- visual field defects

Investigations

Neonates. Hypoglycaemia is the commonest presenting feature as a result of cortisol and growth hormone deficiencies, and the hypoglycaemia screen taken at the time of hypoglycaemia must include:

- glucose (laboratory)—to confirm a true low glucose
- cortisol—should show appropriate stress response to the hypoglycaemia

- growth hormone—should show appropriate stress response to the hypoglycaemia

Thyroid function tests will show an inappropriately low TSH for the prevailing Free T4. An initial cranial ultrasound may show abnormalities such as an absent septum pellucidum or other midline anomalies, and an MRI scan will provide further details. A prolonged conjugated hyperbilirubinaemia may be the result of MPHD.

Older children. The investigation of children with short stature and growth failure due to growth hormone deficiency are outlined in Chapter 4 Growth and Puberty. Involvement of the thyroid axis can be detected from standard tests of Free T4 and TSH, and pubertal development is best assessed clinically rather than by formal LHRH testing. Any child found to be deficient of any pituitary hormone must have an MRI scan and DNA analysis where appropriate.

Associations

Prader-Willi Syndrome is a rare condition with significant hypothalamo-pituitary involvement. Infants have poor suck and other feeding problems, but from the age of 2 years children manifest uncontrolled appetite with rapid development of obesity unless access to food is strictly controlled. Further details on clinical features and management are presented in Chapter 5 Genetics and Chapter 27 Neurodevelopmental Medicine.

Treatment and management

Hormone deficiencies are almost always lifelong chronic conditions and so management must be holistic. The principles are:
- replacement of hormones in doses that vary with age or size
- verbal and written instructions about the management of intercurrent illness in children with ACTH and cortisol deficiency with annual review of competence of carer and child or young person. They also need open access to an acute unit
- regular monitoring of growth and development by a team with specialist expertise
- regular clinical and biochemical surveillance for the emergence of other deficiencies
- regular surveillance for adherence to, and safety of, replacement treatment
- induction of puberty at an appropriate age
- effective transition to adult endocrine services
- counselling and support for families and affected children and young people

Relevant pharmacological agents used

Replacement hormones are almost always biologically identical to the natural hormone but it is often not possible to deliver them in a dose regime that mimics physiological production. For example, growth hormone is given as a single daily injection in contrast to the 3–4 nocturnal peaks and troughs seen physiologically. Steroid replacement tries to mimic the diurnal rhythm of cortisol production but inevitably fails because the lower dose given at night means that levels the following morning may be unrecordably low, but giving a higher dose can affect sleep patterns and growth. Provided doses are appropriate, side effects are rare and parents can be reassured.

However, there are some side effects that are more common and important:
- growth hormone—headache, idiopathic intracranial hypertension, lipohypertrophy
- hydrocortisone—features of Cushing syndrome if doses are consistently too high

- thyroxine—sleep and behaviour problems, headache, idiopathic intracranial hypertension

Inappropriate or excess anterior pituitary hormone production

Any damage to the brain, not just the hypothalamopituitary axis, can lead to inappropriate gonadotrophin production causing early puberty, particularly in girls. Causes include:
- cerebral palsy and metabolic disorders
- low dose cranial irradiation
- optic nerve or hypothalamic gliomas—seen in children with NF1
- hypothalamic hamartomas

Rarely children will present with symptoms suggestive of pituitary hormone excess due to a hormone secreting tumour. Prolactinomas usually present in older children with:
- galactorrhoea
- headache due to raised intracranial pressure
- visual problems
- pubertal delay

They are usually managed very successfully with dopamine agonists such as cabergoline, but children should be screened for other pituitary problems. Prolactin is a stress hormone and levels should be interpreted with caution before concluding they are pathological.

Cushing disease is very rare and in children is usually caused by an ACTH-secreting pituitary adenoma. Pituitary gigantism due to GH excess is even more rare.

Posterior pituitary hormone deficiency

In children, the most common disturbance of posterior pituitary function is diabetes insipidus (DI) which is described as either:
- cranial DI—insufficient antidiuretic hormone (ADH—also known as arginine vasopressin AVP) release—congenital or acquired
- nephrogenic DI—renal resistance to ADH action

Congenital causes of cranial DI include midline anomalies such as holoprosencephaly or septo-optic dysplasia.

Acquired causes include tumours (germinoma), infiltration (histiocytosis), infection, trauma and post neurosurgery (especially for craniopharyngioma).

Cranial DI is rare but life threatening if not identified. The symptoms are polyuria and polydipsia, but the challenge is to distinguish between children with DI and the vast majority with polyuria and polydipsia who have habitual water drinking. The history and examination, plus some simple blood and urine tests, should help distinguish between the two.

Certain features in the history and examination are suggestive of DI:

- presentation in an older school age child or teenager
- inability to sleep through the night due to thirst and needing a drink
- seeking fluid from other sources (flower vases, toilets) if denied a drink
- features suggestive of anterior pituitary involvement such as slow growth
- symptoms of raised intracranial pressure
- developmental problems including vision
- dysmorphic features
- evidence of midline defects

Investigations

These may not be necessary if it is clear from the history and examination that the cause is habitual water drinking. If there is doubt, a fasting serum sodium, potassium, creatinine and osmolality with a paired, fasting urine sodium and osmolality should be requested, but the child must be allowed open access to sugar-free fluids even if they are not encouraged. A normal fasting response will show a serum osmolality of 275–295 mOsmol/kg and a urine osmolality of greater than 850 mOsmol/kg, although the latter may be lower if the child has been allowed fluids.

PRACTICE POINT—Water deprivation test

Must only be performed in a unit that has experience and expertise in both running the tests and interpreting the results. The test is potentially dangerous.

- The child must be supervised at all times by a senior endocrine doctor or specialist nurse who is immediately available
- allow free fluids until the start of fasting
- weigh and calculate weight with 5% loss—and document both
- fluid balance is monitored throughout
- close supervision to avoid inadvertent access to water
- serum and urine electrolytes and osmolality measured at start and at intervals
- child is weighed at regular intervals through the test
- end test if weight loss exceeds 5% or tests confirm presence or absence of DI
- fast should not exceed 8 hours—but the result is usually clear sooner
- if DI is confirmed, a test dose of desmopressin (DDAVP) is given and fluid balance and investigations monitored over the next few hours

---

In DI, there is inappropriately dilute urine (<750 mOsm/kg) despite a serum osmolality >295 mOsm/kg. If the results are not conclusive, a water deprivation test must be undertaken at a centre with expertise as it has potentially dangerous consequences.

Interpretation of the above test: The urine at T = 0 is very dilute and the serum sodium slightly low because the child has been allowed free fluids, but as time progresses the urine concentrates normally; the serum osmolality remains within the reference range and the sodium normalises. There is no significant weight loss. These all confirm a diagnosis of habitual water drinking and the parents can be reassured that it is safe to limit fluids if they wish.

If cranial DI is diagnosed the child needs serum tumour markers beta-HCG and AFP plus MRI scanning of the hypothalamo–pituitary axis to exclude infiltrative disorders. They may also need anterior pituitary function testing.

Treatment and management

Cranial DI is treated with desmopressin (DDAVP) usually given orally but it can be administered nasally to babies and small children or parenterally after neurosurgery. It is introduced slowly and the doses gradually increased to avoid dilutional hyponatraemia that can be more dangerous than untreated DI. The reason to treat is to control unpleasant symptoms and patients with intact thirst can still drink to correct any water depletion whilst the doses are optimised.

Posterior pituitary hormone excess

Syndrome of inappropriate antidiuretic hormone (SIADH)

SIADH is characterised by impaired water excretion leading to hyponatraemia with hypervolaemia or euvolaemia as a result of unsuppressed or increased levels of ADH (vasopressin).

Symptoms are unusual where the sodium is 125–135 mmol/l, but levels below this put a child at risk of cerebral oedema and progressive neurological symptoms. In severe acute hyponatraemia (< 120 mmol/l), the child is at risk of:

- headache
- vomiting
- reduced level of consciousness
- seizures and death

Chronic hyponatraemia, developing over 24 hours or more, may have more subtle features such as restlessness, weakness, fatigue or irritability due to brain adaptation.

Time into fast (mins)	Weight (kg)	Serum osmolality mOsmol/kg (275–295)	Urine osmolality mOsmol/kg (>850 after 12 hour fast)	Serum sodium (mmol/l) (133–146)
0	15.4	276	110	131
30	15.4	278	130	133
60	15.1	282	275	137
90	15.0	287	450	138
120	15.0	290	680	138
180	14.9	293	875	141

Table 25.1 Hypothetical water deprivation test in a toddler with polydipsia and polyuria. Weight at start = 15.4 kg. 95% weight = 14.7 kg—if weight drops to 14.7 kg then the test must stop.

Associated conditions

- respiratory infections—pneumonia, bronchiolitis and TB
- central nervous system infections, trauma, raised intracranial pressure
- drugs that increase ADH release, e.g. cyclophosphamide, carbamazepine, sodium valproate
- pain

Investigations

In addition to serum sodium, samples for paired urine and serum osmolality and urine sodium should be obtained. Characteristically, these will show an inappropriately high urine osmolality (>100 mOsmol/kg) for the low serum osmolality (<275 mOsmol/kg) plus high urine sodium (>10 mOsmol/kg) due to excess ADH causing water, but not solute, retention.

Management and complications

Awareness of the possibility of SIADH and treatment of any underlying cause are the important steps in management. In at-risk patients, strict fluid balance, regular weights and blood and urine electrolytes should be undertaken along with the use of isotonic fluids which are volume restricted to 50% to 66% of calculated requirements to maintain euvolaemia.

Urgent correction of hyponatraemia is rarely necessary and any rapid rises in sodium can cause irreversible osmotic demyelination syndrome—dysarthria, confusion and coma—that can present days after sodium has normalised. Unless the child is seizing, sodium levels should not increase by more than 8 mmol/l in 24 hours. This is usually achieved by treating the underlying cause, restricting fluids as mentioned above and resisting the suggestion to administer hypertonic saline. If the child is fitting, then the sodium can be increased more rapidly using hypertonic saline, but this must be undertaken with caution as rapid rises are potentially harmful.

Adrenal disorders

- adrenal insufficiency
- Cushing syndrome
- phaeochromocytoma

The adrenal cortex produces glucocorticoids (cortisol), mineralocorticoids (aldosterone) and androgens (dehydroepiandrosterone—DHEA).

Adrenal insufficiency

Increased generalised pigmentation of the skin, especially parts of the body which are not exposed to the sun, suggests primary adrenal insufficiency. Characteristic darkening occurs as a consequence of increased ACTH breakdown leading to increased levels of melanocyte stimulating hormone (MSH) and the subsequent skin pigmentation. Pigmentation does not occur in secondary adrenal insufficiency when the ACTH level is low.

The metabolic derangements in primary adrenal insufficiency, as a consequence of both cortisol and aldosterone deficiency, include:
- hyponatraemia
- hyperkalaemia
- metabolic acidosis
- hypoglycaemia

Adrenal insufficiency in the neonate

The most common cause for primary adrenal insufficiency in infancy is congenital adrenal hyperplasia (CAH) which typically presents in the first 2 to 3 weeks of life with:

- poor weight gain
- vomiting
- increased pigmentation of mucous membranes, scrotum, palmar creases, nipples
- eventual adrenal crisis—with tachycardia and hypotension

The most common enzyme deficiency causing CAH is 21-hydroxylase deficiency, which occurs in 90 percent of all patients. Affected females with CAH are usually identified earlier than males by varying degrees of clitoromegaly and virilisation leading to diagnostic evaluation, even before the onset of an adrenal crisis.

Adrenal insufficiency in the older child and adolescent

Causes include:
- Addison disease (autoimmune adrenalitis) which may be part of the autoimmune polyendocrinopathy syndromes and can present with:
  - nonspecific symptoms (vomiting, lethargy, malaise, anorexia)
  - significant weight loss
  - hyperpigmentation
  - hypoglycaemia
  - shock
- secondary adrenal insufficiency
  - congenital hypopituitarism (septo-optic dysplasia; isolated ACTH deficiency)
  - surgery for suprasellar tumours
  - cranial irradiation
  - pituitary dysfunction from trauma or meningitis
- exogenous use of steroids
  - results in iatrogenic Cushing syndrome and can also cause secondary adrenal insufficiency.

Alternative diagnoses and differing features

Differential diagnoses to consider for primary adrenal insufficiency depend on the presenting feature. Severe hyponatremia can also occur in pseudohypoaldosteronism (PHA), a condition which mimics hypoaldosteronism. However, PHA is due to a failure of response to aldosterone, and the aldosterone levels are significantly elevated. In contrast to primary adrenal insufficiency, patients with PHA do not have hyperpigmentation (as the ACTH level is not elevated) and they do not suffer from hypoglycaemia (as there is no cortisol deficiency).

Investigations and expected results in primary adrenal insufficiency

- electrolytes—hyponatraemia, hyperkalaemia
- glucose—hypoglycaemia

- blood gas—metabolic acidosis
- short synacthen stimulation test suboptimal cortisol levels despite stimulation
- ACTH—elevated in primary adrenal insufficiency
- urinary steroids—elevated serum 17-hydroxyprogesterone and serum testosterone levels in females would indicate the diagnosis of 21-hydroxylase deficiency

Treatment and management

In acute adrenal crisis, the patient is often in shock and needs urgent administration of:
- hydrocortisone—IV or IM
- fluid resuscitation with 0.9% saline
- 10% dextrose IV to correct hypoglycaemia
  For ongoing maintenance:
- oral hydrocortisone to replace glucocorticoid deficiency
- oral fludrocortisone to replace mineralocorticoid deficiency
- young infants also require oral sodium chloride supplementation

Excessive dosage of hydrocortisone will result in iatrogenic Cushing syndrome whilst inadequate hydrocortisone replacement dose can lead to tiredness, malaise with poor weight gain and increased pigmentation. Girls with salt-wasting CAH who have inadequate glucocorticoid replacement may experience increasing androgenisation with progressive clitoromegaly and acne. In both boys and girls with salt-wasting CAH and inadequate glucocorticoid replacement, the excessive androgen levels can induce a growth spurt and early growth plate fusion, which may limit the final height.

CLINICAL SCENARIO

A 9-year-old boy with type 1 diabetes has the following results in his annual review blood tests, and these were confirmed on repeat. The bloods were taken after clinic when he was reportedly well with normal growth and weight gain. His near-patient HbA1c was 52 mmol/mol (20–42).

Sodium	128 mmol/l	(133–146)
Potassium	5.3 mmol/l	(3.5–5.5)
Urea	8.2 mmol/l	(2.5–6.5)
Creatinine	58 µmol/l	(29–53)
Glucose	7.4 mmol/l	(Target range 4.0–7.0)

In the absence of evidence of DKA, significant hyperglycaemia or renal impairment the sodium and potassium results are suggestive of aldosterone deficiency. The elevated urea reflects the associated volume depletion and vasoconstriction. Primary adrenal failure (Addison disease) must be excluded with a short Synacthen test. All patients with type 1 diabetes are at risk of other autoimmune conditions.

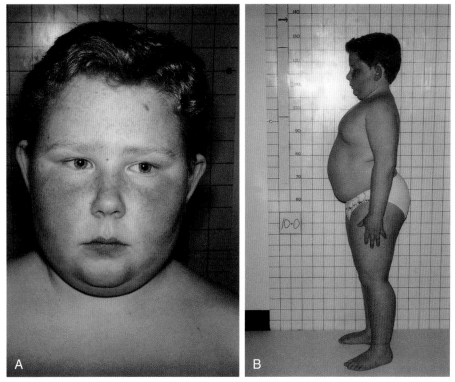

Fig. 25.2 A 13-year-old boy with Cushing disease showing central obesity, striae, plethoric facies and short stature.

Cushing syndrome

Increased levels of serum cortisol can be due to:
- ACTH-secreting pituitary tumour—Cushing disease (Figure 25.2)
- Cortisol-secreting adrenal tumour or ectopic site or exogenous source—Cushing syndrome

The commonest cause of Cushing syndrome in childhood is iatrogenic use of exogenous steroids (oral, inhaled, topical) and the guidelines in the UK are that all children on regular inhaled steroids should have their height and weight measured and plotted every 6 months.

Cardinal features of Cushing syndrome are:
- excessive weight gain with falling height centiles
- hypertension
- proximal myopathy

Some characteristic adult features of Cushing syndrome are much less common in children. These include:
- excessive fat on the face ('moon face')
- excessive fat at the base of the neck ('buffalo hump')
- disproportionate centripetal distribution of fat on the trunk

- facial plethora
- hypertrichosis with hirsutism
- thick violaceous striae over the trunk, back and limbs (cortisol-induced atrophic skin)

Alternative diagnoses

Children with simple obesity are often tall with normal height velocity and the fat is generally distributed over both the limbs and trunk. The striae in obesity are stretch-marks, which are thin and skin coloured, in contrast to the thicker violaceous coloured striae of hypercortisolism.

Investigations

Initial tests aim to confirm hypercortisolism and subsequent tests to identify the source of the increased cortisol.
Test to confirm hypercortisolism:
- urinary free-cortisol excretion (24-hour urine collection)
- serum cortisol circadian rhythm study (0900 h, 1800 h and midnight when asleep)
- overnight dexamethasone suppression test with 1 mg dexamethasone

- low-dose dexamethasone suppression test (LDDST) with 0.5 mg dexamethasone administered 6-hourly for 48 hours with cortisol measured at 0 hr, 24 hr and 48 hr

Hypercortisolism is present if the 24-hour urine cortisol is elevated, if there is loss of the normal circadian rhythm of cortisol secretion or if the serum cortisol is not suppressed after dexamethasone.

Subsequent tests aim to identify the source of increased cortisol and include:
- CRH test—corticotrophin-releasing hormone is injected and sequential bloods for ACTH and cortisol taken
- diagnostic imaging studies
  In ACTH-dependent pituitary Cushing disease:
- the ACTH level is in the normal range or is elevated
- there is a marked increase in cortisol with the CRH test
- suppression of serum cortisol during the LDDST strongly supports Cushing disease (due to negative feedback from dexamethasone)

In ACTH-independent Cushing syndrome (adrenal or ectopic):
- the ACTH is low or undetectable (negative feedback)
- there will always be no significant suppression of cortisol with the LDDST
  Diagnostic imaging will further define the cause of Cushing syndrome with MRI of the pituitary gland for suspected Cushing disease and MRI of the adrenal glands for Cushing syndrome.

Treatment and management

The management of ACTH-dependent Cushing disease from a pituitary adenoma requires trans-sphenoidal surgery whilst benign adrenal tumours require abdominal surgical resection. Adrenal carcinoma carries a poor prognosis but is initially treated with chemotherapy. Those children receiving chronic, low-dose steroid treatment who are at risk of developing Cushing syndrome should be managed on the lowest dose and the least damaging regimen as possible to control their disease.

Phaeochromocytoma

Phaeochromocytoma is a neuroendocrine tumour arising from adrenal medulla or sympathetic chain. Although uncommon in childhood, it is an important differential for hypertension. Further details can be found in Chapter 20 Nephro-urology.

Thyroid disorders

Hypothyroidism

As part of the Newborn Screening Programme, all babies in the UK are screened for congenital hypothyroidism due to gland dysgenesis or dyshormonogenesis. The test looks for high TSH and so it will not pick up congenital hypopituitarism. In neonates and infants, delayed treatment of thyroid dysfunction may cause permanent nervous system damage and developmental delay whilst early treatment with thyroxine can optimise growth and mental development. Hypothyroidism results in clinical features associated with a decreased metabolic rate.

Hypothyroidism is more common in children with Down syndrome and type 1 diabetes mellitus and assessment is therefore part of the annual screening for both conditions.

Congenital hypothyroidism can be due to defective thyroid development as a result of:
- thyroid agenesis
- thyroid hypoplasia
- ectopic thyroid gland
- dyshormonogenesis (gene mutations for thyroid hormones enzymes and proteins)
  Congenital hypothyroidism detected by the newborn screening programme allows adequate treatment to begin within 2 weeks of life and can optimise a child's growth and development.

Infants who are not diagnosed and treated early can present with:
- decreased activity and excessive weight gain
- constipation
- coarse facies
- dry skin
- bradycardia
- delayed developmental milestones
  Detection of a goitre in congenital hypothyroidism suggests the possibility of dyshormonogenesis, which can be associated with deafness in Pendred syndrome.

Acquired hypothyroidism usually presents in the older child and it may be due to:
- iodine deficiency
- autoimmunity (Hashimoto's thyroiditis)
- thyroidectomy or irradiation
- anti-thyroid drugs
- diseases of the pituitary and hypothalamus

Presenting features in this age group include:
- suboptimal height velocity—peer group or sibs overtaking is a common presentation
- excessive weight gain

- constipation
- deteriorating school progress from slowed mentation
- cold intolerance
- delayed puberty
- dry skin and sparse hair
- goitre
- bradycardia
- proximal muscle weakness

Investigations

In the UK, the first newborn bloodspot sample is taken at 5 days of age in all babies. Babies born at less than 32 weeks' gestation also have a second (repeat) blood spot sample at 28 days of age or on the day of discharge home as immaturity may mask congenital hypothyroidism.

An elevated TSH concentration on the newborn blood spot sample or a second 'borderline' result requires referral for diagnostic investigation. If primary congenital hypothyroidism is considered, then thyroid ultrasonography and a technetium thyroid scan must be undertaken to clarify if the thyroid gland is absent, hypoplastic or ectopic.

Acquired hypothyroidism from a central cause will lead to low TSH and free T4 whilst a peripheral cause will identify a raised TSH and low levels of free T4. Initial screening bloods should also include thyroid peroxidase antibodies, as these will be elevated in Hashimoto's thyroiditis.

Treatment and management

The aim of therapy for congenital hypothyroidism is to normalise free T4 within 2 weeks and TSH within the first month of life and an optimal cognitive outcome depends on both the adequacy and timing of postnatal therapy. The free T4 level should subsequently be maintained within the upper quartile of the reference range with a low normal TSH.

With a later presentation, treatment is with thyroxine replacement at a dose that increases with body size. Schoolteachers might notice that the previously quiet child is more animated and active but all can be reassured that treatment is simply restoring the child to normal. In those with severe disease, starting thyroxine treatment during the pubertal years can accelerate puberty with a potential to reduce final height and therefore puberty may need to be delayed with gonadotrophin-releasing hormone analogues whilst catch-up growth is maximised.

The presence of normal serum thyroxine with inappropriately elevated TSH levels during treatment may suggest an inadequate thyroxine dose or nonadherence to treatment.

CLINICAL SCENARIO

A 20-month-old child with congenital hypothyroidism due to gland aplasia was reviewed in outpatients and the following series of blood tests observed. The prescribed dose of thyroxine was appropriate for body size.

Age Fre	T4 (pmol/l)	TSH mU/l
Normal range	(21–24)	(0.5–4.5)
15 m	21.3	0.8
18 m	22.5	44.8
20 m	22.1	1.2

These results are highly suggestive of poor adherence. Replacement thyroxine aims for a free T4 in the upper quartile meaning the TSH is usually at the lower end of the normal range. The result at 15 months is ideal but at 18 months the TSH has risen, but the free T4 has not dropped as would be expected if a dose increase was needed. If the prescribed dose is fine for body size it is important to explore if doses are being missed before increasing the dose. Toddlers may start refusing their tablets, spitting them out or hiding them as was the case in this child. Poor adherence is common at any age but, in children under 3 years, persistent abnormal thyroid tests will have a deleterious effect on cognitive development and may be a safeguarding concern.

Hyperthyroidism

Graves' disease (thyrotoxicosis), the most common cause in childhood, is characterised by a diffuse goitre, hyperthyroidism and ophthalmopathy and is the result of elevated levels of TSH receptor antibody.

Children with hyperthyroidism may present with:
- weight loss
- increased sweatiness and heat intolerance
- tachycardia and palpitations
- decreased concentration and falling school performance
- goitre (Figure 25.3)
- exophthalmos
- fine finger tremors
- proximal myopathy
- lid lag

Investigations

Hyperthyroidism can be diagnosed with elevated serum free T4 levels, suppressed TSH and elevated TSH receptor antibodies.

Treatment and management

The management of Graves' disease in children encompasses three therapeutic options:

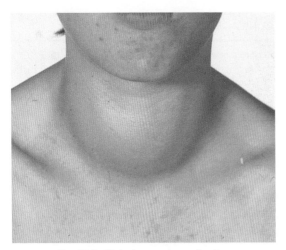

Fig. 25.3 Clinical appearance of goitre.

- antithyroid medication
- radioiodine therapy
- thyroidectomy

Initial treatment with antithyroid medication is generally preferred in children and long-term remission rates are around 50% to 60% after several years of therapy.

Antithyroid medication

The thionamide derivatives (carbimazole, methimazole, thiamazole) effectively block the synthesis of thyroxine. Propylthiouracil is not usually used for Graves' disease in children as they are at higher risk of liver failure than adults. While the thionamides and propylthiouracil can promptly inhibit thyroid hormone formation, they do not inhibit thyroid hormone release. Until levels of circulating thyroid hormones normalise, the symptoms and signs of hyperthyroidism are controlled with beta blockers such as propranolol or atenolol. Thyrotoxicosis can also be controlled more quickly with Lugol's iodine, which blocks the release of stored hormones and is useful in a thyroid storm.

Radioiodine

The combination of a higher rate of side effects with the use of antithyroid drugs in children, a lower remission rate and longer treatment period to remission in prepubertal children has led to the use of radioiodine earlier in the course of the disease. Radioiodine can achieve high remission rates, but there is a small risk of thyroid cancer if the thyroid gland is not fully ablated after radioiodine therapy.

Thyroidectomy

Thyroidectomy, which can also achieve high rates of remission, can result in hypoparathyroidism or dysphonia due to damage of the recurrent laryngeal nerves.

Potential complications

Thionamides can occasionally be associated with side effects including urticaria, Stevens Johnson syndrome, arthralgia and an increase in liver enzymes. Although rare, agranulocytosis is the most severe side effect of antithyroid drugs occurring within the first 100 days of treatment in 95% of patients.

Neonatal Graves' disease is caused by transplacental passage of high titres of TSH receptor stimulating IgG antibodies in mothers with a current or previous history of Graves' disease. Neonates born to thyrotoxic mothers who have been treated with thionamides in the third trimester of pregnancy may initially have hypothyroidism from the effect of maternal medication, but after the drug has been metabolised and cleared, features of hyperthyroidism may appear in the neonate, as a result of continued action of the maternal TSH receptor stimulating IgG antibodies.

Neonates with hyperthyroidism may present with goitre, poor weight gain and irritability. Those with severe disease may present with cardiac failure and respiratory distress from tracheal compression by the large goitre. In severe disease, neonates may require Lugol's iodine whilst those with milder disease would require carbimazole and propranolol. The medication can be gradually weaned after about 8–24 weeks.

Disorders affecting calcium regulation

- disorders resulting in hypocalcaemia
- disorders resulting in hypercalcaemia
- rickets

Ionic calcium is tightly regulated within very narrow limits and this is vital for normal cellular activity, normal signal transduction and normal neuromuscular activity. This delicate calcium balance is achieved by calcium transport across three organ systems namely, the intestines, the kidneys and bones, through the effects of two principal hormones—parathyroid hormone (PTH) and 1,25-dihydroxyvitamin D (1,25-(OH)2D). The calcium-sensing receptors (CaSR) in the parathyroid glands and renal tubules monitor the serum calcium level and integrate the hormonal response,

A fall in the ionic calcium level is detected in the parathyroid glands and renal tubules and causes an increase in PTH and active vitamin D secretion. This leads to:
- increased renal tubular reabsorption of calcium and decreased tubular reabsorption of phosphate and increased phosphate excretion (the "phosphaturic effect")

- increased bone resorption, leading to calcium release from bone into the circulation
- stimulation of 1 alpha-hydroxylase activity at the proximal renal tubule, which results in increased secretion of 1,25-(OH)2D and increased reabsorption of intestinal calcium

All these changes restore the ionic calcium level to normal. Conversely, when the serum calcium ion is elevated, PTH secretion is reduced which results in inhibition of calcium reabsorption at the kidneys and decreased bone resorption.

Disorders resulting in hypocalcaemia

Hypocalcaemia can result from three categories of disorders, which reflect the three main components in the regulation of serum calcium:
- Disorders of PTH secretion and action
  - familial hypoparathyroidism
  - congenital hypoparathyroidism
  - Chromosome 22q11.2 deletion (DiGeorge syndrome)
  - pseudohypoparathyroidism
  - acquired causes include parathyroidectomy or auto-immune poly-endocrinopathy
- Disorders of vitamin D deficiency or action:
  - 1 alpha-hydroxylase deficiency or renal disease
  - 25-hydroxylase deficiency or liver disease
  - vitamin D resistance
- Abnormality of the Calcium-sensing receptor (CaSR)
  - activating mutations of the CaSR gene

Low serum calcium levels cause:
- increased neuromuscular excitability
- paraesthesia and tingling sensation around the mouth, fingers and toes
- tetany with carpopedal spasms
- seizures
- Chvostek's sign (tapping of facial nerve over cheek gives twitching of mouth)
- Trousseau's sign (carpal spasm with inflated blood pressure cuff)

Investigations

In a child with hypocalcaemia, the following parameters should be checked:
- serum calcium (corrected for any elevated albumin level)
- serum phosphate (index of PTH activity when there is hypocalcaemia)
  - low serum phosphate level reflects increased PTH activity
  - high serum phosphate reflects reduced PTH activity
- serum magnesium (as hypomagnesaemia inhibits PTH release)
- serum alkaline phosphatase (marker of bone turnover)
  - levels are raised when hypocalcaemia is secondary to a disorder of vitamin D
  - levels in the normal range when secondary to hypoparathyroidism
- 25-hydroxyvitamin D reflects vitamin D disorders
- serum electrolytes and creatinine will help in determining renal disease
- x-rays of the metaphyses of long bones can help in the diagnosis of rickets
- ECG for prolongation of the QT interval
- chest x-ray for thymic shadows
- chromosomal analysis for 22q11.2 deletion

Alternative diagnoses

The disorders resulting in hypocalcaemia can be differentiated based on the clinical findings (specific phenotypic features for 22q11.2 deletion (DiGeorge syndrome) and pseudohypoparathyroidism) and the biochemistry.

Treatment and management

Treatment of acute severe hypocalcaemia requires urgent correction of hypocalcaemia:
- intravenous bolus of 10% calcium gluconate over 10 minutes, diluted to 1 in 10
- subsequent calcium infusion that is repeated if symptoms persist or serum calcium remains low

Table 25.2 Characteristic biochemical results seen with hypocalcaemic disorders				
	Serum calcium	Serum phosphate	Serum PTH levels	Serum alkaline phosphatase
hypoparathyroidism	↓	↑	↓	normal
pseudohypoparathyroidism 1a	↓	↑	↑↑	normal
vitamin D deficiency	↓	↓	↑	↑↑↑

Oral calcium supplements should replace intravenous administration once the severe symptoms have resolved.

Management of hypoparathyroidism or pseudohypoparathyroidism is with a vitamin D analogue such as calcitriol to increase intestinal calcium absorption. Hypomagnesaemia will respond to oral magnesium supplement and vitamin D deficiency should be treated with cholecalciferol.

Disorders resulting in hypercalcaemia

The hypercalcaemic disorders can be divided into primary or secondary hypercalcaemia. The primary hypercalcaemic disorders can be grouped into the disorders associated with elevated, normal or suppressed PTH levels:
- Disorders associated with raised PTH levels:
  - severe neonatal hyperparathyroidism
  - multiple endocrine neoplasia
  - parathyroid adenomas
- Disorders associated with normal PTH levels:
  - familial hypocalciuric hypercalcaemia—due mutations of CaSR gene
- Disorders associated with suppressed PTH levels:
  - Williams syndrome

The secondary causes of hypercalcaemia include the following:
- malignancy (acute leukaemia, hepatoblastoma, medulloblastoma)
- chronic renal failure
- immobilisation
- drug induced (vitamin D intoxication, thiazides)
Parathyroid tumours occur in 90% of patients with multiple endocrine neoplasia type I.

The clinical features associated with hypercalcaemia are nonspecific and include:
- headache, irritability, nausea and vomiting
- abdominal cramps and constipation
- proximal muscle weakness or generalised myopathy (when severe)
- dehydration and polyuria (when severe)

Treatment and management

The management of hypercalcaemia is to lower the serum calcium levels and correct the underlying disease. General measures include:
- reducing calcium in parenteral feeds
- discontinuing medications which lead to hypercalcaemia (thiazides, vitamin D)

Other specific measures include:

Increasing the urinary calcium excretion by volume expansion with intravenous saline infusion and the administration of a loop diuretic (furosemide) which blocks reabsorption of calcium at the loop of Henle.

Rickets

Rickets is a condition in which there is failure of normal mineralisation of growing bone. It is generally caused by a lack of mineral supply, which can be due to:
- deficiency of calcium
- vitamin D deficiency—most common
- disorders of vitamin D metabolism (deficiency of 1 alpha-hydroxylase or 25-hydroxylase)
- vitamin D receptor resistance
- deficiency of phosphate—x-linked hypophosphataemic rickets most common
Rickets can present as congenital rickets at birth, as a result of maternal vitamin D deficiency. The poor bone mineralisation results in craniotabes, a rachitic rosary and a bell-shaped chest.

Classical rickets presents in the toddler age group with:
- bow legs (genu varus—Figure 25.4) or knock knees (genu valgus) when child starts to walk
- delayed motor development
- bone pain and muscle weakness
- flared wrists and ankles
Radiologically, there may be metaphyseal cupping and fraying, where the metaphyses are replaced by a concave 'moth eaten' appearance, which is best seen at the radius and ulna, lower end of the femur and upper end of the tibia (Figure 25.5).

TABLE 25.3 Characteristic biochemical results seen with hyperparathyroidism

	Serum calcium	Serum phosphate	Serum PTH levels	Serum alkaline phosphatase
hyperparathyroidism	↑	↓	↑↑	normal

Table 25.4 Characteristic biochemical results which differentiate causes of rickets

	Serum calcium	25-hydroxy vitamin D	Serum phosphate	Serum PTH levels	Serum alkaline phosphatase
nutritional rickets (vitamin D deficiency)	initially normal low at later stage	↓	↓	↑↑	↑↑
vitamin D resistant rickets		marked elevation ⬆	↓	↑↑	↑↑

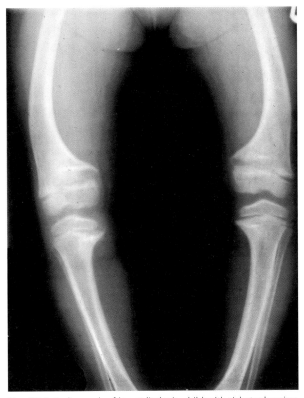

Fig. 25.4 Radiograph of lower limbs in child with rickets showing obvious bowing and ragged metaphyseal areas.

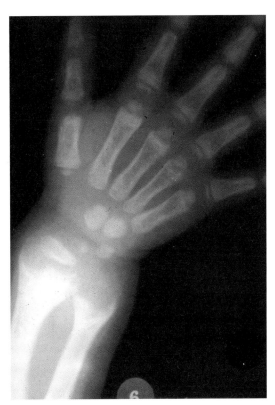

Fig. 25.5 Wrist radiograph showing the changes of rickets—metaphyseal cupping and splaying.

More severe forms of rickets can present as hypocalcaemic seizures in infants and tetany with carpopedal spasms in older children.

Investigations

In a child with clinical signs of rickets, the following investigations are essential:
- x-rays of the wrists and knees to assess epiphyseal growth plates
- serum total calcium, phosphate and alkaline phosphatase
- serum 25-hydroxyvitamin D level
- PTH
- albumin
- creatinine

Urine should be assessed for calcium, phosphate and creatinine, so that the fractional excretion of phosphate, tubular reabsorption and tubular threshold for phosphate can be calculated to establish a diagnosis of x-linked hypophosphataemic rickets.

Treatment and management

The treatment of choice for vitamin D deficiency is vitamin D (2000 U/day for at least 3 months), either in the form of cholecalciferol or ergocalciferol, with oral calcium in the diet or as a supplement. In the UK all children up to 5 years have free access to Healthy Start vitamin supplements that contain vitamin D.

Endocrine complications of other diseases

Many conditions and their treatment can lead to endocrine complications and examples include:

Chronic disease

Any chronic disease can impair growth and delay puberty partly due to downregulation of growth hormone production, and this would include children who are subject to prolonged abuse, particularly emotional. Growth will improve once the underlying cause is identified and managed, and sometimes, in psychosocial dwarfism, this reversal may aid the diagnosis.

Complications of steroid treatment

Children and young people prescribed high-dose steroids, such as those with acute lymphoblastic leukaemia or nephrotic syndrome, are at risk of developing glucose intolerance that may need—usually temporary—treatment with insulin. The more common scenario is seen in children receiving long-term treatment with lower doses administered by any route—including nasal—that can lead to two potential complications:
- iatrogenic Cushing syndrome
- inability to mount the usual cortisol response during intercurrent illness

Iatrogenic Cushing syndrome presents with growth failure and weight gain. Facial swelling is quite common but the other classic features are much less frequent. All children receiving chronic steroid treatment should be managed on the lowest dose and least damaging route and regime possible to control their disease. Steroid sparing agents such as tacrolimus may be considered. Such children need careful monitoring that includes plotting their height and weight at regular intervals on an appropriate growth chart.

Coexisting with iatrogenic Cushing syndrome is the risk of an adrenal crisis where the children may be unable to mount the usual cortisol response during intercurrent illness or following an accident. It is important that such a child is recognised and appropriate tests undertaken to confirm the risk. This may not always be possible and, if there is any doubt, children and their families should be provided with written advice about managing acute illness including immediate telephone advice and open access to a local hospital unit. They will need to know how to increase their baseline dose or, preferably, be prescribed a physiological replacement steroid such as hydrocortisone to take in these circumstances. Parents or carers should be confident about giving parenteral steroids if the child is vomiting and cannot tolerate oral steroids, and schools should also have a written care plan.

Endocrine problems in childhood cancer

Some children with cancer present with an endocrinopathy, particularly those with tumours in or around the hypothalamopituitary axis. These children can present with:
- isolated growth hormone deficiency
- multiple pituitary hormone deficiency (MPHD) including diabetes insipidus
- growth hormone excess
- gonadotrophin dependent sexual precocity
- pathological pubertal delay

Girls with androgen-secreting ovarian tumours are likely to present with growth acceleration, virilisation and voice changes.

All children who have undergone treatment for childhood cancer should be monitored for potential late effects, and this must include measuring their height and weight and plotting on a growth chart. Those where growth becomes a concern and those who have a known risk of endocrine problems should be managed by a multidisciplinary late effects team that includes a paediatric endocrinologist. Lifetime surveillance for those known to be at risk is recommended.

Radiotherapy is the single most important risk factor for endocrine late effects as it causes age-, dose- and site-dependent damage—direct or collateral—to any tissue caught in the field.

The most common late endocrine effects from radiotherapy include:
- hypothalamopituitary dysfunction
  - develops after cranial or total body irradiation used in stem cell transplantation Growth hormone deficiency develops following relatively low doses of radiotherapy whilst other deficiencies (LH, FSH, TSH

and ACTH) are largely confined to children who have received higher doses
- primary thyroid deficiency
  - common following mantle radiotherapy for Hodgkin lymphoma
- gonadotrophin-dependent sexual precocity
  - common in children who receive low-dose radiotherapy for brain tumours especially, but not specifically, if located near the hypothalamopituitary axis
- primary gonadal failure leading to infertility
  - direct radiotherapy to the gonads or total body irradiation may affect ovarian and testicular function causing failure to enter or complete puberty

The most common late endocrine effects from chemotherapy include:
- infertility
  - certain agents lead to loss of gonadal tissue and, where predictable, both boys and girls will be offered treatment modalities to preserve eggs or sperm
- reduced bone mineral density
  - a particular problem for survivors of ALL and brain tumours for a variety of reasons including steroid treatment, poor nutrition, immobility and hormone deficiencies. Prevention with a healthy calcium-containing diet, regular exercise and avoiding smoking and excess alcohol is best, plus treatment of any vitamin D deficiency
- obesity
  - a significant problem for survivors of childhood cancer and almost 50% of children with ALL are obese after 10 years of follow up for reasons that are not clear. Children who have damage to the hypothalamopituitary axis from a tumour or local surgery are at high risk of hypothalamic obesity which can be severe and intractable and appetite control can be a significant problem for these patients.

IMPORTANT CLINICAL POINTS

Anterior pituitary hormone deficiency
- growth hormone deficiency is the most common axis to be affected
- slow growth is almost always the presenting problem in children over the age of 2
- hypoglycaemia is the commonest presenting feature in neonates

Posterior pituitary hormone deficiency
- most common disturbance is diabetes insipidus
- normal response to fluid restriction will show a serum osmolality of 275–295 mOsmol/kg and a urine osmolality of greater than 850 mOsmol/kg
- In DI there is inappropriately dilute urine of less than 750 mOsm/kg despite a serum osmolality of greater than 295 mOsm/kg
- cranial DI is treated with desmopressin (DDAVP) usually given orally

Posterior pituitary hormone excess
- SIADH leads to impaired water excretion with hyponatraemia and hypervolaemia

Primary adrenal insufficiency leads to
- hyponatraemia hyperkalaemia metabolic acidosis hypoglycaemia increased generalised pigmentation of skin
- most common enzyme deficiency causing CAH is 21-hydroxylase deficiency

Cushing syndrome
- Initial investigations are 24-hour urine for free-cortisol excretion, serum cortisol circadian rhythm study and overnight dexamethasone suppression test

Thyroid disorders
- Newborn screening looks for high TSH but will not detect congenital hypopituitarism
  Calcium disorders treatment of acute severe hypocalcaemia requires IV bolus of diluted 10% calcium

Further reading

Donaldson MC,; Gregory JW,; Van-Vliet G,; Wolfsdorf JI. Practical Endocrinology and Diabetes in Children. Wiley. 4th Edition. April 2019.

Royal Children's Hospital Melbourne. Clinical Practice Guidelines: Hyponatraemia. Revised August 2018. https://www.rch.org.au/clinicalguide/guideline_index/Hyponatraemia/.

Chapter | 26 |

Neurology

Shakti Agrawal, Amitav Parida

After reading this chapter you should be able to:
- understand and request suitable neurophysiological and neuroimaging studies.
- assess and diagnose abnormalities in skull development.
- investigate and manage headache.
- assess, diagnose, investigate and manage seizure disorders.
- assess, diagnose and manage muscular dystrophies, neuropathies, myopathies and myalgia.
- assess, diagnose and manage ataxia.
- assess, diagnose and manage stroke.

Neurological investigations

Neurophysiological investigations
Electroencephalogram (EEG)

EEG is used in the assessment and diagnosis of seizure disorders, encephalopathy and sleep disorders.

The commonly used EEG investigations are:
- standard awake EEG—usually requested after a second seizure but may also be considered after a cluster of seizures, focal seizures or a prolonged seizure. The interpretation should recognise that the interictal EEG may be normal in a child with epilepsy and abnormal in children who do not have epilepsy
- sleep-deprived EEG—useful in the diagnosis of conditions where abnormalities are likely to be seen in sleep such as epileptic spasms with hypsarrhythmia or structural focal epilepsy
- awake EEG with photic stimulation and hyperventilation—useful in diagnosing childhood absence epilepsy
- ambulatory EEG—used to capture suspected seizures where there is significant uncertainty about the diagnosis of epilepsy after standard awake and sleep EEG
- video telemetry—requires an inpatient stay and uses multiple-angle video recording to characterise the seizure and correlate it with the parallel EEG recording

Cerebral function monitoring

The most common application is in the NICU to assess babies with suspected hypoxic ischaemic encephalopathy where it is used to detect electrical seizures and suppressed brain activity.

In PICU, cerebral function monitoring may be used in children with status epilepticus or acquired brain injury, as seizures cannot be detected clinically if the child is paralysed and ventilated.

Nerve conduction studies and electromyography

These investigations help define the pathophysiological process seen with neuromuscular disorders such as Guillain Barre syndrome. They can assess function at different locations on the neural conduction pathway. These are:
- anterior horn cell—spinal muscular atrophy
- peripheral nerves—Guillian-Barre syndrome
- neuromuscular junction—acquired and congenital myasthenia
- muscle—congenital myopathies or muscular dystrophies

Neuroimaging
Cranial ultrasound

Indications
- screening for intraventricular haemorrhage in preterm babies

- measuring the ventricular index in hydrocephalus to guide intervention
- ischaemic injury in the basal ganglia in a term neonate
- detecting arterial ischaemic stroke
- used to detect large structural abnormalities such as agenesis of the corpus callosum
- cerebral calcifications in congenital infection (CMV or toxoplasmosis)

Computed tomography (CT) imaging

CT is commonly used in neurological emergencies as it has a shorter scan time and is better tolerated in children than is MRI. There is, however, a radiation exposure.

Indications:
- traumatic brain injury looking for acute subdural, extradural, parenchymal and subarachnoid bleeds and skull fractures. Cerebral oedema and features of raised intracranial pressure can be seen on CT
- abnormal skull shape where craniosynostosis is suspected as the images allow 3D reconstructions
- acute stroke to identify occlusion of a cerebral artery by thrombus
- ventriculoperitoneal shunt blockage

Magnetic resonance imaging (MRI)

MRI has the advantage of not using ionising radiation and has the ability to use a number of differing sequences to identify a wide range of pathological abnormalities. However, in younger children, it may not be tolerated without sedation or general anaesthesia due to longer scanning times, claustrophobia and the noise within the magnet.

Indications:
- suspected spinal emergencies—spinal cord compression and transverse myelitis
- neurological emergencies—encephalitis or demyelinating conditions
- tumour and abscess assessment
- epilepsy and developmental impairment or regression

The most common sequences are T1 and T2 weighted images, where water appears bright on T2 sequences but dark on T1 sequences. Diffusion weighted images help to identify areas of cytotoxic damage to the brain, for instance an acute arterial ischemic stroke.

Magnetic resonance spectroscopy acquires signal from a single localised area and measures the concentration and physical properties of cell metabolites such as choline (elevated in some tumours) or lactate (elevated in hypoxic ischaemic injury and stroke).

Abnormal head shape

Microcephaly

Microcephaly is generally defined as an occipito-frontal head circumference (OFC) greater than 3 standard deviations **below** the mean for the age and sex. Causes include:
- hypoxic ischaemic insult at birth
- congenital infection
- foetal alcohol syndrome
- genetic disorders
- structural brain abnormalities

Macrocephaly

Macrocephaly is an OFC greater than 3 standard deviations **above** the mean for the age and sex. Causes include:
- familial—important to measure and plot parental OFC
- hydrocephalus
- neurogenetic conditions including neurometabolic and neurocutaneous disorders

Plagiocephaly

The most common cause of abnormal head shape in infants is positional plagiocephaly, which results from a baby lying on the back for long periods with the head on one side. If development and neurological examination is normal, then no investigations are necessary. Parents may be advised to implement supervised 'tummy time' to allow time without pressure on the skull bones. Preterm babies classically have a scaphocephalic head shape for similar reasons.

Craniosynostosis

Craniosynostosis describes an abnormal and premature fusion of the skull bones and may involve one or multiple sutures (Figure 26.1). Multiple-suture craniosynostosis is more likely to be associated with underlying genetic conditions such as Crouzon, Apert or Pfeiffer syndrome.

Abnormal fusion of the skull sutures may result in scaphocephaly (fusion of the sagittal suture), trigonocephaly (metopic suture synostosis), nonpositional plagiocephaly (unilateral coronal synostosis) and bilateral lambdoid synostosis.

Multiple suture craniosynostosis is more likely to result in complications such as raised intracranial pressure, and these children may require neurosurgical intervention at a recognised craniofacial centre.

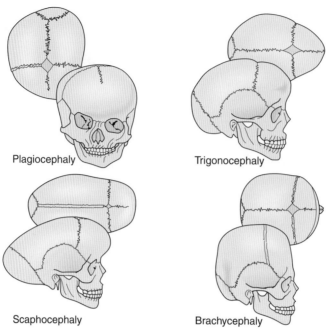

Plagiocephaly

Trigonocephaly

Scaphocephaly

Brachycephaly

Fig. 26.1 Premature fusion of cranial sutures leading to abnormal shapes of skull (Image used with permission from Principles of Neurological Surgery. Ed. Kitchen ND et al. 4th edition. Chapter 9. Tushar Jha R et al. Elsevier Inc.)

Epilepsy

Epilepsy is a clinical diagnosis that is usually based on the description or video recording of two unprovoked seizures which are 24 hours apart. Seizures are described as either focal or generalised and they may be associated with impairment of awareness (dyscognitive seizures) or preserved awareness. Motor manifestations include tonic stiffening, clonic jerking, dystonic posturing, loss of tone, myoclonus and forced head version. Nonmotor manifestations may include emotional disturbance, visual hallucinations, loss of speech, sensory changes or aura.

Epilepsy syndromes are determined by age of onset of the seizures, ictal manifestations and neurodevelopment of a child in the context of the abnormalities present on an electroencephalogram (EEG). Reaching an electroclinical diagnosis is crucial in helping to guide treatment and determine the aetiology and prognosis.

Neonatal seizures

These are described in Chapter 2 Neonatology.

Epilepsies of infancy

Epilepsies presenting beyond the neonatal period in infancy are more likely to result from a monogenic

disorder or a structural brain malformation rather a postnatal acquired insult.

Many neurogenetic conditions associated with early developmental impairment may present or be associated with epilepsy. There may be characteristic dysmorphic features that will help point towards a specific diagnosis such as Rett's syndrome or Angelman syndrome.

Epileptic spasms (ES)

These were previously known as **infantile spasms,** and they tend to present between 3 and 24 months of life but can be present from the neonatal period. They are characterised by recurrent brief, stereotypical movements occurring in clusters, with extension or flexion of both arms and sudden flexion of the head. The majority of infants presenting with ES will ultimately develop intellectual and motor disability.

The EEG in ES shows a chaotic background activity known as hypsarrhythmia (Figure 26.2) that is evident particularly during a period of sleep. West syndrome describes the characteristic triad of the characteristic epileptic spasms, developmental regression and hypsarrhythmia on EEG. Epileptic spasms are also associated with many conditions including tuberous sclerosis where cortical tubers are the epileptogenic foci.

Treatment of epileptic spasms usually involves the combination of steroids and vigabatrin, although in tuberous sclerosis treatment is initially with vigabatrin alone. The

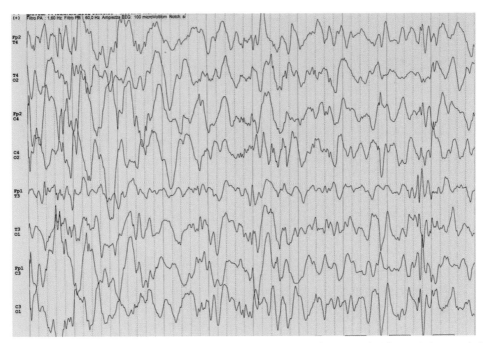

Fig. 26.2 EEG of 3-year-old boy with tuberous sclerosis showing hypsarrhythmia. (Image used with permission Metabolic Epilepsy: An update. Nicita F et al. Jap Soc Ch Neurol. 2013: 35.9)

aim of treatment is to control the epileptic encephalopathy and so improve the developmental potential of the child.

Epilepsies in young children
Childhood absence epilepsy

Typically presents between 4–8 years of age with multiple, abrupt-onset absences lasting 20–30 seconds. There may be eyelid flickering, head deviation, subtle lip twitching or hand automatisms. Seizures can be induced by hyperventilation. The EEG will show the typical pattern of three per second spike and wave activity (Figure 26.3). Treatment is with either ethosuximide or sodium valproate and most children respond well.

Myoclonic atonic and myoclonic absence epilepsy

The condition presents in the preschool years and differs from absence epilepsy by the presence of myoclonic jerks and atonic head drops accompanying the absence episode. The seizures are typically more refractory to treatment, and developmental impairment is common. Batten's disease, a neurodegenerative lysosomal storage disease, may present in a child with developmental regression associated with myoclonic seizures. Treatment with carbamazepine and phenytoin may make absence epilepsy worse.

Childhood epilepsy with centrotemporal spikes

This condition was previously known as **benign Rolandic epilepsy** and presents with focal, often nocturnal, seizures sometimes with secondary generalisation. The focal seizures are typically associated with speech arrest and facial twitching. Many children will only have one or two seizures and so treatment may not be required.

Lennox Gastaut syndrome

A condition that is commonly associated with drug refractory epilepsy as well as early developmental impairment. The hallmark seizure types are nocturnal tonic seizures although atypical absences, drop attacks, myoclonic jerks and focal seizures can be seen. The most common cause is a structural brain abnormality such as hypoxic ischaemic injury from the neonatal period. Treatment of this condition is difficult and usually involves the use of multiple antiepileptic medications as well as nondrug options such as the ketogenic diet, vagal nerve stimulation and, in suitable children, epilepsy surgery.

Epilepsies of adolescence
Juvenile absence epilepsy

Patients present normally after 8 years of age, and the EEG will often demonstrate photosensitivity along with

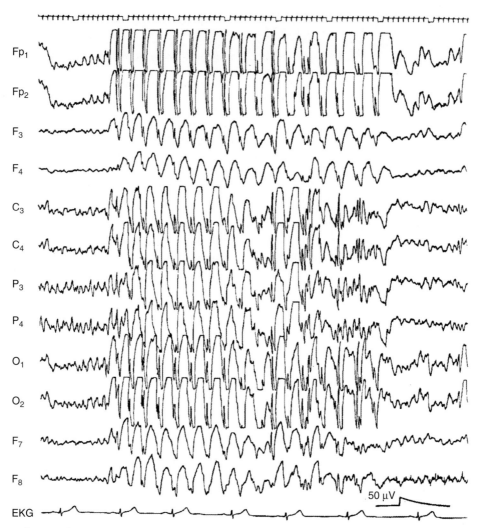

Fig. 26.3 EEG of 3-year-old boy with absence seizures showing 3 per second spike and wave activity. (Image used with permission from Pädiatrie hoch2. Ed. Muntau AC and Driemeyer J. Chapter 19. Elsevier GmbH.)

a polyspike and wave pattern. Most will go on to have generalised convulsive seizures that may persist into adulthood, and so treatment with a broad-spectrum anticonvulsant such as levetiracetam, lamotrigine or sodium valproate is usually recommended.

Juvenile myoclonic epilepsy

This may present initially with absence seizures followed by the onset of myoclonic jerks and generalised tonic clonic seizures in the later teenage years. Lifelong treatment with sodium valproate, lamotrigine or levetiracetam is recommended whilst carbamazepine may make seizure control worse.

Structural focal epilepsies (temporal, frontal and occipital lobe epilepsy)

These result from areas of structurally abnormal brain tissue such as an area of cortical dysplasia, and the most common areas of abnormality are the temporal lobes followed by the frontal lobes.

Temporal lobe epilepsy is most typically associated with mesial temporal sclerosis where there may have been a history of prior febrile convulsions in infancy. Temporal lobe seizures may manifest in an aura such as a feeling or fear, déjà vu or jamais vu (never seen) or a rising epigastric sensation prior to the onset of a focal motor seizure which may become generalised.

Frontal lobe seizures are often nocturnal and frequently present a diagnostic challenge. They may manifest in a dystonic posturing, salivation and rapid thrashing movements (hyper motor seizures), and there are often several short seizures in a night.

Occipital lobe seizures may manifest in multicoloured visual hallucinations particularly shapes such as circles or flashes.

Anticonvulsant treatment can be effective, but epilepsy surgery should be considered early in children under 2 years and in those children where seizures do not respond to two appropriately chosen antiepileptics.

Outcomes

Around 50% to 60% of children and young people with epilepsy will have complete seizure remission during their childhood. The presence of ongoing seizures and intellectual disability are associated with worse social outcomes in adulthood for children with epilepsy.

Treatment and management

Seizure disorders are usually treated with single-agent, antiepileptic medications in the first instance, but some may require the addition of further drugs if control is poor. Many commonly used antiepileptic medications need to be started at a low dose and increased slowly over a few weeks to avoid excessive side effects, particularly sedation. Children with drug refractory epilepsy should be referred to paediatric neurology services for further assessment and consideration of other treatment options including a ketogenic diet, vagal nerve stimulation or even epilepsy surgery.

Table 26.1 **Epilepsy syndromes and commonly used antiepileptic drugs**

Epilepsy syndrome	Commonly used AEDs	Common AEDs which may make epilepsy worse
neonatal acute seizures	levetiracetam, phenobarbitone	
infantile spasms	prednisolone vigabatrin	
child absence epilepsy	sodium valproate ethosuximide	carbamazepine
benign focal epilepsies of childhood	levetiracetam sodium valproate carbamazepine	
Lennox Gastaut syndrome	sodium valproate lamotrigine clobazam	carbamazepine, phenobarbitone
structural focal epilepsy	carbamazepine lamotrigine levetiracetam	
juvenile absence epilepsy juvenile myoclonic epilepsy	sodium valproate levetiracetam lamotrigine	carbamazepine

Table 26.2 **Common pharmacological agents used in the treatment of epilepsy**

	Common side effects	Cautions
sodium valproate	abnormal behaviour hepatic disorders thrombocytopenia weight increase	liver dysfunction especially in children under 3 years and usually in first 6 months
carbamazepine	Leucopenia thrombocytopenia liver dysfunction cutaneous drug reactions	withdraw immediately if liver dysfunction or leucopenia
levetiracetam	Anxiety depression insomnia skin reactions	
lamotrigine	Agitation dry mouth sleep disorders cutaneous drug reactions	Brugada syndrome myoclonic seizures may be exacerbated
phenytoin (now mainly used in status)	gingival hyperplasia hepatic disorders megaloblastic anaemia arrhythmias if IV cutaneous drug reactions	
ethosuxamide	Agranulocytosis leucopenia Stevens-Johnson syndrome	

Seizure-like disorders

Normal and abnormal paroxysmal events

Neonatal tremor (jitteriness) is a common benign movement disorder in the term neonate, and the tremor can always be stopped by holding the baby. Tactile stimulation and loud noise may provoke the jitteriness. Neonatal abstinence syndrome occurs in the days after birth and is due to the withdrawal of drugs such as opioids or antidepressants, particularly selective serotonin reuptake inhibitors, that were taken by the mother.

Severe gastro-oesophageal reflux in babies and infants may result in back arching, torticollis and sometimes tonic stiffening of the arms and legs and the episodes are often associated with feeds.

Spasmus nutans is an idiopathic condition with torticollis, nystagmus and characteristic head nodding. The diagnosis is one of exclusion, and therefore ophthalmic assessment and neuroimaging is mandatory as optic nerve lesions and brain tumours can present in a similar way.

Breath holding spells tend to occur in infancy when a traumatic or emotional event upsets the child who starts to cry, pauses and then becomes pale or cyanosed. In more severe episodes, the child then loses consciousness, stiffens and sometimes jerks.

Reflex anoxic seizures are similar in presentation to breath holding attacks, but the primary event is not associated with breath holding. A classical description is of a child falling over and losing consciousness in response to a surprising or painful stimulus. The child will be pale and there may be tonic stiffening and clonic jerking. The events tend to last less than a minute and, in most children, no treatment is required and parental reassurance can be given. Iron deficiency is associated with these episodes and assessment of the iron status should be considered in a child with multiple episodes.

Motor stereotypies are typically involuntary, repetitive, purposeless movements such as body rocking, hand flapping, head banging and teeth clenching. The child can be distracted to terminate a motor stereotypy.

Infantile gratification disorder results from stimulation of the genitalia by the infant who will be exhibit rocking movements and grunting noises and may stiffen the legs or stare into space.

Night terrors and parasomnias tend to start around 3 to 7 years of age and do not usually occur more than twice each night. Sleepwalking is common.

Daydreaming is usually seen in situations where a child is bored, but the appearance may raise the possibility of absence seizures. It is usually possible to distract the child out of the former but not the latter.

Vasovagal syncope is a transient impairment of awareness and is common in adolescents, particularly girls. There is often a history of presyncopal symptoms such as feeling hot, nauseous and dizzy before a collapse. All children with syncope should have a 12-lead ECG and serial lying and standing blood pressures to exclude an arrhythmias or orthostatic hypotension as causes.

Nonepileptic seizures are variably referred to as nonepileptic attacks, functional seizures, pseudo-seizures, hysterical seizures or dissociative seizures. There are episodes of motor, sensory and cognitive symptoms and are not associated with epileptiform EEG changes. The episodes are described by observers as variable thrashing with side-to-side head and body movements. Eyes are usually closed and there will be resistance to eye opening. Psychological comorbidities such as depression and anxiety are common and a referral to psychology services is recommended.

Habit spasms or tics are common and tend to occur from 4 to 8 years of age, particularly in boys. Eye blinking, facial grimacing and shoulder shrugging are common whilst vocal tics such as throat clearing and coughing may also be present. Tics will often wax and wane in their frequency and most children do not need any investigation or treatment. A diagnosis of Tourette syndrome may be made if at least one vocal and one motor tic have been observed and the tics have lasted for more than one year with no alternative medical explanation present.

Narcolepsy. This is a rare neurological condition characterised by excessive daytime somnolence and can be associated with cataplexy (drop attacks on laughing and suddenly falling asleep). Diagnosis is made with a multi-latency sleep test and possibly a lumbar puncture to look at the level of orexin (a neuropeptide that regulates awakened state) in CSF.

Headache

Primary headache disorders include tension-type headaches, cluster headaches and migraine whilst secondary headaches are the consequence of recognised and identified causes such as meningitis, brain tumours and idiopathic intracranial hypertension.

Certain features in the history suggest pathological causes for the headaches and indicate a need for further investigations. These features include:
- atypical migraine variants
- cluster headache
- personality change
- headaches present on waking from sleep
- rapidly progressive chronic headache

Primary headache disorders

Tension-type headaches present with a mild to moderate tightening sensation round the head without any obvious specific triggers. Paracetamol or ibuprofen are usually effective for acute treatment whilst acupuncture or amitriptyline may be used for prophylaxis.

Migraine headaches are usually moderate to severe, unilateral or bilateral throbbing headaches with associated nausea, vomiting, photophobia and phonophobia.

Cyclical vomiting syndrome is a recognised migraine variant, and the patient experiences severe attacks of nausea and vomiting over a period of 1 to 10 days.

Hemiplegic migraine is another migraine variant presenting with unilateral weakness, ipsilateral sensory and visual symptoms and dysarthria associated with a migraine headache. The symptoms can persist for a few hours to a few days.

Cluster headaches are extremely rare in childhood, are classically unilateral around the eye and temporal areas and are described as sharp and burning in quality. They are usually associated with unilateral lacrimation, periorbital erythema, nasal congestion, ptosis and pupil constriction. An acute episode may need treatment with subcutaneous or intranasal triptan whilst verapamil can be used for prophylaxis.

Treatment and management

Simple migraine headaches can be treated effectively with paracetamol or ibuprofen. Triptans can also be used at the onset of headache and then repeated after 2 hours if symptoms have not resolved.

Lifestyle factors such as encouraging good sleep hygiene, limiting screen time, staying well hydrated, avoiding caffeine, alcohol and other food triggers should also be stressed.

For children with frequent episodes of migraine regular prophylactic medication may be required. Propranolol or topiramate are suggested as the first-line prophylactic agent and amitriptyline may also be considered. Pizotifen is often used in clinical practice for migraine prophylaxis although there is a lack of evidence about its efficacy in children.

Secondary headache disorders

Some headaches may have a relatively obvious secondary cause such as trauma or infections of sinuses, middle ear or teeth. Other causes would include:

Intracranial bleeds that often produce a sudden-onset, severe, 'thunderclap' headache. An urgent CT scan should be performed with this presentation.

Hypertension may lead to headaches as a presenting feature.

Idiopathic intracranial hypertension presents with a progressive headache, visual symptoms such as blurring or diplopia and papilloedema often in patients who are overweight. Neuroimaging is mandatory to exclude a space-occupying lesion or a cerebral venous sinus thrombosis. If neuroimaging does not demonstrate a cause for raised intracranial pressure, then an LP should be undertaken and an opening pressure above 280 mmH$_2$O would be consistent with the diagnosis.

If visual failure is identified then treatment must be undertaken as there is a risk of permanent sight loss, and urgent referral to the neurosurgical team for CSF diversion should be undertaken. When the vision is not threatened, treatment with acetazolamide is offered along with advice to lose weight.

Medication overuse headache can lead to chronic headaches in young people. These headaches are the result of excessive use of analgesia (use of paracetamol, ibuprofen, codeine or triptans three or more times a week) and an abrupt withdrawal should be considered. Symptoms may then improve.

Ataxia

Acute ataxia

The child with acute ataxia presents with unsteady, broad-based gait, slurred speech and a tremor.

Causes include:
- **para infectious cerebellitis**—post-varicella ataxia typically occurs 5–14 days after the onset of vesicles and, in most children, the ataxia is mild. Cerebellitis may also occur due to other viruses. MRI neuroimaging and, if safe, lumbar puncture is recommended in patients with more severe symptoms
- **demyelinating conditions**—these may be isolated episodes following some infections whilst recurrent episodes can be seen with conditions such multiple sclerosis
- **metabolic disorders**—ornithine transcarbamylase deficiency, maple syrup urine disease or mitochondrial disorders
- **brain tumours**—posterior fossa tumours

- **opsoclonus myoclonus ataxia syndrome** (OMAS)—an immune-mediated condition which may be associated with a neuroblastoma
- **labyrinthitis**—vertigo, nausea, dizziness and an unsteady gait suggest middle ear infection

Episodic ataxias

Presentation with recurrent acute, episodic ataxia and the causes include:
- toxic or metabolic
- basilar migraine

Chronic ataxia

Chronic nonprogressive ataxia in children may be caused by posterior fossa brain malformations such as Dandy Walker or Arnold Chiari malformations

Progressive ataxias

- Friederich's ataxia presents with pes cavus, absent tendon reflexes in addition to a slowly progressive ataxia
- ataxic telangiectasia—telangiectasia of the sclera and immune deficiency
- abetalipoproteinemia—identified by low levels of cholesterol and triglycerides
- metachromatic leukodystrophy—younger children with developmental regression and ataxia

Neurocutaneous syndromes

Several genetic disorders involve abnormalities of the skin, brain and spine. Clinical examination of any child referred for suspected developmental impairment, seizures or any other neurological concerns should involve inspection of the skin. Images of dermatological features can be seen in Chapter 23 Dermatology.

Neurofibromatosis type 1 (NF1)

NF1 is the most common neurocutaneous disorder and has an autosomal dominant inheritance. Children with the condition may present with the characteristic skin stigmata or concerns about development. Intellectual disability, autism spectrum disorders and attention deficit hyperactivity disorder are all significantly more common in children with NF1. The diagnosis is made if two of the following features are present:
- six or more café au lait spots
- dermal neurofibromas

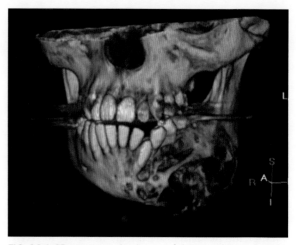

FIG. 26.4 3D reconstruction image of the jaw of a 12-year-old girl with neurofibromatosis type 1 showing bone destruction from neurofibroma extension

- freckles in axillary and inguinal areas
- Lish nodules in the iris
- family history of NF1
- optic glioma
- invasive osseous lesions (Figure 26.4)

Treatment and management

Annual review of child with NF1 should involve:
- ophthalmology assessment
- blood pressure measurement—may develop hypertension from renal artery stenosis or pheochromocytoma
- assessment for new neurological symptoms—high risk of developing low-grade gliomas and astrocytomas
- assessment for skeletal abnormalities—leg length discrepancy, pseudo-arthrosis and scoliosis

Neurofibromatosis type 2 (NF2)

NF2 is much rarer than NF1 with the average age at diagnosis of 18–24 years, but its features may be underrecognised in the paediatric age group. Inheritance is autosomal dominant, but almost half of the children present de novo. Individuals can present with:
- palpable intradermal schwannomas
- mononeuropathy (particularly oculomotor, facial, radial and fibular nerve palsies)
- cataracts
- retinal hamartomas

Treatment and management

Once the diagnosis is made, annual surveillance is recommended with annual MRI scans, audiology and ophthalmology assessments.

Tuberous sclerosis

Inheritance is autosomal dominant but around two-thirds occur spontaneously. Infants may present with epileptic spasms or focal seizures due to associated intracranial tubers. Some may present with early developmental impairment or features of a pervasive developmental disorder such as autism spectrum disorders or attentional deficit hyperactivity disorders. Over half of children will have some form of intellectual disability. Ash leaf macules may not be visible on an initial external examination, and assessment using Wood's light should be performed.

Skin findings (see Ch 23 Dermatology) include:
- facial angiofibromas
- ash leaf macules
- shagreen patches
- subungual fibromas

Treatment and management

Epileptic spasms respond best to vigabatrin although epilepsy can be drug refractory, and so nondrug treatments such the ketogenic diet, epilepsy surgery, vagal nerve stimulation and everolimus should be considered.

All children with tuberous sclerosis should have annual surveillance, including:
- renal imaging—may show angiomyolipomas, multiple renal cysts or polycystic kidney disease
- MRI brain scan initially every 1–2 years to identify subependymal giant cell astrocytoma (SEGA)
- ophthalmology assessment—assess for retinal hamartomas

Sturge Weber syndrome (SWS)

The condition is identified by the presence of a port-wine stain in the distribution of the trigeminal nerve and is often suspected at birth. The majority of children will develop structural focal epilepsy that can be refractory to medical treatment. If SWS is suspected, an MRI of the brain should be performed and this may show evidence of leptomeningeal angiomatosis.

Treatment and management

Over half of the children will have learning disabilities. Children might need antiplatelet therapy due to risk of stroke, and epilepsy surgery may need to be considered in children with drug resistant seizures.

Neuromuscular disorders

Floppy infant syndrome
Central hypotonia

The majority of infants with low tone will have a central neurogenetic cause such as Down syndrome or Prader-Willi syndrome. Examination of such children will reveal that the axial body tone is likely to be low, but peripheral tone and antigravity limb movements may be normal. Deep tendon reflexes are preserved or increased.

Peripheral hypotonia

Peripheral hypotonia may be the result of abnormalities at different levels. These would be:
- anterior horn cell—spinal muscular atrophy
- neuromuscular junction—congenital myasthenic syndrome
- muscle—congenital myopathies and muscular dystrophies
- nerves—congenital neuropathies

Where a peripheral cause of hypotonia is seen, the baby is likely to be floppy both centrally and peripherally with a paucity of peripheral limb antigravity movements. Reflexes may be depressed, particularly in congenital neuropathies, and tongue fasciculations may be present. The baby, however, is likely to be bright and alert with no features of encephalopathy. Contractures and arthrogryposis may be evident. Examination of the parents, particularly the mother, may provide further information as the presence of ptosis may point towards myasthenia whilst a facial weakness and may be seen in congenital myotonic dystrophy.

Investigations will include nerve conduction studies, electromyography and genetic studies. A markedly raised creatinine kinase should be indicative of a congenital muscular dystrophy. The determination of particular diagnosis by a histological review of a muscle biopsy sample is becoming increasing replaced by the use of genomics.

Spinal muscular atrophy (SMA)

Spinal muscular atrophy is the second most common autosomal recessive genetic condition in the UK population after cystic fibrosis. The child with SMA type 1 will typically appear to have normal tone at birth but within the first 6 months shows increasing hypotonia. The diaphragm is spared and consequently, a diaphragmatic pattern of breathing is observed. Tongue fasciculations may be present, peripheral movements are reduced and reflexes may be depressed. The natural history of SMA 1 is progressive respiratory failure and often death before the two years of life. Those children with SMA type 2 and type 3 can live into adulthood. Children with SMA do not have any cognitive difficulties but develop orthopaedic complications over time such as scoliosis.

Treatment and management

Prompt diagnosis of SMA is now essential as new therapeutic agents can dramatically change the disease course for some. Nusinersan may lead to normal motor development in children when treatment is given soon after birth.

Duchenne muscular dystrophy (DMD)
Becker muscular dystrophy (BMD)

Both DMD and BMD are x-linked recessive disorders. Boys present with delayed motor development, calf pseudohypertrophy and a positive Gower's signs, although those with BMD tend to have weaknesses more in the upper limbs rather than the lower limbs. Some patients may present with speech delay or communication difficulties. Motor symptoms tend to be evident before 6 years of age with increased proximal weakness, and most boys with DMD will lose the ability to walk by 12 years of age. Girls tend to be asymptomatic carriers but exceptionally have symptoms.

Investigation

A markedly elevated creatinine kinase level is indicative of both DMD and BMD and a normal value effectively excludes the diagnoses. The conditions are caused by mutations in the dystrophin gene. Muscle biopsy and EMG will show features consistent with a myopathy. ECG and echocardiography are necessary as arrhythmias and cardiomyopathy are frequently seen.

Treatment and management

Physiotherapy and steroids have been shown to delay loss of strength and ambulation of over time. Adolescents with DMD develop respiratory failure due to respiratory muscle weakness that is often made worse by an evolving scoliosis. Respiratory physiotherapy, noninvasive ventilation and appropriately timed scoliosis surgery can improve survival. Life expectancy is 36 years on average in males although most require noninvasive ventilation. Those with BMD seem to have a slower deterioration and can usually maintain a more normal lifestyle.

Progressive muscular conditions

Limb girdle muscular dystrophies present with a pattern of weakness greater in proximal rather than distal muscle groups and over time may develop scapular winging and contractures.

Facio-scapulo-humeral muscular dystrophy is a slowly progressive disorder that often presents in teenage years with facial and shoulder weakness, and scapular winging is a common sign. Life expectancy is often normal.

Metabolic myopathies

Inherited metabolic disorders such as glycogen storage and mitochondrial disorders may present with exercise intolerance, muscle cramps, progressive muscle weakness or episodes of rhabdomyolysis.

Myasthenia

Myasthenia in childhood results either from an acquired autoimmune disorder or a congenital myasthenic syndrome. It is a disorder of neuromuscular junction transmission characterised by muscle fatigue and weakness which may be limited to the extraocular muscles or involve the facial, bulbar and proximal muscles groups. Single fibre electromyography or repetitive nerve stimulation can demonstrate impaired neuromuscular transmission. The condition may be congenital or acquired.

Acquired myasthenia gravis Newborn babies born to mothers with myasthenia gravis may be affected due to transplacental transfer of antibodies and treatment is with pyridostigmine or steroids. All children should have a CT or MRI scan of the thorax to look for a thymoma.

Peripheral neuropathies
Guillain Barre syndrome (GBS)

This condition is an immune-mediated neuropathy that can occur in the context of a recent infection. It presents acutely with sensory changes and motor weakness spreading from the lower to the upper extremities over hours, days or weeks. The weaknesses can progress to involve the muscles of the trunk and lead to respiratory failure and may even involve the cranial nerves producing diplopia or problems with swallowing. Tendon reflexes are depressed or absent although plantar reflexes will remain flexor.

Investigations

GBS is primarily a clinical diagnosis, but nerve conduction studies will provide supportive information. MRI of the spine can be helpful in differentiating the condition from acute flaccid myelitis, transverse myelitis and spinal cord compression. CSF protein is significantly raised.

Treatment and management

The child presenting with these symptoms must be monitored closely to identify respiratory compromise and, in children who are old enough to comply, regular monitoring with forced vital capacity testing can help to detect impending respiratory failure.

Treatment may need to be initiated urgently if there are signs of rapid deterioration. Intravenous immunoglobin or plasma exchange and respiratory support, including intubation and ventilation, may be required for those with the most severe disease.

Rare causes of peripheral neuropathy

- vincristine used in treatment of malignant disease
- lead, mercury, organophosphate ingestion, glue sniffing
- uraemic polyneuropathy with chronic kidney disease

Hereditary sensory and motor neuropathy (HMSN)

This group of conditions show autosomal dominant inheritance and cause progressive neuromuscular impairment over the first 2 decades of life. Both motor and sensory nerve dysfunction are evident and classically produce pes cavus and claw toes as well as wasting of the intrinsic muscles of the hand. Sensation may be impaired and tendon reflexes depressed. Supportive treatment will focus on pain management and physiotherapy.

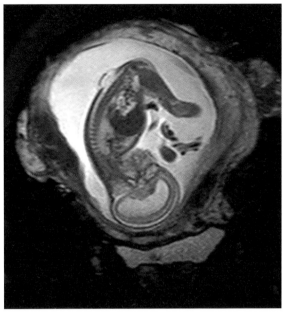

Fig. 26.6 MRI in utero scan showing fetus with lumbo-sacral meningomyelocoele

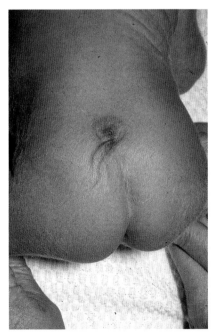

Fig. 26.5 Newborn baby with midline neurocutaneous marker suggesting spinal dysraphism

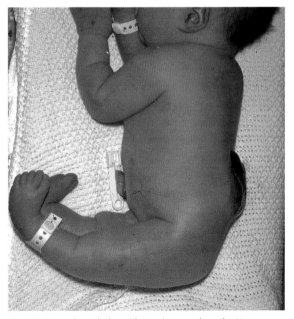

Fig. 26.7 Newborn baby with meningomyelocoele. Note hypoplastic lower limbs, genu recurvatum and talipes that have occurred as a result of in utero neural dysfunction

Spina bifida

Spina bifida describes a congenital malformation where the vertebral column is open. Spinal dysraphism is the term used for the spectrum of congenital anomalies associated with defects in the neural arch that cause herniation of neural tissue or the meninges. Where a defect is not visible, there may be neurocutaneous markers on the skin in the midline such as a tuft of hair (Figure 26.5), dermal sinus, lipoma or a patch of dysplastic skin.

The most common and clinically important manifestation is myelomeningocele leading to postnatal exposure of neural tissue. The condition is commonly detected antenatally on routine ultrasonography and further assessed by foetal MRI imaging (Figure 26.6).

Many babies born with myelomeningocele will also have a coexisting Arnold-Chiari malformation resulting in cerebellar tonsillar herniation through the foramen magnum. Hydrocephalus due to obstruction of cerebrospinal fluid at the level of fourth ventricle may occur and requires the insertion of a ventriculoperitoneal shunt.

Children with myelomeningocele will have motor and sensory deficits below the level of the lesion (Figure 26.7) with a lower-level lesion being associated with an improved motor outcome. Intellectual disability may be associated with complications of hydrocephalus.

Treatment and management

Foetal repair for open spina bifida has recently become available. Immediate postnatal management requires the defect to be wrapped in plastic wrap film to prevent infection and surgical repair is then undertaken in the first few days of life. CSF diversion surgery with a ventriculoperitoneal shunt may also be required.

Urodynamic studies will frequently show evidence of urinary retention, overflow and ureteric reflux and consequently intermittent catheterisation is often necessary. Orthopaedic surveillance and intervention may be necessary for spinal, hip, leg and foot deformities.

Stroke

Stroke can be classified as:
- ischaemic stroke—arterial ischaemic stroke or cerebral venous sinus thrombosis
- haemorrhagic stroke—due to bleeding

Perinatal arterial ischaemic stroke

The term describes a stroke occurring from 20 weeks' gestation to day 28 of life and thus may occur in utero or in postnatal life. Risk factors in the baby include the presence of congenital heart disease, infection and asphyxia. Most babies present acutely with focal motor seizures, apnoeas and poor feeding although some present in infancy or childhood with focal epilepsy or hemiplegia. Treatment is largely supportive and affected children are at risk of developing cerebral palsy, structural focal epilepsy and learning difficulties.

Arterial ischaemic stroke

Some preexisting conditions may predispose to stroke and include Down syndrome, sickle cell disease and NF1. The

---

IMPORTANT CLINICAL POINTS

Abnormal head shape
- microcephaly may be caused by
  - acquired brain injury
  - congenital infection
  - inherited metabolic disorders
  - nonprogressive neurogenetic disorders
- macrocephaly is often familial
- macrocephaly with early developmental impairment may be due to hydrocephalus or an underlying neurogenetic condition

Headaches
- most common are migraine and tension-type headaches
- secondary headache disorders include idiopathic intracranial hypertension, space occupying lesions, subarachnoid haemorrhage, meningitis and cerebral abscess

Acute ataxia
- causes include
  - infection
  - demyelinating conditions
  - toxins and metabolic conditions
  - stroke
  - brain tumours

Stroke
- ischaemic
- haemorrhagic

child can present with acute hemiparesis, slurred speech, ataxia, dysarthria or even focal seizures. A number of conditions can appear similar to stroke and include hemiplegic migraine, postictal Todd's paresis and medically unexplained neurological presentations. Urgent MRI or CT brain with angiography should be conducted within an hour of presentation. All children should have an echocardiogram to exclude structural problems such as a patent foramen ovale.

Treatment and management

Under expert supervision thrombolysis may be considered in children over 2 years of age. A child with sickle cell disease may need an urgent exchange transfusion. Anticoagulation with high dose aspirin for 2 weeks followed by prophylactic aspirin is recommended.

Haemorrhagic stroke

Children with cerebral haemorrhage should be evaluated for an underlying vascular anomaly such as an arteriovenous malformation, intracranial aneurysm or cavernous malformation. Acute surgical intervention such as evacuation of a haematoma may be required to help manage raised intracranial pressure.

Further reading

Epilepsies: diagnosis and management. NICE guideline [CG137]. Published January 2012. https://www.nice.org.uk/guidance/cg137

Headaches in over 12s: diagnosis and management. NICE guideline [CG150]. Published September 2012. https://www.nice.org.uk/guidance/cg150

Stroke in childhood: Royal College of Paediatrics and Child Health. RCPCH May 2017. http://www.rcpch.ac.uk/stroke-guideline

Chapter 27

Neurodevelopmental medicine

Katherine Martin, Nadya James

After reading this chapter you should be able to assess, diagnose and manage:
- developmental disorders and learning difficulties
- speech and language disorders including autism spectrum disorder
- neurodevelopmental disorders
- a child with neurodisability

The care of children with neurodevelopmental disorders covers a range of skills provided by different members of a large multidisciplinary team. The prime objectives of this team are the initial identification of areas of concern for the family, exploration of any underlying pathology, quantifying the extent of any disability and guiding families on how to support the child. Medical assessment, genetic counselling, physiotherapy, occupational therapy, speech and language support, vision and hearing review, education and social support are all needed.

Intellectual disability

Intellectual disability (ID), also referred to as learning disability (LD), indicates a cognitive testing result that is 2 standard deviations below the mean. This is equivalent to an IQ of 70.

A more useful definition, however, is:
- a significantly reduced ability to understand new or complex information or to learn new skills
- a reduced ability to cope independently

The majority of individuals with an ID do not have an identified underlying medical diagnosis. It is recognised that those infants born preterm (under 37 weeks' gestation) are at increased risk of developmental concerns in later life, and the greater the prematurity the greater the risk of significant developmental issues. Children who

present with developmental regression are of particular concern and need urgent review (Table 27.1).

Important areas of assessment for potential developmental impairment include:
- prenatal and perinatal history—maternal alcohol consumption, smoking, medication, illicit drugs, gestation, birth and postnatal complications
- family history—consanguinity, family history of ID or neurological disorders
- early milestones
- age when concerns first noted and any regression
- current school/nursery progress and learning styles
- life skills (e.g. dressing, toileting, crossing a road, making a snack, negotiating friendships, understanding daily routines)
- growth including head circumference (compared with OFC of parents)
- features of any underlying syndrome
- issues with hearing, vision, sleep and continence
- school or nursery information of degree of impairment

There are situations where the clinical picture of ID is evident but where a more remedial issue is identified. These include:
- significant neglect or emotional abuse
- unrecognised sensory impairment—poor vision or hearing
- motor dysfunction impacting on interaction and communication
- untreated medical illness
- mental and emotional health concerns

Associations

Some of the problems associated with ID are related to the underlying causes, but others are seen independent of whether any cause is identified. The following are more common in individuals with ID:
- epilepsy (approximately 30 times more likely)

Table 27.1 Developmental warning signs	
Age	**Identified feature**
at any age	maternal concern
	regression of previously acquired skills
at 10 weeks	not smiling
at 6 months	persistent primitive reflexes
	persistent squint
	hand preference
	little interest in people, toys, noises
at 10–12 months	not sitting
	no double syllable babble
	no pincer grip
at 18 months	not walking independently
	fewer than 6 words
	persistent mouthing and drooling
at 2½ years	no 2–3 word sentences
at 4 years	unintelligible speech

- constipation (approximately 11 times more likely)
- visual impairment (approximately 8 times more likely)
- obesity
- mental health disorder, particularly depression and anxiety
- hearing loss
- reflux and heartburn
- some forms of dementia

Investigations

Investigations must be tailored to the individual child and clinical judgement used as to which, if any, are required. Investigations to consider would aim to identify any underlying pathology and would include:
- genetic analysis
- metabolic screen
- MRI imaging
- EEG
- skeletal survey
- congenital infection screen

Treatment and management

For some with ID, there are specific management issues related to an underlying diagnosis. The majority with ID will not need long-term paediatric care unless there

are allied medical concerns that require management in their own right. For most children and young people with ID, management is based around some guiding principles:

Development.
- early referral to support teams such as Portage, preschool support or the school Special Educational Needs Coordinator (SENCO) and Specialist Teachers for vision/hearing impairment is important
- Education and Health Care Plan (EHCP) should be provided that accurately reflects the needs and strengths of the young person and is made available, with parents' permission, to the education team to help secure funding for ongoing support
- EHCP continues until age 25 if still in education and many young people can go on to college or an employment placement. The young person may live in supported or independent accommodation with support

Medical.
- early referral to any required allied health teams such as Speech and Language Therapy, Physiotherapy and Occupational Therapy
- GP is made aware that the young person has been diagnosed with ID as they will be required to undertake annual reviews from age 14 years
- transition to adult care should commence by about 14 years of age and involvement of the following teams should be considered:
  - community mental health services
  - adult ID teams
  - adult specialists
  - dedicated transition clinics

Social and well-being
- young people with ID are vulnerable to childhood abuse, exploitation (sexual, financial, criminal) and bullying and discrimination. It is therefore important to be aware of the features of emotional and mental health concerns that include an inability to fully express their feelings, manifesting as withdrawal, lethargy, distressed behaviour and anxiety.
- at age 18, young people are assumed competent irrespective of ID or other factors. As they enter adult life, they may be unaware of how to ask for help when needed for issues including medical review, financial advice, mental health support, legal advice and accessing facilities and services

Cerebral palsy

Cerebral palsy is defined as 'a group of permanent neurological disorders resulting from non-progressive brain injury or malformation that occurred in the developing foetal or infant brain and primarily affecting body movement, posture and muscle coordination. The motor dysfunction in cerebral palsy is often associated with abnormal cognitive abilities including communication and behaviour disturbance'.

Cerebral palsy should be considered a description of clinical findings rather than a definitive diagnosis in itself as there are many aetiologies that result in the clinical picture of cerebral palsy. The movement disorder is often accompanied by other issues which may include:

- intellectual disability
- vision and/or hearing impairment
- dysphagia, excessive drooling
- gastro-oesophageal reflux
- bladder and bowel issues
- communication difficulties
- epilepsy
- recurrent respiratory illnesses
- secondary musculoskeletal complications

Classification

Cerebral palsy can be classified in a number of different ways:

Type of movement disorder:
- spastic (motor cortex damage)
- dyskinetic (basal ganglia damage—resulting in additional involuntary movements)
- ataxic (cerebellar damage affects proprioception)
- mixed pattern (damage to a combination of areas)
Distribution of the effects on the limbs:
- bilateral (diplegia or quadriplegia)
- unilateral (hemiplegia or monoplegia)
Severity of impact on functional abilities:
- clinical scales have developed to describe levels of motor skills, communication and functional capacity

Use of the appropriate terminology not only facilitates communication between professionals but can also help discuss a child's broad prognosis and potential comorbidities.

Cerebral palsy may present with:
- tonal abnormalities (a stiff irritable baby)
- asymmetry of movements (early hand preference)
- atypical or late motor development (delayed walking, persistent toe walking)

In the mildly affected child, issues may not become apparent until the child is independently mobile and starts to show more subtle differences such as toe walking. Clinical signs will depend on the nature and severity of the cerebral palsy but will include abnormalities of muscle tone, posture and reflexes, together with any developmental impact these may have.

Alternative diagnoses

Many other disorders may have an initial presentation similar to cerebral palsy and include:
- inborn errors of metabolism—citrullinaemia and biotinidase deficiency
- mitochondrial disorders—Leigh's disease (though these features progress)
- genetic dystonias, hereditary spastic paraparesis—children may have a family history of 'cerebral palsy'

Associations

- gastro-oesophageal reflux
- sialorrhoea (drooling) due to bulbar dysfunction and poor oro-motor control
- bowel and bladder dysfunction
- epilepsy
- sleep disorders due to pain and musculoskeletal discomfort
- respiratory illnesses from aspiration of food or gastric contents and inadequate cough
- postural issues can cause restrictive respiratory difficulties

Investigations

All children with a clinical picture of cerebral palsy should have neuroimaging (preferably MRI) performed. This will often confirm underlying aetiological changes such as periventricular leukomalacia or a large middle cerebral artery infarct

Treatment and management

A coordinated multiagency approach is essential. Growing knowledge and understanding of the developing brain supports the need for early targeted intervention coordinated by a paediatrician who can make appropriate assessment and involve the appropriate members of the multidisciplinary team.
- **physiotherapy**—to support and promote development of motor skills, maintain ranges of movement and minimise deformities and other complications of tonal and postural abnormalities
- **occupational therapy**—to support development in play and self-care skills and participation needs in school/nursery
- **orthotics**—provide a range of aids such as splints and gaiters to support a child's posture and development
- **speech and language therapy**—to address communication, feeding and swallowing difficulties
- **visual impairment**—70% of children with cerebral palsy are thought to have some degree of strabismus, visual field loss, difficulties with eye movements, reduced

visual acuity or cerebral visual impairment in which the eye has good visual acuity but the brain is not able to process the images seen

- **hearing impairment**—an estimated 10% to 20% of children with cerebral palsy have some degree of hearing impairment
- **intellectual disability**—affects around 50% of people with cerebral palsy and is moderate or severe in around 20%. Involvement of the early-years education team (Portage) may be appropriate depending on likely cognitive level or developmental trajectory.

Relevant pharmacological agents used

Medication may be required to manage hypertonia or symptoms of associated issues including gastro-oesophageal reflux disease, constipation, neuropathic bladder, drooling and epilepsy (Table 27.2).

Table 27.2 **Oral treatments for hypertonia**		
Drug	**Adverse effects**	**Notes**
Baclofen	Constipation	poor diffusion into brain
	urinary retention	can be given intrathecally
	Confusion	
	Paraesthesia	
Diazepam	Sleepiness	dependence may occur with prolonged usage
	respiratory depression	
	paradoxical agitation	
Tizanidine	Arrhythmias	unlicensed in children
	drowsiness	blood monitoring in those on high doses
	hepatic enzyme elevation	
Dantrolene	hepatic enzyme disorder	monitoring of liver function advised
	confusion	
	skin reaction	

Botulinum toxin A is a treatment for focal hypertonia (spasticity or dystonia) and the toxin is injected directly into the muscles needing treatment. The effect lasts around 4–6 months. It is contraindicated in patients receiving aminoglycoside treatment due to potentiation of the action of the toxin.

Two main surgical treatments are available for spasticity associated with cerebral palsy.

Intrathecal baclofen pumps provide a continuous low dose of baclofen directly into the intrathecal space. This produces a global effect on an individual's hypertonia and, since much lower doses are required than when used orally, the risk of adverse drug-related effects is much lower. The reservoir of drug within the pump system needs refilling every 3 months.

Selective dorsal rhizotomy is a procedure in which a proportion of the sensory nerve roots at one or more spinal levels are cut, reducing the sensory feedback within the spinal reflex and thus reducing the spasticity. The current availability on the NHS is limited to a specific group of children who are already walking with a degree of independence and who have particular changes on their MRI brain scan.

Complications and sequelae

Hip subluxation, which may progress to complete dislocation, is a common complication. Approaches to control or reduce the progression of subluxation include a postural management programme, use of botulinum toxin A, oral medication and tendon lengthening surgery.

Scoliosis is frequently, but not exclusively, related to pelvic obliquity or hip subluxation. The availability of 'growing rods' (implanted rods that can be extended as the child grows) allows earlier surgical intervention for those in whom progression of the curvature is rapid or is causing other issues such as respiratory difficulties.

Specific syndromes

As knowledge of genetics advances, more and more clinical syndromes are being identified. Many of the children and young people diagnosed with these conditions will have varying degrees of intellectual disability and an understanding of how these issues can be managed is presented here. Details of the phenotypic features for each of these conditions are outlined in Chapter 5 Genetics and should be reviewed together with this section. Affected families will benefit from expertise from community paediatrics, geneticists and other clinical specialities as indicated (e.g. cardiology and ENT) along with allied health professionals (dieticians, physiotherapy, etc.) and agencies such as education and child and adolescent mental health services. Genetic counselling for the parents and the young person themselves when older, is important.

Down syndrome

Relevant features that may impact on development:
- hypotonia and hypermobility
- intellectual disability common (usually mild–moderate)
- respiratory and ENT infections—glue ear common giving hearing problems
- obstructive sleep apnoea
- hypothyroidism
- coeliac disease—increased risk
- diabetes mellitus type 1—increased risk
- leukaemia—increased risk of acute myeloid and lymphoid leukaemia

Treatment and management. It is important that the family have early support and information about Down syndrome and are referred to a support team experienced in providing the required care. The child will require annual reviews throughout life including screening for complications (hypothyroidism, coeliac disease, atlanto-axial instability, obstructive sleep apnoea). Physiotherapy and orthotics input is essential for motor skills development whilst support for development and education needs is important. Some complications such as structural cardiac abnormalities, visual problems and hearing difficulties may be identified at an early age and required involvement of specialist teams. The child with Down syndrome has a high risk of respiratory infection due to immune-compromise and may need antibiotic prophylaxis.

Complications and sequelae.
- most will have a degree of intellectual disability
- cervical atlantoaxial instability and risk of subluxation
- reduced fertility is common, but contraception is still important
- life expectancy is shorter with approximate age at death of 55–60 years

Fetal alcohol syndrome disorder

Relevant features that may impact on development:
- growth restriction
- clear evidence of brain involvement (microcephaly or behavioural impairment)
- skeletal abnormalities—chest wall, joint contractures
- behavioural problems (Autism spectrum disorders, ADHD, higher functions affected)

Alternative diagnoses and differing features.
- Williams syndrome—has hypercalcaemia and aortic stenosis
- Noonan syndrome—often macrocephaly and lymphoedema

- Cornelia de Lange syndrome—microcephaly and limb abnormalities
- chromosome 22q11.2 deletion—hypocalcaemia and often cleft lip and palate

Treatment and management. Behavioural and educational difficulties due to reduced attention and increased impulsivity are often significant and support is invariably required.

Rett syndrome

Relevant features that may impact on development:
- growth failure, progressive microcephaly
- initial normal development but then regression and withdrawn
- low tone, motor delay, feeding problems, speech delay and loss of motor function
- stereotypical midline hand movements and unprovoked screaming episodes
- seizures
- bruxism (teeth grinding)

Treatment and management. The early features of this condition may resemble autism spectrum disorder or metabolic disorders due to the presence of stereotypical movements, bruxism and then developmental regression. Particular attention is directed at ensuring optimal nutrition and support for feeding, ensuring physiotherapy for spasticity and scoliosis, support in education and daily activities and assessment for appropriate support with communication.

Williams syndrome

Relevant features that may impact on development:
- intellectual disability
- sociable and language skills comparatively good ('Cocktail Party Chatter')
- hypercalcaemia
- hypothyroidism

Alternative diagnoses and differing features.
- Fetal alcohol syndrome disorder—characteristic facies
- Noonan syndrome—often macrocephaly and lymphoedema
- Chromosome 22q11.2 deletion—hypocalcaemia and often cleft lip and palate
- ADHD and autism spectrum disorder

Treatment and management. Calcium levels and thyroid function need close monitoring and, as children may develop joint contractures, they need physiotherapy support. Dental caries are a recognised complication and regular review is necessary. Social and educational difficulties are likely and will be the main focus for support. The sociable nature and good verbal skills of young people with Williams syndrome can make them vulnerable to exploitation

Chromosome 22q11.2 deletion (Di George syndrome, velocardiofacial syndrome)

Relevant features that may impact on development:
- hypoplastic thymus—immunodeficiency through leucopenia and recurrent infections
- hypocalcaemia—parathyroid hypoplasia—present with seizures
- speech and developmental delay
- cleft lip and palate

Treatment and management. Children need regular review with feeding support in infancy some will require lifelong supplementation with vitamin D and calcium if hypoparathyroidism leads to hypocalcaemia. Immunology advice is important particularly before administering any live vaccine.

Prader Willi syndrome (PWS)

Relevant features that may impact on development:
- low tone and poor suck and poor feeding with a weak cry
- lack of satiety cues that leads to increasing obesity from 2 years of age
- learning impairment common
- hypermobile and late motor milestones
- short stature
- rigid behaviour with obsessions, autism-like features and temper outbursts

Alternative diagnoses and differing features.
- 'simple' obesity
- hypothyroidism
- Laurence-Moon-Biedl syndrome—digital and dental abnormalities

Treatment and management. Children with PWS need NG tube feeds in infancy and strict restriction of access to food when older along exercise planning. Physiotherapy support is usually needed to address hypotonia and to increase the ability to exercise. Growth hormone is licensed for use in PWS without formal testing and increases muscle mass, improves bone mineral density and decreases body fat as well as beneficial effects on linear growth so may be started in a toddler. However, it has been linked to worsening of respiratory function so is contraindicated in severely obese children and until

polysomnography has excluded evidence of central sleep apnoea.

Angelman syndrome

Relevant features that may impact on development:
- manifests between 6 and 12 months of age
- significant developmental delay and later microcephaly
- motor features include ataxia, fine tremors, stiff-legged gait
- described as happy with laughter and hand flapping
- epilepsy common association
- particular impact on speech
- excitable, poor attention, poor sleep
- fascination with water, mirrors, balloons

Treatment and management. Support is required for social and educational delay with particular help with nonverbal communication aids. Specific advice to families will be necessary for sleep problems.

Complications and sequelae.
- generally healthy from a systemic view and compatible with a healthy life
- sociable and friendly, making young person vulnerable
- obesity in adult life

Communication disorders

Speech (verbal expression) and language (expression and reception of information) issues are the most commonly reported developmental concerns. Such difficulties may be isolated or seen as one element of a more global developmental disorder.

A number of environmental factors are associated with delays in acquisition of spoken language:
- significant neglect reduces a child's opportunities to mix and socially interact with others is associated with speech delay.
- exposure to more than one spoken language may appear to cause a mild delay in a preschool child. Other areas of the child's development will follow the expected course and the language delay usually resolves by school age.
- 'screen time' (the amount of time a child spends watching any form of screen entertainment) in excess of 2 hours per day has been found to be linked to speech delay, although direct causation has not been proven.
- prolonged use of dummies or thumb sucking has also been associated with delayed speech development.

Children with selective mutism, a form of anxiety disorder, have normal language and communication development and may have no apparent problems in the home environment. However, in certain settings such as at school or in other social settings, they are unwilling to speak and may 'freeze'. If this is not managed appropriately, it may continue into adulthood.

A mild–moderate hearing loss can cause speech and language impairment and early identification and management will optimise the child's future development of language skills. In the UK, all infants are offered screening for hearing loss shortly after birth and where the hearing impairment is more significant, early intervention will maximise the child's language and communication development.

Specific language impairment is an impairment in the acquisition and use of language that is:
- persistent
- affects the child's everyday functioning
- occurs in the absence of other contributing factors
- social interaction skills are all typical for age

Treatment and management

When assessing a child with a potential communication disorder the following points are important to consider:
- whether the difficulties are solely related to speech and language or represent wider communication difficulties. They may even be a presenting feature of global developmental impairment
- whether the child's hearing is normal
- presence of factors that would put the child at an increased risk of speech and language delay or impairment (prematurity, neglect, bilingualism)
- presence of conditions that may be associated with speech and language difficulties

In addition to a hearing test, referral to speech and language therapy should be undertaken. This assessment will identify the specific types of difficulties and support the future language development of the child.

Complications and sequelae

Children and young people with communication difficulties can show a delay in social skills, leading to frustration and challenging behaviour.

Neurodevelopmental disorders

Neurodevelopmental disorders refer to a group of conditions with the following features in common:
- delayed or impaired development of the central nervous system
- onset during infancy or early childhood
- steady course with potential for gradual improvement over the lifespan

- usually involve more than one aspect of higher brain functioning (higher communication, visuospatial, motor planning, emotional regulation)

The main disorders which fall into this category include:
- autism spectrum disorder (ASD)
- attention deficit hyperactivity disorder (ADHD)
- developmental coordination disorder (DCD)

All three of these disorders have a significant degree of overlap with each other and also with symptoms of other difficulties such as:
- tics and Tourette syndrome
- sensory processing problems
- difficulties with emotional regulation
- impaired executive function (see later)

The exact cause of these disorders is unknown, but genetic factors are likely, as one or more of the three main disorders are frequently found in the same extended family. The main difficulty in identifying and diagnosing neurodevelopmental disorders is that many of the symptoms are part of normal human experience (Table 27.3).

Executive function

Impairment of executive function is part of ADHD, ASD and DCD and leads to some of the biggest difficulties in daily life. In normal situations, it is the higher brain processing activity that governs how we process and act upon things in order to achieve a goal or to cope with the new or unexpected. Disorders of executive function can produce the following symptoms:
- poor self-organisation
- difficulty following multistep instructions
- reduced ability to judge time
- poor forward planning
- impaired memory

Table 27.3 Symptoms that may indicate a neurodevelopmental disorder

Symptom	May be normal	May be abnormal
playing alongside rather than with peers	aged 2	aged 7
taking things literally and not understanding metaphor	aged 5	aged 14
cannot concentrate for over 10 minutes	aged 3	aged 10
uses adult-style interaction	aged 15	aged 6
cannot use a knife and fork	aged 4	aged 10

Treatment and management. The mainstay of treatment for all the neurodevelopmental disorders is via education and behavioural intervention. In some areas there are established parental courses and access to specialist nurses, but there are also extensive local and national organisations for ASD and ADHD. Sleep problems are common and melatonin is used in some children.

Autism spectrum disorder (ASD)

Autism spectrum disorder is a lifelong neurodevelopmental disorder that encompasses a wide variety of presentations and phenotypes including:
- impairment in social communication and interaction
- rigid or repetitive patterns of thought and behaviour
- frequently includes unusual motor patterns (mannerisms and stereotypies) and sensory sensitivity

Due to the wide range of severity of ASD, diagnosis requires historical as well as current information, combined with detailed observation and examination of the child. Diagnosis can be made as young as 18 months or may not be formally diagnosed until adolescence or even adulthood. There is no set test for ASD, although structured assessment tools are available (Table 27.4).

Other alternative diagnoses include:
- attachment disorder and neglect
- developmental delay with intellectual disability
- specific language impairment
- visual impairment
- obsessive-compulsive disorder
- anxiety, social phobia, elective mutism and formal mood disorder
- ADHD, DCD and tics

Table 27.4 Some of the recognised features of ASD

Social communication and interaction	Rigidity/repetitive of thoughts and behaviour	Allied symptoms
Parental report		
language delay/regression	repeated lining up/sorting behaviour	fascination with things that spin/make noise/lights
words used out of context/without correct meaning	highly restricted diet	sensory difficulties with socks, seams, waistbands
lack of pointing	echolalia	
does not understand body language/tone of voice	rituals that must be followed	
	adverse reaction to change	
	very literal, struggles with sarcasm or metaphor	
School report		
not interested in peers	distress if routines alter	may sniff or lick objects when exploring
friendship on own terms	concrete or 'black and white' thinking	seeks out sensations such as rocking or spinning
difficulty taking turns	specific topics of interest	overwhelmed by busy and noisy places
difficulty with compromise	difficult to move child from one task to another	
Direct observation		
eye contact poor or over-intense	repetitive behaviour—flicking switches, turning taps	hand flapping
reduced awareness of personal space	conversation returns to fixed topics	toe walking
does not pick up on social cues or facial expression	'factual' conversation rather than 'chit-chat'	over-reaction to noise
describes self by name or 'he/she' rather than 'I'	difficulty with pretend play or using imagination	unusual gait or repetitive movements

Treatment and management

Supportive treatment uses educational and behavioural techniques and each child should have an allocated key worker. Examples of such techniques include:
- visual timetables and 'now and next' boards
- social stories (teaches about the appropriate actions in different situations)
- use of clear and concrete instructions in smaller steps
- vocalising feelings and emotions (e.g. I am feeling sad because of X)
- use of a child's name to cue them into a group instruction
- negotiation—offering choices rather than orders
- providing routine and preparing a child in advance for unusual events
- options for when overwhelmed such as a quiet place to eat lunch

Complications and sequelae

There are particular time points that are challenging for the child with ASD. These include:
- school transition from primary to secondary that may be overwhelming
- adolescence and changes of puberty introducing socially confusing events
- anxiety and mental health disorders needing active treatment
- difficulty in understanding the intentions of others, making a young person with ASD more vulnerable to sexual and criminal exploitation.

Attention deficit hyperactivity disorder (ADHD)

This condition is difficult to diagnose under 5 years of age as many of the symptoms are normal in younger children. Individuals have difficulties in controlling impulsive behaviour and are often described as 'challenging'. The presentation is different in girls and is therefore under-recognised and usually diagnosed later than in boys.

Children and young people present with concerns about difficult behaviour that is inconsistent with the child's developmental level. The behaviour has been present for at least 6 months and has had a negative impact on social and academic activities.

Different subtypes of ADHD are recognised and are:
- inattentive subtype
  - poor attention to detail and so presenting as making careless mistakes
  - does not follow through on instructions and fails to finish tasks
  - reluctant to engage in tasks that require sustained mental effort
  - easily distracted by extraneous stimuli

- hyperactive-impulsive
  - fidgets, taps hands and feet or squirms in seat
  - leaves seat in situations when remaining seated is expected
  - unable to play or engage in leisure activities quietly
  - difficulty waiting his or her turn
- combined subtype

Associations

ADHD is linked to:
- autism spectrum disorder (ASD)
- developmental coordination disorder (DCD)
- tic disorder and Tourette syndrome
- sensory difficulties
- poor sleep

Investigations

Formal assessment and diagnosis comes from a detailed family history, observation in school or nursery settings and questionnaires targeted towards symptoms of ADHD. Invasive investigations are usually unnecessary.

Treatment and management

The most important part of managing ADHD in a child is helping the family, young person and school understand the individual symptom profile. This involves introducing learning strategies that will aid focus and concentration, sensory techniques for hyperactivity, developing emotional awareness, risk analysis and realistic expectations of behaviour. Examples of this approach will include:
- sitting with peers who will not distract
- ensuring that the teacher can make frequent eye contact
- providing information in small 'chunks' at a time
- using the child's name to cue them into an instruction
- offering regular physical exercise and a space to 'unwind' after school

Relevant pharmacological agents used

Methylphenidate should be initiated under specialist supervision and produces an increase dopamine levels in the prefrontal cortex and, in most children, improves symptoms. It can lead to a loss of appetite, weight loss and sleep disruption. Hypertension and palpitations can be induced and a family history of cardiac disorders should be excluded. Methylphenidate may trigger anger, anxiety or tics.

Dexamfetamine has similar effects to methylphenidate but is short acting and so multiple daily doses are needed.

Complications and sequelae

Medication can lead to poor growth, weight gain, hypertension and sleep and mood disturbances, and all need monitoring. ADHD itself is linked to complications such as mood disturbance and low self-esteem and an increase in risk-taking behaviours. This can include alcohol or drugs misuse, unsafe sex and the failure to see the long-term implications of life choices.

Developmental coordination disorder (DCD)

This is primarily a disorder of motor skills that are substantially below that expected given the child's age and experience and would include the descriptions of clumsy child syndrome and developmental dyspraxia or apraxia. Sensory symptoms are, however, also common.

Parental concerns arise because of:
- poor coordination of both gross and fine motor skills
- reduced spatial awareness and difficulty of judging distances
- postural instability

The child will be described as clumsy with frequent falls, having poor pencil control and difficulty with buttons and laces, may be a messy eater and have poor balance. They may be sensitive to touch, sound and noise and be 'forgetful' or 'disorganised'.

Investigations

These are tailored towards a formal assessment of movement skills using recognised assessment tools and will be undertaken by an occupational therapist or physiotherapist.

Treatment and management. The mainstay of management is adaptation and adjustment and involves:
- teaching exercises to improve core stability, balance and gross and fine motor skills
- adapting surroundings such as elastic shoelaces, adapted cutlery and writing material
- extra time in exams or situations where significant motor skills are needed

Complications and sequelae

Those with DCD may be more liable to accidents and mishaps, but the main complication is the impact on self-esteem and confidence. Symptoms do persist into adulthood and can impact long term on career choices and psychosocial well-being.

IMPORTANT CLINICAL POINTS

Intellectual disability
- a significantly reduced ability to understand new or complex information or to learn new skills
- some children with clinical picture of ID may have a remedial explanation
- early referral to support teams is important

Cerebral palsy
- permanent motor dysfunction associated with abnormal cognitive abilities
- types—spastic, dyskinetic, ataxic and mixed pattern
- all with a clinical picture of CP should have neuroimaging (preferably MRI)
- botulinum toxin A is a treatment for focal hypertonia
- Education and Health Care Plan continues until age 25

Communication disorders
- speech and language issues are most common developmental concerns
- number of environmental factors associated with delays in spoken language
- communication difficulties can lead to challenging behaviour

Neurodevelopmental disorders
- ASD, ADHD and DCD have significant overlap
- exact cause of these disorders is unknown
- ASD—features include language delay, ritualistic behaviour, poor eye contact
- ADHD—features include behaviour that has negative impact on social activities
- DCD—disorder of motor skills that are substantially below expected for age

---

Further reading

Down Syndrome medical interest group. https://www.dsmig.org.uk/. Accessed March 2021 Horridge K. Assessment and investigation of the child with disordered development. *Arch Dis Child Educ Pract Ed*. October 6, 2010.

Cerebral palsy in under 25s: assessment and management. NICE Guideline [NG62]. Published 25 January 2017. NICE Guideline [NG62]. Accessed February 2021.
Developmental follow-up of children and young people born preterm. NICE Guideline [NG72]. Published date: 09 August 2017.

Chapter 28

Ophthalmology

Louise Allen

After reading this chapter you should be able to assess, diagnose and manage:
- visual impairment
- proptosis and ptosis
- strabismus and nystagmus
- glaucoma, papilloedema, eye tumours and cataract

Eye and vision disorders affect 10% of otherwise healthy UK children but are much more prevalent in children with underlying neurological or systemic conditions. Eye anomalies often occur as part of a genetic syndrome and may aid recognition of an underlying systemic diagnosis. The early detection and management of childhood ophthalmic conditions is important to prevent lifelong visual impairment.

Vision in childhood

Eye and vision screening programmes

Visual neuroplasticity is at its most critical and malleable in the first 3 months of life and gradually declines over the first decade. Unless rapidly addressed, poor quality visual input during this period will result in abnormal neuronal development and permanent visual impairment due to amblyopia.

The impairment can be caused by:
- visual deprivation—as seen with infantile cataract or ptosis
- retinal image blur—if there are uncorrected refractive errors
- visual suppression from one eye—due to strabismus-producing diplopia

The eye and vision screening programmes in the UK are designed to detect the conditions that cause amblyopia at two time points:
- newborn and infant physical examination (NIPE)
This checks for the presence of the red reflex within 72 hours of birth and at 6–8 weeks, primarily to enable management of congenital cataract within the critical period.
- 4- to 5-year school vision screening—test of each eye to enable management of amblyopia within the period of neuroplasticity

Visual development and visual impairment

Vision is a multifaceted sense comprising:
- visual acuity (resolving power)
- peripheral vision
- colour and contrast sensitivity

The neuronal cells forming the visual pathway continue to mature after birth and visual function reaches adult levels by 4–5 years of age. In the U.K., nearly 4% of the childhood population are registered severely visually impaired or blind (compared to 12% in resource-poor countries), and half these children will have additional motor, sensory, learning impairments or systemic disease. The screening programmes, and access to specialist paediatric ophthalmic care, prevent many children from developing severe visual impairment, and consequently the majority (75%) of those who are registered blind have an unpreventable and untreatable cause. The most common cause of childhood visual impairment in resource-rich countries is cerebral visual impairment and in resource-poor countries is cataract. Visual impairment certification may be based on reduced visual acuity, restricted visual field or a combination of the two (Table 28.1).

Table 28.1 Assessment of children presenting with ophthalmic signs

Structure	Features to assess
orbits and eyelids	- symmetry of the orbits and presence of proptosis which is more obvious if viewed from above symmetry of the eyelid height - a ptosis that covers half or more of the pupil will be amblyogenic
eye alignment and movement	- symmetry of the corneal light reflections to a pen torch - elicited eye movements to a toy or torch - cover test for near and distant targets - assessment of nystagmus
globe and pupil	- symmetry of globe size, assessment of corneal diameter and clarity - pupil symmetry, shape and response to light - presence of a relative afferent pupillary defect
ocular media	- red reflex assessment with ophthalmoscope
fundus	- ophthalmoscopy of the optic nerve head and macula

Testing visual function

Most children over 6 years old can use an adult visual acuity chart such as a Snellen chart. Viewing distance is important; standard Snellen charts are viewed from 6 metres, and at this distance the child should be able to resolve letters down to line 6 (6/6 or 20/20 vision). The child who is only able to resolve the top letter will have 6/60 vision (a person with "normal vision" would be able to see this letter from 60 metres away).

Many specialists now use logMAR visual acuity notation, and 0.00 logMAR is equivalent to 6/6 visual acuity and 1.00 logMAR is equivalent to 6/60. Specialist charts are usually required for visual acuity testing in young children, although digital apps using symbol charts can be helpful.

Assessment of the red reflex

This examination should be performed whenever a child is seen with visual symptoms or ocular signs. Its prime function is to detect treatable opacities in the ocular media such as cataract and retinoblastoma.

Abnormal ophthalmic findings

Proptosis

Proptosis is abnormal forward displacement of the globe and indicates either insufficient space within the orbit or an acquired increase in the volume of intraorbital tissue. The globe may be nonaxially displaced away by an orbital mass, whereas an axial proptosis suggests a mass within the muscle cone of the orbit. Proptosis may be easier to detect if the child's face is viewed from above, and objective assessment is possible by measuring the horizontal distance from the lateral orbital ridge to the corneal surface of each eye using a ruler.

Causes of proptosis

- congenital—craniosynostosis; encephalocele; dermoid
- inflammatory—orbital cellulitis; myositis
- neoplastic—haemangioma; rhabomyosarcoma; neuroblastoma; optic nerve glioma
- traumatic—orbital haematoma; complex orbital facture

Orbital cellulitis requires urgent intravenous antibiotic therapy and treatment should not be delayed, but an atypical presentation or failure to improve on antibiotics warrants orbital imaging and further investigation. Rhabdomyosarcoma causes a rapidly progressive, nonaxial proptosis, associated with pain and inflammation of the periocular tissues which may mimic orbital cellulitis. Orbital biopsy may be required if neoplasm is suspected. Proptosis can lead to a compressive optic neuropathy or amblyopia, given that many of the patients present at a young age.

Treatment and management

All children should have specialist referral since proptosis can lead to corneal exposure which, if untreated, can lead to corneal ulceration and perforation. Regular lubrication, lid taping or a tarsorrhaphy may be necessary to protect the cornea

Ptosis

Ptosis is drooping of the upper eyelid which may be unilateral, bilateral and asymmetrical and can be congenital or acquired.

Causes of ptosis.

- congenital
  - isolated congenital levator muscle dysgenesis (most common cause)
  - congenital myasthenic syndromes

A 3-year-old girl presented with a 4 day history of headache, polydipsia and polyuria and 1 day history of bulging of her right eye. She had previously been well and there was no history of trauma. Past medical and family history revealed nothing of relevance. Immunisations were up to date.

Examination showed that she was quiet and withdrawn but responsive to her parents' commands. She was apyrexial, heart rate 100 and BP 90/65. She had an obvious proptosis to her right eye which was evident when viewed from above. There was no obvious orbital erythema. Her pupils were equal and reactive to light, there was no relative afferent pupillary defect.

An urgent referral was made to paediatric ophthalmology. A nonaxial proptosis and limitation of ocular motility was identified. Formal visual acuity assessment was not possible but the child could fixate and follow small toys when the left eye was occluded. Fundoscopy was difficult and inconclusive.

Initial investigations including urea and electrolytes were undertaken and showed:

sodium	148	(135–146 mmol/l)
potassium	4.9	(3.5–5.3 mmol/l)
urea	5.5	(2.5–6.5 mmol/l)
creatinine	85	(13–39 µmol/l)
glucose	5.2	(3.0–6.0 mmol/l)

Serum osmolality was 295 mOsmol/kg and urine osmolality 130 mOsmol/kg. These findings indicate diabetes insipidus. An urgent MRI scan was obtained and demonstrated a mass in the pituitary fossa extending into the orbit and multiple lytic lesions in the skull.

These findings suggested a diagnosis of Langerhans cell histiocytosis, and biopsy of the orbital mass confirmed this. Further staging was undertaken and the child started on intensive systemic therapy. A full recovery was obtained. The absence of a relative afferent pupillary defect suggested a good visual prognosis, and full visual function was reestablished following a period of amblyopia therapy.

- syndromic—Noonan syndrome, Turner syndrome
- acquired
  - myotonic dystrophy
  - myasthenia gravis
  - Horner syndrome

Clinical presentation

The drooping of the upper eyelid is usually obvious. Bilateral ptosis will often result in the child adopting a chin-up head posture and recruiting the frontalis muscle to improve lid opening. This leads to the brows being arched and elevated. Amblyopia is more likely to occur with unilateral ptosis because the adaptive chin-up mechanism, seen in bilateral ptosis, does not occur. Interruption of the **sympathetic chain** will cause a 2–3 mm ptosis and smaller pupil in the affected eye and produce Horner syndrome, whilst interruption of the **parasympathetic fibres**, which travel alongside the third cranial nerve, will cause a dilated pupil, usually accompanied by evidence of third cranial nerve dysfunction (ptosis, ocular motility disturbance).

Treatment and management

Children with ptosis should be referred for specialist review to aid diagnosis and ensure amblyopia is adequately managed. Further management includes occlusion therapy for amblyogenic ptosis, with the aim to delay surgery until 4 years of age to improve the long-term cosmetic result.

Strabismus (squint)

Strabismus is a misalignment of the visual axes. Whilst acute onset strabismus will provoke a complaint of diplopia in older children, symptoms are less frequent in younger children who are able to suppress the vision in the squinting eye and who then rapidly develop amblyopia. It is important to ascertain that the eye movements are full and that the eyes track together in all nine positions of gaze (by moving an interesting toy in a large H pattern centred at the midline). Pseudo-squint is common in infants and describes the appearance of eye misalignment due to epicanthic folds or broad nasal bridge (Figure 28.1).

- esotropia—eye turns inwards
- exotropia—eye turns outwards
- hypertropia—eye turns upwards
- hypotropia—eye turns downwards

Causes of strabismus.

- **concomitant**—the ocular misalignment is similar in all positions of gaze. It is the result of refractive or accommodative problems or reduced vision in one or both eyes as in cataract or retinoblastoma (Figure 28.2).
- **incomitant**—the ocular misalignment changes markedly depending on the position of gaze and can be the result of cranial neuropathy, orbital cellulitis, myositis or myasthenia gravis (Figures 28.3 and 28.4).

Acute onset squint presents with diplopia, but younger children may not develop any symptoms. The corneal light reflections will be asymmetrical and the cover test will identify the movement of the squinting eye to take up visual fixation when the other is occluded. All children presenting with strabismus should have red reflex assessment and fundoscopy, if possible, to exclude a sensory cause or papilloedema when raised ICP can cause bilateral sixth nerve palsies.

Treatment and management

Children with intermittent or constant concomitant strabismus and normal red reflex assessment should be referred routinely to eye clinic for refraction and possible amblyopia therapy. Children with an abnormal red reflex or with a recent onset of incomitant strabismus need urgent referral and investigation.

Nystagmus

Nystagmus can be physiological, as at the extreme periphery of gaze, but can also be an important sign of ocular, neurological or vestibular abnormalities.

Causes of nystagmus.

* sensory—due to poor vision such as aniridia and albinism

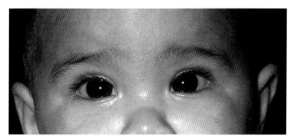

Fig 28.1 Pseudo squint. Appearance of eye misalignment due to broad nasal bridge but the symmetry of the corneal light reflections in each eye with respect to the anatomical landmarks of the pupil and corneal limbus indicates the eyes are aligned. (Copyright - Ms Louise Allen - used with permission)

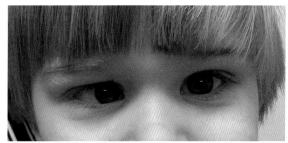

Fig 28.2 Right esotropia in a child with full eye movements: a concomitant squint. (Copyright - Ms Louise Allen - used with permission)

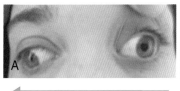 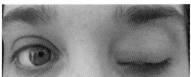 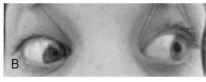

Fig 28.3 Left complete 3rd nerve palsy (arrows indicate the direction of gaze). Manual elevation of the ptotic left upper lid would show the left eye to be rotated 'down and out' due to the unopposed action of the lateral rectus (6th nerve) and superior oblique muscles (4th nerve). Involvement of adjacent parasympathetic neurons causes a dilated pupil. Examination of eye movements show limited adduction (a) but full abduction (b). Elevation and depression of the left eye would also be limited. (Used with permission. Adapted. Sayadi J et al. J Fran Ophth. 2019: 42;9. Elsevier Masson SAS)

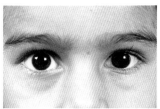 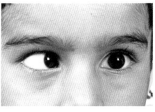

Fig 28.4 Left 6th nerve palsy (arrow indicates the direction of gaze). The eyes appear aligned in central gaze, but an esotropia develops in left gaze due to limited abduction of the left eye. (Image used with permission and adapted from Taylor and Hoyt's Pediatric Ophthalmology and Strabismus. Ed. Lyons CJ and Lambert SR. 5th edition. Chapter 83. Kekunnaya R and Sachdeva V. Elsevier Ltd.)

- idiopathic motor—most common form found with normal ocular and neurological function
- acquired—secondary to neurological disease or vestibular dysfunction

Specific ophthalmic disorders

Optic nerve head swelling

The optic nerve head can appear swollen on ophthalmoscopy for many reasons. The term papilloedema is reserved for swelling secondary to raised intracranial pressure (ICP).

Causes of optic nerve head swelling

- inflammation—multiple sclerosis; neuromyelitis optica
- compression—optic nerve glioma; neurofibroma
- infiltration—leukaemia; granulomatous disease
- infection—bartonella or borrelia infection; toxoplasmosis
- papilloedema—intracranial tumour; idiopathic intracranial hypertension (Figure 28.5)
- malignant hypertension
- pseudo-papilloedema—congenital anomalous optic nerve head; optic disc drusen

Optic disc swelling due to optic neuropathy will present as rapid visual loss in one or both eyes, often with associated systemic signs suggesting the cause. A relative afferent pupillary defect will be present if the neuropathy is unilateral or asymmetrical.

Optic disc swelling due to raised ICP does not initially cause reduced visual acuity, but if left untreated, cumulative neural cell death will lead to permanently reduced visual acuity, constricted visual fields and optic atrophy.

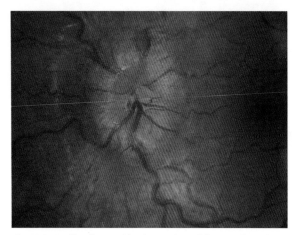

Fig 28.5 Papilloedema with obscuration of the vessels at the disc rim.

Symptoms of raised intracranial pressure include:
- headache worse in the morning or on lying down or bending over
- nausea and vomiting
- pulsatile "whooshing" tinnitus
- visual obscurations particularly on bending over or coughing
- diplopia or esotropia secondary to bilateral 6th nerve palsies
- localising neurological signs

Treatment and management

Early referral should be made to determine the nature of the disc swelling, test optic nerve function and perform optic nerve head imaging and ultrasonography to detect the presence of disc drusen. Blood pressure should be assessed. Other investigations including neuroimaging, and autoantibody screen (for multiple sclerosis or infection) should be tailored to the circumstances.

Cataract

Cataract prevalence is 4/10,000 children but is twice as common in resource-poor countries, where it is the most frequent cause of childhood blindness.

Causes of childhood cataract

- syndromic—Down syndrome, Alport syndrome
- disorders of eye development—aniridia, persistent foetal vasculature
- metabolic—diabetes, galactosaemia
- infective—congenital rubella, measles
- inflammatory—secondary to JIA-related uveitis
- iatrogenic—radiotherapy, steroid therapy, intraocular surgery
- traumatic, penetrating or blunt injury

Cataracts may be congenital (Figure 28.6) or develop subsequently, but the earlier the onset of the cataract, the more significant the effect on visual development. Approximately 50% of early onset cataracts are detected at newborn and infant physical examination (NIPE) red reflex screening, but if missed, sensory nystagmus and strabismus will develop. Older children may not complain of reduced vision if a developing cataract is unilateral or asymmetrical in severity, and the problem may only be detected on the 4- to 5-year-old screening or routine optometric assessment.

Treatment and management

A systemic cause or syndrome should be sought for all children with bilateral cataract, whatever the age of presentation. Full paediatric and ophthalmic examination would include

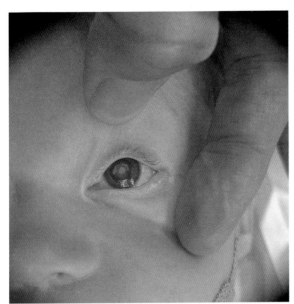

Fig 28.6 Cataract of left lens in a newborn baby. (Copyright - Ms Louise Allen - used with permission)

- congenital infection screen to exclude congenital cataract
- karyotype, microarray and cataract gene panel

All children newly diagnosed with cataracts require urgent referral, but infants must have a specialist opinion without delay due to the narrow surgical time window. Those with bilateral, visually significant, congenital cataracts require urgent surgery, with the best visual outcome being contingent on surgery by 8 weeks of age. Mydriatics or occlusion therapy are warranted if the cataracts are mild or asymmetrical. Following surgery, infants under one require contact lenses or thick glasses to correct their aphakia (absence of a lens) until an artificial lens is implanted as a secondary procedure at a year of age. Early onset unilateral cataract results in severe amblyopia in the affected eye and has a poor visual prognosis, even after surgical correction.

Glaucoma

Aqueous fluid fills the anterior segment and is constantly produced by the ciliary body and drained through the angle located at the root of the iris. Abnormal resistance to aqueous outflow results in increased intraocular pressure and pressure injury to optic nerve axons. This cumulative axonal cell death results in optic disc cupping and peripheral visual field loss.

Causes of childhood glaucoma

- syndromic—Alport syndrome; Sturge-Weber syndrome
- disorders of eye development—aniridia
- inflammatory—secondary to JIA related uveitis
- iatrogenic—steroid therapy; previous intraocular surgery
- traumatic—following penetrating or blunt injury

In infantile glaucoma, the infant sclera can be stretched and the increased intraocular pressure will result in globe enlargement known as buphthalmos. The cornea is less elastic than the sclera and, as it enlarges beyond its normal 11mm diameter, it develops cracks within its structure causing corneal oedema (cloudiness). Corneal oedema is painful and the infant will become light sensitive with conjunctival reddening and epiphora (watering). In children, after the age of 3 years, eye enlargement does not occur due to glaucoma and the child is asymptomatic.

Treatment and management

Regular eye pressure and eye growth measurements are required for children with glaucoma and the following medications may be used in combination to treat the condition:

- topical prostaglandin analogues—bimatoprost
- topical B-blockers—timolol
- topical cholinergic agents—pilocarpine

Surgery is often needed to improve or divert aqueous outflow and reduce intraocular pressure whilst laser ablation of the ciliary body may be used to decrease aqueous production.

Optic nerve hypoplasia (ONH)

This is a nonprogressive, congenital underdevelopment of one or both optic nerves. It is bilateral in the majority of children and accounts for approximately 20% of severe visual impairment in resource-rich countries.

Up to 80% of infants with this condition will have associated pituitary or hypothalamic dysfunction or midline defects, and these may become apparent before concerns are raised about visual function. Sporadic ONH may only be diagnosed during ophthalmoscopy of an infant with poor visual behaviour, nystagmus or strabismus.

Investigations

Infants with endocrine abnormalities should have ophthalmoscopy by a paediatric ophthalmologist whilst those who present at a later stage with ONH should be investigated with neuroimaging and an endocrine work-up.

IMPORTANT CLINICAL POINTS

Vision in childhood

- visual neuroplasticity—most malleable in the first 3 months of life
- visual function reaches adult levels by 4–5 years of age

Proptosis

- causes congenital, inflammatory, neoplastic, traumatic

Ptosis

- acquired conditions include myotonic dystrophy, myasthenia gravis, Horner syndrome

strabismus

- intermittent or constant concomitant strabismus—refer routinely to eye clinic
- recent onset of incomitant strabismus—urgent referral and investigation

Nystagmus

- sensory—poor vision such as aniridia and albinism
- idiopathic motor—with normal ocular and neurological function
- acquired—secondary to neurological disease or vestibular dysfunction

Cataract

- systemic cause or syndrome sought if bilateral cataract
- bilateral congenital cataracts require urgent surgery by 8 weeks of age

Glaucoma

- in infant, the increased ocular pressure results in globe enlargement (buphthalmos)

Further Reading

American Academy of Pediatrics. Eye examination and vision screening in Infants, Children and Young Adults. *Pediatrics*. 1996; 98(1):153–7. https://pediatrics.aappublications.org/content/pediatrics/98/1/153.full.pdf. Accessed: February 2021.

American Academy of Pediatrics. Red reflex examination in infants. *Pediatrics*. 2002; 109: 980. https://pediatrics.aappublications.org/content/pediatrics/109/5/980.full.pdf.

Chapter | 29 |

Musculoskeletal disorders

Flora McErlane, Roshan Adappa

After reading this chapter you should be able to assess, diagnose and manage:
- acute and chronic musculoskeletal disease
- musculoskeletal inflammatory diseases
- common vasculitic disorders
- common inherited bone disorders
- developmental bone disorders—scoliosis, hip dysplasia, Perthes disease

Musculoskeletal **symptoms**, particularly pain, are common in children and usually relate to injury, overuse, rapid growth, biomechanical or postural abnormalities. Musculoskeletal **disorders** are less common and they are usually rheumatological or orthopaedic in origin.

Acute and chronic arthritis

Arthritis is the inflammation of joints and usually presents with pain, swelling, erythema and a reduction in the movement of the affected joints. Children who present acutely need prompt diagnosis and management, especially if an infective cause is suspected.

Causes and associations of arthritis include:
- infection
  - bacterial—*Staphylococcus aureus, Group A beta-haemolytic streptococcus, Streptococcus pneumoniae,* rarely TB
  - viral—mumps, rubella, parvovirus, adenovirus, coxsackie B
  - other organisms—mycoplasma, *Borrelia burgdorferi,* rickettsia
- juvenile idiopathic arthritis
- connective tissue disorders—SLE, dermatomyositis, polyarteritis nodosa (PAN)
- vasculitides—Henoch-Schönlein purpura, Kawasaki disease
- inflammatory bowel disease
- haematological—haemophilia, sickle cell disease, leukaemia

Septic arthritis

Septic arthritis is a significant infection of the joints especially in children under 2 years of age. It usually involves a single joint and the infection is commonly acquired via haematological spread rather than local injury. The most common bacterial organism is *Staphylococcus aureus,* followed by Streptococcus.

Localised symptoms such as pain, restricted movement, swelling and redness are common presenting features and children are usually systemically unwell with pyrexia and elevated inflammatory markers. In young infants, there may be pain on moving the limb and therefore the limb is kept in a neutral position when at rest. Infants with hip involvement hold their legs flexed, externally rotated and abducted whilst older children may limp while walking or even refuse to weight bear due to pain.

Suspected septic arthritis requires an urgent orthopaedic opinion as joint aspiration can provide key information informing diagnosis and choice of antimicrobial therapy.

Investigations

- full blood count—elevated white cell and platelet counts
- ESR and CRP—usually raised
- blood culture—to identify organism and ensure appropriate antibiotic treatment
- joint aspiration—for culture
- joint USS—to identify any effusion
- x-ray—initially normal but established disease results in increased joint space and soft tissue swelling

335

Management and treatment

Antibiotic treatment must be commenced promptly following blood cultures and joint aspiration. It is reasonable to start flucloxacillin and cefotaxime in children below 2 years and flucloxacillin and ampicillin in older children. Antibiotic regimes, however, should be discussed with local microbiologists and schedules tailored in response to the results of cultures and sensitivities. The duration of antibiotics is usually between 4 and 6 weeks.

Reactive arthritis

Reactive arthritis a term used to describe joint pain and swelling triggered by an infection in another part of the body. It usually presents within 6 weeks of the initial infection and often involves the knee or ankle joints. Reactive arthritis commonly follows infection such as salmonella, shigella or campylobacter gut infections. Sexually transmitted infections such as chlamydia must be considered in the differential diagnosis.

Reactive arthritis can be associated with an acute anterior uveitis or urinary tract inflammation. Although any individual can present with an episode of reactive arthritis, it occurs more commonly in individuals who are HLA B27 positive.

Common presenting features will include transient joint swelling, pain and restriction of movement. The joints of the lower limbs, particularly the hip, are often involved although the interphalangeal joints can also be affected.

Treatment and management

Acute inflammation is usually treated with nonsteroidal antiinflammatory drugs such as ibuprofen, naproxen or diclofenac. Rarely, reactive arthritis can become chronic and children may require intraarticular corticosteroid injection or systemic immunosuppressive medication such as methotrexate.

Juvenile idiopathic arthritis (JIA)

JIA is an umbrella term for a heterogeneous group of chronic inflammatory arthritides with onset before the age of 16 years and lasting for at least 6 weeks. The cause of the condition is unknown although a combination of genetic and environmental factors is likely. It is a diagnosis of exclusion but is the most common cause of chronic joint disease in children. Children and young people where this diagnosis is suspected should be referred to paediatric rheumatology services for review and confirmation.

JIA includes seven disease subtypes with each having markedly different characteristics. There is also clinical

Table 29.1 Current accepted classification of juvenile idiopathic arthritis International League of Associations for Rheumatology (2001)

JIA subtype	Joints involved
oligoarticular JIA	1–4
systemic onset JIA	1 or more
polyarticular (RF-negative) JIA	5 or more
polyarticular (RF-positive) JIA	5 or more
psoriatic JIA	multiple
enthesitis*-related JIA	multiple
undifferentiated JIA	multiple

*Point of muscle tendon insertion.

heterogeneity within each of the JIA subtypes that reflects a probable variability in disease pathogenesis. Girls are more commonly affected than boys and there are two peak ages of onset at 1–3 years and 8–9 years (Table 29.1).

Investigations

- full blood count—normochromic, normocytic anaemia with occasional haemolysis Platelets and white cells are usually elevated, although thrombocytopaenia may occur
- blood film at diagnosis—to rule out malignancies
- ESR and CRP—usually raised at presentation and suggest a more severe disease course
- antinuclear antibodies (ANA)—seen in oligoarthritis and are risk factor for uveitis
- Rheumatoid factor (RF) and anti-CCP antibodies (anticyclic citrullinated peptide) are both autoantibodies found in JIA
- HLA B27 positivity—common in enthesitis-related and psoriatic arthritis

Treatment and management

Children with JIA should be managed by a paediatric rheumatology multidisciplinary team with the aim of achieving complete disease control.

Adequate control of pain is crucial to the initial management plan and NSAIDs are usually prescribed. Corticosteroids will modify the disease process and contribute to the analgesic effect but with recognised side effects. Consequently, other disease-modifying medications are used to reduce exposure to corticosteroids. They are commenced soon after diagnosis in children with polyarthritis and later in the disease course in those with oligoarthritis that is unresponsive to joint injections. Methotrexate would usually be the first-choice disease-modifying medication and is usually administered subcutaneously in children. There are a wider range of newer biologic medications that can be used in children whose disease does not respond completely to methotrexate.

Oligoarticular JIA

Oligoarthritis is the most common subtype of JIA, and although it can present at any age, it is most commonly seen in girls in the 1- to 3-year age group. Less than four joints are involved, but these may not be painful and so presentation may be late in the disease course. Parents often notice swelling and limping rather than the child complaining of pain. Uveitis is common, particularly in preschool girls with a positive ANA and is usually asymptomatic, so early and regular slit lamp examinations are essential.

Treatment and management

Synovitis is initially managed with NSAIDs and intraarticular corticosteroid injections. If children require frequent injections or develop features suggestive of joint damage, then they will need systemic immunosuppression with drugs such as methotrexate.

Systemic onset JIA

Systemic onset JIA is a rare autoinflammatory disease. Children are often unwell at presentation and may need extensive investigations to exclude sepsis or malignancy. The condition is characterised by:

- recurrent daily fevers that spike in the morning and early evening
- salmon-pink urticarial rash
- polyarthritis affecting the knees, wrists and ankles is very common
- lymphadenopathy, splenomegaly and hepatomegaly Uveitis is rarely associated with systemic onset JIA.

Polyarticular JIA

Polyarthritis affecting more than four joints is uncommon, and the majority of children have a negative rheumatoid factor test. Presentation can occur at any age and joint involvement may involve the cervical spine, temporomandibular and hands (Figure 29.1). Axial, large joint involvement is more common in children who are HLA B27 positive. IgM rheumatoid factor positive disease is rare and usually occurs in adolescent girls who present with a symmetrical, small joint polyarthritis that behaves in a similar way to rheumatoid arthritis.

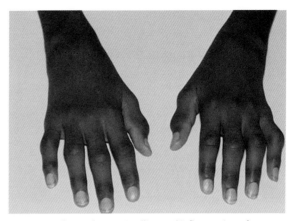

Fig. 29.1 Polyarticular JIA. Swelling and inflammation of the small joints of the hands. (Image use with permission and adapted from Zitelli and Davis' Atlas of Pediatric Physical Diagnosis, Zitelli BJ et al. Ed Zitelli BJ et al 7th. Edition. Chapter 7. Authors Torok K, Cassidy E, Rosenkratz M. Elsevier Inc.)

Psoriatic JIA

Individuals with this subtype will have psoriasis and usually dactylitis and pitting of the nails.

Enthesitis-related JIA

Enthesitis-related JIA describes an arthritis with associated enthesitis (points of tendon insertion) and often involves the sacroiliac joint. These individuals are usually HLA B27 positive and may develop acute anterior uveitis.

Relevant pharmacological agents used

Methotrexate. Blocks the conversion of dihydrofolate to the tetrahydrofolate that is needed in DNA duplication and may be given orally or subcutaneously. The most common side effect is nausea although this is reported less frequently if methotrexate is given subcutaneously. Neutropenia, thrombocytopenia and abnormal liver function tests are all recognised consequences of methotrexate and should be monitored routinely or clinically indicated.

Vasculitic disorders

Juvenile systemic lupus erythematosus (jSLE)

SLE is a multisystem autoimmune disorder, and approximately 15% to 20% of all individuals with this diagnosis will present during childhood or adolescence. Children of any age can develop lupus, although it is very rare in those under the age of 5. Younger children presenting with phenotypic lupus often have an underlying immunological disorder.

jSLE may have a more aggressive disease course than SLE presenting during the adult years. The disease and its treatments can have a significant effect on the life of the child and their family.

The clinical presentation of jSLE is heterogeneous and ranges from a mild disease, characterised by skin rashes, joint pains and fatigue, to life-threatening, multisystem inflammation. The differential diagnosis is wide, including infection, malignancy and other auto-inflammatory or vasculitic conditions. Diagnosis and long-term management should be led by a paediatric rheumatology team.

Common presenting features include:

- nonspecific symptoms—fever, lethargy, headaches, lymphadenopathy, hepatosplenomegaly
- skin—lupus malar rash ('butterfly rash'), discoid facial rash. Skin rashes are often photosensitive
- arthralgia—joint and muscle pain and early morning stiffness. A nonerosive symmetrical polyarthritis may occur
- nephritis—common presenting feature in paediatric-onset disease

Investigations

- full blood count—normochromic, normocytic anaemia with occasional haemolysis. Platelets and white cells are usually elevated, although thrombocytopaenia may occur
- acute phase reactants—usually raised at presentation
- antinuclear antibody (ANA)—directed against the nuclear contents, and children are almost always ANA positive. However, a positive ANA can be found in up to 15% of normal children and can occur as a consequence of viral infection, malignancy or IgA deficiency
- anti-double-stranded DNA are highly specific for jSLE and are seen in the majority of children with lupus nephritis. Titres can correlate with disease activity in some children
- other extractable nuclear antigens (anti RNP, anti-Sm, anti-Ro and anti-La) occur with variable frequencies in children with jSLE and related connective tissue disorders
- antiphospholipid antibodies are autoantibodies which bind to phospholipids in the cell membrane. These antibodies may occur in primary antiphospholipid syndrome, SLE and some vasculitides
- serum immunoglobulins and C4 complement factor reflect the acute phase reactants and can be markedly elevated in children with very active inflammatory disease. Low C3 or C4 complement factors can suggest active jSLE

Treatment and management

The majority of children with jSLE require steroids at the time of diagnosis or for episodes of disease flare. Children with mild disease can be treated with hydroxychloroquine or methotrexate whilst those who are more unwell at the time of presentation may require cyclophosphamide. Modern biologic medications, such as rituximab, can be very effective.

Other systemic rheumatic diseases

A wide range of multisystem autoimmune conditions can affect the musculoskeletal system in children. Examples include drug-induced lupus, undifferentiated connective tissue disease, Sjogren's syndrome, juvenile dermatomyositis, scleroderma and systemic sclerosis (further details can be found in Chapter 23 Dermatology).

Chronic rheumatic diseases of childhood are rare and the diagnosis can be complex. Many of the conditions do not have confirmatory diagnostic tests or simple, reliable measures of disease activity. They require a high index of suspicion following a full history and examination and will invariably require early referral to specialist teams.

Rheumatic fever

Rheumatic fever is a vasculitic reaction to Group A beta haemolytic *Streptococcus pyogenes* infection. Arthritis is the most common presentation and typically the pain is polyarticular, migratory, nondeforming and affecting primarily large joints. The vasculitis also affects other organs including heart, skin and brain.

The diagnosis of rheumatic fever is made by meeting the clinical features listed in the Modified Jones criteria. Further details of the presentation, diagnosis and management are presented in Chapter 16 Cardiology.

Henoch-Schonlein purpura (HSP)

HSP is the most common vasculitic disorder affecting children and mainly involves the skin, kidneys, joints and bowel. It may be triggered by an upper respiratory tract infection. Joint involvement usually presents with swelling and arthralgia involving the ankles or the knees. Further details are presented in Chapter 20 Nephro-urology and Chapter 23 Dermatology.

Treatment and management

Management is mainly symptomatic as the disease is usually self-limiting, frequently resolving within 4 to 6 weeks. If synovitis is severe or persistent, a short course of corticosteroids may be indicated.

Common inherited bone disorders

Osteogenesis imperfecta (OI)

The term describes a group of inherited conditions that are the result of defective collagen production leading to an increased bone fragility and connective tissue abnormalities in other systems. There are over 15 phenotypes and the most common ones are inherited in an autosomal dominant pattern whilst the less common ones are autosomal recessive. There is a wide range of clinical presentations ranging from mild (Type I) through to severe (Type II). The remaining types produce clinical types that are between these two forms.

Clinical presentation

Type I—the classical presentation of this group is with the triad of bone fractures, blue sclera and hearing loss. The fractures are usually to long bones and develop following minimal or insignificant trauma. Infants and young children who initially present with fractures may have a nonaccidental cause in the differential but a positive family history of OI may make this less likely. The defective collagen can also impact on other structures such as the eye where thinning of the sclera reveals the pigmented choroid beneath and so produces the blue appearance to the eye. Hearing loss may be sensorineural, conductive or a mixture and develops from the second decade of life whilst the inability to produce dentine leads to dentinogenesis imperfecta. Other recognised features of Type I disease are thin skin, easy bruising and joint laxity.

    Type II—invariably presents at birth with abnormal limb length or positioning due to in utero or perinatal fractures (Figure 29.2). Infants usually die within the first year due to cardiorespiratory compromise.

    Type III—a severe progressive and deforming phenotype leading to significant physical disability. Although appearing normal at birth, the fractures develop over time and heal with obvious deformity.

Investigation

X-rays will outline obvious fractures and healing callus. Gene analysis is now able to identify the specific mutations found in most of the phenotypes and therefore allow screening of family members.

Treatment and management

There is no cure for osteogenesis imperfecta and therefore management is aimed at anticipating potential complications and minimising their impact where possible. Families can be guided to minimise the risks of potential

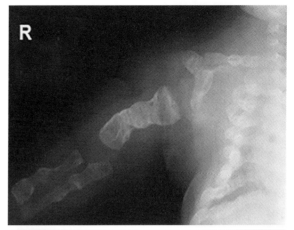
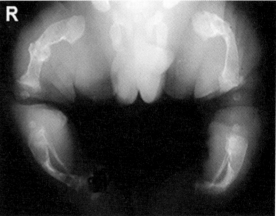

Fig. 29.2 Osteogenesis imperfecta Type II. X-ray images of newborn child showing fracture deformities and healing callus. Bones shortened and abnormal in shape.

fractures where possible and physiotherapy input would help recovery from any fractures sustained. The parents should be referred to genetic services for advice on future pregnancies along with assessment and advice for the wider family if found necessary. Hearing assessment should start from around 10 years of age and then 3 yearly thereafter whilst dental assessment should start as soon as the first teeth appear.

Achondroplasia

This is an autosomal dominant skeletal dysplasia where there is disproportionate short stature with reduced limb and spinal growth. Children usually have characteristic facial features including macrocephaly, frontal bossing and nasal flattening. Reduced pulmonary function and sleep apnoea are recognised findings.

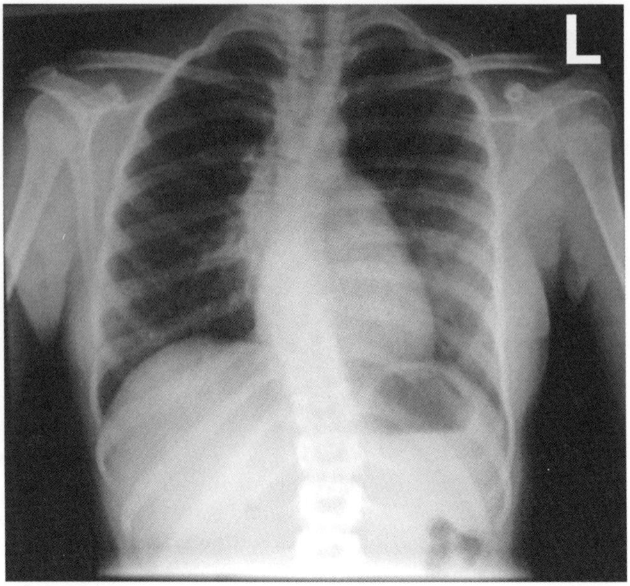

Fig. 29.3 X-ray of spine of 13-year-old girl showing significant scoliosis.

Marfan syndrome

Details of presentation and management are presented in Chapter 4 Growth and Puberty.

Developmental bone disorders

Scoliosis

Scoliosis describes the development of a lateral curvature and rotation of the spine (Figure 29.3). This rotation of the vertebral bodies causes a prominence of the spine, and an asymmetrical appearance to the back and consequently the scoliosis is more obvious when the child bends forward.

Causes include:

- idiopathic—the most common and has two age peaks of under 5 years and 10–14 years
- congenital—due to spine defects—spina bifida, hemi vertebra and VACTERL association
- secondary—to other conditions such as cerebral palsy

The condition is usually identified incidentally and individuals with a slight curvature may be asymptomatic. Those with a more significant curvature can develop some degree of a cardiorespiratory compromise.

Treatment and management

Mild scoliosis needs close monitoring and the abnormality will not progress in many of those affected. Almost all are referred to specialist spinal teams for observation and management until growth is complete. Significant scoliosis impacting on cardiorespiratory function may need braces or the surgical insertion of rods.

Developmental dysplasia of the hip (DDH)

DDH is a disorder of the hip which could be present at birth or become apparent over the first few months of life. Risk factors include breech presentation, female infant, a positive family history and oligohydramnios. Screening includes clinical examination after birth with Ortolani and Barlow tests, hip USS if risk factors are present and subsequent screening examinations of the hips by medical professionals at 6 weeks and at 6 months.

Infants with DDH will present with:

- unequal gluteal folds
- unequal limb lengths
- inability to fully abduct the hip
- Barlow's test—downward pressure through femur is exerted, and if the hip is dislocatable, then the head of femur is felt to move out of the acetabulum
- Ortolani's test—if the hip cannot be dislocated, then an attempt is made to relocate the head of femur back into the acetabulum and this forced movement can be felt

Investigations

USS of hip joint is the most appropriate and reliable investigation in the first 6 months but after this time it is difficult to interpret and x-rays of the pelvis may be needed (Figure 29.4).

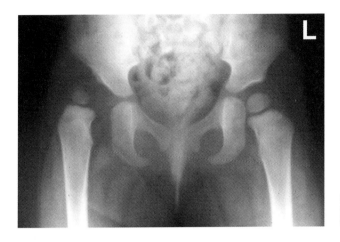

Fig. 29.4 X-ray of 8-month-old child with late presentation of DDH showing displaced head of right femur and acetabular deformity.

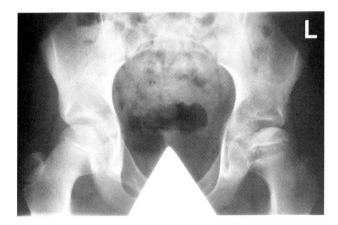

Fig. 29.5 X-ray of 10-year-old male with Perthes disease of the left hip showing distorted femoral head.

Treatment and management

In the newborn with dislocatable or dislocated hip, stabilisation of the hip is attempted using double nappies or using the Pavlick harness. Regular assessments and evaluation are necessary to ensure that the hip is stabilised and maintained in position that allows the acetabulum to develop. In older children, specialist orthopaedic intervention may be needed using traction or surgery. Avascular necrosis of the head of femur is the most significant complication that can occur.

Perthes disease

Perthes disease is a rare condition where the blood supply to the head of the femur is disrupted due to an unknown cause and consequently the head of femur becomes completely or partially misshapen. It usually affects children between the ages of 4 and 10 years and is most commonly seen in boys.

Children with Perthes disease present with:
- pain in the groin, hip, thighs or knees especially after exercise
- limping
- stiffness and restricted movements
- waxing and waning of symptoms

Investigation

An x-ray of the hip joint shows the misshapen head of femur (Figure 29.5) and regular x-rays may be needed to follow the progress.

Treatment and management

In most children, the symptoms subside on their own with supportive management, although regular physiotherapy along with crutches and casts may be needed

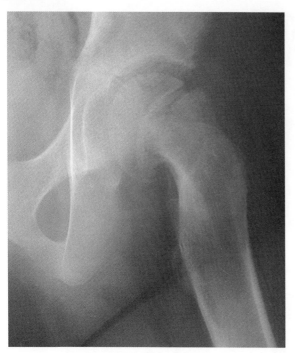

Fig. 29.6 X-ray of 11-year-old overweight boy with slipped femoral caput epiphysis. (Image use with permission Radiographic Essentials for Limited Practice. Ed. Ehrlich RA, Long BW, Frand ED. 6th edition. Chapter 18. Elsevier Inc.)

when the symptoms are severe. If the femoral head is significantly damaged, children may develop persistent joint pain and surgical intervention would be indicated.

Slipped femoral caput epiphysis

Slipped femoral caput epiphysis describes an abnormality of the hip that classically affects adolescents between the ages of 11 and 16 years. The femoral head is displaced from the neck of the femur and symptoms may be acute or chronic in their development. The patients are often obese and will present with groin or hip pain that may radiate to the thigh and knee. Examination reveals marked limitation in movement at the hip.

Investigation

An x-ray of the hip joint shows displacement of the head of femur (Figure 29.6) although this can be subtle and expert radiological opinion should be sought.

Treatment and management

If the diagnosis is confirmed then the patient needs admission, complete bed rest and an orthopaedic opinion. Surgical pinning of the slipped head is likely.

CLINICAL SCENARIO

A 3-year-old girl presented to outpatient clinic with a 3 month history of limping on exertion. The parents reported that the limping had started after a fall from a climbing frame in the local park. She was otherwise well with no significant past medical history. Development was completely normal and the family was not known to social services. Mum had type 1 diabetes and maternal grandmother had Crohn's disease.

The only abnormalities identified on examination were warm swollen knees and restricted movement of the right ankle.

The differential diagnosis would include infection (septic or reactive arthritis), malignancy (leukaemia) or autoimmunity (juvenile idiopathic arthritis).

Key investigations include FBC and film (normal), acute phase reactants (normal) and ANA (1:640).

In the presence of a well child with normal FBC and inflammatory markers, oligoarticular JIA is the most likely diagnosis. The child was referred urgently to paediatric ophthalmology as there is a high risk of chronic anterior uveitis which is potentially blinding. This was identified and she was started on topical steroid drops. She was also referred to paediatric rheumatology where she was treated with intraarticular corticosteroid injections initially. The inflammation did not settle with this treatment and she was started on systemic immunosuppression with methotrexate. The presence of uveitis supported the need for systemic treatment.

Important clinical points

Septic arthritis

- common organisms—*Staphylococcus aureus;* Streptococcus
- joint aspiration provides key information
- antibiotics—under 2 years flucloxacillin and cefotaxime
- over 2 years flucloxacillin and ampicillin

Oligoarticular JIA

- presentation may be late
- uveitis common

Systemic onset JIA

- exclude sepsis or malignancy
- uveitis rare

Polyarthritis

- majority are RF negative

Enthesitis-related JIA

- individuals usually HLA B27 positive
- may develop acute uveitis

jSLE

- joint and muscle pain and early morning stiffness
- nonerosive symmetrical polyarthritis may occur
- almost always ANA positive
- anti-double-stranded DNA are highly specific for jSLE

Perthes disease

- head of femur becomes misshapen

Further reading

Petty RE, Southwood TR, Manners P, et al. International League of Associations for Rheumatology classification of juvenile idiopathic arthritis: second revision, Edmonton, 2001. *J Rheumatol.* 2004; 31(2):390–2.

Chapter | 30 |

Metabolic medicine

Elisabeth Jameson

After reading this chapter you should:
- know the biochemical features of metabolic diseases
- be able to undertake and interpret relevant metabolic investigations
- understand the clinical presentation and prognosis of metabolic diseases
- know the screening procedures for inherited metabolic conditions

Metabolic medicine cares for those children who present with conditions resulting from absence or disruption of metabolic cellular processes. These processes are dependent upon the specific actions of enzymes and, if these are deficient or absent, then cell activity becomes dysfunctional. Conditions which are the result of defective enzymes are usually the result of single gene abnormalities and are known as 'Inborn Errors of Metabolism'.

In clinical terms, inborn errors of metabolism can present at any age with varying degrees of severity depending upon the degree of enzymatic dysfunction. In broad terms, the more enzymatic dysfunction present, the earlier and more severe the presentation. A total absence of enzymatic function may not be compatible with life. Children with metabolic disease often present acutely with poor feeding, altered conscious states or seizure activity or, on investigation, are found to have hypoglycaemia or a metabolic acidosis. However, there are a significant number where presentation is more insidious with growth failure, developmental delay, learning disability or dysmorphism.

The management of such children requires an understanding of the underlying abnormality and the effect of the defect on the body. It will be important for the clinician to know how to address any immediate problems along with management of short-term and long-term consequences of the illness. Most children will be under the care of specially trained paediatricians in tertiary centres or general paediatricians with further training in metabolic medicine who work closely with a tertiary team.

Biochemical features of metabolic diseases

Modes of presentation for metabolic disease:
- hypoglycaemia
- metabolic acidosis
- altered consciousness

Hypoglycaemia

Hypoglycaemia is a common finding in children and is seen in many clinical scenarios. It is seen in the immediate newborn period, particularly in infants who are preterm or growth restricted or who are infants of diabetic mothers and those who are seriously ill with sepsis. If significant hypoglycaemia occurs within the first 72 hours after birth or is recurrent in older infants and children, then investigations should be undertaken to identify an underlying metabolic condition.

Glucose homeostasis is vital in maintaining health. The body generates glucose by the process of gluconeogenesis whereby the body can generate glucose from nonglucose precursors. Glycolysis is the process of the conversion of glucose to pyruvate which enters the tricarboxylic acid cycle to produce ATP. When there is excess glucose available, glycogenesis converts glucose to glycogen for storage in the liver and muscles. At times of increased glucose demand, as in illness, fasting or exercise, the glycogen is converted to glucose by the process of glycogenolysis. If the demand for glucose cannot be met through glycogenolysis alone the body switches to fat metabolism with the subsequent production of free fatty acids and the ketone bodies beta-hydroxybutyrate and acetoacetate (Table 30.1).

Table 30.1 Definitions of terms relating to glucose metabolism

Term	Definition
Hypoglycaemia	a true blood glucose <2.6 mmol/l
Gluconeogenesis	synthesis of glucose from nonglucose precursors in liver, kidney and intestinal epithelium
Glycolysis	oxidation of glucose to pyruvate with generation of ATP
Glycogenesis	conversion of excess glucose to glycogen
Glycogenolysis	degradation of glycogen to glucose

Hypoglycaemia may produce pallor, sweating and irritability in babies and infants prior to being fed. In older children, who have a relatively long overnight fast, early morning lethargy or bad moods should lead to the assessment of a blood glucose. Any baby or child with a profound hypoglycaemia may present with seizures.

Investigations

When a metabolic cause is considered in the differential diagnosis a range of investigations to investigate the cause of the hypoglycaemia will be needed and are outlined below (Tables 30.2 and 30.3).

Treatment and management

Immediate management should aim to correct the hypoglycaemia by the administration of glucose or dextrose following APLS protocols. The route of administration will be dictated by the conscious level of the child, the age of the child and whether the child can tolerate oral administration. Underlying causes may become evident when results of investigations are available and will direct further management.

Metabolic acidosis

Acidosis is a common finding in the acutely unwell baby or child and it is important to determine if this has a metabolic or respiratory cause. Many such children will have a degree of circulatory failure due to sepsis and the diagnosis and management will follow the usual course, but it is important to investigate alternative causes of an acidosis if it is persistent and unresolved (Table 30.4).

Table 30.2 Investigations to be undertaken when patient is hypoglycaemic

Investigation	Rationale for investigation
Insulin	should reflect the expected normal pattern in response to hypoglycaemia—low with low blood glucose. High levels indicate pathological production
C-peptide	C-peptide connects the two insulin sections together in the pre-insulin molecule and is cleaved from each endogenous insulin molecule. Measured values should be the same as measured insulin values and, if significantly lower, indicates administration of exogenous insulin
Growth hormone	promotes gluconeogenesis in the liver so elevated levels can induce hypoglycaemia
Free fatty acids	produced in lipolysis and increases with prolonged hypoglycaemia
Ketone bodies	should be produced when child becomes hypoglycaemic as an alternative energy source for brain and other tissues. A non-ketotic hypoglycaemia requires more detailed investigation
Cortisol	has an effect on gluconeogenesis and aims to increase glucose

Table 30.3 Investigations that can be done when patient is normoglycaemic

Investigation	Rationale for investigation
Acylcarnitine	specific patterns seen in fatty acid oxidation disorders, e.g. raised C8:C10 ratio in MCADD
Ammonia	raised in hepatic encephalopathy which may lead to hypoglycaemia
Lactate	produced in excess when body unable to mobilise stored glycogen

Children with a metabolic acidosis can present with a combination of:
- vomiting
- poor feeding
- reduced conscious level
- tachypnoea (hyperventilation to reduce CO_2 levels)

Table 30.4 Plasma responses seen in primary changes of carbon dioxide and bicarbonate

Abnormality	Primary disturbance	Effect on		Base excess	Compensatory response
		pH	pCO2		
respiratory acidosis	↑ pCO2	↓	↑	negative	↑ [HCO3-]
metabolic acidosis	↓ [HCO3-]	↓	N or ↓	negative	↓pCO2
respiratory alkalosis	↓ pCO2	↑	N or ↓	positive	↓[HCO3-]
metabolic alkalosis	↑ [HCO3-]	↑	N or ↑	positive	↑pCO2

Table 30.5 Interpretation of the anion gap

Metabolic acidosis with raised anion gap (due to addition of 'acids' to plasma)	Metabolic acidosis with normal anion gap (due to loss of bicarbonate—renal or GI)
lactic acidosis	renal tubular acidosis
ingestion, e.g. ethanol, salicylate	Addison disease acetazolamide
renal failure	severe diarrhoea
acid-producing metabolic disorder	post-ureteric diversion into large bowel
diabetic ketoacidosis	

Table 30.6 Investigations required in assessment of abnormal anion gap

Investigation	Rationale for investigation
blood gas	identifies metabolic acidosis
ammonia	can be raised in organic acidaemia, hepatic encephalopathy and urea cycle disorders
lactate	raised in any acutely unwell child. In congenital lactic acidosis may improve but fails to entirely resolve
ketone bodies	present if child hypoglycaemic but level out of keeping with the degree of hypoglycaemia
acylcarnitine	abnormal in organic acidaemias and fatty acid oxidation disorders
plasma amino acids	indicative of mitochondrial disease, amino acidaemia and urea cycle disorders
urine organic acids	identifies organic acidaemias

Investigations

An initial calculation of the anion gap will indicate if there is an excess acid present and, if raised, the acid must be identified. This may be obvious, for example in DKA where a ketoacidosis is present, but in metabolic disease specialist tests will be required (Table 30.5).

> **PRACTICE POINT**
>
> anion gap = [Na+] + [K+] – [HCO$_3^-$] + [Cl-]
>   Normal value = less than 10–14
> - although there may be some small variations in this range between laboratories

Further investigations will be needed to clarify the underlying metabolic cause identified at presentation. The tests would include (Table 30.6):

Treatment and management

Children who are unwell at presentation will require standard APLS resuscitation. If a metabolic cause is considered, then the child should be placed nil by mouth and intravenous dextrose commenced. Dextrose stops catabolism by relieving stress on metabolic pathways and so stopping metabolic decompensation. In severe acidosis there may be a need for sodium bicarbonate although administration of this needs to be undertaken after consultation and with caution.

Metabolic diseases

Idiopathic ketotic hypoglycaemia

Idiopathic ketotic hypoglycaemia is the commonest cause of hypoglycaemia in children. It is a recognised condition with uncertain aetiology although inadequate carbohydrate intake or excessive level of exercise may contribute to the problem. It is, however, a diagnosis of exclusion and an underlying metabolic or endocrine cause must be sought in the first instance.

The condition typically presents between 1–3 years of age with an episode of hypoglycaemia either during an intercurrent illness with reduced oral intake or on waking after the long overnight fast. The crucial finding is the presence of ketones in the urine as the body turns to ketogenesis as an energy source. Children may have a single episode or recurrent episodes but, in the majority, the condition improves between the ages of 5–8 years.

Treatment and management

Carers of the children should be provided with an emergency regimen for use at times of illness. This consists of a glucose polymer drink they must take every 2 hours during the day and every 3 hours at night. The children must avoid long periods of fasting and some may require a long-acting carbohydrate to be taken before sleep.

Glycogen storage disease (GSD)

Glycogen storage disorders are a diverse group of conditions which are the result of dysfunctional or absent enzymes in the glucogenesis, glycolysis or gluconeogenesis pathways. They can be divided into two broad groups, those affecting the liver and those affecting the muscles. The result is an inability to metabolise, mobilise or store glucose which then impacts on blood glucose levels. Stored glycogen in organs and tissues, particularly liver, kidneys and small intestines, will accumulate over time and disrupt their normal function.

Glycogen storage disease type 1 (GSD type 1) is the most common GSD of the hepatic group and is an autosomal recessively inherited condition. The underlying abnormality is a deficiency of glucose-6-phosphatase which facilitates the conversion of glycogen to glucose.

A child with GSD type 1 will usually present before the age of 2 years with the consequences of recurrent and prolonged episodes of hypoglycaemia—seizures, growth retardation or developmental concerns. There are two recognised subtypes—GSD-1a and GSD-1b—and both will present in similar ways although children in the latter group also have chronic neutropenia and suffer with recurrent infections, typically of the skin. Examination of the child will identify a distended abdomen due to hepatomegaly caused by the increasing stores of glycogen. The hepatomegaly can be easily missed as the liver feels very soft.

Investigations

Classical laboratory findings are:
- episodic hypoglycaemia

- persistently raised lactate—anaerobic activities due to low supply of glucose
- raised ketones
- raised lipid levels
- neutropenia—in type 1b but can by cyclical

The raised lactate and ketones can produce a metabolic acidosis and consequently, the child may be hyperventilating when seen.

Treatment and management

The aim of treatment for children with GSD type 1 is to maintain normoglycaemia. This is achieved by the administration of frequent feeds during the day and often continuous gastric feeds overnight. This will allow the child to grow and prevent further accumulation of glycogen. At times of illness the child will have an emergency regime. Children with GSD type 1 may have normal growth and development if periods of profound hypoglycaemia can be avoided. Those with some of the other GSD variants may experience growth failure and developmental delay but only if not treated.

Galactosaemia

Lactose (milk disaccharide) is formed of glucose and galactose. Once cleaved the galactose is converted to UDP-galactose by the enzyme galactose-1-phosphate uridyl transferase (GALT) and then to glucose. It is the absence of this enzyme which leads to classical galactosaemia. There is therefore an accumulation of galactose which is converted to a toxic alcohol-based molecule.

Classical galactosaemia presents in the first week of life as milk feeds are introduced although it can present at a slightly later stage. It is associated with *Escherichia coli* sepsis and this may be the main presenting problem although the explanation for this association is unclear. The condition is inherited in an autosomal recessive manner and is known to be more common within certain populations—Irish travelling families being one such group.

The majority of babies present with:
- jaundice
- poor feeding
- oozing from venepuncture sites due to coagulopathy
- cataracts (in some children though most will develop them if left untreated)

Investigations

Initial investigations will show:
- conjugated hyperbilirubinaemia—liver failure
- abnormal coagulation studies—liver failure
- metabolic acidosis
- urinary reducing substances—galactose
- glycosuria, aminoaciduria and albuminuria

A more detailed assessment will show near complete absence of galactose-1-phosphate uridyl transferase (GALT) activity in red blood cells and the consequent elevated levels of galactose-1-phosphate in plasma and red blood cell.

Treatment and management

Immediate treatment must address the acute problems of liver failure, coagulopathy and sepsis but must also remove galactose-containing formula feeds from the diet. All children who have survived the acute metabolic decompensation must adhere to a lifelong diet with minimal galactose although many will have learning disabilities despite treatment. Any cataracts which have formed will usually resolve with treatment. The majority of females with galactosaemia will be infertile due to ovarian dysgenesis and must be referred to a paediatric endocrinologist at around 10 years of age.

Medium chain acyl-CoA dehydrogenase deficiency (MCADD)

This is the result of a deficiency in the enzyme medium chain acyl-CoA dehydrogenase, which is responsible for the breakdown of stored medium chain fats to create the energy source Acyl-CoA. This leads to affected individuals being unable to meet an increase in energy demands after glycogen stores are depleted. The consequence is the characteristic findings of hypoglycaemia with very low or absent ketones.

Most infants are identified through the UK neonatal screening programme and consequently acute presentations are now uncommon. They may, however, present before they have undergone screening due to a failure to establish breast feeding and classically are nonspecifically unwell with hypoglycaemia and possible seizures. There is the possibility of coma or sudden death if profound hypoglycaemia develops.

Investigations

Investigations will reveal a hypoglycaemia without the expected elevation of ketones (non-ketotic hypoglycaemia).

Treatment and management

Avoidance of long periods of fasting, particularly overnight or during intercurrent illness, is important. As the child grows, they will be able to tolerate a longer fast, but the maximum time allowed should be 12 hours. Families must be given a written emergency regimen which can be shown to medical staff at times of illness. Children with MCADD who are identified on neonatal screening and treated appropriately can expect normal development and growth.

Mucopolysaccharidoses

This is a group of disorders that arise due to the absence or dysfunction of lysosomal enzymes. These enzymes break down molecules known as glycosaminoglycans (GAGs—previously known as mucopolysaccharides) which are found in cells forming bone, cartilage, tendons, connective tissue and corneas. Currently, seven different clinical types are recognised and each has a different presentation and prognosis. Most are recessively inherited although MPS type II is x-linked.

The clinical features are similar across the different types of the disease although they may differ in severity. The symptoms may not be evident in the first few months of life, but concerns about early developmental may lead to referral. Characteristic signs include:
- coarse facial features with corneal clouding (Figures 30.1 and 30.2)
- short trunk
- dysplastic bone development—spinal gibbus
- progressive joint stiffness
- shortened hands
- organomegaly
- developmental delay

Investigations

Glycosaminoglycans are raised in the urine and this can be used as a screening tool for high-risk families.

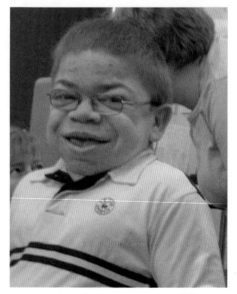

Fig. 30.1 Coarse facial features in a 16-year-old teenager with mucopolysaccharidosis (Image used with permission from Taylor and Hoyt's Pediatric Ophthalmology and Strabismus. Ed. Lyons CJ and Lambert SR. 5th edition. Chapter 65. Ashworth JL and Morris AM. Elsevier Ltd.)

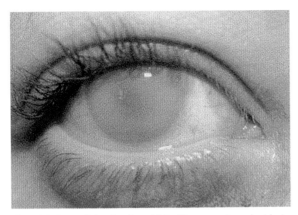

Fig. 30.2 Corneal clouding in a child with mucopolysaccharidosis (Hurlers) (Musculoskeletal Imaging. Ed. Wilson DJ et al. 2nd edition. Chapter 82. Dominguez R et al. Elsevier Inc. Originally from Ashworth JL, Biswas S, Wraith E, et al. Mucopolysaccharidoses and the eye. Surv Ophthalmol. 2006 Jan-Feb;51(1):1-17; with permission.)

Assessment of specific lysosomal enzymes will further clarify the specific enzyme defect followed by genetic testing. Antenatal tissue sampling (chorionic villus or amniocentesis) can allow determination of whether a subsequent foetus carries the specific genetic mutation.

Treatment and management

Most of the treatments which are currently available are aimed at managing the developing symptoms. Enzyme replacement therapy is available for some of the variants of mucopolysaccharidoses and each is specific to one disease type. Prescription and management of these treatments would be under the direction of a paediatrician in metabolic medicine. Some variants may benefit from haematopoietic stem cell transplantation. Long-term outlook is variable and ranges from early death from progressive organ failure to normal development and outlook. Some will have corneal clouding and bone dysplasias.

Urea cycle disorders

Ammonia is produced in the cells from the breakdown of amino acids. It is highly neurotoxic and the urea cycle converts ammonia to urea which is then excreted in the urine.

Neonates with urea cycle disorders classically present in the first 1–5 days of life with:

- vomiting and poor feeding
- irritability
- altered consciousness
- new onset seizures

Babies presenting in this way should have an ammonia level checked urgently as hyperammonaemia is a medical emergency due to its neurotoxic effects. Older children may present with encephalopathy during an episode of intercurrent infection. The neurotoxic effect of high ammonia stimulates respiration leading to a respiratory alkalosis.

Most of the variants of enzyme dysfunction in the urea cycle are recessively inherited but ornithine transaminase deficiency (OTC deficiency) is x-linked. Male infants with OTC deficiency often do not survive the neonatal period whereas index female patients may not present until later in life.

Investigations

Ammonia is a direct stimulant to the respiratory centre and so produces a respiratory alkalosis. Assay of plasma amino acids and urinary organic acids will reveal the presence of orotic acid and are the key to diagnosis. Blood samples taken for ammonia should be free flowing and not capillary samples as haemolysis will cause artefactual elevation of the result.

Treatment and management

Hyperammonaemia is a medical emergency, and where children present with encephalopathy, it is crucial that urgent management of the elevated levels of toxic ammonia is undertaken. Feeds should be stopped and intravenous fluids of 10% dextrose and electrolytes started. 'Scavenger' agents such as sodium benzoate and sodium phenylbutyrate are available and these bind with amino acids (glycine and glutamine) and facilitate excretion of nitrogen, the precursor to ammonia. Patients will usually require haemofiltration.

Longer term management will include a lifelong need for a low protein diet and the administration of ammonia scavengers. Families must be given a written emergency regimen which can be shown to medical staff at times of illness. The most significant complications for these children are seizures and marked learning disability which are both secondary to neurotoxic consequences of hyperammonaemia.

Phenylketonuria (PKU)

Phenylalanine is an essential amino acid and is metabolised by phenylalanine hydroxylase. A deficiency of this enzyme leads to accumulation of toxic levels of phenylalanine in cells which are excreted in the urine.

Untreated PKU is now rarely seen in the UK as it is detected by the newborn screening programme. The baby is normal at birth as the mother has been able to metabolise the phenylalanine that has crossed the placenta during the pregnancy. Babies who are not identified by screening usually present with:

- seizures
- delayed development
- "musty or mousy" odour

Table 30.7 Different features in classical homocystinuria and Marfan syndrome

	Classical homocystinuria	Marfan syndrome
inheritance	autosomal recessive	autosomal dominant
cause	cystathionine beta synthase deficiency	fibrillin defect
musculoskeletal	tall stature, arachnodactyly, high arched palate, kyphoscoliosis pectus excavatum, osteoporosis	tall stature, arachnodactyly, high arched palate, kyphoscoliosis, normal bone density
cardiovascular	aortic and mitral valve regurgitation, risk of venous thrombosis	aortic and mitral valve regurgitation, dilated aortic root with risk of dissection.
ophthalmology	myopia, down-and-out lens dislocation, retinal detachment	myopia, up-and-in lens dislocation, retinal detachment
intellect	learning disability	normal

Progressive signs will include microcephaly, intellectual impairment and behavioural problems.

Investigations

Plasma amino acids are measured to determine the phenylalanine level.

Treatment and management

Involves the introduction of a low protein diet with protein substitutes to ensure nutritional adequacy and regular phenylalanine level monitoring. Poor compliance with treatment results in persistently raised phenylalanine levels and will lead to profound learning difficulties. Females with poorly controlled PKU are at risk of having a baby with learning disability due to intrauterine exposure to elevated phenylalanine levels even if the baby does not have the enzyme deficiency.

Homocystinuria

Classical homocystinuria is due to a deficiency or absence of the enzyme cystathionine beta-synthase which is important in the metabolism of methionine. In the UK, elevated levels of homocysteine are detected by the newborn screening programme.

Those children who are not identified at an early age usually present to a multitude of specialities including:

- orthopaedics for skeletal abnormalities—long limbs, pes cavus, pectus excavatum
- ophthalmology with lens dislocation—(inferior ectopia lentis), glaucoma, cataracts
- community paediatrics for learning disability

Alternative diagnoses

Homocystinuria and Marfan syndrome have many features in common and both should be considered when

such features are identified. Differences are in bold (Table 30.7).

Investigations

Plasma amino acid screen will identify elevated levels of homocysteine.

Treatment and management

Children who are diagnosed with the condition will have a trial of pyridoxine as some will be responsive and they can be treated with high dose vitamin B_6. All children will need a low-protein diet with specialist protein substitutes to ensure adequate nutrition. If untreated, the children will have learning disabilities and seizures and are prone to early death due to thromboembolism events.

Organic acidaemias (acidurias)

These are a group of disorders due to defects within the metabolic pathway of the branch-chain amino acids—leucine, isoleucine and valine. The three most common diseases are methylmalonic acidaemia (MMA), propionic acidaemia (PA) and maple syrup urine disease (MSUD). In the case of MMA and PA, it is the consequent metabolic acidosis and secondary hyperammonaemia that cause illness, whilst in MSUD, it is the raised leucine level which causes an acute encephalopathy.

Methylmalonic acidaemia and propionic acidaemia

Children with MMA and PA typically present within the first week of life with vomiting, irritability, temperature instability and altered levels of consciousness. Routine investigations show a metabolic acidosis with a raised anion gap. The toxic metabolites circulating in the body can suppress the bone marrow leading to a pancytopenia and can affect the urea cycle leading to hyperammonaemia.

Maple syrup urine disease

As the disease name implies, these children produce a sweet-smelling urine. They usually present in the first few days of life with progressive encephalopathy and seizure activity and, if untreated, will progress to coma and death. The diagnosis should be considered in any neonate with encephalopathy who is not improving with standard treatments. It is a difficult diagnosis to make as there are no classical signs or symptoms and can only be made if plasma amino acids are measured. Patients are often diagnosed as having overwhelming sepsis without an offending organism being identified in any samples taken. Measurement of the branched chain amino acids is now a part of the newborn screening programme in the UK.

Treatment and management

The immediate management for these organic acidaemias requires the immediate cessation of feeds and the introduction of intravenous 10% dextrose. The majority of neonates will benefit from haemofiltration to remove ammonia in the case of MMA and PA or leucine in the case of MSUD. Subsequent management requires a strict, lifelong adherence to a low-protein diet and, and in the case of MSUD, a disease-specific protein substitute. Families must be provided with a written copy of their emergency regimen for use at times of illness.

The majority of babies with MSUD have a good neurological outcome despite extremely high levels of leucine at presentation. The long-term prognosis of MMA and PA is generally poor due to their associated complications of cardiomyopathy, long QTc, pancreatitis, optic atrophy and, in the case of MMA, renal failure.

Familial hypercholesterolaemia

Familial hypercholesterolaemia (FH) is due to a defect in the hepatic low-density lipoprotein (LDL) receptor which leads to reduced clearance of LDL from the peripheral circulation. There is also a loss of negative feedback in LDL metabolism which leads to an increased production of LDL. It is the most common inherited disorder in UK and is autosomal dominant in inheritance pattern.

Homozygous individuals can be identified by:
- xanthelasma around the eyes
- xanthoma on the elbows, knees and heels (over the Achilles tendons)

The lesions are pale, nodular and well demarcated. Children or young people who are heterozygote for the gene are usually identified following screening based on an affected close relative (cascade screening) and invariably have no clinical signs. Other secondary causes of hypercholesterolaemia

should be considered in a differential that would include hypothyroidism, Type 1 diabetes mellitus and cholestasis.

Investigations

Lipid profile should be undertaken to confirm the diagnosis, and thyroid function tests, blood glucose and liver function tests are necessary to exclude secondary causes of the abnormal lipid profile results. First degree relatives should be advised to undergo lipid profile screening.

Treatment and management

Current advice for those who are heterozygous is to follow a low-fat diet, to exercise and to consider statin therapy from 8–10 years of age. Those who are homozygous will start this treatment regime as soon as they are diagnosed and will also receive ezetimibe. This medication inhibits intestinal absorption of cholesterol and is used as an adjunct to statin treatment. Many patients with homozygous FH will need lipid apheresis and can be considered for liver transplantation. Patients who are started on statins may experience myalgia and liver dysfunction and therefore need monitoring of creatine kinase and liver function. Patients are at risk of circulatory occlusive disease.

Mitochondrial disease

Mitochondrial diseases are a varied group of conditions where the mitochondria are dysfunctional and fail to generate adequate cellular energy. This dysfunction is very variable and so every person with mitochondrial disease is affected differently, even within the same family.

The conditions are often multisystem in nature and present in many forms and with a huge spectrum of severity. The diagnosis should be considered when there is multisystem disease with no obvious explanation or links between involved systems. Organs most affected tend to be those with highest energy requirements—heart, kidneys, brain, retina and liver.

An example of a mitochondrial disorders would be Leigh syndrome (subacute sclerosing encephalopathy) which has multiple aetiologies. Typically, the child presents between the ages of 3 months to 2 years with:
- progressive neurological deterioration
- developmental regression
- seizures
- altered states of consciousness
- myopathy

Dementia and ultimately ventilatory failure develop as the disease progresses. Investigations show a raised lactate and characteristic MRI scan findings. The child with mitochondrial disease may stabilise and even show some recovery of lost skills but over time will continue to suffer recurrent relapses and ultimately the condition will prove fatal.

CLINICAL SCENARIO

A term female baby who born to Roma parents, presented with tachypnoea at 19 hours of age. She underwent an ABC assessment and was commenced on IV antibiotics as per standard care of the sick neonate. A blood gas revealed a severe lactic acidosis with her lactate level being 25 mmol/l (normal 1–2 mmol/l). This was consistent with a congenital lactic acidosis and supportive care was instituted with the use of sodium bicarbonate to relieve the tachypnoea by reducing the acidosis. Over the course of the next 48 hours, she remained very sick but then her lactate level started to fall. She remained well and was discharged home with a baseline lactate of 7 mmol/l.

Once stabilised, she had investigations for metabolic disease including skin and muscle biopsies for genetics analysis. Ultimately, she was found to have a mutation of the TMEM70 gene which codes for a protein located on the mitochondrial membrane and which is involved in the production of ATP synthase. The abnormality associated with a lactic acidosis, myopathy and hypertrophic cardiomyopathy and consequently she was referred to the cardiology services for further assessment. The cardiomyopathy was confirmed and a management plan was developed.

She has remained well and continues to make developmental progress though does attend a special needs school. She has had episodes of decompensated lactic acidosis associated with intercurrent illness but has made full recoveries each time.

Newborn blood screening programme

Many countries have established a routine screening programme that obtains a blood spot sample from the baby around day 5 of life. Samples are analysed for a range of conditions and any found to be positive or equivocal require a recall for the baby and referral for more detailed investigation.

PRACTICE POINT - UK Newborn Blood Screening Programme

- sickle cell disease (SCD)
- cystic fibrosis (CF)
- hypothyroidism (CHT)
- phenylketonuria (PKU)
- medium-chain acyl CoA dehydrogenase deficiency (MCADD)
- maple syrup urine disease (MSUD)
- isovaleric acidaemia (IVA)
- glutaric aciduria type 1 (GA1)
- homocystinuria (HCU)

IMPORTANT CLINICAL POINTS—metabolic disease

Presentation

- metabolic disease is likely if hepatomegaly
- metabolic disease is likely if ketones absent
- intercurrent illness may lead to metabolic decompensation
- anion gap should be calculated when metabolic acidosis is identified
- source of a raised anion gap must be determined

Specific

- glycogen storage disease—mainly autosomal recessive and hepatomegaly is usual

- galactosaemia—autosomal recessive and can only present once galactose-containing feeds have started
- MCADD—autosomal recessive. Patients must avoid of long periods of fasting
- urea cycle disorders—mostly autosomal recessive (OTC deficiency is x linked)
- markedly raised ammonia indicates a urea cycle disorder
- phenylketonuria—autosomal recessive and lifelong dietary manipulation needed
- homocystinuria—autosomal recessive and lifelong low protein diet needed
- organic acidaemias (acidurias)—autosomal recessive and present with encephalopathy in first few days

Further reading

Emergency Guidelines for Metabolic Conditions. *British Inherited Metabolic Disorders* Group. http://www.bimdg.org.uk/site/guidelines.asp

Chapter |31|

Palliative care

Richard Hain, Timothy Warlow

> After reading this chapter you should understand:
> - the ethics of palliative care in life-limiting conditions and in the withdrawal and withholding of care
> - the application of nonpharmacological and pharmacological interventions in children

Two important aspects of palliative care are ethical issues and symptom control.

Ethical considerations in palliative care involve:

- medical decisions on investigations or treatment that have good and bad consequences
- decision regarding withdrawal or withholding treatment that may prolong life but not offer cure

Symptom control is a key part of palliative care and symptoms are:

- never just a physical event but occurs in a psychosocial and existential context
- unique to the patient and their circumstance and hence needs a holistic approach

At the end of life, it becomes even more important than at other times to preserve the quality of an individual's experience of their life. The purpose of palliative care is not to delay death, but neither must it be to hasten it. The purpose of palliative care is to optimise a child's comfort as far as is possible.

It is vital to remember that the first role of medicine is to care. When health care has no other medical therapies to offer, the child and family should not be abandoned to their experience but rather, as a matter of compassion, continue to accompany them.

Ethics

The principle of double effect

If a treatment is given, knowing beforehand that it could improve the clinical condition or symptom control but an unintended consequence is morbidity or death, then as long as the prime intention was to improve the condition of the patient, the clinician is acting professionally even if the unintended consequence does occur. However, if the intention is to hasten death, then the same treatment would not be acceptable and would be unethical and illegal.

While there is clearly a difference between foreknowledge (knowing that a consequence might happen) and intention (making that consequence the prime aim), in practice it is questionable to rely on that difference in deciding whether an action is right or wrong. Nevertheless, a clinical decision will usually have multiple possible consequences, of which some are more likely than others and it cannot reasonably be denied that it is possible for a doctor to intend only one of them.

Fortunately, in practice the risk of an adverse outcome such as death from medications used in palliative care is remote, providing they are used properly, and it is rarely necessary to have to trade the duration of patient's life against its quality. Occasionally, however, that remote risk will happen and the clinical team may be faced with the knowledge that in intending the care and comfort of their patient, an intervention might have brought the child's death closer. The important point is that prescribing at the end of life recognises hastening death is a possibility but is not the same as acting with an intention to end life.

When making decisions that will affect medical care of a child, parents and doctors have the same moral duty to avoid, as far as possible, inflicting suffering on a child. If the result of a medical decision would be to cause a child suffering that could be avoided, then it is a wrong decision. Parents are living through the darkest time in their lives, and it can be difficult to set aside a primal desire to keep a child alive as long as possible, even in the face of advice that an intervention is likely to do more harm than good. On the other hand, doctors must not confuse what is futile with what is harmful. If doctors feel an

353

intervention should stop even when parents feel strongly that it should continue, they need to show that continuing it will cause more harm to the child than good.

Proportionality and directness

Proportionality

This principle states that any treatment given should be proportional to the stated intention. If morphine is started with intention of pain relief, then it should be at doses that are recommended for pain relief and not at excessively high doses which could suggest an intention to cause respiratory suppression.

Directness

An action cannot be justified if a good outcome is simply a side effect of a bad intention. A doctor could not give a drug that will actively cause a child's death and then claim that by hastening that death, further pain and suffering has been avoided. Sparing suffering would not be the direct intention of the prescription.

Withdrawing versus withholding

There seems an obvious sense in which there can be no moral difference between withdrawing an intervention once it has started and deciding not to offer it in the first place. While that moral equivalence may be enough to help the clinician clarify their thinking, it is important to bear in mind that they are not entirely the same. There is no doubt that the two decisions feel different, and faced with a child who is gasping for breath, the decision not to start invasive ventilation can be difficult, especially if the child's parents have expressed a strong preference that 'everything should be done'. The wider impact on patient and family (and perhaps to the healthcare team too) is also morally relevant.

There can be a temptation to assume that, if withholding treatment would have been a reasonable option in the first place, a decision to withdraw it later is automatically justified. This is not necessarily true, because the circumstances might have changed in the meantime. A decision to withhold treatment should be made on the basis of what is best for the child, and the passage of time can change the balance of probable outcomes. Ventilation should not be withheld, for example, solely because a child is 'palliative' but because, at the moment the decision must be taken, the life-limiting condition means there will be no benefit from ventilation.

Withdrawing treatment that is already in place is always an active decision and is always a moral one, because someone has had to consider whether it was the right action to take. That is not always true when

CLINICAL SCENARIO

Krabbe disease is a progressive neurological condition where a child becomes unaware of their surroundings, and death from respiratory failure typically occurs before the age of 18 months.

A 16-month-old girl is admitted to PICU for mechanical ventilation with increasing frequency over the previous months and each time takes longer for her to regain her baseline level of health. She presents again with signs of infection and respiratory failure and with oxygen saturations of 79% despite maximal face mask oxygen. The blood gas shows a pCO_2 of 11 kPa with a compensated respiratory acidosis. The opinion of the PICU consultant is that the child is dying and that intubation and ventilation are not appropriate, and this is explained to the parents. They respond that they want her to live for as long as is possible and they ask that she is intubated and ventilated.

Despite the fact that the consultant and the clinical team feel that ventilatory support is inappropriate, it is agreed that the young girl should be intubated and ventilated as the parents have not agreed to withhold treatment. While the situation might be futile it is not causing harm to the child and this intervention may prolong life but does not, in itself, result in suffering.

treatments are withheld as this may be done because a reasoned decision has been made or because no decision has been made at all.

The process of making difficult decisions

A particular challenge facing paediatricians is how much authority the preferences of a child's parents should carry when it comes to making medical decisions. Most of the time, parents and paediatricians work together in a collaborative relationship based on mutual trust and respect. Unfortunately, those relationships do not always develop smoothly, or they may be disrupted under the stress of the last phases of a child's life. Parents may express strong preferences for a course of medical action that the doctors feel is not best for the child.

Doctors alone are not able to make a rational decision about what interventions are justified, because there are relevant things about the child that the doctors do not know. It is generally true that doctors know more about a specific illness, and even about the impact the illness on a child at a particular moment. But it is also true that there are other facts about the child that the parents know more about. Parents will typically know more about how much a child enjoys life when well, for example, and even be able to express some of what a child might choose if able to do so. Both sets of knowledge are equally relevant to making a decision about medical intervention that is morally correct.

Furthermore, doctors are not entirely disinterested figures. They have their own beliefs and make their own value judgements. Even when they are able to put those aside (as most do) when they are making a decision, doctors can feel under pressure to balance the needs of the child in front of them against the needs of hypothetical children they will see in the future. Parents are right that when it comes to medical decisions, doctors might be influenced in their decision making by factors that have nothing to do with their child. That is not usually true of parents and it would be hard to expect parents to consider the needs of children other than their own.

The contrary idea that when it comes to medical decision making over children, the role of doctors is simply to carry out parents' preferences, and this usually flows from a certain understanding of autonomy. Again, there is some truth in that claim. It is true that parents have some rights over their children, though parental rights are strictly related to their duty to care.

Many parents assume they have the same sort of authority over decisions in respect of their child. That is not true. Adults are protected from having things done to them without their permission, but the moral imperative in respect of children is different. Children must be protected from interventions that will harm them. The duty to protect children from harm is no less for parents than it is for doctors, and parents are not allowed to want or to permit—still less to require—doctors to do things to their child that will do the child more harm than good. The interests of parents are important, but it is the interests of the child that are paramount, and an action that will cause significant harm to a child does not become a morally right action simply because parents prefer it.

End of life discussions: uncertainty and futility

The goal of discussions about medical interventions at the end of life is to establish what a child's interests are and how they are best served. Parents and doctors each bring certain expertise to the discussion. Each of them knows something about the child's interests and the impact of the disease and interventions. The purpose is to work together to estimate as far as possible what will, as a matter of fact, do the child 'most good and least harm'.

The term 'futile' illustrates an important difference in the perspectives of parents and doctor. Properly understood, describing an intervention as 'futile' simply means it will do no good, but the term does not imply it will do harm. Some doctors might consider that a futile

intervention is always wrong because it uses limited healthcare resources and by doing so harms another child. But, from the perspective of a parent, futility is not a good enough reason to withdraw or withhold an intervention. If parents are to agree with their recommendation, doctors must show that starting or continuing the intervention would harm their child.

Finally, it can be difficult for doctors to know how to balance the needs of the child against those of the parents. For paediatricians, it is the interests of the child that are paramount. If there is a clear and significant conflict between the interests of the child and those of their parents, the default position should always be to decide in favour of a child, and a 'counsel of perfection' would be that no child would ever have a treatment or intervention that was not justified on strictly medical grounds. Some of the harms that arise from a decision about a child might be trivial, but the harms to a family might be severe, and paediatricians do need to consider harm to a parents of the child.

Where the voices of parents and doctors remain at odds, expert mediation services are often able to help narrow the distance between them. In practice, however, the courts are often called upon to adjudicate on what is best for the child and use section 1 of the Children Act 1989:

"… when a court determines any question with respect to the upbringing of a child the child's welfare shall be the court's paramount consideration".

Paediatric Palliative Care (PPC)

'Together for Short Lives' is a UK-based charity and describes palliative care as '...care for children and young people with life-limiting, or life-threatening conditions, and is an active and total approach to care, from the point of diagnosis, throughout the child's life and death. It embraces physical, emotional, social and spiritual elements, and focuses on enhancement of the quality of life for the individual and support for the family. It includes the management of distressing symptoms, provision of short breaks and care through death and bereavement'.

This definition highlights the two key principles of caring for children with life-limiting or life-threatening conditions:

- PPC is **active** care—it does not represent a withdrawal of care
- PPC is **total** care—it does not focus on the medical or physical needs at the expense of nonmedical ones

Active palliative care is the antithesis of the idea that there is 'nothing more we can do' for a child whose life may be short. For the paediatrician, as a child approaches the end of life, symptoms and overall patient care can become increasingly complex, requiring a rigorous, rational approach with extensive planning and anticipation of a constantly evolving clinical picture.

Total palliative care emphasises assessment and management of the whole child—a holistic problem-solving framework in contrast to the more traditional pathophysiological paradigm.

Children who need palliative care

In children, life-limiting conditions (LLC) are conditions which make it likely that a child will not survive into adulthood, either because there is no cure or because there is a significant risk that potentially curative treatment will fail. Asking if one would be surprised if the child died before reaching adulthood may bring clarity to uncertainty, and a negative answer would indicate that the child has a life-limiting condition.

Life-limiting conditions have been grouped together (Table 31.1) into categories to demonstrate the breadth and variety of conditions requiring palliative care in children in contrast with the predominantly cancer focus of the adult specialty.

There are well over 300 life-limiting diagnoses documented and the number is increasing with the expansion of genetic diagnostic techniques. Children may move between groups following disease-modifying therapy, but the categories are a helpful prompt when considering whether a child might benefit from palliative care.

Palliative care and disease-directed treatment

Palliative care planning should be started alongside disease-directed treatment as soon as the diagnosis of a life-limiting condition is made. Timely discussions help prepare everyone for the possibilities both of death and of survival and ensure excellent management of symptoms irrespective of the outcome.

Families—and some professionals—sometimes imagine that palliative care becomes an option only when disease-modifying measures have failed or been ruled out. The assumption is unhelpful and is potentially harmful because it can result in a delay in adequate management of symptoms and reduced likelihood that child and family wishes will be met for the end of life.

Symptoms

Historically, symptoms have been seen essentially as markers of an underlying disorder or as inevitable accompaniments to treatment. Palliative care, however, views a symptom as a problem in its own right—one that is potentially solvable. A symptom is a subjective experience contrasted against the patient's usual functioning; a departure from normal function or feeling. A child's perception of a symptom is partly determined by his or her cognitive and emotional development, and children with severe neurological impairment

Table 31.1 Recognised categories of conditions requiring paediatric palliative care as proposed by Association for Children's Palliative Care (ACT) and RCPCH and which recognise the differing trajectories of illness.	
Category 1	Life-threatening conditions for which curative treatment may be feasible but can fail. Access to palliative care services may be necessary when treatment fails or during an acute crisis, irrespective of the duration of threat to life. On reaching long-term remission or following successful curative treatment there is no longer a need for palliative care services. Examples: cancer, irreversible organ failures of heart, liver, kidney
Category 2	Conditions where premature death is inevitable. There may be long periods of intensive treatment aimed at prolonging life and allowing participation in normal activities. Examples: cystic fibrosis, Duchenne muscular dystrophy
Category 3	Progressive conditions without curative treatment options. Treatment is exclusively palliative and may commonly extend over many years. Examples: Batten disease, mucopolysaccharidoses
Category 4	Irreversible but nonprogressive conditions causing severe disability, leading to susceptibility to health complications and likelihood of premature death. Examples: severe cerebral palsy, multiple disabilities such as following brain or spinal cord injury, complex health care needs, high risk of an unpredictable life-threatening event or episode

Image used with permission from A Core Care Pathway for Children with Life-limiting and Life-threatening Conditions. Ed Woodhead S. 3rd edition. Together for Short Lives. 2013

have particular difficulty in appraising symptom experiences and managing and monitoring their emotional responses.

Use of written symptom management plans communicated to the entire MDT (Figure 31.1) can facilitate adherence to treatment and provide confidence to those in other teams administering medications at doses often outside the range of national formularies and licensing arrangements. Written management plans also empower families with home-based options whilst retaining the option for direct assessment if needed. The plans will include a description of each symptom, the immediate intervention required (e.g. reposition the child, check for wet nappy, suction, use of a fan, massage, music or distraction), instructions for administering 'as needed medications' and finally, whom to call for advice or clinical review if needed. Plans need to be regularly reviewed and shared widely with each iteration.

Effective palliative care requires application of the broad holistic principles to the management of difficult symptoms in children with life-limiting conditions. It is important to see symptom management not as an isolated entity but in the context of the child's disease trajectory, taking into account the ethical issues and need to weigh up the benefit and burdens of all treatments, whether curative or focused on palliating distressing symptoms.

Usually, the lead physician will coordinate the assessment of symptoms although it is often the bedside nurses who have the most valuable professional insight into the daily experience of the child and the role that social interactions have on the overall symptom experience. Others, including religious leaders, may provide understanding of any existential distress or faith-related issues.

General practitioners can offer insight into the family dynamic and illness behaviours that may alter symptom assessment and management. Social workers, teachers and youth workers who know the child and family can also provide context helping to identify anxieties, fears, relationships and behaviours that might exacerbate the symptom. The paediatrician should consider seeking advice in any child with persistent symptoms and ideally from a palliative medicine service.

Psychosocial aspects of the symptom experience

A child's perception of a symptom such as pain is partly determined by cognitive and emotional development. It would be wrong to assume that only patients with fully developed cognition can experience existential distress and this is particularly important for children with severe neurological impairment who make up a significant

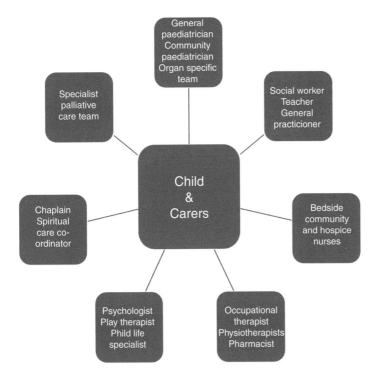

Fig. 31.1 Multidisciplinary teamworking in symptom assessment.

proportion of the children with life-limiting conditions. This latter group are more susceptible to psychosocial problems and some may perceive negative symptoms to be a form of punishment. Chronic or recurrent symptoms can lead to outbursts of aggression, withdrawal from the world socially, reduced adaptive abilities in communication and have a significant impact on function in daily life. These factors all amplify the symptom experience.

Symptoms as spiritual phenomena

Spirituality for the child can be best defined as how they make sense of the world and their place in it. The spiritual experience of symptoms in children is also therefore grounded in their cognitive and emotional development. Parental response not only determines whether the symptom is identified and steps taken to relieve it but also shapes the child's experience and expression of the symptom. It is vital therefore to consider the psychological and existential distress of carers in managing symptoms in their children and addressing this can be the key to gaining control of previously intractable symptoms.

Assessment of symptoms

Symptoms are common in children with life-limiting conditions. A single child can experience many different distressing symptoms simultaneously and the variety, frequency and severity of these increases as a child approaches the end of life.

A broad understanding of symptoms experienced by children with common disease types is a helpful starting point when exploring symptoms with children and their families. For children with cancer, these include pain, poor appetite, fatigue, constipation and headache whilst those with respiratory conditions have dyspnoea, pain, headaches and anxiety. For children with severe cerebral palsy or progressive neurodegenerative conditions, symptoms can include weakness, dysphagia, excessive secretions and seizures, and assessment of such symptoms becomes more complex as they may have more than one cause. Around 90% of these children experience recurrent pain and many have more than one type of pain at any one time.

Listening carefully to the child and parent or carer's description of the symptom experience and exploring their views extensively is important. A thorough examination must be undertaken as well as a medication review, ideally with pharmacist support, looking for side effects and interactions of any medications. Symptom assessment tools (e.g., pain scales) should be used where possible as part of ongoing symptom assessment.

Acknowledgement by a doctor that the symptom exists and of its severity and impact on the life of the child and family can itself offer significant relief of the distress it causes. It is important to be honest from the outset about what can be expected and what should not. Most symptoms can be improved, but in the context of a relentlessly progressing disease, it is often not possible to abolish them completely. Further management should include therapy directed at the disease, other physical interventions aimed at relieving the physical aspects of symptoms (both pharmacological and otherwise) and attention to psychosocial and spiritual issues.

Management of specific symptoms

Pain

Pain occurring in the context of a life-limiting condition is neither wholly acute nor entirely persistent or chronic. The pain usually becomes worse over time, but there is typically an identifiable cause that can theoretically be modified. All the causes of pain occur in a wider psychosocial and spiritual context and are amplified by fear and uncertainty. Table 31.2 describes some of the common sources of pain in children with life-limiting conditions, which are important to consider during history taking. Table 31.3 presents causes of pain that are often overlooked during the clinical examination.

The WHO pain ladder

The WHO pain ladder (Table 31.4) is the template for managing pain in palliative care. It is a simple and rational approach based on three principles:

- management should be simple (for example using the oral route as much as possible)
- as the intensity of pain increases it is necessary to change the type or dosing regimen of analgesic (and not simply to increase the dose or to rotate to another analgesic of the same type)
- it is often possible to identify 'adjuvant' (co-analgesic) interventions that will help relieve pain even though they are not analgesic in their own right (for example, amitriptyline or TENS for neuropathic pain, radiotherapy for bone pain or play therapy for pain amplified by anxiety).

Alongside any of the pharmacological steps, an appropriate co-analgesic should be prescribed. Nonpharmacological options are often effective and are usually nontoxic and include the use of hot packs, massage and hydrotherapy. The correct choice of co-analgesic will also depend on the type of pain as shown by the value of amitriptyline or TENS for neuropathic pain, radiotherapy for bone pain or play therapy if the pain is amplified by anxiety. In some situations, a therapeutic trial on the basis of safety and theoretical benefit for the suspected cause may be appropriate.

Table 31.2 Sources of pain in children with life-limiting conditions

Common	Less common
musculoskeletal (osteopenia, scoliosis, hip subluxation, pathological fractures)	dental caries
	nonspecific back pain
	renal stones and UTI (topiramate, ketogenic diet)
hypertonia (spasticity, dystonia)	pancreatitis (valproate and hypothermia)
muscle fatigue and immobility	cholecystitis (tube feeding)
constipation	ventricular shunt blockage or infection
gastro-oesophageal reflux disease	headache
gastrointestinal dysmotility	
iatrogenic (investigations, surgery)	
sources common to all children (e.g. otitis media, dysmenorrhoea, appendicitis)	

Table 31.3 Other sources of pain in children with severe neurological impairment

eyes—corneal abrasion
mouth, and throat—dental caries and abscess, gingivitis, tonsillitis
central lines, implanted devices, shunt catheter sites—malfunction, infection
gastrostomy tube—gastrostomy tube tension, site infection
abdomen—constipation, distention
skin—hair tourniquet or pressure ulcer
extremities and joints—occult fracture, subluxation

Table 31.4 The WHO pain ladder and analgesia required as pain intensity increases

	Degree of pain	Analgesia to offer
Step 1	Mild pain	simple analgesia (paracetamol, ibuprofen), given 'as needed'
Step 2	Moderate pain	low-dose opioids (equivalent to 0.1 mg/kg oral morphine) given 'as needed'
Step 3	Severe pain	higher-dose opioids (equivalent to 1 mg/kg/24h oral morphine at first, but titrated up in line with increasing pain severity), given regularly and 'as needed'

Opioids, and particularly morphine, are the mainstay of pain management in palliative care, and they are very safe in children providing they are used correctly. Local practice varies between units, but where needed, advice and support on starting these medications, the dose adjustments and any changes in formulations can be obtained from paediatric palliative medicine teams.

Opioids are available in various formulations and the most appropriate should be chosen based on the clinical situation. For most children with moderate pain, occasional oral morphine is easy to take and is effective. It can, however, take 20 minutes to be effective, and if a more rapid onset is needed, a buccal opioid such as diamorphine, fentanyl or alfentanil might

be preferable. A child with severe pain will need regular opioids and will benefit from the convenience of a transcutaneous patch or slow-release formulation. Only fentanyl and buprenorphine are available as transdermal patches.

The correct dose of opioid to prescribe will depend on three factors:
- the weight and age of the child
- the severity of the pain
- the current exposure of the child to opioids

It is not possible to establish a safe dose without knowing all three parameters, and in particular, it is not safe to prescribe opioids on the basis of a child's weight alone. A child who has been on regular opioids for some time will develop physiological tolerance and likely need a larger total daily dose of opioids in order to relieve their pain when compared with an opioid-naive child of the same weight.

Pain strongly counters the side effects of sedation and respiratory depression seen in higher dose opioid analgesics, and a child in very severe pain will benefit from a potent opioid and experience few, if any, of these adverse effects. The child with mild, constant pain will require a much lower dose to adequately treat their pain whilst avoiding toxicity.

The most suitable initial dose of opioids to use in an obese child is best calculated using the ideal body weight for height in combination with the factors described above. Subsequent doses will be guided by the effectiveness of those initial doses and the number of doses required to control the child's pain, rather than anthropometric parameters.

Immediate release opioid preparations are usually used in the first instance except in severe persistent pain where regular dosing is required from the start. Once a 24-hour total dose has been established, then a slow-release preparation with 12- or 24-hour dosing can be introduced. 'Background dosing' needs the parallel prescription of extra doses for 'break-through' pain and if frequent, extra doses are needed, then the 'background' dose must be reviewed and increased.

If control needs to be improved then the dose should be increased and not the frequency of administration. The dose escalation should be in steps of 25% to 33% of the total daily dose (background plus breakthrough amounts). Laxatives should be started at the same time as the opioid.

Buprenorphine or fentanyl can be considered for transdermal administration although, as they are not licensed for use in children, they should only be prescribed by those with experience in their use. Transdermal administration should only be introduced once the effective total daily dose of morphine has been established and should not be used if the pain experienced by the patient is changing relatively frequently. A 'dose conversion' exercise must be undertaken before prescribing from an established morphine dose and it is usual practice to further reduce the calculated transdermal dose to avoid a hyperalgesia effect. Tables of equivalent potency are available in commonly used formularies.

Nausea and vomiting

Diet modification, portion sizes and distraction can be of benefit in the management of nausea and vomiting. Some drugs have a very restricted range of action, such as ondansetron for chemotherapy-induced nausea and vomiting or cyclizine for raised intracranial pressure. Others have a much wider range of action, such as levomepromazine (Nozinan). It is important to avoid co-prescribing medications whose actions duplicate or even counteract one another.

Dyspnoea

Dyspnoea is a subjective experience rather than an observation. A change in respiratory rate might be of concern for the carers of a child, but it does not need to be treated unless distressing for the child. The range of mechanisms that can underlie dyspnoea is extremely wide, and identifying them can suggest specific interventions (e.g. analgesics for pain, anticholinergics for secretions, oxygen for symptomatic hypoxia or NIPPV for hypercarbia).

CLINICAL SCENARIO

An 8-year-old boy has an osteosarcoma of his right femur and is experiencing moderate, persistent pain in that region that is resistant to massage, hot packs, distraction and ibuprofen gel. Paracetamol for the pain has been tried but is not sufficient. The boy weighs 30 kg and has not previously received opioids.

Since the child is opioid naïve and his pain is moderate and not severe, it would be appropriate to start him on morphine sulphate 3 mg (100 mcg/kg/dose) as required for pain.

A review in the following week records that the morphine sulphate has been effective, but as his disease has progressed, his pain has become more severe and the morphine dose is insufficient to manage his symptoms. He therefore started on morphine sulphate 5 mg 4-hourly regularly (1 mg/kg/day) with an additional breakthrough dose of 5mg (1/6 of his total daily background dose) given as required.

A further review at 48 hrs finds that he is much more comfortable but has used three doses of 5 mg morphine sulphate for breakthrough pain each day. The total morphine sulphate use is therefore 45 mg/day (30 mg in regular 'background' doses plus 3 x 5 mg breakthrough doses). The regular dose is therefore increased by 50% to 7.5 mg 4-hourly. This takes his new background opioid dose to 45 mg/day. A further 7.5 mg morphine sulphate dose is prescribed as 1–2 hourly as required for breakthrough pain.

Once regular dosing is commenced, further increases take account of the background and additional breakthrough doses given, ensuring each increase is not more than 50% every 48 hrs.

A review after further 48 hrs finds that his pain is now well controlled on 45 mg morphine sulphate per day. It is now appropriate to switch him to a longer acting preparation such as MST or a transdermal preparation such as fentanyl or buprenorphine. Such conversions should be undertaken with caution and should only be undertaken under the guidance of those with specialist expertise.

There are also generic interventions that will help dyspnoea of any cause. Suction, breathing exercises, a flow of air on the face (e.g. by using a handheld fan) and nebulised saline can all be effective and return a sense of control to child and family. Systemic opioids and benzodiazepines, particularly buccal midazolam, relieve dyspnoea by interaction with receptors in the central nervous system. These are specialist indications and discussion with a palliative care team is advised.

Other symptoms

The range of symptoms that might affect an individual child is wide and encompasses experiences as diverse as constipation, confusion and hypercalcaemia. The same principles, however, apply to all:

- a symptom is a subjective experience
- symptoms occur in a context that is psychosocial and spiritual as well as physical and in a child who is part of a network of relationships
- symptom management demands collaboration with parents and colleagues from many different professional backgrounds and that demands excellent communication and documentation
- symptom management requires meticulous balancing of the benefits and harms of an intervention, whether the intervention is pharmacological or otherwise
- pharmacological management requires specialist understanding of the therapeutics of symptom control in order to minimise risk and maximise effectiveness

When treatment fails

Whilst the goal is complete relief of symptoms, there are situations where this is not possible. As the disease course fluctuates, symptoms can reappear and even treatment that was initially effective can begin to fail. Under these circumstances it becomes important to reexplore the child and family's objectives. Such discussions may result in a shared conclusion to redirect goals and decisions, perhaps accepting drowsiness as inevitable in the name of comfort and reconsidering the role of further investigation, resuscitation and hospitalisation.

At the end of life, it becomes even more important to preserve the quality of an individual's experience of their life. The purpose of palliative care is not to delay death, but neither must it be to hasten it. The purpose of palliative care is to optimise a child's comfort as far as is possible.

Open and unhurried discussion of issues at the end of life reduces the likelihood of conflicts. A systematic approach to end-of-life planning with parents should be introduced in a timely fashion several months or even years before death is expected and should involve both palliative care and intensive care teams as well as the lead paediatric service for the child. Where conflict remains despite those discussions, there are third party mediation services that can help find an acceptable compromise. Ultimately, the courts can reluctantly offer a practical resolution by evaluating all proposed courses of action against the best interests of the child and giving a decision that is binding on all parties.

CLINICAL SCENARIO

A 10-year-old boy with severe cerebral palsy has profound hypotonia and is fed via a gastrostomy. He is registered blind but is able to communicate with single words and gestures. Over the last year his health has started to deteriorate with more frequent chest infections, difficult to manage secretions and periods of not tolerating feeds. He presents to the Children's Assessment Unit with his mother as he has been difficult to console over the past few days and the slightest movement or transfer significantly worsen his distress. When asked if he is in pain, he nods but is unable to explain his experience further.

This is a typical presentation of a child with severe neurological impairment in pain or distress and there are many possible causes for his pain (see Tables 31.2 and 31.3). Enquiring about dentition and gastrostomy site issues are commonly overlooked, as well as consideration of adverse effects of antiepileptic medications. Damage to parts of the somatosensory system in these children can be responsible for generating pain without nociceptive pain input or creating the perception of pain from stimuli such as touch and sound which are normally not painful.

Following assessment, a painful swelling of his right thigh is identified and an x-ray demonstrates a pathological fracture with significant osteopenia. The findings are explained to the young man with the help of the play team and the situation discussed with his mother.

Whilst it may seem that the management of a simple fracture is straightforward involving simple analgesia and orthopaedic management, the presented situation is much broader than this. Disease-directed therapy might include traction and fixation and consideration of bisphosphonates. These carry risks and burdens and, given as the patient is approaching the end of his life, each intervention would need to be carefully considered in terms of the balance of benefit and burden. Addressing the issue of the clinical deterioration and the need for parallel planning for survival or death is important. A professional with good relationship with the family, at an appropriate time, should start these discussions and complete advanced care planning.

IMPORTANT CLINICAL POINTS

Ethical aspects of palliative care

- the decision to withhold an intervention is ethically equivalent to a decision to withdraw it although there may be other morally relevant considerations that mean the two are not equivalent
- neither parents alone nor doctors alone are in a position to know the interests of the child and therefore medical decisions at the end of life must be made in collaboration
- open discussions about end-of-life plans should begin early enough to allow a relationship in which parents and healthcare team bring complementary expertise to bear on what is best for the child
- occasional disagreement is inevitable. The need for medical mediation should be recognised early but healthcare teams might find it necessary to apply to the courts in order to feel confident they are supported in making controversial decisions
- the courts will order parents and doctors to act in accordance with what they conclude is best interests of the child

Practical issues in management of palliative care

- palliative care should be considered for all children at the point at which a diagnosis of a life-limiting or life-threatening condition is made
- successful symptom management requires a compassionate yet rigorous assessment of physical, psychosocial and spiritual factors
- symptoms should be managed alongside the investigation of an underlying cause
- both disease-directed and nonpharmacological strategies should be considered alongside palliative pharmacological treatments
- parent or carer anxiety and distress can significantly impact the expression and experience of symptoms in children and must be acknowledged and addressed

Further reading

Hain, RDW, Goldman A, Rappaport A, Meiring M. Oxford Textbook of Palliative Care in Children. 3rd ed. Oxford University Press. 2021

Making decisions to limit treatment in life-limiting and life-threatening conditions in children. 3rd Ed. RCPCH. 2015 Withholding and withdrawing life-prolonging treatments. General Medical Council. London. 2002

The Core Care Pathway from Together for Short Lives. Together for Short Lives. https://www.togetherforshortlives.org.uk/resource/core-care-pathway/

End of life care for infants, children and young people with life-limiting conditions: management. NICE guideline [NG61]. Published December 2016. Updated July 2019. https://www.nice.org.uk/guidance/ng61

Chapter |32|

Ethics and law

Martin Hewitt

After reading this chapter you should be able to:
- apply legal rights of children and young people within the current UK legal framework

Ethics

Ethics are the principles by which we live our lives. They are defined by many factors including religion, law and custom. Ethical codes define our moral practice and aim to distinguish between right and wrong, good and evil or fair and unfair.

Medical ethics are the principles by which medicine is practiced and they are defined by the same factors as above plus the professional standards and expectations ascribed to medical practitioners. Professional bodies, nonprofessional groups (usually patient groups) and the general expectations of the public are responsible for developing these 'principles of practice'.

The need for a code of conduct of practice has been long recognised. Even before the Hippocratic Oath, there were statements which defined important and agreed principles of medical care. The Hippocratic Oath was sworn by many doctors on qualification and updated versions are still used in many countries today.

The four 'prima facie' principles of medical ethics dictate that the clinician demonstrates and has a respect for autonomy, nonmaleficence, beneficence and justice although further principles have been proposed. The term 'prima facie' indicates that these four core principles should be followed unless they are in conflict with each other. In that situation it is necessary to make a choice between the conflicting principles—and paediatric practice provides many such conflicts!

The core principles are described as:

Autonomy

This is the recognition that a competent adult, with full capacity of understanding, is able to make decisions about their own lives and bodies—even where this may seem counter to their well-being and survival. Failure to respect this fundamental right may lead to the clinician being accused of assault.

Nonmaleficence

There is an understanding that any decision or treatment offered to a patient must not be harmful. The original Hippocratic Oath stated "I will use treatment to help the sick according to my ability and judgment, but never with a view to injury and wrong-doing". Medical intervention, however beneficial to the patient, must balance the possible risk of harm to the patient. Where that risk is significant then intervention needs careful consideration and may even be inappropriate.

Beneficence

The aim and intention of the clinician is to act in the best interests of the patient and ensure that any advice or treatment provided is for the benefit of the patient.

Justice

This principle requires the clinician to be fair and honest in all dealings with their patient.

These four, often quoted, core principles, however, do present difficulties when applied to children and young people at all the stages of their emotional and intellectual development. In the intellectually competent young person, the principle of autonomy has a greater importance and the young person can agree to interventions without the permission of their parents or guardian. When, however, the competent young person refuses an intervention that is thought by others to be in their best interests, then 'beneficence' seems to take precedence and the opinion of the young person can be discounted.

When the child is considered to be 'intellectually immature', decisions will, understandably, be made by their parents or guardians. The principle of autonomy and nonmaleficence then becomes difficult to apply, but there would still be a place for understanding a child's requests and concerns and an aim to respect these where possible. A young child will certainly object to a simple blood test but it would be argued that they are unable to understand the need for the test and the consequences of their objection. The young child is not allowed to make 'unwise' decisions and so it is the parents and clinicians who will agree that the intervention is in the child's best interest—beneficence.

It can be argued that the principle of autonomy does not apply to children and young people. UK law supports this view as '…the child's welfare shall be the court's paramount consideration' and so allows the court to make decisions on behalf of the child.

In practice, those attributes necessary to make informed decisions and act autonomously—to be able to understand the terms used in any information given, to process and rationalise that information and to understand the potential consequences of any decision—evolve over many years. The ability to act in an autonomous way will vary between individuals, between the issues under discussion and the range of potential outcomes for that decision, and this ability will mature over time. This was recognised by the UK courts:

> "As a matter of Law, the parental right to determine whether or not their minor child below the age of sixteen will have medical treatment terminates if and when the child achieves sufficient understanding and intelligence to understand fully what is proposed."

—Lord Scarman (1985)

Confidentiality

The common law in the UK requires doctors to keep all personal information provided by patients as confidential and that an understanding of such an arrangement is essential to the maintenance of trust between the two parties. The General Medical Council, similarly, requires doctors to recognise that confidentiality is central to their interaction with patients. Ensuring patient confidentiality is, therefore, an ethical, professional and a legal requirement.

The principle, however, is not absolute and the doctor may share confidential information in certain circumstances. This would include situations where the patient agrees to the sharing of the information as in an individual with a medical problem asking for some details to be shared with a new employer, or when there is a court order to share the information such as a mental health assessment to place before a court which can then influence any sentence given. A more extreme example would be a need to share information that has a wider public interest such as when a patient makes a credible threat of violence to others.

Confidentiality requires further consideration in paediatric practice. Children and young people are entitled to the same standards of confidentiality as other patients, but their rights are not absolute and can be overridden when there is a clear justification, such as the risk of significant harm. There are situations where a mature, competent teenager would expect their medical information to remain confidential, including keeping that information from their parents. In such a situation, this would include denying parents the right to automatically view the medical records of the young person. If the medical practitioner felt that there was an exceptional reason that justified disclosure without consent, then the young person should be told of the need to break their confidentiality and the reasons fully explained. In the absence of any such reason justifying disclosure, they should be encouraged, but not forced, to share their health information with their parents.

The sharing of information about a child with the parents would, in most situations, be expected practice, but where there is a concern about the welfare of the child then some aspects of the care may be withheld—for example, if a carer is suspected of poisoning a young child—until more information is obtained.

Where there are safeguarding concerns then the paediatrician must share information with other members of the multidisciplinary team involved in child protection—social services and police. It would, however, be considered good practice to advise the parents that this was the intended action.

The four core principles have, however, been expanded and developed by various declarations over many years. Some, such as Declaration of Geneva, Declaration of Human Rights and the UN Rights of the Child, have all contributed to the establishment of codes of practice for the clinician.

CLINICAL SCENARIO

A boy of 14 years was admitted to hospital with difficulty in breathing. Initial imaging had indicated that he had a thoracic lymphoma and he would require a biopsy, insertion of a central venous line and administration of chemotherapy. His prognosis was very good.

His parents asked that he was not told of the underlying diagnosis and that the word 'cancer' was not used as his grandfather had died of 'cancer' some 2 months earlier. They felt that they were acting in his best interests.

The consultant explained that their wish to protect him from the diagnosis was understandable and that it was clear that the parents were acting in his best interests. It was, however, important to consider what was in the best interest [beneficence] of the young man and for all the team members to be truthful and honest [justice].

The consultant explained that it was likely that the patient would work out the diagnosis even if he was not given the full diagnosis or the word 'cancer' not used (he was, after all, to be treated on a paediatric oncology ward). It was then pointed out that when he did find out that he had cancer he would be angry that those around him had not been truthful. If that did happen then it would undermine his trust in his parents and clinical team members and he then may not believe any future explanations provided. Furthermore, there was always the prospect that someone—friend, relative, team member—might inadvertently reveal the diagnosis.

It was suggested that by giving him the words and the understanding of his diagnosis that his fears and concerns may be reduced and such knowledge would allow him to participate fully in conversations about his illness.

After some further thought, both parents agreed to a full and honest discussion. It was agreed that the discussion would include the patient, the parents and members of the medical and nursing staff. The patient understood the information given and had confidence to progress through treatment. When last seen, he was at university and enjoying his life some 7 years after diagnosis.

The General Medical Council of the UK sets expected standards of medical care and training and has produced a series of booklets which outline important issues for the clinician.

GMC Professional Standards requires the doctor to:
- be honest
- be open
- respect confidentiality
- treat patients with respect
- ensure patient safety
- maintain up-to-date clinical knowledge
- ensure good verbal communication
- ensure good recordkeeping
- ensure robust teamwork

The GMC also produces specific standards of best practice for all doctors who have any contact with children and young people under the age of 18 years.

GMC Professional Standards for doctors working with children
- protect children from abuse or neglect
- communicate appropriately with children and YP
- respect their confidentiality
- treat patients with respect
- ensure patient safety
- maintain up-to-date clinical knowledge
- share relevant information with other agencies
- ensure good recordkeeping

Research ethics

Research is a fundamental basis for good clinical practice. It is the bedrock of improved understanding, improved treatment programmes and improved care and support for patients.

"Nothing is more terrible than to see ignorance in action".

—Van Goethe

It is incumbent on any good doctor to support research projects wherever possible, to access research findings whenever available and to implement research findings whenever feasible.

Research may be funded by the government (in the UK—National Institute for Health Research), commercial drug companies, university departments, health organisations and charities.

Medical research in the UK involving NHS patients or adult social care, any of the data or samples from these individuals and, in some cases, their carer, must submit their study to the National Research Ethics Service (NRES). No research on these individuals or data can be undertaken without full approval from an NRES ethics committee.

Research involving children requires the submission of the full protocol to a specific Research Ethics Committee designated to review studies in those under 18 years. Clarification of the process of age-appropriate explanations and the method of obtaining consent and assent will be examined before approval given.

Trials involving medicinal products in children ('drug trials') must go to a committee registered to review both paediatric and medicinal products studies. Such trials must be compliant with the EU Clinical Trials Directive of 2001 which requires written parental consent of any individual under the age of 16 years.

365

Law

The UK law recognises that children are individuals within a family and that parents have prime responsibility for the care and protection of their children. The laws aim to ensure children can grow and develop with the support of their wider family and reach their full potential.

It also understands that children and young people are potentially vulnerable and need protection from adults immaterial of whether they be the parents, relatives or unknown individuals.

There are some differences in the law relating to children between the four countries making up the UK, but in general they all have a similar approach to the legal issues relating to children and young people. The AKP exam will not test a knowledge of the differences in legal practice between the four nations of the UK. In clinical placements, however, it is imperative that all clinicians are aware of the legal directives for the geographical area in which they work.

Definition of a child

The UN Convention on the Rights of the Child defines a child as everyone under 18 unless "under the law applicable to the child, majority is attained earlier" and this definition was incorporated in UK law. This defined age recognises that the vulnerability of a young person persists into later teenage years and there is an ongoing need to protect young people from possible abuse and exploitation. The UK Children Act (1989 and 2004 along with subsequent amendments) applies to all children and young people up to their 18th birthday.

Children in the family

The Children Act (1989 and 2004 along with subsequent amendments) established organisational structures and working arrangements for all those professionals closely involved with children and young people. These professional groups include:
- local authority services
- social services
- health care
- police
- education
- probation services
- young offenders' institutions

The working arrangements between these groups was aimed at supporting the child within the family wherever possible and this was an important goal for any review of a child when welfare concerns had been raised. Those organisations, however, must work together to promote and protect the welfare of all children in situations where it was felt that the normal family arrangements had broken down.

The Act provided a legal framework for protecting children from abuse and required the compulsory intervention in family life for the best interests of a child. Consequently, all those who have contact with children and young people as part of their working practice have a legal obligation to report to the appropriate authorities—either social services or police—any concerns about the welfare and safety of a young person. When abuse is suspected, there is a primary duty of all investigative agencies to cooperate and share relevant information pertaining to their concerns about wider welfare of the child or young person. The doctor has a legal responsibility to assist in this process.

It is now mandatory for all social care staff, health care professionals and teachers in England to report female genital mutilation (FGM) in under 18s to the police.

Welfare of the child is paramount

All paediatricians must act in the best interest of the child, first and foremost. In most situations the intentions of the parents and clinician would be in agreement, but where there is conflict, the clinician must weigh up the implications of both decisions on the welfare of the child or young person. When a serious illness has major implications on the future health of the child, and there is a conflict between parents and clinicians, then the opinion of other senior colleagues should be sought and ultimately the involvement of the law courts.

Parental responsibility

A 'parent' is recognised as the biological or adoptive mother or father to the child. The biological mother has full parental rights and responsibilities and is recognised as the prime carer of the child. The biological father will have equal rights and responsibilities as the biological mother if he was married to the mother at the time of the birth or his name is recorded on the birth certificate of the child. Adoptive parents are given the rights and responsibilities during the legal adoption process.

Both legal parents retain their responsibility throughout any changes to their own circumstances such as major illness, criminal investigations or even imprisonment. A court order may remove that responsibility from either parent and transfer it to other individuals such as another family member or a local authority. The mother or father may also voluntarily surrender their responsibility and transfer it to another individual but again this must be done formally via a court order if it is to be recognised.

Consent

The law on consent for those under 18 years is understandably complex. It recognises that young people do not always have the capacity to absorb and understand complex information. That capacity to understand such information will change over time as the child and young person moves towards adulthood at their 18th birthday. During that time the law looks to the adult with parental responsibility to provide understanding on behalf of the young person. Current acts of Parliament identify those individuals with parental responsibility and directs that they provide the necessary informed consent.

The biological mother must always be approached for consent to any intervention on a young person or child. The biological father can only provide consent if he meets the criteria that gives him full parental responsibility and that responsibility is not lost following a divorce from the mother.

The biological father who was not married to the mother at the time of the birth or whose name is not recorded on the birth certificate may also be able to give consent if there is a formal court-approved agreement between the biological mother and biological father or a court-approved directive that transfers that responsibility to the biological father (for example, if the biological mother had incapacitating mental illness).

Both biological parents retain parental responsibility even if they are under investigation for issues of safeguarding related to the child. The parents still have to give consent for interviewing the child or the taking of images. If they refuse permission for any interaction that is considered important, then a court order would be obtained.

Those who can give consent for a child or a noncompetent young person:
- biological mother
- biological father married to mother at time of birth
- biological father named on birth certificate
- same-sex partner—only if adopted and through a court order
- nonbiological father—only through a formal court order
- adoptive parents—only through a formal court order
- social worker for child in care—through a court order
- medical practitioner—technically does not give consent but acts in the child's best interest in extreme circumstances when parent not available

---

Grandparents cannot give consent unless they have been given parental formal responsibility by a family court.

If the child is in the care of a local authority, as directed by a court order, then a social worker acting for that local authority can give consent.

No individual who is acting in loco parentis (such as teachers, accompanying friend, partner of absent parent) can give consent.

If the child is seriously unwell and no responsible adult available, then a senior doctor can make a decision that is considered to be in the best interests of the child. This would usually be reserved for any emergency situations with potential threat to life of the child or the possibility of long-term injury. It would be usual practice, if time allowed, to discuss the matter with a second senior colleague and record that discussion in the clinical notes along with signatures of the parties involved. Where there is no immediate danger to life or injury, then it would be usual to try and locate the responsible adult.

If the child needs less-immediate treatment that is thought to be in the their best interest and the parents refuse such treatment, then the involvement of mediation services can be beneficial to all parties and failing that the clinician can seek the opinion of the High Court.

Foster parents do not have the right to give consent for any treatments for a child. The child or young person is placed with foster parents by the local authority who have taken over the parental responsibility. The foster parents are therefore acting on behalf of the local authority, and any requests for consent for a medical intervention has to be passed on to a representative social worker. It is they who have to provide consent for the intervention.

In some situations, the child may be temporarily placed with foster parents but the local authority has not taken over legal guardianship. In these situations, the biological mother and possibly the biological father (if the previously stated requirements are met) are still the individuals to needed to provide consent.

Families who adopt children will gain parental responsibility by being the named individuals in the application process.

Same-sex couples within a civil partnership or who are married and who elect to adopt a child will both have equal rights in the same way as heterosexual couples who adopt.

Consent for treatment is not required from both parents although a pragmatic and considerate position for the clinician to take would be to ensure both are fully informed and supportive of any treatment decisions. Where there is a conflict of opinion between both parents, then time should be made to discuss the differing concerns and even offer a second opinion. Ultimately, the courts may be called upon to decide on behalf of the child.

Consent by a young person

The ability to give consent to treatment is dependent on the ability to understand the consequences of receiving that treatment. Such understanding will differ depending upon the complexity of the proposed treatment and the age of the young person involved. It is the responsibility of the clinician to assess whether the patient has the capacity to understand the implications of the proposed treatment. Young children who do not have the capacity to understand cannot give or withhold consent and the legal parent or guardian must be called upon to give consent.

Involving the child or young person in any decisions about health care and health-related interventions is considered good practice. Even very young children will benefit from explanations appropriate to their level of understanding as this will minimise fears and help with compliance. The age of the child and nature of the intervention will influence how the discussion may proceed although some parents may prefer to undertake such discussions themselves. This latter approach should be supported but care taken to ensure that such discussions lead to the young person being fully informed of the proposed treatment.

Young people over the age of 16 years can give valid consent to treatment providing they understand the risks and consequences of such treatment.

Although young people develop the rights to give consent for themselves as they grow older, those with parental responsibility retain the right to give consent on behalf of the young person until they reach the age of 18 years, Therefore, for a period of 2 years, both the young person and the individual with parental responsibility have the right to give consent for treatment. In practice, the clinician should consider seeking consent from the young person in the first instance but then obtain their understanding and approval to also seek consent from the parent or carer unless the treatment under discussion is of a sensitive and private nature.

Young people under the age of 16 years present particular issues with regard to consent, and this needs careful consideration. Clearly as the person matures, issues may develop where the young person does not wish to have a discussion in the presence of their parents. A young person may wish to keep topics such as sexual health, mental health and relationships confidential. The young person may also seek advice about specific treatment and ask that the parents are neither involved nor informed.

The doctor must obviously explore the reasons and concerns of the young person and, where possible, encourage the young person to discuss the matter with the parents in the first instance. If the young person insists on not informing the parents and is felt to have the capacity

to understand the consequences of treatment then the clinician may provide such treatment without seeking the consent or knowledge of the parents.

This was the scenario which provided the legal ruling now known as an assessment of 'Gillick competence'. Mrs Gillick took her health authority to court after a local GP had prescribed oral contraceptive medication to her 15-year-old daughter without seeking parental consent. In 1985, the House of Lords heard the appeals of the lower UK courts and widened the issue away from contraception and ruled on the question of whether a young person under the age of 16 years could consent to treatment without parental involvement.

'Gillick competence' therefore refers to the ability of the young person to consent to any examination, investigation or treatment without involving their parents as long as they fully understand what is being proposed. The legal right to make decisions on treatment moves from parent to child as the young person develops an understanding of the consequences of those decisions. This principle applies to those under the age of 16 years. The law, however, gives very little guidance on the process of assessing competence.

Any consent given following the assessment of competence must be given voluntarily and without pressure or coercion from other individuals and should recognise the possibility of mental health issues that could influence that decision.

'Fraser guidelines' were provided at a later date and are a separate ruling applying specifically to sexual health particularly contraceptive advice and treatment.

A young person can be given contraceptive advice, even under the age of 16 years, if they:
- understand the doctor's advice
- cannot be persuaded to inform parents or to allow the doctor to inform them
- are likely to have sexual intercourse with or without contraception
- are likely to suffer physically or psychologically unless contraception is available

Withholding treatment

An adult with parental responsibility can refuse examination, investigation and treatment of their child. If, however, the clinician feels that this is not in the best interests of the child then legal advice would be sought.

A young person between 16 and 18 year in England and Wales can give consent to treatment but may not be able to refuse treatment. If the clinician and the parents agree that any such treatment is potentially able to save "life or limb" and therefore considered to be in the best interests of the young person, then they can request a court to overrule the opinion of the young person. Previous examples include issues of mental health and heart lung transplant. The practicalities of how such a decision can be implemented, however, will require a great deal of thought and consideration. In Scotland, the legal approach differs and a young person aged between 16 and 18 years is regarded as having full competence and can both consent and decline treatment.

Mental Capacity Act

Children and young people do present with significant mental health illness and may reject clinical decisions regarding their health but which are thought to be in their best interests. The Mental Capacity Act (2005) applies to those over the age of 16 years and provides a framework which allows decisions to be made on their behalf by another individual. The person making the decision will usually be a parent or carer but may also be a doctor or a social worker. In some circumstances, the court may appoint a person to represent the young person and make the necessary decisions. Core principles of the Act require that any decisions made are in the best interest of the young person and it should not be assumed that a young person lacks capacity simply because they make an unwise decision.

CLINICAL SCENARIO

A 17-year-old boy had been treated at a hospital in England for his Ewing sarcoma some 2 years previously. He had had a very difficult time during treatment with major problems with emesis and life-threatening infections. Since his treatment had finished, he had returned to a full and very active life. Unfortunately, he presented again with shortness of breath and was found to have multiple pulmonary metastases. He was offered second-line combination of chemotherapy which had some evidence of inducing a further remission. He declined further treatment and his decision was supported by his parents. There were no concerns about his mental state.

Further discussions were had with the patient and his parents outlining the details of the treatment and the chances of disease remission. He still declined the treatment. His likely progress without treatment was explained—first in discussion and then explicitly in a letter. He still declined treatment.

It was decided that he fully understood the consequence of refusing treatment and remained determined that that was his wish. He wished to enjoy his final days with friends and family. His parents fully supported his decision. His wishes were respected and he died at home some weeks later.

The child under arrest

If a young person under the age of 18 years is arrested and held in custody then the police have a legal obligation to ensure an appropriate adult is present throughout the time they are held. The appropriate adult is usually the next of kin. The police have the legal power to collect evidence and protect against loss of evidence. If a young person is arrested who is designated as being under the care of the Local Authority ('Looked-After' status) then the local authority—usually through the duty social work team—must be informed.

Discrimination and protected status

The UK government introduced the Equality Act in 2010. This identified nine protected characteristics, introduced them into UK law and established that it was illegal to discriminate against individuals—directly or indirectly—on the basis of any of these attributes.

Protected characteristics covered by the Equality Act 2010:
- age
- disability
- gender reassignment
- marriage and civil partnership
- pregnancy
- race
- religion
- sex
- sexual identity

Duty of candour

A further act of Parliament (Health and Social Care Act 2008—Regulated Activities—Regulations 2014) required all health care professionals to be truthful and honest with patients in the event of an error in their treatment or care. The doctor is required to tell the patient (or their relatives) when there has been an adverse event in the provided care and they must apologise for that shortfall. The clinician must try and correct the error and explain fully to the patient about any short-term or long-term potential problems. Any apology should occur as soon as possible after the event. In practice, most significant errors will be investigated by the institution as a formal 'Serious Untoward Incident'—SUI—but this should not be used as a reason to delay an apology.

The clinician must also actively support the principle of duty of candour when dealing with colleagues and must never try and suppress attempts to honestly explain the sequence of events by colleagues.

That need for openness and honesty by the clinician must also be extended to individuals from the organisation who may be investigating any such incident. Their investigation will identify aspects of practice which need to change and thereby protect future patients.

IMPORTANT CLINICAL POINTS

Confidentiality

- children and young people are entitled to the same standards of confidentiality as other patients
- confidentiality can be overridden if there is a clear justification
- if there are safeguarding concerns, then information must be shared with other members of the safeguarding MDT

Law

- welfare of the child is first and foremost action
- welfare of child may override parent decision

Consent

- child under 16 years may give valid consent if they understand the implications

- young people over 16 years can give consent to treatment
- decision of young person over 16 years may be overruled if they decline treatment
- 'Fraser guidelines' and 'Gillick competence' are not the same
- biological father can give consent only if named on birth certificate

Honesty

- required all health care professionals to be truthful and honest with patients in the event of an error in their treatment or care

Further reading

Working Together to Safeguard Children. HM Government. Published July 2018. Accessed: March 2021. https://assets.publishing.service.gov.uk/government/uploads/system/uploads/attachment_data/file/942454/Working_together_to_safeguard_children_inter_agency_guidance.pdf.

Ethical Guidance for doctors. General Medical Council. Accessed March 2021. https://www.gmc-uk.org/ethical-guidance/ethical-guidance-for-doctors

Chapter 33

Patient safety and clinical governance

Martin Hewitt

After reading this chapter you should:
- be able to apply patient safety thinking
- understand how human factors detrimental to care can be minimised
- be able to lead a safe and effective handover

Clinical governance

This term describes the framework of practice that ensures patients receive the highest possible care from the NHS. All staff—whatever their role and whatever their grade—are required to contribute to the continued improvement in the quality of individual patient care. This can be achieved through staff education and development, continuous review of practice, a culture of openness and honesty on practice issues and full and clear communication with individual patients.

Practical aspects of clinical governance

Clinical effectiveness

This can be achieved by ensuring that the care provided is, where possible, based on sound evidence from research and subsequently improved through audit and performance review. The National Institute for Health and Care Excellence (NICE) provides national guidance on the prevention and treatment of many conditions after reviewing all available evidence. All published information is reviewed and updated at regular intervals.

Multidisciplinary teams

High-quality patient care requires the skills, experience and training of many individuals. This is best achieved by incorporating staff into multidisciplinary teams and ensuring that all members communicate effectively on behalf of the patient.

Clinical audit

This is part of the process of reviewing the clinical performance of a team and is now well-established in clinical care. Audit requires the identification of important standards of excellent practice, review of the practice of the team against those standards, the presentation of results to the relevant teams and introducing a change in practice to ensure all meet the standards.

Near misses and mistakes

Clinical practice is complex and difficult and sadly mistakes do occur. The impact of any mistake can be devastating for the patients and families and can also impact on clinicians involved. It behoves all clinicians to strive to avoid mistakes in their practice but if they do occur, it is then the responsibility of the clinicians and the institution to help understand and explain the issue. There is no place for hiding, disguising or obfuscating the events. Being open and honest is hard to do but it does benefit all involved. The law on Duty of Candour has already been presented (Chapter 32 Ethics and Law) and clearly indicates that any attempts to hide the truth constitutes a criminal offence.

The term 'clinical incidents' is used to describe any event relating to the patient and his or her clinical care which results in harm, or which could have led to harm had the events been allowed to progress. Clinical incidents—actual or potential—must be reported to the institution for assessment so that clinical risks can be identified and reduced. Such clinical incident reporting is not part of a disciplinary process and team members are encouraged to view it as part of a reflective system that supports improvement.

All institutions provide opportunities for patients and families to submit comments and complaints on any aspect of the care they receive. Although complaints can be difficult to receive by the individual or team, it is important to recognise that they may highlight an aspect of care which does not meet the needs of patients and which is not recognised by team members. They should be seen as an opportunity to learn about the impact of practice on the care provided. All hospitals have a Patient Advice and Liaison Service (PALS) which offers confidential advice, support and information on health-related matters to patients and families and can often act as an intermediary in some situations.

PRACTICE POINT—actions to be considered if a clinical incident occurs

- ensure patient is safe and effects of incident addressed immediately
- ensure ongoing review of patient
- inform senior colleague
- be honest with patient and family in a timely manner
- apologise for events and avoid blaming individuals
- record details of event fully in notes—including date and time of event
- record details of discussions with patient and carer
- complete a clinical incident form
- • support any assessment process

Risk management

The process which looks at clinical situations and tries to identify possible problems before they occur. It recognises that in complex care, there are many areas where errors are made and a review of practice aims to break down the process to component elements and identify potential problems. Having identified any areas where the safety of the patient—or staff—could be compromised, it is then possible to introduce checks of, and changes to, practice so as to minimise or remove risks in care.

Effective communication

It is important to ensure that patients and their carers have an understanding of the various aspects of the care being provided to them. Knowledge and understanding of the problem, the management options and the potential outcomes are all important for the patient and will reduce the fears and worries brought about by ignorance. It is imperative that members of the MDT take time to address these concerns and present the information in an understandable manner that is devoid of jargon. It is also imperative that effective verbal and written communication takes place between members of the MDT.

PRACTICE POINT—risk assessment of administration of vincristine

Children and adults diagnosed with acute lymphoblastic leukaemia receive multiple chemotherapy drugs orally, intravenously (IV) and intrathecally (IT).

Historical protocols required the administration of intrathecal methotrexate and intravenous vincristine on the same day. Sadly, there were some patients who were erroneously given vincristine intrathecally and died from vincristine neurotoxicity.

Following one such event, the Chief Medical Officer in the UK appointed an external and independent assessor to look at the events surrounding the practice. Evidence was taken and the series of events which led to the death of a patient following vincristine given into the intrathecal space were reviewed in detail. National mandatory guidelines were produced and strict changes to practice were required in all centres providing intrathecal chemotherapy. These included:
- only approved centres treating appropriate numbers of patients allowed to administer IT chemotherapy
- national protocol changed so IV vincristine and IT methotrexate to be given on separate days
- only fully trained medical staff to prescribe IT chemotherapy
- only fully trained pharmacy staff allowed to dispense IV and IT chemotherapy
- only fully trained staff in designated centres allowed to administer intrathecal drugs
- all intrathecal needles in the institution use connector which is incompatible with standard syringe fittings
- drugs for intravenous administration dispensed in syringes incompatible with intrathecal needle connector or in infusion bags

These changes and others were introduced and aimed to remove all risk to patients receiving treatment.

Engaging with public and users

Most aspects of clinical care are improved by seeking the opinions and experiences of patients and carers. They offer a unique insight into all aspects of care and often identify issues which the clinical team may have failed to recognise. Changes based on patient experience can lead to significant improvements in patient care.

Information governance

All who work in the NHS have a legal responsibility to protect the personal and clinical details of patients. The importance of patient confidentiality cannot be overemphasized, and restricting access to clinical information to only those who have a need to know should be at the centre of any health care service. All UK institutions require their staff to attend courses on information governance and to realise the many ways—often inadvertent—where patient details can be shared with inappropriate individuals. Examples would include:

- overheard corridor conversations
- computer terminals left open and showing patient details
- medical notes left in public places
- handover sheets being lost
- emails shared with inappropriate individuals
- clinical letters sent to wrong addresses
- clinical details left on answerphones

Apply patient safety thinking

Clinical team leaders have a responsibility to ensure that the care provided is appropriate for the individual patient and their particular circumstances. All clinicians must ensure that they apply up-to-date understanding of all the problems that is effective and safe. Examples would include checking:

- patient details are correct and refer to the patient being assessed
- the treatment proposed is the most up-to-date and appropriate for that patient
- any drug doses are appropriate for age and clinical condition
- patient and carer have an appropriate understanding of the intended intervention and consent has been obtained from the patient and carer

A further example of the need to consider patient safely was the introduction a Paediatric Early Warning Score (PEWS) system. This technique is designed to identify children who may be unstable and at risk of a clinical deterioration. It uses age-appropriate sheets to record standard core observations and identify whether these parameters together indicate an adverse trend. Some systems use coloured banding for observations to ensure all values are recognised as abnormal but all will produce an overall score of the clinical status of the patient. It provided a visual and graded aid to staff that forewarned of a clinical deterioration in the patient and prompted the need to seek more senior review and advice in a timely manner. There is an aim to produce a single PEWS system and charts for all health care institutions in the UK.

Human factors in patient care

Providing high-quality patient care is a complex and demanding practice involving many individuals at many levels of experience. Those who have a role in reviewing clinical problems recognise that many errors are not the result of one individual—they are often the result of a series of small but accumulating mistakes at many levels. Examples of contributing factors would include:

Health care institution

There is a need for a safety culture where all employers recognise that they have a prominent role in protecting patients from potential harm.

Communication

Robust methods of communication are vital for excellent patient care and communication failures are a leading cause of inadvertent patient harm. Failure to hand over important details of patient management, failure to record details of event in the notes or the 'status effect' where a junior team member feels unable to challenge the actions of a senior are all examples of sources of communication failure.

Team structure

Rigorous introduction of the concept that teams anticipate complex issues and undertake pretask briefings. One such example is the WHO Surgical Safety checklist to be used with an operating team prior to surgery where every member is introduced and their roles clarified, patient details are checked and the planned operation details are confirmed. The process also ensures all relevant equipment and team members are available and creates opportunities for all team members to speak up if concerns are identified.

Team leadership (supervisors)

Team members need to understand the team structure and be clear in their mind who is responsible for specific patients and for certain decisions on care. Team leaders need to be available for advice and to guide the team in establishing priorities in patient care.

Decision making

Standard patient care produces multiple occasions where decisions are required and some may be made outside the experience of the team member. A culture where the seeking of support and guidance is important and to be encouraged.

Stress

Clinical work with often complex and demanding problems can lead to significant mental and physical pressures

CLINICAL SCENARIO

A 7-year-old boy was admitted for a planned repair of a scoliosis under the care of the adult spinal surgical team. The operation proved difficult and the patient was managed in the paediatric intensive care for 48 hours. Due to pressure on the beds in the intensive care unit the boy was transferred back to the surgical ward at 03:00 hrs. Over the following 3 days, the boy was reviewed by senior spinal surgical team members accompanied by the ward-based doctor. An ongoing diarrhoeal illness was recorded each day in the notes and fluid adjustments made. A sudden collapse occurred on the third ward day and the emergency paediatric medical team was called. Assessment of fluid status and associated hypotension was corrected and the child made a full recovery.

A serious untoward incident review was undertaken. It identified that poor communication between clinical teams resulted in the avoidable incident. The spinal surgical team had assumed that the senior medical team was reviewing the child each day. The review also noted the transfer of the child from the PICU had been arranged by ward-based teams and senior medical staff were unaware of the presence of the child until the acute event.

Following the SUI review, new policies were introduced to address these issues. Clarity of regular senior involvement in patient reviews along with clear and direct communication between clinical teams on patient transfers was established as a hospital-wide policy.

on team members. Reactions to stress can vary between individuals and range from impacting on mood to impacting on health. On occasions the stress and pressures can be so great as to lead to suicide. It is imperative that colleagues try and be aware of the stresses in others and aim to mitigate and support where possible.

Fatigue

Most individuals work in a shift pattern but fatigue is always possible. Long and demanding shifts can bring emotional fatigue whilst personal or domestic problems can all impact on the ability of the clinician to act effectively. Colleagues must aim to support wherever possible.

Work environment

Some clinical settings are not appropriate for the tasks allocated to that area and consequently increase the risk of patient harm. Inadequate information systems, rooms that are not private such that conversations are overheard or examinations observed and lack of availability of appropriate equipment.

Education and training

Lifelong learning and regular appraisal are part of normal practice and should be part of established practice for all clinical staff.

Safe and effective handover

The current practice for providing clinical care for patients requires multiple clinical teams and their members to transfer both the responsibility of care and the attendant clinical information, in a safe and clearly understood manner. All members of those disparate teams, whether they have direct contact with patients or are involved in supporting the contact team, will provide care during differing parts of the day and different parts of the week. It is therefore vital that there are effective and robust systems in place to share and hand on clinical information. Both verbal and written information relating to patient management occur many times each day and robust systems are needed to eliminate errors and misunderstanding in such handovers.

Formal handover sessions are now well established for most teams providing direct patient care. The exact format of that event will differ between different institutions and the clinical teams working there and no single structure applies to all teams. There are, however, some core features for handover meetings to ensure that safe and comprehensive information is passed to colleagues. These include:

- agreed fixed times for the handover (usually morning, late afternoon, evening)
- adequate time allowed for meeting but focussed and time-limited
- adequate location to accommodate all participants and allow for confidentiality
- all team members to attend except if an emergency occurs
- senior clinician attends meetings
- adequate information technology to access lab results and radiology
- all patients listed with their identification and location
- unstable patients and those with concerns are presented in detail
- focused presentation of information on all other patients
- presentation of tasks to be completed
- provision of a full list of results that need to be reviewed
- action plans developed and clearly communicated in meeting
- clear allocation of responsibilities

Formal structure to the handover and clear team leadership has obvious benefits for all under the care of the team. The brief and focussed meeting will also have a benefit for the clinical staff by:

- promoting the culture of seeking senior advice
- providing support to senior and junior colleagues
- providing professional protection by clarifying roles and responsibilities
- generating opportunities for education and understanding

Interactions between individuals lies at the core of effective team working and mutual support. The need to ensure that the transfer of requests or instruction between colleagues will also benefit from a more formalised approach particularly if there is a difference in seniority between individuals. One such recognised structure uses an acronym—SBAR (Situation, Background, Assessment, Recommendation)—and is used to provide safe, effective and agreed understanding for the sharing of information between team members such as in telephone contacts (Tables 33.1 and 33.2).

Table 33.1 Example of SBAR in conversation between junior doctor and consultant

S	Situation	"Hello. Is that Dr Jones and are you the on-call consultant for paediatric medicine? Thank you. I'm Dr Wilson, ST1 doctor covering E38 paediatric ward tonight, and I've been asked to see Daniel Smith, a 2-month-old boy who was admitted tonight with vomiting.
B	Background	Daniel was born at term by normal delivery and was well until yesterday. He had been bottle fed until then but started to vomit small amounts. There is no associated diarrhoea and all other family members are well. Examination showed him to be mildly dehydrated and anxious looking. The vomiting has become more frequent and forceful. Examination showed no abnormalities. Blood and urine samples have been sent and results awaited.
A	Assessment	I think he may have pyloric stenosis but am also considering a urinary tract infection.
R	Recommendation	You suggest we stop oral fluids, start IV fluids and await blood and urine results. You want me to contact you again in about an hour following a patient review and with the results. Thank you."

Table 33.2 Example of SBAR in conversation between doctor and a young patient with asthma

S	Situation	"Hello. I'm Dr Green and I am one of the paediatric doctors. Can I just confirm that you are Michelle Thompson and you are 13 years old? And that this is your mum. Thank you. My colleague Dr Wilson saw you earlier today when you came into hospital and she asked me to come and check how you are.
B	Background	I know that you have asthma and have had this since you were much younger and that you are usually well. You use a blue inhaler when you are feeling tight chested or before any sport sessions at school. I gather it was very cold today at the start of your football training and your inhaler wasn't helpful so you came to the emergency department.
A	Assessment	When Dr Wilson saw you earlier, she decided that you needed added oxygen and the salbutamol by a nebuliser and asked me to come and see you to check that things are improving. All your observations recorded on this chart are much better and that suggests that you are improving. With your permission, I would like to listen to your chest to be sure all is well.
R	Recommendation	I think we should keep the oxygen going for the time being but we can reduce how often we give you salbutamol by a nebuliser and let's see how you cope with that. We will come back and see you again in about an hour to be sure things continue to improve. Does that make sense? And have you or your mum got any questions?"

Further reading

Acute care toolkit: Handover. Royal College of Physicians (UK). Published September 2015. https://www.rcplondon.ac.uk/guidelines-policy/acute-care-toolkit-1-handover

Clinical governance. Public Health England. Updated March 2021. https://www.gov.uk/government/publications/newborn-hearing-screening-programme-nhsp-operational-guidance/4-clinical-governance

Chapter | 34 |

Evidence-based paediatrics

Lucy Foard, Agnieszka Jaworska-Ganly

After reading this chapter you should be able to:
- apply evidence-based medicine to clinical practice
- interpret a research paper or systematic review appropriately

Evidence-based paediatrics requires the paediatrician to use the current best evidence in the assessment of clinical conditions and treatment options and to apply that to the specific needs of the individual young patient. Consequently, an understanding of the scientific evidence that supports clinical practice is one of the many important skills for the paediatrician to master, in particular the ability to read and understand both the strengths and the limitations of published studies and so identify the most appropriate management plan.

It is appropriate to develop an open and critical approach to any published work and to develop a structured review of any an article. The essence of scientific publication has always been to seek input and opinion from colleagues with knowledge and understanding of the study topic and to allow any conclusions to be supported or challenged.

A structured review used in the assessment of published research
- the relevance of the research question to current clinical practice
- clear definitions provided for study groups and parameters
- study topics stated clearly at the start of the trial
- changes to study protocol are presented and implications considered
- study population relevant to current clinical practice
- study population correctly identified, recruited and recruitment bias avoided
- presence of appropriate controls
- sample size correctly calculated to answer the initial question
- appropriate outcomes measured rather than surrogate markers
- appropriate statistical tests used
- appropriate conclusions drawn

Study design

Publications of studies follow a standard format and present the background to the issue of interest, the methodology to be used, the results obtained, the outcomes discussed and the references used.

A recognition of the numerous formats that are used in obtaining data in a published study is an important first step in understanding the strengths of the conclusions drawn. The 'Hierarchy of Evidence' ranks study design formats and their potential for bias or systematic error.

Systematic Reviews are a collation and summary of all evidence in a particular area and include metaanalyses where results from different studies are reanalysed together. They provide an improvement in the assessment of a topic

Table 34.1 Hierarchy of Evidence as proposed by Professor Greenhalgh. This sets out the most common study design formats and ranks the potential for bias or systematic error

Level	Type of evidence
I	Systematic reviews and metaanalyses of RCTs with definitive results
II	RCTs with definitive results (confidence intervals that do not overlap)
III	RCTs with nondefinitive results (clinically significant effect but with confidence intervals overlapping the threshold for this effect)
IV	Cohort studies
V	Case-control studies
VI	Cross sectional surveys
VII	Case reports

RCT = Randomised controlled trial.

of interest by increasing the size of the populations studied and thereby provide a greater precision and generalisability than single studies. They also use predefined and transparent criteria in the collection and analysis of the combined information. The quality—that is the risk bias—of included studies is evaluated, with particular assessment of the methods of subject selection, randomisation and blinding.

Randomised control trial (RCT). Subjects are randomly assigned to one of two groups (experimental versus control) with the only expected difference being the outcome studied, and consequently these types of studies provide the most reliable evidence on the effectiveness of interventions. In a blind RCT study, the participants in the clinical trial do not know if they are receiving the placebo or the real treatment, whilst in a double-blind study, neither the participants nor the researchers are aware of which group of individuals are to receive the placebo and which are to receive the experimental treatment. This aims to minimise the placebo effect and bias.

Crossover study. This is a variation of the RCT where all subjects receive all treatment options consecutively but the order in which these treatments are offered is randomised. There may even be multiple phases in the study with differing treatment options, and in such studies each patient will act as their own control. Crossover studies are useful when recruitment to a trial may leave some participants not being offered a new trial medication and so making recruitment difficult.

Cohort studies are used to study incidence, causes and prognosis. They are usually prospective in nature and follow individuals with a particular condition or who receive a particular treatment and they are compared with another group of people who are not affected by the condition or who did not receive the treatment. Longitudinal studies are required for questions about prognosis.

Case-control studies can be considered retrospective. They begin with the outcomes and do not follow people over time. Researchers choose individuals with a particular characteristic (the cases) and compare features of interest with a control group of individuals who do not have the characteristic. This type of study is required for questions around causation.

Lower-level designs include cross-sectional studies where a defined population is observed at a single point in time or at certain time intervals, case reports and expert opinions.

Methods

Statistical and sample size

Statistical power refers to the ability to identify an effect that is present in a population using a test based on a sample from that population. It is directly linked to sample size and too few patients may mean there is not enough power to detect a difference of interest. Complex and formal power calculations need to be undertaken prior to the start of a study to ensure that it has sufficient statistical power to determine any differences between groups.

Table 34.2 Factors that determine statistical power

incidence	an outcome that occurs infrequently requires many more patients in order to detect a difference
population variance	the greater the variance (standard deviation) in the population then the more patients are needed to demonstrate a significant difference
treatment effect size	a small difference in any effect between groups or treatments needs a higher number of subjects to allow identification of those differences. the opposite is true
alpha type-I error	refers to the probability of finding a difference when a difference does not exist. The most common alpha cut-off used is 5% (often seen as $p \leq 0.05$), indicating a 5% chance that a significant difference is actually due to chance and is not a true difference
beta type-II error	refers to the probability of not detecting a difference when one actually exists. Beta is directly related to study power. Most research uses a beta cutoff of 20% (0.2), indicating a 20% chance that a significant difference is missed

Bias

The interpretation or appraisal of outcomes requires consideration as to whether the outcome is truly due to the treatment or intervention or whether other explanations are possible. Systematic errors may be introduced into sampling or testing and lead to various types of bias.

Research bias can compromise the validity of the interpretation of outcomes, leading to the exclusion of a true effect or the acceptance of a false one. Bias can be divided into:
- selection bias
- information bias
- confounding variables

Selection bias is linked to the recruitment of patients; a cohort of individuals deciding not to participate in the study could lead to under- or overestimation of a particular effect or risk. Patients lost to follow-up, self-selection into a study and lack of randomisation are further examples.

Information bias occurs when patients are misclassified, for example, when individuals with a particular disease or exposure are classified as nondiseased or nonexposed due to an inaccuracy of diagnostic tests. Such a problem will invalidate outcomes.

Confounders are variables that influence both the dependent variable and independent variable, causing a spurious association. Confounding variables are those that may compete with the exposure of interest (e.g. treatment) in explaining the outcome of a study. For example, in a study about whether a lack of exercise (independent variable) leads to weight gain (dependent variable) in children, the number of calories consumed would be a confounding variable. Identifying possible confounders early on and controlling for them will assist in eliminating bias.

> **PRACTICE POINT—considerations for reducing bias in research studies**
>
> - well-designed research protocols
> - randomised selection of patients
> - random allocation to groups
> - blind or double blind
> - balance confounding variable across groups
> - maximising follow up
> - analysing randomised controlled trial data on 'intention to treat' principle

Data analysis

Statistical tests

The most commonly used statistical tests are shown along with the appropriate conditions under which they should be used. They can generally split into:
- tests of difference—comparing means
- tests of relationships—strength of correlations between variables

It is important to understand the basis and appropriateness of tests used in analysing the collected data.

The chi-squared (χ^2) test falls outside of the above categories and is a test of association. The test is designed for use with nominal data (named categories), and the frequency of such data is presented in a contingency table. Chi-squared tests are commonly performed on 2 x 2 data, for example, to investigate if there is an association between maternal smoking (yes or no) and child's asthma status (asthmatic or not asthmatic) in a given population. Larger chi-squared tables can be used.

Values of statistical test outcomes are not useful on their own, and the drawing of conclusions relies on interpretation of the associated confidence intervals and p-values. The correlation R-value would be an exception to this as its value indicates the strength of the correlation.

The summary statistics that are usually used to measure treatment effect mostly include odds ratios (OR), relative risks (RR) and mean differences (from tests such as t-tests and ANOVA). This data is commonly expressed as a value, followed by a confidence interval in brackets.

Data outcomes

The results of studies will show the summarised data with calculated values of means and ranges along with assessments of the strength of this data. Confidence intervals

Table 34.3 Statistical tests and their application to data types

Tests of difference		
Tests used to:	**Parametric data**	**Non-parametric data**
compare two paired (related) groups	t-test (paired)	Wilcoxon signed rank
compare three or more unmatched (independent) groups	ANOVA	Kruskal–Wallis
compare three or more matched (related) groups/conditions	ANOVA (repeated measures)	Friedman's ANOVA
investigate relationship between two variables	Pearson's correlation	Spearman's rank

Tests of relationship		
Tests should	**Parametric data**	**Non-parametric data**
investigate relationship between two variables	Pearson's correlation	Spearman's rank
predict a value from other measured variables (relationships between)	Logistic regression (category variable) or Linear regression (continuous variable)	Nonparametric regression (less used)

and p-values are the usual additions to help the reader understand the provided values.

Interpretation of confidence intervals and p-values

- a confidence interval is calculated as a measure of treatment effect and shows the range within which the true treatment effect is likely to lie (subject to a number of assumptions)
- a p-value is calculated to assess whether trial results are likely to have occurred simply through chance
- confidence intervals are preferable to p-values, as they tell us the range of possible effect sizes compatible with the data
- p-values simply provide a cutoff beyond which it can be asserted that the findings are 'statistically significant' (most commonly, this cutoff is $p < 0.05$)

379

Confidence intervals

For most research, it is usually impossible to study every individual within a population. Researchers therefore can only estimate the parameters of a population by calculating an estimated range for those parameters using a select sample of this population. The confidence interval is a way of measuring how well values from this sample represent the values of the greater population.

The 'confidence interval' defines the range of values, expressed as upper and lower confidence limits, within which the 'true' population mean is **likely** to lie (given that only using a sample of this population is studied). Most research studies report a 95% confidence interval (95% CI). It is important to emphasise that there is a 5% chance that the 'true' population mean lies outside the quoted range.

If a confidence interval is narrow, more precise population estimates can be made, but if the interval is wider, then the uncertainty is greater, although there may still be enough precision to make decisions about the efficacy of an intervention. Sample size affects the width of the confidence interval and, in normal circumstances, as the sample size increases, the range of the interval will narrow.

The confidence interval alone can indicate whether a result is significant but the p-value is required to confirm the statistical strength of this significance.

Example 1: Study that uses confidence intervals

Study: Activity levels in children following a school exercise programme
(This is a fictitious study to demonstrate statistical interpretation)
Objective: To detect changes in levels of activity in year 8 teenagers (12–13 years old) following a school-delivered fitness and exercise programme in one town in the UK and to assess whether the normal level of parental exercise influenced any changes.
Design: A cross-sectional study carried out in the same school classes before and after the introduction of the fitness and exercise programme. Participants and their carers were given fitness tracker devices to wear for 1 full week before and after the exercise programme. Devices recorded daily steps taken but the devices did not display the results. Parents were split into those who achieved an average of more than 10k steps per day and those who achieved less.
Participants: 1356 children, mean age 12.6 years, surveyed 2 months before introduction of the exercise programme and 1176 in the same school classes surveyed 2 months later.
Outcome measures: Data analysis using combination of steps taken and distance covered when walking, running or cycling. The device was able to exclude motorised journeys.
Results:
- the overall geometric mean of daily steps undertaken by the teenagers increased from 12.3k (95% confidence intervals (CI) 7.5 to 14.1) to 17.7k (95% CI 15.2 to 20.3) after the exercise programme
- for children whose mother figure achieved more than 10k daily steps, there was an increase in the mean number of daily steps taken from 11.4k (95% 10.9 to 12.1) to 13.5k (95% CI 11.6 to 14.3) after the exercise programme
- for children whose mother figure did not achieve more than 10k daily steps, there was an increase in the mean number of daily steps taken from 8.7k (95% 7.2 to 11.7) to 11.2k (95% CI 11.3 to 13.2) after the exercise programme
- for children whose father figure achieved more than 10k daily steps, there was an increase in the mean number of daily steps taken from 11.9k (95% CI 10.4 to 12.5) to 15.3k (95% CI 13.2 to 16.4) after the exercise programme
- for children whose father figure did not achieve more than 10k daily steps, there was an increase in the mean number of daily steps taken from 10.8k (95% CI 9.7 to 12.5) to 13.9k (95% CI 11.3 to 15.8) after the exercise programme

Which of the following statements are correct?
Select two answers only

A   children in the study whose father figure achieved more than 10k daily steps showed a significant increase in the number of daily steps taken after the exercise programme
B   children in the study whose father figure did not achieve more than 10k daily steps showed a significant increase in the number of daily steps taken after the exercise programme
C   children in the study whose mother figure achieved more than 10k daily steps showed a significant increase in the number of daily steps taken after the exercise programme
D   children in the study whose mother figure achieved more than 10k daily steps showed a significant increase in the number of daily steps taken after the exercise programme
E   the fitness and exercise programme should be introduced into all schools in the UK
F   the fitness and exercise programme was effective in producing an increase in activity in this age group

Source: Fictitious study

Explanation of answers for Example 1.

The study compares the overall geometric mean of daily steps before and after the exercise programme in a group of teenagers and their carers and aims to identify any differences. The best way to determine this would be to use the CI of the difference between the two means (before and after), and if the exercise programme had had no effect, then the mean number of steps taken at each time point would be similar and the 95% confidence interval for the before and after results would overlap. If the exercise programme had produced a significant difference between the mean values for daily steps, then the 95% confidence intervals would not overlap (although by definition, there is an outside possibility that mean values were outside the 95% range).

Interpretation of confidence intervals: difference between the means

Where a research study looks for **differences** in stated outcomes then the usual approach will be to compare the mean values of the feature of interest in the different study groups. If the two groups are very similar then the observations will be in the same range and the difference between the calculated means will be close to zero. Confidence intervals for the difference between group means can then be interpreted as follows:

Interpreting a 95% CI for difference between the means

CI crosses zero	the studied effect is not significant as zero indicates no difference between means
All CI values on same side of zero (all positive or all negative)	the studied effect is significant as the 95% confidence interval does not cross zero

Interpretation of confidence intervals: ratios
When confidence intervals are applied to ratios (OR, RR etc.), then the calculated ratio will be 1 or close to 1 if the two groups under study are the same or very similar. Confidence intervals for the ratios can then be interpreted as follows:

Interpreting a 95% CI for ratios (OR, RR etc)

CI crosses 1	there is no difference between arms of the study and the outcome of the study can be interpreted as not statistically significant

The overall mean number of steps taken is 12.3k before and 17.7k after and the 95% CI do not overlap (7.5 to 14.1 before and 15.2 to 20.3 after the exercise programme). The programme has produced the change (if it was the only intervention) so answer F is correct.

Similarly, the children whose father figure was active (achieved more that 10k daily steps) had an increase in the mean number of daily steps taken from 11.9k to 15.3k and the 95% CI do not overlap (10.4 to 12.5 before and 13.2 to 16.4 after the exercise programme) so answer A is correct.

Although the results of the study are encouraging, the study cannot dictate whether the programme should be introduced. There will be many other factors which would need to be considered including applicability of the programme to all schools.

Interpreting a 95% CI for ratios (OR, RR etc)

CI is less than 1	the intervention is likely to be less effective and, as the ratio does not cross 1, the findings are statistically significant
CI is greater than 1	the intervention is likely to be more effective and, as the ratio does not cross 1, the findings are statistically significant

P-values

P-values are used less frequently and most studies will present confidence intervals in their publications. P-values are used when there is a 'null hypothesis' and direct whether the evidence presented should lead to the 'null hypothesis' being rejected or accepted. P-values help clarify whether the results of a comparison between two forms of treatment are there because of a real difference or whether the difference is due to chance.

The common threshold for p-values is 0.05 which indicates that there is a 1 in 20 chance that there is a real difference between the two arms of a study.

Interpreting a p-value at 0.05 level

$p > 0.05$	the test result is not statistically significant, and therefore the null hypothesis—that no statistical significance or effect between variables will be found—is accepted
$p < 0.05$	the evidence against the null hypothesis is sufficiently strong and the result can be interpreted as statistically significant

The lower the p-value, the higher the significance of the finding.

Data interpretation

Odds

The term 'odds' describes the number of events observed in a particular group against the number of nonevents in the same group. If 12 children in a class of 30 develop a parvovirus infection then the odds of a single child having the infection will be 12:18. Probability is different, though related, and in this same example the probability of a child developing parvovirus infection would be 12/30 or 2/5 (40%).

Odds ratio

An odds ratio (OR) takes this concept further and is a measure of association. It presents the odds of an association between two events such as the patient response using a new medication compared to the odds of the response occurring in those who were not exposed to the intervention (the control group).

The odds ratio can also be used to determine whether a particular exposure is a risk factor for a particular outcome and to compare the magnitude of various risk factors for that outcome.

In the odds ratio:
- the numerator is the odds (number of events/number of no events) in the intervention group
- the denominator is the odds (number of events/number of no events) in the control group

Interpreting an odds ratio

OR = 1	observed outcome is the same in the two groups
OR = <1	intervention gives a poorer outcome
OR = >1	intervention gives a better outcome

Example 2. Study that uses odds ratios

Study: Radiological features in abusive and nonabusive injury
(This is a fictitious study to demonstrate statistical interpretation)

Objective: To identify the evidence base behind the radiological features that differentiate abusive trauma (AT) from nonabusive head trauma (non-AT)

Setting: Metaanalysis of radiological diagnostic databases from 10 major paediatric trauma centres over a 10-year period and including 4392 patients.

Patients: Primary comparative studies of children less than 7 years old attending the trauma centre with final coded radiological features identified as AT and non-AT. Findings were referenced to any safeguarding team conclusions. Main outcome measure are radiological features that differentiate AT from non-AT.

Results: The odds ratio (OR) and 95% confidence intervals (95% CI) for various factors associated with AT were as follows:
- parietal skull: OR 0.6 (95% CI 0.3–0.7)
- proximal dislocation of ulnar: OR 0.8 (95% CI 0.4–2.1)
- transverse fracture femur: OR 0.45 (95% CI 0.1–0.8)
- spiral fracture humerus: OR 0.55 (95% CI 0.3–0.8)
- posterior fractured ribs: OR 4.2 (95% CI 1.2–8.1)

Which of the following statements is correct?
Select one answer only

A   posterior fractured ribs are more commonly associated with AT than non-AT

B   a parietal fracture is significantly more likely to occur in AT than non-AT

C   proximal dislocation of ulnar is significantly more likely due to abuse

D   the finding of a spiral fracture humerus requires referral to social services

E   interpretation is limited by the lack of control subjects

Source: Fictitious study

Explanation of answers to Example 2.

The odds ratio in this question describes a relationship between the observed events and the two different groups surveyed (abusive trauma versus nonabusive trauma). It is important to be clear which group is identified as the 'intervention group' and which is the 'non-intervention group'. In this example those children subject to abusive trauma are the 'intervention group' and those with 'non-abusive' trauma are the 'control group'.

If the values of the observations for each fracture type were exactly the same in each group—AT and non-AT—then the ratio estimate would equal 1. If the ratio estimate was less than 1, then the outcome of interest (e.g. fracture A) occurred less frequently in the intervention group (AT individuals) than in the control group (non-AT individuals). Similarly, if the ratio estimate is greater than 1 then the outcome of interest (e.g. Fracture A) occurred more frequently in the intervention group than in the control group.

Further information comes from the calculated confidence intervals which describe the range within which the true observed ratio may lie. The study results can be displayed graphically in a forest plot to help explain the point further.

If the ratio estimate was to the left of 1 on a forest plot, the outcome of interest (e.g. fracture A) occurred **less frequently** in the intervention group (AT individuals), and if the ratio estimate is located to the right, then the outcome of interest (e.g. fracture A) occurred **more frequently** in the intervention group than in the control group (Figure 34.1).

Only the value and range for fractured ribs is associated with abusive trauma (answer A is correct) and the value does not cross 1 and so makes it a significant observation. The value range for dislocation of the ulnar crosses 1 and therefore the findings for that injury are inconclusive. The other three values indicate that they occur less frequently in AT. This study structure cannot use control subjects—the trauma is either AT or non-AT.

Relative risk (RR)

In statistical terms, risk refers simply to the probability that an event will occur, whether it be a desirable or undesirable event. It explains how many times more likely that an event will occur in the treatment/intervention group, relative to the control group. Relative risk can be calculated by dividing the risk of the event occurring in the intervention group by the risk of it occurring in the control group. For example, a RR of 0.33 would suggest that the intervention group would have a third of the chance of developing Disease X (as compared to the control group) whilst a RR of 10 would indicate that the intervention group would be 10 times more likely to develop the disease compared with the control group.

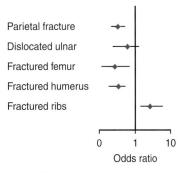

Fig. 34.1 Plot of odds ratio from study of fractures associated with abusive trauma (AT—intervention) and non-abusive trauma (non-AT—control)

Interpreting a relative risk statistic

RR = 1	exposure does not affect outcome
RR = <1	exposure group less at risk of developing problem

Interpreting a relative risk statistic

RR = >1	exposure group at increased risk of developing problem

Example 3. Study that uses relative risk

Study question: Risk of recognised complications with high- and low-dose prednisolone as part of treatment protocol for childhood acute lymphoblastic leukaemia
(This is a fictitious study to demonstrate statistical interpretation)

Objective: To identify the impact of an increased dose of prednisolone used as part of treatment protocol for childhood acute lymphoblastic leukaemia on the survival, risk of clinical obesity and risk of developing hip dysplasia.

Methods: Database interrogation of four international randomised control trials where low-dose and high-dose prednisolone was used as part of the trial treatment in children under 14 years with acute lymphoblastic leukaemia.

Outcome measures:
Incidence of known complications of steroid use including clinical obesity (BMI greater than 95th centile for age) and hip dysplasia.

Results:
A total of 1340 children were recruited.

- Rates of death in the lower and higher dose groups were 27.2% and 19.6%, respectively
- Relative risk of death in the lower dose group was 1.45 (95% CI 1.15 to 1.84)

In 1340 children, when the lower dose option group was compared to the higher dose group and the rates and relative risks were:
for clinical obesity—20.6% versus 23.5%; relative risk 0.77 (95% CI 0.62 to 1.1)
for hip dysplasia—8.4% versus 11.3%; relative risk 1.43 (95% CI 0.98 to 1.77)

What is the most appropriate change of clinical practice to be drawn from the results presented above? Select one answer only

A   change in practice to give low-dose prednisolone to minimise the risk of hip dysplasia

B   change in practice to give high-dose prednisolone because of concerns about increased mortality in lower dose groups

C   the relative risk of death in the lower dose group is not significant and the findings would not support a change in the dose of prednisolone to become standard treatment

D   Population studies with large numbers do not need calculated confidence intervals

E   Change in practice to doses of low-dose prednisolone to minimise the risk of clinical obesity

Source: Fictitious study

Explanation of answers to Example 3.

The relative risk in this question describes the impact of dose changes of prednisolone on risk of death, development of clinical obesity and hip dysplasia. If the risks of the complication (death, obesity, hip dysplasia) were similar from the two interventions (high- and low-dose prednisolone) then the confidence intervals would include

1. Confidence interval ranges below and not including 1 would indicate an advantage of the low-dose treatment whilst those greater than and not including 1 would indicate a disadvantage of the low-dose treatment.

- the CI for the risk of developing hip dysplasia crosses 1 and therefore it is not possible to conclude that there is an advantage to the low-dose prednisolone—answer A is incorrect.

Example 4. Study that uses risk difference

Objective and design:

A cohort study investigated the incidence of strokes in adult life for those children given cranial irradiation for tinea compared with a control group who did not receive cranial irradiation.

Results:

During the study period, 112 adults were found to have had a stroke from the cohort of 6227 who had received cranial irradiation in childhood, and 21 adults had had a stroke from a cohort of 11592 age-matched controls who had not received cranial irradiation. The risk difference is RR1 (112/6227 = 0.018) - RR2 (21/11590 = 0.002) = 0.016.

Explanation:

The risk difference of 0.016 suggests that there is a 1.6% increased risk of developing a stroke if exposed to radiation.

Source: Fictitious study

- the relative risk for the low-dose group is greater than 1 and therefore is an adverse outcome—answer B is correct.
- the relative risk of death in the low dose is increased and is significant—answer C is incorrect.
- confidence intervals are crucial in large numbered studies to help define the likely population mean—answer D is incorrect.
- clinical obesity is certainly less prevalent in the low-dose group but the CI do not confirm that the difference is significant—answer E is incorrect.

Risk difference

Risk difference (RD) (often called attributable risk or excessive risk) can be defined as the difference in risk of a condition, such as a disease, between an exposed group and an unexposed group.

If RR1 is the disease risk in an exposed population and RR2 is the disease risk in a nonexposed population then the risk difference (RD) equals RR1–RR2. RD can therefore be a number between -1 and +1.

Interpreting a risk difference statistic

RD = zero   no difference in risk between groups

Interpreting a risk difference statistic

RD = less than zero (negative)   decreased risk in exposed group

RD = greater than zero (positive)   increased risk in exposed group

Number needed to treat

The number needed to treat (NNT) can be understood as the number of patients that need to be treated in order for one to benefit. For example, an NNT of 20 would be interpreted as '20 patients need to be treated to avoid one additional death'.

If the NNT was 1, then all patients in the treatment group will have benefitted, but no one in the control arm will have benefitted. Generally, the higher the NNT, the less effective the treatment, because more people need to receive the treatment for one person to benefit. Any clinically observed benefit, however, could make the intervention worthwhile, and an NNT of 30 could still be beneficial if the outcome was life threatening.

Further reading

Greenhalgh T: How to read a paper. *Getting your bearings* (deciding what the paper is about). BMJ. 1997;315(7102):243–246.

Goldacre, B. *Bad Science*. Harper Collins. 2008

Makin TR, Orban de Xivry JJ: *Ten common statistical mistakes to watch out for when writing or reviewing a manuscript.* https://elifesciences.org/articles/48175.

Chapter | 35 |

Exam questions and answers

Martin Hewitt

This chapter contains 50 questions in the style and format of the MRCPCH AKP examination. A single exam paper would contain 60 questions and take 150 minutes (2½ hours) to complete. These 50 questions would therefore take 125 mins to complete if you choose to run the questions as a practice exam.

Questions

Question 1
A 14-year-old male was brought to the emergency department by his mother who found him collapsed in his bedroom. He had admitted to taking a large quantity of his mother's antidepressant medication in the morning with the intention of taking his life.

Which of the following features in a history would indicate an increased risk of later successful suicide? (Select one answer only).
A. diagnosis of depression
B. early morning timing
C. finding a letter explaining reasons
D. recent death of father
E. recent parental separation

Question 2
A 9-year-old boy was referred by his GP following parental concerns about his behaviour. He was described as aggressive at times and prone to temper tantrums. He would often leave things behind at school and then suggest that this was due to instructions from his teacher. His teachers described him as intelligent and although easily distracted, he could be absorbed in some of his work. His mother acted as a single parent as his father was in prison for armed robbery. He was born at 34 weeks' gestation but required no intensive neonatal interventions.

His height and weight followed the 75th centile and there were no abnormal findings on examination.

What is the most likely explanation for his presenting problems? (Select one answer only)
A. attention deficit disorder
B. autism spectrum disorder
C. disruptive domestic circumstances
D. hyperactivity disorder
E. oppositional defiant disorder

Question 3
The 19-year-old mother and her 1-year-old daughter attend paediatric outpatients' clinic following a referral for advice about a family condition. The brother of the mother is now 18 years old and requires full support at home having been diagnosed with Wiskott-Aldrich syndrome. Mother is well without any health issues.

What is the chance of the 1-year-old daughter inheriting Wiskott-Aldrich syndrome? (Select one answer only)
A. 1 in 2 chance of inheriting
B. 1 in 4 chance of inheriting
C. 2 in 3 chance of inheriting
D. No chance of inheriting
E. Unable to say as mother of baby needs assessment

Question 4
A 14-month-old boy was referred from the emergency department with a 3-day history of vomiting and constipation. Concerns were also raised about his growth. His parents were asylum seekers having recently arrived in the UK. He was born at term, weighed approximately 3 kg and appeared normal at that time. He had never been able to weight bear or walk but his speech, vision and hearing were thought to be normal. His parents were first cousins and they had three children alive and well but two others had died when under 2 years old with vomiting illnesses.

On examination, his weight and length were below the <0.4 centile and head circumference was on the 50th centre. He was extremely wasted and dehydrated and had swelling of the wrists and bowing of the lower limbs. He had reduced tone but no focal neurological signs. Rest of examination was normal.

The initial results show:

Full blood count normal

Sodium	126 mmol/l	(133–146)
Potassium	1.4 mmol/l	(3.5–5.5)
Bicarbonate	11 mmol/l	(19–28)
Urea	7.2 mmol/l	(2.5–6.5)
Glucose	3.2 mmol/l	(3.0–6.0)
Calcium	2.1 mmol/l	(2.2–2.7)
Phosphate	0.9 mmol/l	(0.9–1.8)
ALP	1560 U/l	(76–308)

Urine in pH 6; protein plus; glucose trace

What is the most likely explanation for these findings? (Select one answer only)
A. Bartter syndrome
B. Fanconi syndrome
C. Galactosaemia
D. MCAD deficiency
E. Mucopolysaccharidoses

Question 5
A 3-year-old boy was brought to the emergency department following the development of a rash on his face, trunk and limbs. His family was originally from the Egypt and he had recently eaten a cracker with tahini (sesame) and immediately felt an itching sensation on his tongue. A rash had developed within 30 minutes but there were no associated difficulties with his breathing. He responded to chlorphenamine. He had previously been diagnosed with eczema and mild hay fever but there was no family history of atopy.

On examination he had a widespread urticarial rash.

Which investigation is the most appropriate to identify the cause of his presentation? (Select one answer only)
A. C1 esterase inhibitor levels
B. Food challenge test with sesame
C. Serum IgE levels
D. Serum tryptase levels
E. Skin prick testing with sesame

Question 6
A 14-year-old boy has had a second relapse of his osteosarcoma and has developed pulmonary metastases. Following discussions with him and his parents it is agreed that further curative treatment will not be offered and active management of his palliative needs will be introduced. He currently an in-patient whilst the plan for his pain management is established.

His current symptom is that of bone pain and this requires oral morphine at a dose of 5 mg every 4 hours.

What would be the appropriate next step to improve his pain control should the current regime fail? (Select one answer only)
A. Convert to a fentanyl patch at an adjusted higher dose
B. Increase frequency to every 2–3 hourly
C. Increase morphine dose but continue at every 4 hours
D. Start intravenous diamorphine as patient-controlled analgesia
E. Start subcutaneous diamorphine infusion

Question 7
A 3-year-old boy was brought to the emergency department by his father. He had been with his grandmother for the day and she had reported that he had not been 'his usual self' for about an hour before his father picked him up. Over the following 2 hours at home, he became agitated and then increasingly drowsy. His father noted he had some jerking movements whilst being brought to hospital.

On examination in hospital, his observations are pulse 124/minute, respiratory rate 24/minute and temperature 37.3°C. His oxygen saturations are 98% with face mask oxygen. He has normal volume pulses, normal heart sounds and a capillary refill of <2 seconds. His chest is clear and there is no increased respiratory effort. Examination of the abdomen is normal. He opens his eyes to painful stimuli and has some abnormal flexion movements. He is only making mumbling sounds.

What is the next most important response? (Select one answer only)
A. Administer IV ceftriaxone
B. Administer IV mannitol
C. Arrange urgent CT scan of head
D. Collect urine for toxicology
E. Intubation and ventilation

Question 8
You are a junior doctor who has started working on the oncology ward in the last week. You are asked by the new registrar to prescribe an intrathecal methotrexate dose for a patient who is due to receive the dose whilst under anaesthesia for the insertion of a central venous line.

What is the most appropriate response? (Select one answer only)
A. Advise delay administration of dose until next anaesthesia
B. Check protocol to confirm dose and timing of methotrexate
C. Discuss with oncology pharmacist
D. Indicate that you are unable to prescribe the dose
E. Prescribe the intrathecal dose

Question 9
You will be presented with a list of ECG findings and three scenarios.

Which of the following ECG abnormalities is the most likely cause of the presentations described? (One answer only for each scenario).
A. axis deviated to right
B. axis—superior
C. P wave peaked
D. Prolonged PR interval
E. QRS complex widened
F. QT interval prolonged
G. QT interval shortened
H. T wave flattened
I. T wave inverted in V6
J. T wave upright in V1

Scenario 1
A 6-week-old boy presented with cardiac failure and echocardiogram showed a partial atrioventricular septal defect.

Scenario 2
A 7-year-old girl had started chemotherapy having been diagnosed with high white count acute lymphoblastic leukaemia. Examination undertaken at 12 hours after starting treatment described her as 'twitchy' and revealed positive Chvostek and Trousseau signs.

Scenario 3
A 2-year-old girl was found to have a cardiac murmur during examination for a chest infection. Further examination revealed a carotid thrill and a 4/6 ejection systolic murmur in the upper right sternal edge.

Question 10
A 15-year-old girl was referred to out-patients and attended with her mother. Her father had been diagnosed with Huntington disease and was advising all his family to be tested for the condition. The girl was well without any symptoms and both she and her mother were requesting that she was 'tested for the gene' for Huntington disease.

Which is the most appropriate action for managing this request? (Select one answer only)
A. Advise waiting until she is over 18 before undertaking any testing
B. Arrange testing for the Huntington disease gene
C. Obtain more details of the results of the father
D. Reassure her that females cannot develop Huntington disease
E. Refer to genetics for counselling

Question 11
A 2-year-old girl was referred to out-patients for review of recurrent coughs, temperatures and poor speech. She was born at term but spent 3 days in the neonatal unit due to an oxygen requirement and was discharged home without need for respiratory support. Throughout her first year of life, she had recurrent chest infections that were treated with antibiotics. She failed a routine screening test for hearing at 12 months but was not brought for further investigation until she was 18 months old when bilateral grommets were inserted and her hearing improved considerably. Height and weight were following the 2nd centile.

Examination identified tachypnoea, hyperinflation of the chest, Harrison's sulci and bilateral coarse crepitations in both lung fields. The chest x-ray taken in clinic is shown below (Figure 35.1).

Which of the following investigations will identify the underlying cause for this presentation? (Select one answer only)
A. Bronchoscopy
B. Echocardiography
C. High resolution CT chest
D. Nasal brush biopsy
E. Sweat test

Question 12
A 4-year-old girl was brought to the emergency department by her grandparents who had been looking after her for the day. She had been found collapsed in the house whilst out of their sight for only a few minutes. She had been perfectly well before wandering into the kitchen on her own. There was no suggestion of trauma or a fall. The grandparents were worried that she may have eaten peanuts as these were found scattered on the floor. She was known to have asthma and eczema and the child's parents were concerned that she may have food allergies.

Examination found her to be pale and floppy, responding poorly to stimuli. Her pulse was 160/minute, capillary refill was 5 seconds, systolic blood pressure was 75mmHg. Oxygen saturation was 90% in air.

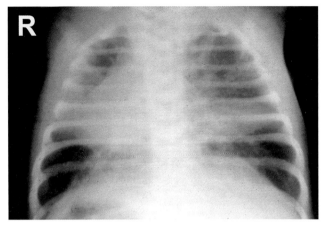

Fig. 35.1 Question 11.

What is the next most important step in her management? (Select one answer only)
A. Give 0.9% saline bolus 20 ml/kg
B. Give adrenaline 1:1000 150 mcg IM
C. Give adrenaline 1:1000 150 mcg IV
D. Give adrenaline 1:1000 300 mcg IM
E. Give hydrocortisone 100 mg IV

Question 13

A 7-year-old girl was referred with concerns about adult sweat odour, acne and pubic hair. Her mother was worried that this was early puberty and that she would start her periods very soon. There was no obvious history of growth acceleration and she was otherwise well with no significant past medical or drug history. Her mother had had gestational diabetes in all three of her pregnancies and her paternal grandfather and his sister had type 2 diabetes. Her mother started her periods at 11 years and her father's voice broke at about 15 years.

On examination her height is on the 75th centile which is tall for family size with the mid-parental centile 25th–50th. Her weight is on 99.6th and her calculated BMI >99.6th centile for age. Breast development is difficult to score due to her body habitus but is assessed as B1. Examination of the perineum shows sparse long pubic hair confined to the vulva and is otherwise normal. The remainder of the examination is unremarkable.

What is the most likely diagnosis? (Select one answer only)
A. Androgen secreting ovarian tumour
B. Congenital adrenal hyperplasia
C. Cushing disease
D. Exaggerated adrenarche
E. Gonadotrophin dependent sexual precocity

Question 14

A 6-year-old boy was seen in the emergency department with pyrexia and lethargy. He was recently diagnosed with asthma and was started on inhaled budesonide the week before this attendance. His mother had gestational diabetes whilst his maternal grandma was on metformin.

On examination, his height and weight are on the 9th centile. He is apyrexial, clinically well and no abnormalities are found on examination.

Initial urinalysis showed:

Blood	negative
Protein	negative
Ketones	negative
Nitrites	negative
Glucose	++

Further investigations showed:

Random blood sugar	8.8 mmol/l	3.0–6.0 mmol/l
HbA1c	54 mmol/mmol	20–42 mmol/mol
Fasting blood sugar	6.7 mmol/l	3.0–6.0 mmol/l

What is the most likely cause for his glycosuria? (Select one answer only)
A. Monogenic diabetes
B. Renal glycosuria
C. Steroid induced glycosuria
D. Type 2 diabetes
E. Urinary tract infection

Question 15

A 3-week-old boy was admitted with vomiting up to 4 times daily for the last 2 days. The vomiting was not related to feeding and was not projectile. His bowel frequency had reduced but the stools were normal. He was born at term and was discharged home the following day. His birth weight was 3.6 kg.

On examination the baby weighed 3.7 kg and is clinically undernourished with redundant skin folds. He is drowsy, clinically dehydrated with cool peripheries and he has a sunken fontanelle. His temperature is 37.8°C, pulse 176/minute and BP 75/30. The remainder of the examination was unremarkable.

The initial results show:

Sodium	119 mmol/l	(135–146)
Potassium	7.8 mmol/l	(3.5–5.3)
Bicarbonate	13 mmol/l	(19–28)
Urea	15.3 mmol/l	(0.8–5.5)
Creatinine	96 μmol/l	(21–75)
Glucose	1.9 mmol/l	(2.5–5.5)

Which investigation is most likely to lead to the underlying diagnosis? (Select one answer only)
A. CT Scan
B. Plasma insulin
C. Blood cultures
D. Serum 17-hydroxyprogesterone
E. Serum testosterone

Question 16

A 3-year-old girl is seen in the emergency department with her grandmother who was concerned about bruising to her buttocks. The grandmother explains that the child had been left with her that morning by the boyfriend of the child's mother who had gone to work. The bruising was discovered when grandmother went to change the child's clothing. The new boyfriend of the mother appears in the emergency department.

Examination records a distressed child with bruises to her buttocks, arms and backs of thighs.

The paediatric registrar requests blood tests.

Who is able to give legally accepted permission for the blood tests? (Select one answer only)
A. Boyfriend of mother
B. Duty Social Worker
C. ED Consultant
D. Grandmother
E. Mother

Question 17

A 14-year-old female was admitted to hospital with parental concerns about food intake and her severe underweight. She was diagnosed with anorexia nervosa about 18 months previously and had been under the care of the eating disorders team. Her parents expressed concerns about recent changes in her diet with nothing consumed for the preceding 4 days.

Examination identified that she was cachectic but more detailed assessment was limited as she refused further examination.

A refeeding programme was agreed with the girl and included daily blood tests. The results of investigations at 48 hours after starting feeds showed:

Sodium	136 mmol/l	(135–146)
Potassium	3.2 mmol/l	(3.5–5.3)
Urea	4.2 mmol/l	(2.5–6.5)
Creatinine	75 μmol /l	(40–90)
Glucose	2.8 mmol/l	(3.0–6.0)
Calcium	2.6 mmol/l	(2.2–2.7)
Phosphate	0.7 mmol/l	(0.9–1.8)
ALP	322 mmol/l	(49–242)

What is the next most appropriate action required in view of these results? (Select one answer only)
A. Give IV bolus 10% glucose
B. Obtain ECG
C. Pause reintroduction of calories for 24 hours
D. Start oral phosphate supplementation
E. Start oral potassium supplementation

Question 18

A 6-year-old boy weighing 20 kg was admitted with acute abdominal pain and a diagnosis of appendicitis with peritonitis was made. He was taken to theatre where a perforated appendix was identified and resected.

There were no immediate postoperative problems although he remained nil by mouth and received intravenous dextrose/saline 4%/0.18% at a rate of 75 mls/hr. On the second day after surgery, he had a short, generalised convulsion of 2 minutes duration.

Initial blood results were:

Sodium	128 mmol/l	(135–146)
Potassium	3.6 mmol/l	(3.5–5.3)
Bicarbonate	12 mmol/l	(22–29)

Urea	2.4 mmol/l	(2.5–6.5)
Creatinine	32 µmol/l	(29–53)
Glucose	5.2 mmol/l	(3.0–6.0)
Calcium	2.3 mmol/l	(2.2–2.7)

What is the most appropriate next step in his management? (Select one answer only)
A. Administer slow IV sodium chloride infusion (40 mmol over 30 minutes)
B. Restrict IV fluids to 65% maintenance using 0.9% saline
C. Restrict IV fluids to 65% maintenance using dextrose/saline 4%/0.18%
D. Restrict IV fluids to 65% maintenance using dextrose/saline 5%/0.45%
E. Start oral sodium chloride supplements (2 mmol/kg/day)

Question 19
A 4-year-old boy was referred for assessment of chronic diarrhoea and recent poor weight gain over the last 6 months. He would pass soft, occasionally liquid, stool on 2 to 3 occasions per day although there was no report of blood in the stool. His appetite was generally good and he was usually active. He was born at 30 weeks' gestation and required ventilatory support for 7 days. He developed necrotising enterocolitis at that time and was managed with antibiotics, parenteral feeding and bowel rest and made a full recovery.

On examination his height is on the 9th centile whilst his weight is on the 0.4 centile. His temperature is 37.3°C, pulse 100/minute, capillary refill 3 seconds, blood pressure 95/75. His abdomen is soft and there are no palpable masses or organomegaly. Examination of both respiratory and neurological systems shows no abnormalities. A range of investigations were undertaken and the results are shown below.

Haemoglobin	135 g/l	(115–140)
White cell count	4.8 x 10^9/l	(3.0–10.0 x 10^9/l)
Neutrophils	2.1 x 10^9/l	(2.0–6.0 x 10^9/l)
Lymphocytes	0.7 x 10^9/l	(1.5–9.5 x 10^9/l)
Platelets	167 x 10^9/l	(150–400 x 10^9/l)
ESR	16 mm/hr	(< 20)
Electrolytes	Normal	
Urea & creatinine	Normal	
Liver function tests	Normal	
IgG	2.9 g/l	(3.1–16.1)
IgA	0.1 g/l	(0.3–2.8)

IgM	0.4 g/l	(0.5–2.2)
Stool culture	no ova, cysts or parasites	

What is the most likely diagnosis? (Select one answer only)
A. Alpha-1-antitrypsin deficiency
B. Chronic giardia lamblia infection
C. Inflammatory bowel disease
D. Intestinal lymphangiectasia
E. Short bowel syndrome

Question 20
A 2-year-old child had been assessed in the ED after a reported fall down the stairs. The ED team were concerned that the injuries may be nonaccidental.

Which of the following observations support the explanation of an accidental fall? (Select one answer only)
A. Bruising over the abdomen with liver laceration
B. Fractures to both humerus and femur
C. Single transverse femur fracture
D. Single fracture to the tibia
E. Vertebral fracture at T11

Question 21
A practice nurse contacts the on-call registrar for advice on immunisation. She plans to administer the routine MMR vaccine to a 15-month-old boy but has been told by the mother that the child has an egg allergy. A widespread rash developed after eating a boiled egg when he was 7 months old. There is a strong family history of atopy.

What is the most appropriate advice to give to the practice nurse? (Select one answer only)
A. Administer separate mumps, measles and rubella vaccine
B. Admit to the Day Care Unit and give MMR
C. Give MMR at GP practice
D. Omit MMR
E. Refer to OP for further review

Question 22
A 3-year-old girl with Down syndrome attends the outpatients department for her annual review.

Which of the following screening investigations should be undertaken at this visit? (Select one answer only)
A. Alpha fetoprotein
B. Antinuclear antibodies
C. Coeliac screen
D. Growth hormone assay
E. Urinary catecholamines

Question 23

A 14-year-old boy who is known to have sickle cell disease, presented to the emergency department with fever, breathing difficulties and pains in his limbs and back.

On examination, he is pale and finds it difficult to be comfortable. His temperature was 38.2°C, pulse 160/minute, systolic blood pressure 110/65, but cardiac auscultation finds no abnormalities. His respiratory rate was 40, O_2 saturations 91% in air, no recession evident and breath sounds were normal and equal. Examination of the abdomen identified a 3 cm liver edge. Remaining examination was normal.

The initial results show:

Haemoglobin	66 g/l	(110–140)
MCV	53 fl	(70–86)
MCH	17 pg	(23–31)
White cell count	8.3 x 10⁹/l	(5.0–12.0)
Platelets	320 x 10⁹/l	(150–400)

What is the next most important step in his management? (Select one answer only)
A. Blood sample for culture
B. Blood transfusion
C. Intranasal diamorphine
D. IV antibiotics
E. IV dextrose saline maintenance fluids

Question 24

A 5-week-old baby boy was referred by the GP with episodes of 'twitching' and a temperature of 38.3°C despite being given a dose of paracetamol. There is a history of penicillin allergy in the mother.

On presentation in hospital, he is miserable and only wakes when stimulated. His pulse is 166/minute, respiratory rate 54/minute, capillary refill time 2 seconds and temperature of 37.9°C. He has dry mucous membranes but good skin turgor and his fontanelle is flat. There are no abnormal findings from the rest of the systems.

Investigations are undertaken and then antibiotics started.

Haemoglobin	124 g/l	(95–125)
White cell count	4.1 x 10⁹/l	(6.0–15.0)
Platelets	375 x 10⁹/l	(150–450)

Electrolytes, urea and creatinine—normal

Glucose	4.8 mmol/l	(2.5–5.5)
Bilirubin	23 µmol/l	(<21)
Albumin	36 g/l	(30–45)
ALT	52 U/l	(0–41)
CRP	34 mg/l	(< 5)

Urine dip negative, microscopy awaited.
CSF:

Glucose	3.2 mmol/l	(2.2–4.4)
Protein	0.98 g/l	(0.15–1.2)
WCC	50 x 10⁶/l	(0–30)
Lymphocytes	45 x 10⁶/l	(<30)
Neutrophils	15 x 10⁶/l	(0)

Which of the following IV treatments is most appropriate for this baby? (Select one answer only)
A. acyclovir
B. benzylpenicillin and gentamicin
C. benzylpenicillin, gentamicin and acyclovir
D. cefotaxime and amoxicillin
E. cefotaxime, amoxicillin and acyclovir

Question 25

A 12-year-old boy presented to the emergency department with three episodes of rapid heartbeat that had occurred over the previous four weeks. The episodes were of sudden onset, lasted about 5 minutes and terminated spontaneously. He was anxious, lightheaded and slightly breathless during these episodes. He was otherwise well. There was nothing of relevance in the past medical or family history.

Examination was normal. His ECG is shown below (Figure 35.2).

What is the most likely cause of his episodes of fast heartbeat? (Select one answer only)
A. First degree heart block
B. Hypertrophic cardiomyopathy
C. Right bundle branch block
D. Short QT syndrome
E. Wolff-Parkinson-White syndrome

Question 26

A 3-month-old boy is one of nonidentical twins and has recently been diagnosed with severe combined immunodeficiency. Neither of the twins have yet received any of their planned immunisations. The parents ask for advice on immunisation of the child and other family members.

Which of the following is appropriate advice for this family? (Select one answer only)
A. 4-year-old sibling can have preschool immunisations
B. 8-year-old sibling can receive intranasal influenza vaccination
C. 13-year-old sibling can receive her HPV vaccine
D. the nonidentical twin can have all first-year vaccines
E. the patient can receive all first-year vaccines

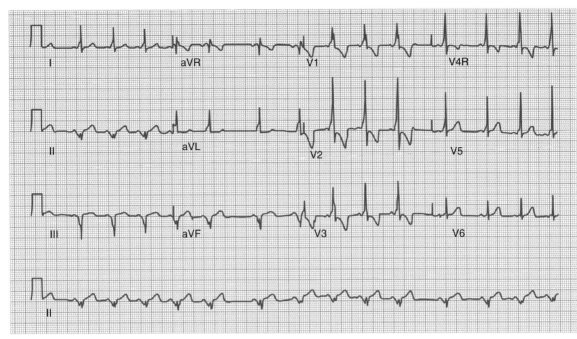

Fig. 35.2 Question 25.

Question 27

A 9-year-old boy presented with pallor, bruising and temperatures. There was nothing abnormal in the past medical or family history.

Examination found him to be pale with obvious ecchymoses on his trunk and limbs and with widespread lymphadenopathy. His temperature was 39.3°C, pulse 120/minute, blood pressure was 70/55. Examination of the abdomen revealed a 3 cm liver and a 2 cm spleen. Remaining examination was normal.

Initial investigations showed:

Haemoglobin	64 g/l	(115–140)
White cell count	346 x 10⁹/l	(5.0–12.0)
Platelets	12 x 10⁹/l	(150–400)
Sodium	147 mmol/l	(135–146)
Potassium	6.6 mmol/l	(3.5–5.3)
Urea	12.2 mmol/l	(2.5–6.5)
Creatinine	77 µmol/l	(29–53)

Which two actions must be undertaken immediately? (Select two answers only)
A. administer bolus 0.9% saline at 10 ml/kg
B. administer platelet transfusion
C. administer red cell transfusion
D. commence fluids—0.9% saline with potassium
E. commence IV antibiotics
F. IV calcium gluconate
G. nebulised salbutamol

Question 28

An 18-month-old girl attended the emergency department following a generalised seizure which lasted 3 minutes. She had been unwell with a coryzal illness over the previous 48 hours and had refused her morning milk. The family were asylum seekers from a war-torn area and had recently moved to the UK. There was no relevant past medical or family history.

Examination revealed her to be drowsy with limited response to stimuli. Her temperature was 37.2°C, pulse 120/minute, capillary refill was 3 seconds, blood pressure was 95/65. Abdomen was soft with no organomegaly and there were no focal abnormalities identified on examination of her neurological system. Rest of the examination was normal.

Initial blood tests were undertaken.

Full blood count

Sodium	143 mmol/l	(135–146)
Potassium	3.9 mmol/l	(3.5–5.3)
Bicarbonate	18 mmol/l	(19–28)
Urea	7.2 mmol/l	(2.5–6.5)
Creatinine	85 µmol/l	(13–39l)
Glucose	1.1 mmol/l	(3.0–6.0)
ALT	65 U/l	(0–28)
AST	112 U/l	(8–60)
Bilirubin	12 µmol/l	(< 17)
Ammonia	52 µmol/l	(30–60)

Capillary gas

pH	7.21	(7.35–7.45)
pCO_2	3.2 kPa	(4.6–6.0)
Base excess	-7 mmol/l	(-2 to +2)

What is the most likely diagnosis? (Select one answer only)
A. A. Ornithine transaminase deficiency
B. B. Galactosaemia
C. C. Glycogen storage disease
D. D. Medium chain acyl-CoA dehydrogenase deficiency
E. E. Organic acidaemias

Question 29

A 15-year-old girl was referred with concerns about short stature and delayed puberty. She had always been one of the shortest in her peer group but this had become more marked in the past 4 years as her friends have progressed through puberty. She had noticed some breast development for about 2 years and had had a few brief episodes of vaginal bleeding but no pubic hair or growth spurt. Apart from constipation which responded to laxatives she had no other significant medical history. Her school progress had dropped off in the past couple of years which upset her parents. Her father's height was on the 50th centile and he reported puberty at a normal age. Her mother was on 9th centile for height and she started her periods age 15 years. A maternal aunt had rheumatoid arthritis.

On examination she has no obvious dysmorphic features but is slightly pale. Her height is on the 0.4th centile and her weight the 50th centile for her age. She has reached Tanner Stage 3 breast development but is Tanner Stage 1 for pubic hair. The remainder of the examination is unremarkable.

What is the most likely diagnosis? (Select one answer only)
A. Coeliac disease
B. Constitutional delay of growth and puberty
C. Pituitary tumour
D. Primary hypothyroidism
E. Turner syndrome

Question 30

A 3-year-old boy had been admitted to the ward for observation after a seizure caused by tricyclic antidepressant ingestion whilst visiting his grandmother. He has not attended hospital previously and was happy and playing with his father.

What action should be put in place for safe discharge? (Select one answer only)
A. Ask the health visitor to visit and discuss safe medicine storage
B. Arrange for his 6-month-old sister to be seen for a child protection medical
C. Ask GP to review child after discharge for late effects of tricyclic medication
D. Delay discharge until a safeguarding strategy meeting has taken place
E. Make a safeguarding referral to the local social services team

Question 31

A 4-month-old baby girl was brought to the paediatric assessment unit by her father because she felt hot at home.

At triage her temperature was 37.2°C, pulse 135/minute, respiratory rate 36/minute saturations of 99% in air.

One hour later on your review she is alert and smiling. She has some nasal secretions but no recession and a clear chest on auscultation. She is well perfused with normal heart sounds and pulses. Her abdomen is soft and nontender. She has a rash within the nappy area which spares the creases and some mild erythematous areas in her antecubital and popliteal fossae. She takes a bottle of milk whilst in the observation area. There has been no change in her observations since she was seen in triage. The urine sample taken was negative on dipstick testing.

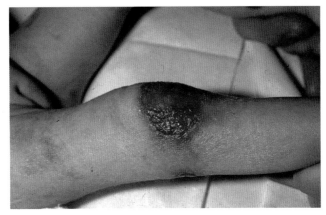

Fig. 35.3 Question 33.

Which of the following is the most appropriate action at this stage? (Select one answer only)

A. Admit for a period of observation of 6 hours
B. Discharge home with safety—net advice
C. Start oral antibiotics for a presumed upper respiratory tract infection
D. Take a FBC and CRP and await the results to guide management
E. Take a FBC and CRP and start antibiotics whilst waiting for results

Question 32

A 10-year-old boy who has cystic fibrosis was admitted as his coughing had become more intense and productive and he had developed a fever over the last 4 days. He also had nasal congestion and a dark-coloured discharge. His cystic fibrosis was diagnosed by the neonatal screening programme and had been well managed by his parents. He was performing well at school.

On examination his temperature is 37.9°C, pulse 110/minute, respiratory rate 36/minute and oxygen saturations are 92% in air. Examination of his chest shows equal expansion, equal air entry with widespread, episodic wheeze along with course crackles on the whole of the left lung field. He has a 4 cm palpable liver but no splenomegaly.

His FEV1 had fallen significantly since his previous clinic visit. The initial results show:

Haemoglobin	132 g/l	(115–140)
White cell count	15.2 x 10⁹/l	(5.0–12.0)
Lymphocytes	4.2 x 10⁹/l	(1.5–7.0)
Neutrophils	7.8 x 10⁹/l	(2.0–6.0)
Eosinophils	3.2 x 10⁹/l	(0.1–0.8)
Platelets	238 x 10⁹/l	(150–400)

Electrolytes	normal	
LFT	normal	
IgA	1.8 g/l	(0.3–2.8)
IgG	26.3 g/l	(3.1–16.1)
IgE	98 kU/l	(<63)

CXR = Widespread areas of opacity indicative of mucus plugging.

Which investigation is most likely to lead to the underlying diagnosis? (Select one answer only)

A. Aspergillus antibody assay
B. Blood culture
C. CO transfer factor
D. High resolution CT of chest
E. PCR assay for mycobacterium

Question 33

A 17-month-old girl was referred to the paediatric assessment unit by her GP with concerns about a lesion on there right knee (Figure 35.3). This seemed to have developed over last few days and was initially treated with topical Fucidin but had increased in size. The child seemed to be in some discomfort and she had a temperature of 37.4°C. Her mother had regular follow-up assessments with the dermatology outpatient department.

What is the most likely diagnosis? (Select one answer only)

A. Discoid eczema
B. Discoid lupus erythematosus
C. Epidermolysis bullosa
D. Nonaccidental scald injury
E. Staphylococcal infection (scalded skin syndrome)

Question 34

A 6-year-old girl was referred by her GP with concerns about her growth. Her height was below the 0.4th and her weight and head circumference were on the 9th centile. She was otherwise well and in year 2 at school. No illnesses in the immediate family and both parents are of normal height.

Examination identifies bilateral ptosis that her mother says has been present for some years. There was no other visible abnormality of her eyes, she had normal visual acuity and a normal range of movements. Examination of the central and peripheral nervous systems was normal.

Which investigation is most likely to determine the cause of the ptosis? (Select one answer only)
A. Antibodies to acetylcholine receptors
B. Fundoscopy
C. Karyotype
D. MRI brain
E. Urinary catecholamines

Question 35

A 11-month-old baby boy presented with delay in gross motor development. He was born at term following a difficult pregnancy as his mother had felt constantly tired and had had long periods off work. Delivery had been normal and there were no dysmorphic features noted in the boy at birth and examination was normal at that time. There were no initial concerns about his development but he was unable to sit independently until 8 months of age and was currently unable to stand unsupported. He was initially breast fed before weaning onto the family diet at 6 months of age. He was the second child of non-consanguineous Asian parents.

Examination shows him to be pale but alert and smiling when engaged. His vision and hearing seem to be intact. Spontaneous movement of all four limbs is noted but not against gravity. He is able to transfer objects between his hands. He was not able to maintain a sitting position and could not weight bear. His overall tone was reduced and all reflexes were difficult to elicit. Rest of examination was normal.

Initial investigations were undertaken.

Haemoglobin	98 g/l	(110–140)
MCV	91 fl	(70–86)
MCH	32 pg	(23–31)
White cell count	5.8 x 10^9/l	(5.0–12.0)
Platelets	167 x 10^9/l	(150–400)
Electrolytes	Normal	

Calcium	2.6 mmol/l	(2.2–2.7)
Phosphate	1.2 mmol/l	(0.9–1.8)
ALP	322 U/l	(76–308)

What is the most likely diagnosis? (Select one answer only)
A. Alpha-thalassaemia trait
B. Folate deficiency
C. Hypothyroidism
D. Iron deficiency anaemia
E. Vitamin B12 deficiency

Question 36

A 12-year-old boy attended ED with a 2-day history of increasing frequency of falls. He had been previously well with only an URTI some 10 days previously but only required one day off school. He described a feeling of numbness in his feet and a weakness in his legs such that he had taken to his bed. He had been well up to this event, took no regular medications and there were no relevant features in the family history.

On examination he is quiet but alert and spoke clearly and appropriately. Vital signs were normal and he was apyrexial. Neurological examination of the lower limbs showed reduced power bilaterally in quadricep and calf muscles. Reflexes were absent in knee, ankle and plantars.

MRI of spine and brain and subsequent CSF findings supported a diagnosis of Guillain-Barré syndrome.

What is the most significant complication in next few days that needs close monitoring? (Select one answer only)
A. Brain stem herniation
B. Hearing deficit
C. Permanent loss of vision
D. Respiratory hypoventilation
E. Spinal cord compression

Question 37

A 4-year-old boy presented to the surgical team with abdominal pain and vomiting and is diagnosed with appendicitis. He was thought to look pale and bloods were undertaken prior to theatre and during his postoperative stay. The family had recently arrived in the UK from the Sudan as father is studying at the local university. Mother's pregnancy and delivery were normal.

On examination his temperature is 37.8°C, pulse 140/minute, blood pressure was 95/76. Examination of the abdomen identified tenderness in the right iliac fossa. Remaining examination was normal.

The initial results show:

Haemoglobin	101 g/l	(110–140)
MCV	50 fl	(70–86)
MCH	21 pg	(23–31)
White cell count	14.3 x 10^9/l	(5.0–12.0)
Platelets	360 x 10^9/l	(150–400)
Electrolytes	normal	
Ferritin	19 µg/l	(12–200)
ALT	27U/l	(0–41)
AST	45 U/l	(18–92)
Bilirubin total	26 µmol/l)	(<21)
Bilirubin conjugated	1 µmol/l)	(<2)
Haemoglobin electrophoresis		
HbA_2	9%	
HbF	6%	

What is the likely diagnosis? (Select one answer only)
A. Alpha thalassaemia major
B. Alpha thalassaemia trait
C. Beta thalassaemia major
D. Beta thalassaemia trait
E. HbH disease

Question 38
You will be presented with a list of diseases and three scenarios.

Which of the following diagnoses best explains the presentations described? (One answer only for each scenario).
A. Drug-related eruption
B. Group A Streptococcus
C. Hand foot and mouth
D. Human herpes virus 6B
E. Kawasaki disease
F. Measles
G. Parvovirus B19
H. Pityriasis rosea
I. Rubella

Scenario 1
A 2-year-old girl was seen in the paediatric assessment unit with a 24-hour history of high fever and minor coryzal symptoms. There were no red flag symptoms, and she was discharged home after assessment with safety netting advice. The parents contacted the unit some 72 hours later to say that the girl now has a rash mostly on her trunk, multiple nonitchy pink dots that 'go away with the glass test'. She is now afebrile.

Scenario 2
A 2-year-old girl was seen in the paediatric assessment unit with fever, cough and sore throat. Her fluid intake had reduced. The family had recently arrived in the UK from a war-torn country and were currently housed in an asylum centre. Examination revealed a macular rash on her head, face, trunk and arms. She had seen a GP the day before and started on penicillin. She appeared unwell, was pyrexial at 38.2°C and had a conjunctivitis.

Scenario 3
A 2-year-old girl was seen in the paediatric assessment unit with a 24-hour history of fever, anorexia, erythematous rash and difficulty in swallowing. On examination she was pyrexial at 37.8°C with a widespread, deep red, macular rash which gave a coarse feel to the skin along with circumoral pallor on face, trunk and limbs. She had erythematous tonsils with white plaques and cervical lymphadenopathy.

Question 39
A 15-year-old boy who had been diagnosed with Type 1 diabetes some 12 months previously was referred by his GP with concerns about lethargy. This had become more evident over the preceding 3 months and was beginning to impact on his school attendance and performance. He was taking 18 units of a long-acting insulin in the evening and used an Insulin:CHO ratio of 1:10 to calculate premeal insulin dosage.

On examination, his height was on the 25th centile and his weight on the 75th centile although his weight had been on the 50th centile some 6 months previously. He was noted to be quiet and withdrawn in clinic and slightly pale. No abnormalities were found on further examination.

The initial results show:

Haemoglobin	112 g/l	(110–140)
MCV	74 fl	(70–86)
White cell count	7.5 x 10^9/l	(5.0–12.0)
Platelets	340 x 10^9/l	(150–400)
HbA1c	47 mmol/mmol	(20–42)
Random blood sugar	7.8 mmol/l	(3.0–6.0)

What is the most likely cause for his recent lethargy?
A. Coeliac disease
B. Depressive illness
C. Hypothyroidism
D. Inadequate insulin dose
E. School refusal

Question 40

A 3-day old baby boy was admitted from the postnatal ward following a generalised seizure following a 24-hour period of lethargy, irritability and poor feeding. He had a birthweight of 3.3 kg and was bottle fed without problems. There were no adverse conditions identified in the family history.

Examination found him to be lethargic and responding poorly to stimuli. He looked pale and his temperature was 37.3°C, pulse 140/minute, respiratory rate 52/minute and capillary refill was 4 seconds, systolic blood pressure was 85. He was hypotonic but reflexes were present and equal. The remaining examination was normal.

A full infection screen was undertaken. CSF microscopy showed no cells but culture result awaited. Urgent CT scan was normal. Intravenous fluids and antibiotics were started.

Full blood count

Sodium	143 mmol/l	(135–146)
Potassium	3.9 mmol/l	(3.5–5.3)
Bicarbonate	26 mmol/l	(19–28)
Urea	0.5 mmol/l	(0.8–5.5)
Creatinine	78 µmol/l	(21–75)
Glucose	2.6 mmol/l	(2.5–5.5)
ALT	56 U/l	(0–41 U/l)
AST	112 U/l	(18–92 U/l)
Bilirubin	109 µmol/l	(<21)
Ammonia	312 µmol/l	(<100 µmol/l)

Capillary gas

pH	7.48	(7.35–7.45)
pCO2	3.4	(4.6–6.0 kPa)
Base excess	+3	(-2 to +2 mmol/l)

What is the most likely diagnosis? (Select one answer only)

A. A. Ornithine transaminase deficiency
B. B. Galactosaemia
C. C. Glycogen storage disease
D. D. Medium chain acyl-CoA dehydrogenase deficiency (MCADD)
E. E. Organic acidaemia

Question 41

A 7-month-old boy was referred by his health visitor to the emergency department due to concerns about poor feeding and breathlessness. The family had recently arrived in the UK and were seeking refugee status. Mother's pregnancy and delivery were normal.

On examination, he is pale and has icteric sclera. His temperature is 37.1°C, pulse 140/minute, systolic blood pressure was 80 and he had a gallop rhythm detectable on cardiac auscultation. His respiratory rate was 40, no recession and breath sounds were normal and equal. Examination of the abdomen identified a 3 cm liver edge and a 2 cm palpable spleen. Remaining examination was normal.

The initial results show:

Haemoglobin	64 g/l	(110–140)
MCV	55 fl	(70–86)
MCH	16 pg	(23–31)
White cell count	11.2 x 10⁹/l	(5.0–12.0)
Platelets	240 x 10⁹/l	(150–400)
Film	target cells seen	
Electrolytes	normal	
ALT	27 U/l	(0–41)
AST	45 U/l	(18–92)
Bilirubin total	86 µmol/l	(<21)

Which investigation is most likely to lead to the underlying diagnosis? (One answer)

A. Bone marrow aspirate
B. Ferritin
C. Glucose-6-phosphate dehydrogenase assay
D. Haemoglobin electrophoresis
E. Liver biopsy

Question 42

A baby boy was admitted to the NICU at 4 hours of age with vomiting and tachypnoea. He was born at term by vaginal delivery with meconium-stained liquor, had APGARS of 8 at 1 and 10 at 5 and weighed 3.2 kg. On the postnatal ward he had fed by bottle but had promptly vomited the full amount and then developed a persistent cough.

Examination showed him to be centrally pink, pulse 120/minute and respiratory rate 46/minute. Heart sounds were normal and auscultation identified basal crackles on the right lung field. The remaining examination was normal.

What is the most likely diagnosis? (Select one answer only)
A. Congenital lobar emphysema
B. Meconium aspiration
C. Oesophageal atresia
D. Persistent tachypnoea of the newborn
E. Volvulus

Question 43

A 2-year-old girl was admitted with pallor and bruising and a diagnosis of acute lymphoblastic leukaemia was made. She was started on the appropriate chemotherapy regime and bloods taken some 8 hours later are shown. (A repeat sample confirmed results.) Peaked T waves are noted on the ECG monitor.

Initial blood results were:

Sodium	128 mmol/l	(135–146)
Potassium	7.4 mmol/l	(3.5–5.3)
Bicarbonate	12 mmol/l	(22–29)
Urea	2.4 mmol/l	(2.5–6.5)
Creatinine	32 µmol/l	(29–53)
Glucose	5.2 mmol/l	(3.0–6.0)
Calcium	2.3 mmol/l	(2.2–2.7)

What is the next immediate step in her management? (Select one answer only)
A. Administration of IV insulin and glucose
B. Infusion of 8.4% sodium bicarbonate
C. Infusion of IV 10% calcium gluconate
D. Infusion of IV salbutamol
E. Nebulised salbutamol

Question 44

A 6-day-old baby was reviewed on the postnatal ward following concerns raised about poor feeding and vomiting since birth. He was born at 36 weeks following a normal pregnancy and there were no abnormalities detected on his first examination. He was being breast fed. His parents were from an Irish travelling community.

On examination, he is jaundiced, hypotonic and has small bruises on trunk and limbs. He has a respiratory rate 40/minute, normal chest movements, normal breath sounds and hepatomegaly of 2 cm. Rest of the examination is normal.

The initial results show:

Haemoglobin	162 g/l	(145–220)
White cell count	15.3 x 10^9/l	(10.0–26.0)
Platelets	260 x 10^9/l	(150–400)

Electrolytes	normal	
Glucose	2.2 mmol/l	(2.5–5.5)
ALT	72 U/l	(0–41)
AST	123 U/l	(18–92)
Bilirubin total	82 µmol/l	(<21)
Bilirubin conjugated	14 µmol/l	(<2)
PT	32 secs	(10–12)
aPTT	75 secs	(28–55)

What investigation is likely to provide the underlying diagnosis? (Select one answer only)
A. PCR of urine for CMV
B. Plasma alpha-1-antitrypsin level
C. Plasma ammonia level
D. Plasma galactose level
E. Syphilis serology

Question 45

A 6-year-old girl presents with drooping of both eyelids. She was diagnosed with acute lymphoblastic leukaemia some 6 months previously and has been treated with chemotherapy following the national protocol.

She was quiet but had obvious bilateral ptosis. Examination of the CNS identified full range of eye movements, normal pupillary reflexes and seemingly normal vision. Examination of peripheral nervous system identified normal muscle bulk, reduced power in all four limbs and absent reflexes at all points. Remaining examination was normal.

What is the most likely cause of her presenting features? (Select one answer only)
A. Cervical transverse myelitis
B. CNS relapse of leukaemia
C. Horner syndrome
D. Myasthenia gravis
E. Vincristine toxicity

Question 46

A 12-week-old baby boy was referred to the acute admissions unit with concerns of lethargy, poor feeding and weight loss. He was born at term by a normal delivery and had a birthweight of 3.3 kg. He was bottle fed but initially had small vomits after feeds which increased in volume until the last week. He gradually became less interested in feeds and the volume taken gradually decreased until he was only taking 60 mls of formula on 4 occasions each day. He was the first child of parents who were 18 and 19 years old.

On examination he was quiet and anxious and weighed 3.6 kg (<0.4 centile). He had extensive nappy rash in the perineal area. His temperature was 36.2°C, pulse 180/minute, capillary refill 4 seconds, BP 65/45. respiratory rate 32/minute and breath sounds normal. Abdomen was soft and no palpable masses.

Full blood count	Normal for age	
Sodium	133 mmol/l	(135–146)
Potassium	3.1 mmol/l	(3.5–5.3)
Chloride	89 mmol/l	(95–106)
Bicarbonate	34 mmol/l	(19–28)
Urea	7.5 mmol/l	(0.8–5.5)
Creatinine	82 μmol/l	(21–75)
Glucose	3.8 mmol/l	(2.5–5.5)

Blood gas (capillary)

pH	7.48	(7.35–7.45)
pCO2	5.8	(4.6–6.0 kPa)
Base excess	+7	(-2 to +2 mmol/l)
Lactate	4.3	(1–2 mmol/l)
Urine dipstick analysis	negative for red cells, leucocytes, nitrites	

What is the most likely diagnosis? (Select one answer only)
A. Achalasia
B. Hiatus hernia
C. Parental neglect
D. Pyloric stenosis
E. Congenital adrenal hyperplasia

Question 47

A 17-year-old girl living in London was diagnosed with anorexia nervosa. Clinical examination and investigations indicated that her physiological status was poor and electrolyte abnormalities were significantly deranged. A treatment plan was proposed which included admission to a local hospital and the instigation of graded nasogastric feeding. Her parents supported this plan. The girl, however, refuses nasogastric feeding but agreed to the admission.

What is the next step in addressing her refusal of nasogastric feeding? (Select one answer only)
A. Accept decision of patient
B. Act on permission from parents
C. Request psychiatrist to assess mental capacity
D. Seek court order to start treatment
E. Start treatment without consent

Question 48

A 9-year-old boy presented to the emergency department with bleeding from the gums following a dental extraction procedure on the previous day. He had been previously well and was not known to bruise easily or to bleed excessively when injured. He was described as 'double jointed'. He attended hospital clinics for his severe eczema and asthma but both were well controlled. Both parents were well with no history of excessive bruising or bleeding although mother is also 'double jointed'. A maternal grandfather was known to bruise easily.

On examination, the boy looked well but had obvious oozing of blood from the dental extraction sites.

Haemoglobin	98 g/l	(110–140)
MCV	72 fl	(70–86)
MCH	27 pg	(23–31)
White cell count	7.2 x 10⁹/l	(5.0–12.0)
Platelets	240 x 10⁹/l	(150–400)
PT	12 secs	(10–12)
aPTT	62 secs	(28–45)

What is the likely diagnosis? (Select one answer only)
A. Ehlers-Danlos syndrome
B. Haemophilia A
C. Haemophilia B
D. Protein C deficiency
E. Wiskott-Aldrich syndrome

Question 49

A 10-month-old boy presented to the emergency department with abnormal movements. His mother described that when waking from a sleep he will suddenly bend forward, his head flicks forward and down and his arms appear to push out forward. She is unsure of movements in his legs. He seems startled and cries after the event. The episodes can occur in clusters but he seems well between episodes. The pregnancy, delivery and early course of life were normal though he seemed to have lost some of the skills he had earlier such as transferring objects in his hands. His immunisations are up to date and he had recently been given his MMR vaccine. Review of his 'Red Book' showed that his length, weight and OFC were following the 50th centile.

He is alert and smiling appropriately with no abnormalities noted on examination of his cardiovascular, respiratory or neurological systems. He had three pale skin lesions on his back, each about 3.5 cm in size.

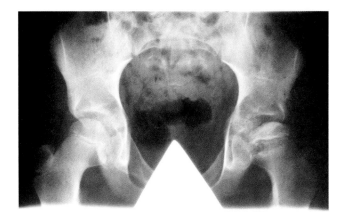

Fig. 35.4 Question 50.

Neurological opinion is sought and further investigations undertaken.

An EEG shows hypsarrhythmia.

What is the most appropriate first-line treatment for this child? (Select one answer only)

A. Clonazepam
B. Ketogenic diet
C. Pyridoxine
D. Topiramate
E. Vigabactrin

Question 50

A 9-year-old boy attended the emergency department with a 12-hour history of pain in the left hip. The pain was worse on standing and he was now unable to weight bear. There was no history of recent trauma. He recently had been referred for review as he experienced frequent loose stool without blood.

On examination he is in discomfort. His temperature was 37.4°C, pulse 110/minute and BP 120/85. His height is on the 75th centile and his weight on the 98th. He has no obvious rashes and no obvious swelling over the left hip. He has obvious pain on moving his hip and knee joint and reduced movement at the hip. There was no swelling of any other joint and all have full movement.

An x-ray of the pelvis and hips was undertaken (Figure 35.4).

What is the most likely diagnosis? (Select one answer only)

A. Inflammatory bowel reactive arthritis
B. Juvenile idiopathic arthritis
C. Osteosarcoma
D. Perthes disease
E. Slipped capital epiphysis

ANSWERS

In the real examination, every question has an added weighting that makes marking a more complex process than simply adding the number of correct answers obtained. Complex and long questions will provide more marks that a "spot diagnosis question". It is not possible to reproduce this approach for the answers presented here.

Answer 1
Correct answer: C—finding a letter explaining reasons
A. recent diagnosis of depression—a recognised cause of self-harm behaviour but not indicative of increased later risk of successful suicide
B. early morning timing—is unusual but is not indicative of increased later risk
C. finding a letter explaining reasons—implies planned action and is related to future intent
D. recent death of father—a recognised cause of self-harm behaviour but not indicative of increased later risk
E. recent parental separation—a recognised cause of self-harm behaviour but not indicative of increased later risk

Answer 2
Correct answer: E—oppositional defiant disorder
This boy is under 12 years of age, presents with symptoms of aggression and defiance.
A. attention deficit disorder—although distractible he is able to concentrate on issues
B. autism spectrum disorder—no repetitive or social awkward behaviours
C. disruptive domestic circumstances—doesn't explain aggression and lying
D. hyperactivity disorder—no history of hyperactive behaviour
E. oppositional defiant disorder—correct answer

Answer 3
Correct answer: D—No chance of inheriting
Wiskott-Aldrich syndrome is X-linked recessive and is only passed on to male descendants although females may be carriers.

Answer 4
Correct answer: B—Fanconi syndrome
The child presents with vomiting, growth retardation, clinical features of rickets, acidosis and low sodium and potassium. Fanconi syndrome consists of renal tubular acidosis affecting the proximal tubule together with a minor aciduria, glycosuria, phosphaturia and hypokalaemia.

Cystinosis is the most likely cause given the family history that suggests an autosomal recessive inheritance.
A. Bartter syndrome—usually polydipsia, low sodium and potassium and alkalosis
B. Fanconi syndrome—correct answer
C. Galactosaemia—usually presents in first weeks of life with jaundice
D. MCAD deficiency—hypoglycaemia main feature and would not lead explain rickets
E. Mucopolysaccharidoses—developmental delay main feature and would not explain rickets

Answer 5
Correct answer: E—Skin prick testing with sesame
This young boy presents with an acute onset of symptoms following the ingestion of a foodstuff known to cause urticarial reactions—sesame. He had an immediate reaction of local sensation changes and urticarial rash. This suggests IgE-mediated food allergy to sesame.
A. C1 esterase inhibitor levels—deficiency is an autosomal dominant condition
B. Food challenge test with sesame—would not be appropriate as first investigation
C. Serum IgE levels—will be raised as atopic
D. Serum tryptase levels—released by mast cells in anaphylaxis but would not clarify diagnosis
E. Skin prick testing with sesame—correct answer

Answer 6
Correct answer: C—Increase morphine dose but continue at every 4 hours
This is an acute situation and gaining control of the young person's pain is vitally important. The initial control may change over the following weeks but current management requires pain control.
A. Control of the pain with immediate release morphine is required before an appropriate dose of fentanyl can be calculated.
A. B Increasing frequency before increasing the dose is inappropriate.
B. Correct answer
C. PCA may have a place but requires the effective daily dose to be determined first.
D. Subcutaneous diamorphine requires the effective daily dose to be determined first.

Answer 7
Correct answer: E—Intubation and ventilation
The clinical history is in keeping with a tricyclic overdose—drowsy, agitated, decreased GCS of 7 and a seizure. He also had time with an elderly relative who may not have appropriate safety measures around tablet storage. Priority is to protect airway.

A. Administer IV ceftriaxone—no features to suggest meningitis
B. Administer IV mannitol—clinical features do not suggest raised ICP
C. Arrange urgent CT scan of head—no suggestion of trauma or raised ICP
D. Collect urine for toxicology—important but not a priority
E. Intubation and ventilation—correct answer—a priority

Answer 8
Correct answer: D—Indicate that you are unable to prescribe the dose
Strict UK guidelines indicate that only staff who have been appropriately trained and who appear on the Trust register are allowed to prescribe, check, handle or administer intrathecal chemotherapy.

Answer 9
Scenario 1
Correct answer is B—superior axis
Partial atrioventricular septal defect produces a superior axis on ECG.
Scenario 2
Correct answer is F—Prolonged QT interval—hypocalcaemia
This girl has symptoms of hypocalcaemia and would display a prolonged QT interval on ECG.
Scenario 3
Correct answer is I—T wave inverted in V6
This girl has aortic stenosis causing left ventricular hypertrophy. The ECG would show T wave inverted in V6.

Answer 10
Correct answer: A—Advise waiting until she is over 18 before undertaking any testing
Huntington's disease is inherited as an autosomal dominant condition with onset of symptoms in adult life. Undertaking the testing in a 15-year-old will deny her the opportunity to make her own decision as an adult and lose her right to confidentiality.
A. Advise waiting until she is over 18 before undertaking any testing—correct answer
B. Arrange testing for the Huntington's disease gene—inappropriate
C. Obtain more details of the results of the father—would not change advice
D. Reassure her that females cannot develop Huntington's disease—autosomal dominant
E. Refer to genetics for counselling—appropriate but only delays the initial advice

Answer 11
Correct answer: D—nasal brush biopsy

This young girl has hearing difficulties, recurrent chest infections, dextrocardia and situs inversus. This suggests Kartagener syndrome—primary ciliary dyskinesia and dextrocardia. Cilia line the epithelium of the eustachian tube, sinuses, trachea, bronchi and nasopharynx.
A. Bronchoscopy—would not find cause of hearing and cardiac abnormalities
B. Echocardiography—would not find cause of hearing difficulties
C. High resolution CT chest—would not find cause of situs inversus
D. Nasal brush biopsy—correct answer
E. Sweat test—would not find cause of situs inversus

Answer 12
Correct answer: C—Administer adrenaline 150 mcg IM
The history is highly suggestive of an acute anaphylactic reaction and this child is in extremis and is likely to deteriorate. Administration of adrenaline is the crucial first action whilst other actions are initiated.
A. 0.9% saline bolus 20 ml/kg—needed but obtaining IV access will create a delay
B. Administer adrenaline 150 mcg IM—correct answer
C. Administer adrenaline 150 mcg IV—would not administer IV in first instance as likely delay in obtaining IV access.
D. Administer adrenaline 300 mcg IM—dose for those over 6 years
E. Administer hydrocortisone 100 mg IV—given after IM adrenaline and with IV access

Answer 13
Correct answer: D—Exaggerated adrenarche
This girl has evidence of mild androgen production with no significant growth acceleration or virilisation such as clitoromegaly. She is tall for her parents due to obesity which is common in this condition. It is a marker of insulin resistance and she is at risk of developing metabolic syndrome as an adult similar to other family members.
A. Androgen secreting ovarian tumour—there is no significant growth acceleration or virilisation
B. CAH—there is no significant growth acceleration or virilisation
C. Cushing disease—cardinal feature is growth cessation
D. Exaggerated adrenarche—correct answer
E. Gonadotrophin dependent sexual precocity—there is no obvious breast development

Answer 14
Correct answer: A—Monogenic diabetes
Apart from her urinary symptoms, this young boy is well. A strong family history, raised HBA1c and only slightly raised fasting glucose would indicate monogenic diabetes.

A. Monogenic diabetes—correct answer
B. Renal glycosuria—would not explain raised HBA1c or raised fasting glucose
C. Steroid induced—short exposure time and would not explain blood results
D. Type 2 diabetes—would expect normal urinary ketones
E. Urinary tract infection—would not explain abnormal blood results

Answer 15
Correct answer: D—Serum 17-hydroxyprogesterone

This baby boy presents with poor weight gain, vomiting and evidence of dehydration and shock with a metabolic acidosis. The hyponatraemia, hyperkalaemia and hypoglycaemia are all consistent with primary adrenal insufficiency and at this age the likeliest diagnosis is congenital adrenal hyperplasia (CAH).
A. Cranial CT—no evidence of an acute brain injury
B. Plasma insulin—hyperinsulinaemic hypoglycaemia is not associated with these electrolyte abnormalities
C. Blood cultures—sepsis would not explain this electrolyte pattern
D. Serum 17-hydroxyprogesterone—correct answer
E. Serum testosterone—will be raised but would not confirm diagnosis

Answer 16
Correct answer: E—Mother
A. Boyfriend—a recent boyfriend is not the biological father and has no legal right to give consent
B. Duty Social Worker—does not have legal right to give consent
C. ED Consultant—can make decisions in life-threatening situations only and therefore in the child's best interest
D. Grandmother—does not have legal right to give consent
E. Mother—correct answer

Answer 17
Correct answer: D—start oral phosphate supplementation

This girl is at risk of refeeding syndrome as she has had a negligible intake of calories. It is characterised by hypophosphatemia, associated with fluid and electrolyte shifts. The problems result from the sudden increase in insulin released when feeding occurs.
A. give IV bolus 10% glucose—asymptomatic hypoglycaemia that needs close monitoring but does not require bolus dose of glucose
B. obtain ECG—monitoring for ECG changes is important but not first priority
C. pause reintroduction of calories for 24 hours—pace of refeeding may need review but is not the immediate concern

D. Start oral phosphate supplementation—correct answer
E. Start oral potassium supplementation—may be required but not before giving phosphate

Answer 18
Correct answer: B—Restrict IV fluids to 65% maintenance using 0.9% saline

The seizures experienced by this boy are the result of the identified hyponatraemia. Review of his fluid regime shows that he has received dextrose/saline 4%/0.18% which should never be used in otherwise healthy children needing intravenous fluids. This is iatrogenic hyponatraemia. Adding extra sodium to his fluids is inappropriate as the prime problem is that of excess water administration. A normal healthy child without evidence of renal disease will be able to excrete any sodium in excess of requirements.

Answer 19
Correct answer: D—intestinal lymphangiectasia

This boy has protracted diarrhoea and apparent poor weight gain. Examination showed no abnormalities. His height and weight were on the lower centiles but more measurements would be needed to ascertain if they reflected unexpected growth. Investigations showed lymphopenia, low immunoglobulins, particularly IgA, and low albumin indicating protein loss from the GI tract as seen in intestinal lymphangiectasia.
A. Alpha-1-antitrypsin deficiency—would not explain blood results
B. Chronic giardia lamblia infection—excluded by normal stool culture
C. Inflammatory bowel disease—no blood in stool reported and normal ESR
D. Intestinal lymphangiectasia—correct answer
E. short bowel syndrome—did not have surgery for NEC

Answer 20
Correct answer: A—Single fracture to the tibia

Minor soft tissue injuries (abrasions and bruises) occur in most accidental falls, but internal organ damage is extremely rare.
A. Bruising over the abdomen with liver laceration—highly suggestive of abusive trauma
B. Fractures to both humerus and femur—highly suggestive of abusive trauma
C. Single transverse femur fracture—highly suggestive of abusive trauma
D. Single fracture to the tibia—correct answer
E. Vertebral fracture at T11—highly suggestive of abusive trauma

Answer 21
Correct answer: C—Give MMR at GP practice
Egg allergy is not a contraindication for MMR vaccine. Studies have shown that those with proven egg allergy do

not have significant adverse reactions. The full immunisation should be given at the GP practice in the usual way.

Answer 22
Correct answer: C—Coeliac screen

Children with Down syndrome are at higher risk of developing coeliac disease and the onset may be insidious. Screening may identify the issue at an early stage.
A. Alpha fetoprotein—raised in germ cell and liver tumours but not an increased risk
B. Antinuclear antibodies—joint problems are a potential problem but not autoimmune
C. Coeliac screen—correct answer
D. Growth hormone assay—assessed only if a clinical indication
E. Urinary catecholamines—at increased risk of leukaemia but not neuroblastoma

Answer 23
Correct answer: C—Intranasal diamorphine

This boy presents with history and examination features indicating that he has an acute chest syndrome. The control of pain must be the priority—all the other interventions will follow quickly after. Hyperhydration is to be avoided as that can lead to fluid overload and respiratory failure.
A. Blood sample for culture—part of infection screen
B. Blood transfusion—needed but not the first priority
C. Intranasal diamorphine—correct answer
D. IV antibiotics—needed but not the first priority
E. IV dextrose saline maintenance fluids—needed but not the first priority

Answer 24
Correct answer: E—IV cefotaxime, amoxicillin and acyclovir

This baby is under 3 months old and in the NICE red category for risk of serious illness. Although the temperature is <38°C, the baby was given paracetamol.

It is possible that the baby had focal seizures and, with a mild raise in ALT, along with a CSF consistent with early viral encephalitis, the appropriate choice is a third-generation cephalosporin, plus listeria cover (amoxicillin) plus cover for possible herpes simplex encephalitis. The penicillin allergy in the mother does not play a role in antibiotic choice for this baby.
A. acyclovir—only covers for encephalitis
B. benzylpenicillin and gentamicin—inadequate bacterial and viral cover
C. benzylpenicillin, gentamicin and acyclovir—inadequate broad antibiotic cover
D. cefotaxime and amoxicillin—does not cover organisms causing encephalitis
E. cefotaxime, amoxicillin and acyclovir—correct answer

Answer 25
Correct answer: E—Wolff-Parkinson-White syndrome
A. First degree heart block—no electrical disassociation
B. Hypertrophic cardiomyopathy—QRS complexes not consistent
C. Right bundle branch block—not evident on ECG
D. Short QT syndrome—not evident on ECG
E. Wolff-Parkinson-White syndrome—correct answer

Answer 26
Correct answer: E—13-year-old sibling can receive her HPV vaccine

This baby should not be given any live vaccines and close family members should also avoid live vaccines.
A. 4-year-old sibling can have preschool immunisations—MMR is a live vaccine
B. 8-year-old sibling can receive intranasal influenza vaccination—live vaccine
C. 13-year-old sibling should decline HPV vaccine—correct answer—HPV not live vaccine
D. the nonidentical twin can have all first-year vaccines—rotavirus is a live vaccine
E. the patient can receive all first-year vaccines—rotavirus is a live vaccine

Answer 27
Correct answer: A—administer bolus 0.9% saline at 10 ml/kg
Correct answer: E—commence IV antibiotics

This young boy has acute leukaemia and there is hyperkalaemia, renal compromise and hyperuricaemia. He is also pyrexial and hypotensive—likely septicaemic shock. The priority is to support his circulating volume and protect against infections as he is immunocompromised.
A. administer bolus 0.9% saline at 10 ml/kg—correct answer
B. administer platelet transfusion—these should be requested but antibiotics administration must take precedence
C. administer red cell transfusion—this should be requested but antibiotics administration must take precedence
D. commence fluids—0.9% saline with potassium—needed but should not contain potassium
E. commence IV antibiotics—correct answer
F. IV calcium gluconate—only if potassium above 7.0 mmol/l
G. nebulised salbutamol—only if potassium level unresponsive to first-line treatment

Answer 28
Correct answer: D—Medium chain acyl-CoA dehydrogenase deficiency (MCADD)

This child presents with a seizure after a period of fasting due to a mild intercurrent illness. As the child was from a resource-poor country, she would not have been part of a neonatal screening programme. Initial investigations indicate a mild dehydration, hypoglycaemia and a metabolic acidosis with a low bicarbonate. The required compensation of the metabolic acidosis by increasing bicarbonate is not present and reflects the acute onset of the illness. Her liver function tests are mildly abnormal.

A. A. Ornithine transaminase deficiency—would not explain hypoglycaemia
B. B. Galactosaemia—presents in first week of life and usually have jaundice
C. C. Glycogen storage disease—present with hypoglycaemia but have hepatomegaly
D. D. Medium chain acyl-CoA dehydrogenase deficiency (MCADD)—correct answer
E. E. Organic acidaemias—usually present in first few days of life with encephalopathy

Answer 29
Correct answer: D—Primary hypothyroidism
This girl has normal timing but an abnormal sequence of puberty. This scenario is typical of primary hypothyroidism. The high TSH mimics FSH and the oestrogen produced by the ovaries leads to breast development and some bleeding but no growth due to low thyroxine. Although rare, it illustrates the importance of timing and sequence when assessing puberty.

A. Coeliac disease—delayed puberty but the sequence is normal
B. Constitutional delay of growth and puberty—sequence is normal but late
C. Pituitary tumour—puberty may be early or delayed but the sequence is normal
D. Primary hypothyroidism—correct answer
E. Turner syndrome—no obvious dysmorphic features and primary ovarian failure leads to no development

Answer 30
Correct answer: A—Ask the health visitor to visit and discuss safe medicine storage
Safeguarding is everyone's responsibility and information sharing is important; however, not every situation where the child has had a harm results in full child protection or safeguarding proceedings. An isolated incident of accidental ingestion of a prescribed medicine is not of sufficient concern to require full safeguarding processes. There is no additional information given to suggest this would be necessary in this situation.

Answer 31
Correct answer: B—discharge home with safety—net advice
Whilst parental perception of fever is important and should not be dismissed without consideration, in this child there are no amber or red symptoms to suggest moderate or high risk of serious illness. NICE guidance suggests that in this group of children (those who had fever and no focus), only a urine sample and examination to rule out pneumonia is required.

A. No evidence that a specific period of observation is helpful in a well child
B. Correct answer
C. Nasal secretions with no other respiratory signs do not warrant antibiotics
D. FBC and CRP are unlikely to be helpful in the context of a well
E. Fever without source should not be treated with antibiotics in a well child

Answer 32
Correct answer: A—Aspergillus antibody assay
The clinical story and blood results suggest allergic bronchopulmonary aspergillosis which is an immune-mediated response to environmental aspergillus fumigatus in the airways of children with cystic fibrosis. A fever, raised IgE and new radiological changes are consistent with the diagnosis.

A. Aspergillus antibody assay—correct answer
B. Blood culture—likely to be culture negative
C. CO transfer factor—would not determine the cause of any lung damage
D. High-resolution CT of chest—would not determine the cause of any lung damage
E. PCR assay for mycobacterium—would not explain raised IgE

Answer 33
Correct answer: C—Epidermolysis bullosa
The lesion is well demarcated on a site common for epidermolysis bullosa due to local trauma. Appearance suggests a junctional injury between epidermis and dermis.

A. Discoid eczema—gives red scaling rash
B. Discoid erythematosus—gives red scaly rash to face and scalp
C. Epidermolysis bullosa—correct answer
D. Nonaccidental scald injury—nothing in history and odd place for such an injury
E. Staphylococcal infection—low temperature, discrete edges without extending erythema

Answer 34
Correct answer: C—Karyotype
Short stature and a long-standing bilateral ptosis in a girl suggest an underlying genetic cause with Turner syndrome the most likely explanation.

A. Antibodies to acetylcholine receptors—myasthenia would not impact on height

B. Fundoscopy—no history to suggest raised intracranial pressure
C. Karyotype—correct answer
D. MRI brain—no history or examination to suggest intracranial pathology
E. Urinary catecholamines—neuroblastoma can cause proptosis, Horner's syndrome and "dancing eye" syndrome but not ptosis. Also, history too long.

Answer 35
Correct answer: E—Vitamin B12 deficiency
This child presents with gross motor delay and a macrocytic anaemia. The mother was a strict vegetarian and she had symptoms of vitamin B12 deficiency during pregnancy. The child was B12 deficient at birth. Examination indicates motor regression (was sitting, now not sitting).
A. Alpha-thalassaemia trait—produces a microcytic anaemia
B. Folate deficiency—in extreme deficiency can produce thrombocytopenia and neurological features
C. Hypothyroidism—bright and smiling
D. Iron deficiency anaemia—produces microcytic anaemia
E. Vitamin B12 deficiency—macrocytic anaemia and gross motor delay

Answer 36
Correct answer: D—Respiratory hypoventilation
Guillain-Barré syndrome is a progressive ascending neuropathy that may ultimately lead to involve innervation of respiratory muscles. Monitoring includes frequent peak flow assessment.
A. Brain stem herniation—increase in intracranial pressure does not occur
B. Hearing deficit—cranial nerve involvement is an adverse feature but rare finding
C. Permanent loss of vision—optic nerves are not involved although eye movements may be affected
D. Respiratory hypoventilation—correct answer
E. Spinal cord compression—mild inflammation occurs but does not lead to compression

Answer 37
Correct answer: B—Beta-thalassaemia trait
This child has abnormal haematological results identified incidentally when presenting with abdominal pain. He has, therefore, been generally well until this presentation. The family is from the Africa where haemoglobinopathies are more common.
Investigations show a moderate anaemia with microcytic, hypochromic indices. Ferritin is normal and so excludes iron deficiency as a cause of the anaemia. Raised bilirubin indicates haemolysis. Haemoglobin electrophoresis shows that the normal haemoglobin production is compromised and the persistence and increased

production of HbA$_2$ and HbF is part of that compensation.
A. Alpha thalassaemia major—is incompatible with postnatal life
B. Alpha thalassaemia trait—raised HbA$_2$ not usually seen in alpha thalassaemia trait
C. Beta thalassaemia major—usually identified earlier and often transfusion dependant.
D. Beta thalassaemia trait—correct answer
E. HbH Disease—HbH would be identified on electrophoresis

Answer 38
Scenario 1
Correct answer is D—HHV 6B
Scenario 2
Correct answer is F—measles
Scenario 3
Correct answer is B—Group A streptococcus

Answer 39
Correct answer: C—Hypothyroidism
The main symptom for this boy is lethargy and examination identified he is withdrawn and pale. He had had significant weight gain over the previous 6 months. HbA1c was only marginally out of target range and he was not anaemic.
A. Coeliac disease—no features in the history, not anaemic, weight gain not expected
B. Depressive illness—would need further clinical details in the history
C. Hypothyroidism—correct answer
D. Inadequate insulin dose—would expect higher HBA1c from hyperglycaemia
E. School refusal—would need further clinical details in the history

Answer 40
Correct answer: A—Ornithine transaminase deficiency
This baby presents at a few days of age and initial blood samples indicate a respiratory alkalosis along with a markedly raised ammonia. The liver enzymes are normal indicating that the high ammonia is not due to a primary liver dysfunction and suggest a primary metabolic problem—a urea cycle defect. Ornithine transaminase deficiency is the most common urea cycle defects and it is x-linked.
A. Ornithine transaminase deficiency—correct answer
B. Galactosaemia—would not explain raised ammonia
C. Glycogen storage disease—excluded by normal glucose and would not explain raised ammonia
D. MCADD deficiency—would not explain raised ammonia
E. Organic acidaemias—would give a metabolic acidosis

Answer 41
Correct answer: D—Haemoglobin electrophoresis

This child presents with history and findings suggestive of cardiac failure. The family is from the Middle East where haemoglobinopathies are more common and antenatal screening less likely to have occurred. He has hepatosplenomegaly.

Investigations show marked anaemia with microcytic, hypochromic indices. White cell and platelet counts are normal. Target cells are the result of a reduced red cell volume indicative of defective red cell production. Raised bilirubin indicates haemolysis but liver function tests are normal. A haemoglobinopathy is the likely explanation.

A. Bone marrow aspirate—no evidence of white cell or platelet abnormality
B. Ferritin—iron deficiency would not produce haemolysis
C. G6PD deficiency—he is generally well and would not explain abnormal LFTs
D. Haemoglobin electrophoresis—indices suggest abnormal red cell production
E. Liver biopsy—liver enzymes are normal

Answer 42
Correct answer: C—Oesophageal atresia

A. Congenital lobar emphysema—respiratory features more evident and would not explain vomiting
B. Meconium aspiration—would expect more history aspiration of meconium and early respiratory symptoms
C. Oesophageal atresia—correct answer
D. Persistent tachypnoea of the newborn - would expect early respiratory symptoms
E. Volvulus—vomiting usually bile stained and not immediate

Answer 43
Correct answer: C—infusion of IV 10% calcium gluconate

This young girl has hyperkalaemia at the start of chemotherapy as part of a tumour lysis syndrome. This is checked and is not an artefact. The patient is at risk of cardiac arrhythmia and IV calcium gluconate will have an immediate cardioprotective effect. Administration of insulin/glucose, nebulised salbutamol and IV salbutamol will facilitate the transfer of potassium into the cells but their effect takes some time to appear. Sodium bicarbonate does not have a role.

Answer 44
Correct answer: D—plasma galactose level

This child presents in the first week of life with poor feeding and vomiting and is found to be jaundiced and tachypnoeic. Abnormal glucose, liver function and clotting tests are noted. Tachypnoea suggested compensating acidosis. These findings suggest galactosaemia and is confirmed by demonstrating raised levels of galactose and absent galactose-1-phosphate uridyl transferase activity. Galactosaemia is seen more commonly in children of Irish travellers.

A. PCR of urine for CMV—congenital CMV usually asymptomatic but have thrombocytopenia and anaemia
B. Plasma alpha-1-antitrypsin level—can give deranged LFT but presents later in life
C. Plasma ammonia level—urea cycle disorders present with irritability and seizures
D. Plasma galactose level—correct answer
E. Syphilis serology—expect thrombocytopaenia

Answer 45
Correct answer: E—vincristine toxicity

A. Cervical transverse myelitis—would not explain ptosis
B. CNS relapse of leukaemia—would expect single nerve involvement and pain
C. Horner syndrome—no evidence of miosis
D. Myasthenia gravis—no preceding or family history
E. Vincristine toxicity—gives peripheral neuropathy after frequent doses

Answer 46
Correct answer: D—Pyloric stenosis

This baby presents with dehydration, hypovolaemia and poor weight gain. His history indicates a long history of vomiting which is evident when on full feeds. Investigations show hypochloraemic, hypokalaemic alkalosis.

A. Achalasia—would not give abnormal biochemistry
B. Hiatus hernia—does not give abnormal biochemistry
C. Parental neglect—would not explain abnormal blood results
D. Pyloric stenosis—correct answer
E. Congenital adrenal hyperplasia—gives low sodium and high potassium

Answer 47
Correct answer: D—Request psychiatrist to assess mental capacity

If left untreated, this girl will die from her electrolyte derangement but she is of an age where her decision to reject the proposed treatment needs careful consideration. The Mental Capacity Act covers this age group and requires an assessment of mental capacity to decide whether her illness is affecting her ability to make rational decisions about her health. Application to the courts would require proof of an attempt to assess mental capacity. Starting treatment without consent is a criminal assault

Answer 48
Correct answer: B—Haemophilia A

This boy presents with epistaxis and no past history of bleeding problems although he is 'double jointed'. The family history indicates maternal grandfather may have had a clotting problem and so raises the possibility of an x-linked condition. Laboratory results indicate a clotting problem consistent with haemophilia but it is not possible to distinguish between haemophilia A and haemophilia B on the results given. However, haemophilia B would usually have presented earlier in life with bleeding problems and is much less common than haemophilia A.

A. Ehlers-Danlos syndrome would not explain abnormal clotting
B. Haemophilia A—correct answer
C. Haemophilia B—less common than haemophilia A
D. Protein C deficiency—produces thrombotic episodes
E. Wiskott-Aldrich syndrome—platelets are normal

Answer 49
Correct answer: E—vigabatrin

The description is consistent with infantile spasms in a child who may have developmental delay. The cutaneous features suggest that this boy has tuberous sclerosis. Current UK treatment would use vigabatrin from the list of medications.

A. Clonazepam
B. Ketogenic diet
C. Pyridoxine
D. Topiramate
E. Vigabatrin

Answer 50
Correct answer: D—Perthes disease

The boy is 9 years old which is in the common age range for Perthes and he has acute onset and localised pain with no other joints involved. He is overweight. X-ray shows distortion of the left femoral head.

A. Inflammatory bowel reactive arthritis—would not explain changes on x-ray
B. Juvenile idiopathic arthritis—would not explain changes on x-ray
C. Osteosarcoma—x-ray does not show localised expanding lesion
D. Perthes disease—correct answer
E. Slipped capital epiphysis—the head has not slipped from the neck of the femur

Index

Note: Page numbers followed by '*f*' indicate figures those followed by '*t*' indicate tables and '*b*' indicate boxes.